DATE DUE

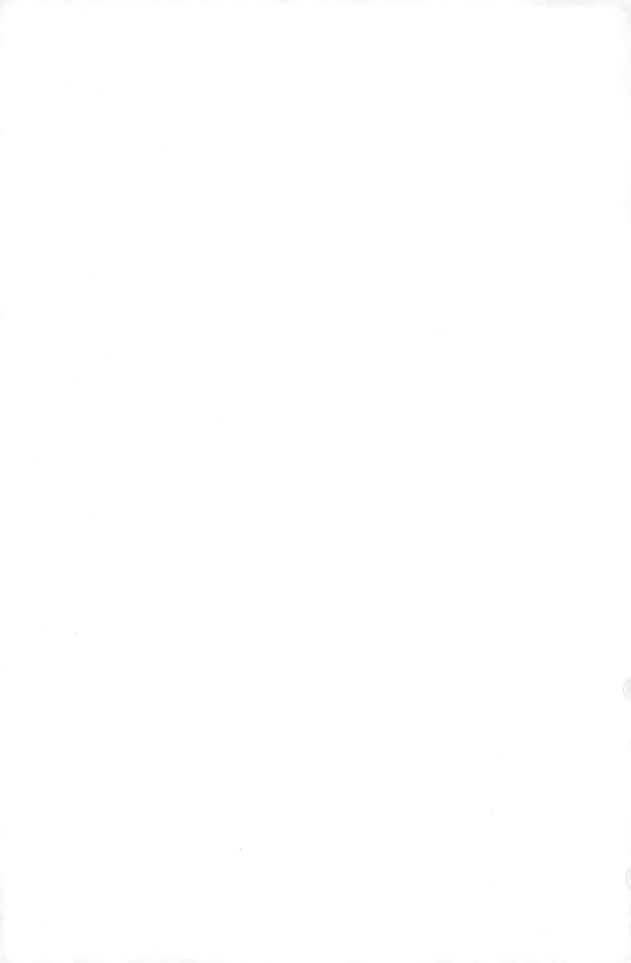

Springer Series on Epidemiology and Public Health

Series Editors: Wolfgang Ahrens, Iris Pigeot

For other titles published in this series, go to
www.springer.com/series/7251

Luis A. Moreno • Iris Pigeot • Wolfgang Ahrens
Editors

Epidemiology of Obesity in Children and Adolescents

Prevalence and Etiology

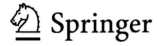 Springer

Editors
Luis A. Moreno
GENUD (Growth, Exercise, Nutrition
and Development) Research Group
E.U. Ciencias de la Salud
Universidad de Zaragoza
Zaragoza
Spain
lmoreno@unizar.es

Wolfgang Ahrens
Bremen Institute for
Prevention Research and Social Medicine (BIPS)
University Bremen
Achterstrasse 30
28359, Bremen
Germany
ahrens@bips.uni-bremen.de

Iris Pigeot
Bremen Institute for Prevention Research
and Social Medicine (BIPS)
University Bremen
Achterstrasse 30
28359, Bremen
Germany
pigeot@bips.uni-bremen.de

ISBN 978-1-4419-6038-2   e-ISBN 978-1-4419-6039-9
DOI 10.1007/978-1-4419-6039-9
Springer New York Dordrecht Heidelberg London

Printed on acid-free paper

Springer is part of Springer Science+Business Media (www.springer.com)

Preface

The societal and scientific concerns related to the worldwide obesity epidemic have grown continuously. Scientists and actors in the field of public health not only aim at assessing the size of the problem but also they strive to better understand its causes. *Epidemiology of Obesity in Children and Adolescents* addresses both aspects from an epidemiological perspective while acknowledging that any approach to tackling obesity at a young age by primary prevention is most promising when based on a complete knowledge of its causes and characteristics, as well as a thorough understanding of mechanisms leading to this epidemic.

Part I of this book provides a comprehensive worldwide description of obesity in children and adolescents and the time trends surrounding this situation. It will also describe the known determinants of this condition in various areas of the world. This ecological perspective will give an up-to-date overview of the magnitude of the problem. It will also provide clues towards understanding the association between major lifestyle, social, and economic changes and the geographic/temporal variations of the prevalence of obesity.

As obesity has a multifactor origin, Part II of this book will address the contribution of the known and suspected risk factors involved in weight gain and the etiology of obesity. Each chapter in Part II addresses a specific causal pathway and provides a comprehensive overview of the current knowledge. The epidemiological perspective of this book is broadened by the inclusion of chapters that describe basic biological mechanisms.

Thus, *Epidemiology of Obesity in Children and Adolescents* serves two purposes. First, it gives a global overview of the obesity epidemic and second, it provides an in-depth insight into its causes and mechanisms: the understanding of which may help to develop more effective prevention measures.

With these goals in mind, we invited key experts and leaders in the corresponding fields to explain and summarize the current knowledge. We had the opportunity to work together with many of these experts in the framework of two large-scale epidemiological studies investigating the etiology of obesity and the development and evaluation of interventions, namely the IDEFICS study addressing children and the HELENA study addressing adolescents. Both projects were supported within the 6th EU Framework Programme. We would like to acknowledge the outstanding expertise of all contributors and their effort in providing the best available knowledge.

We hope that this book will be useful for a broader readership of professionals dealing with childhood obesity, such as: public health specialists, epidemiologists, pediatricians, nurses, dieticians, psychologists, health educators, health services experts, other health professionals, and policy makers.

Son Antem, Mallorca, March 4th 2009   Luis A. Moreno
                                                                                                        Iris Pigeot
                                                                                                        Wolfgang Ahrens

Contents

Chapter 1
Introduction

Iris Pigeot, Luis A. Moreno, and Wolfgang Ahrens

Obesity has become a major determinant of morbidity and mortality in many areas of the world, the most important diseases being type 2 diabetes, hypertension, cardiovascular diseases, musculoskeletal and psychological disorders as well as several types of cancer. For example, the relative risk of contracting disease among obese was estimated to be in the order of 6.74 in males and 12.41 in females for type 2 diabetes, 1.84 in males and 2.42 in females for hypertension, 1.72 in males and 3.10 in females for coronary artery disease, 4.20 in males and 1.96 in females for osteoarthritis, 1.82 in males and 2.64 in females for kidney cancer and 3.22 for endometrial cancer (Guh et al. 2009).

The prevalence of obesity has increased dramatically in the last few decades, with rising trends in almost all developed countries in spite of institutional prevention efforts (Hedley et al. 2004; Pratt et al. 2008). Primary prevention efforts in adults were mostly disappointing (McKinnon et al. 2009) and there is increasing evidence that the manifestation of obesity and its co-morbidities starts from early childhood onwards (Franks et al. 2010). Therefore, there has been growing interest to better understand the mechanisms acting during the developmental stages from gestation through childhood to adolescence. The prevalence of obesity in children is on the rise in most parts of the world (Flodmark et al. 2004; Hedley et al. 2004; McArthur et al. 2003) and although there is recent evidence that this trend may be leveling off in some developed countries like the US, Australia, and some European countries (Ogden et al. 2008; Olds et al. 2009; Péneau et al. 2009; Stamatakis et al. 2009; Sundblom et al. 2008) the level is still unacceptably high. Also, the obesity-related hospital discharges in youth (6–17 years) increased from 1979–1981 to 1997–1999. The discharges of diabetes nearly doubled (from 1.43 to 2.36%), gallbladder diseases tripled (from 0.18 to 0.59%) and sleep apnea increased fivefold (from 0.14 to 0.75%) (Wang and Dietz 2002).

The definition of obesity in children is typically based on percentile curves of the body mass index (BMI) and therefore it might be argued that the rising trend in obesity is more an artifact than a real problem. For this reason, it is necessary to investigate whether children who have been classified as obese will be also classified as obese later in life. In this regard, tracking is defined as the persistence

I. Pigeot (✉) and W. Ahrens
Bremen Institute for Prevention Research and Social Medicine (BIPS), University Bremen,
Achterstrasse 30, 28359, Bremen, Germany
e-mail: pigeot@bips.uni-bremen.de

L.A. Moreno
GENUD (Growth, Exercise, Nutrition and Development) Research Group,
E.U. Ciencias de la Salud, Universidad de Zaragoza, Zaragoza, Spain

L.A. Moreno et al. (eds.), *Epidemiology of Obesity in Children and Adolescents*,
Springer Series on Epidemiology and Public Health 2, DOI 10.1007/978-1-4419-6039-9_1,
© Springer Science+Business Media, LLC 2011

of a relative position in a population over time. Several longitudinal studies have shown that around half of obese children in school age continued to be obese during adulthood and this tracking has also been observed in pre-school children (Freedman et al. 2005; Martínez Vizcaíno et al. 2002; Vogels et al. 2006). Although there is some concern that not only obesity but also related co-morbid conditions track from childhood into adulthood, the evidence for the tracking of cardiovascular risk factors has not yet been proven. This lack of evidence may be due to methodological weaknesses inherent in the assessment of physiological states like hypertension that have much higher day-to-day variation and are less stable than body composition. However, there is moderate evidence that these risk factors track from adolescence onwards, too (Eisenmann et al. 2004; Morrison et al. 2005).

Also, the treatment costs of obesity and its related morbidities are a growing concern. According to Wolf and Colditz (1998) the total economic cost attributable to obesity in the US was estimated at 99 billion USD in the year 1995. About 52 billion USD of this amount were direct medical costs. The economic burden of obesity in Canada in 2001 was 4.3 billion CAD, of which 1.6 billion CAD were direct costs and 2.7 billion CAD were indirect. The total economic cost of obesity represented 2.2% of the total health care costs in Canada (Katzmarzyk and Janssen 2004). Müller-Riemenschneider et al. (2008) estimated that the relative economic burden in ten Western European countries ranges from 0.09 to 0.61% of each country's gross domestic product and judged this to be a conservative estimate. For example, for the UK it was estimated that direct costs of overweight and obesity to the National Health Service were about 3.2 billion GBP (Allender and Rayner 2007). The authors mentioned that the obesity-related costs range from 480 million GBP in 1998 to 1.1 billion GBP in 2004. For the US it was estimated that the total health care costs attributable to obesity/overweight would double every decade to 861 to 957 billion USD by 2030 accounting for 16 to 18% of the total US health care costs (Wang et al. 2008). Although knowledge about economic costs of obesity in children is scarce, it has been estimated that annual hospital costs in the US (based on 2001 constant USD value) increased more than threefold from 35 million USD in 1979–1981 to 127 million USD in 1997–1999 (Wang and Dietz 2002).

As obesity develops already early in life it is important to understand the causes and mechanisms leading to this disorder in children. The first part of this book gives a comprehensive overview of the descriptive data worldwide to describe the size of the problem and the distribution of potential risk factors. This may give a first idea of the etiology which is then analyzed in detail in the second part of this book. The knowledge about the main drivers of obesity can help to identify the most promising targets amenable to primary prevention rather than the mere treatment of the disorder. Lifestyle develops during childhood and adult behavioral patterns are already established at the end of this life period. This and our inclination towards primary prevention are the reasons why this book focuses on children and adolescents, since we assume that any interventions will have the biggest impact if applied in these age groups.

The serious health issues and the economic implications of the rising prevalence of childhood and adolescent obesity raise ethical and public policy questions regarding the responsibility for health, food production and consumption, for an obesogenic environment and patterns of physical activity, the role of the state, and the rights and duties of parenthood. These aspects are discussed before the first part of this book describes the worldwide distribution of overweight and obesity in children and adolescents, its time trends and main risk factors where each chapter is devoted to a continent or otherwise defined geographic area. The data are discussed in view of the socio-demographic and socio-economic profile of each geographic area.

The aim to give a worldwide picture was challenging since data are very scarce for some areas and not always publicly available. Thanks to the engagement of distinguished experts it was possible to retrieve data sources that would otherwise not easily become available to the reader and to collate these data in comprehensive chapters. However, after several attempts the editors decided to no longer search for such data for Sub-Saharan Africa except those provided by the WHO Global Database on Child Growth and Malnutrition for pre-school children (WHO 2009).

Although each expert sought to include the most recent and nationally representative data, in some countries large scale systematic surveys were lacking and often data referred to restricted study populations. It may be considered a strength that most experts succeeded in providing actual data, i.e., data collected after the year 2000 while only in rare cases they had to revert to data from the 1990s. Comparability of data across countries is hampered by the fact that the available reports are sometimes based on different age groups or used differing age categorizations. The most important limitation, however, roots in the different reference systems used to classify overweight and obesity during growth, which lead to varying prevalence estimates if applied to the same population (see synthesis of Part I, Chapter 13). This problem is aggravated by the use of different anthropometric methodologies in the absence of a commonly accepted standard protocol (Chapter 3).

While Part I of this book gives a descriptive overview of the prevalence of overweight and obesity as well as of some selected risk factors that are considered relevant for a given area, the mechanisms that link a given risk factor to the development of these disorders are presented in detail in Part II.

It may be considered a simple fact that obesity develops when energy intake exceeds energy expenditure. However, the complex interplay of various risk factors in the etiology of obesity in childhood and adolescence is still not fully understood. These factors range from biological determinants like genetic polymorphisms, epigenetic changes, and early nutrition factors, over behavioral characteristics including food patterns and eating behavior, physical activity and sedentary behavior to psychological, social, and environmental factors. During growth weight is regulated by numerous physiological mechanisms that have evolved to maintain the balance between nutrient supply and energy consumption on the one hand and growth and energy expenditure on the other. Easy access to tasty, energy dense foods as well as the decreased need and opportunity for physical exertion create a positive energy balance and are considered to be the driving forces of the obesity pandemic.

In Part II of this book leading experts highlight the current knowledge on these factors and give an assessment of their evidence by summarizing the state-of-the art in etiological obesity research. Only a better understanding of the complex etiology of obesity and related disorders will pave the way for better and more effective primary prevention interventions.

As described above, one major problem that impairs the comparability of prevalence data across several countries is related to the use of different reference systems and the lack of a standardized protocol to measure anthropometric variables. Two multicenter studies funded in the 6th EU Framework Programme, namely HELENA (Moreno et al. 2008a, b) and IDEFICS (Ahrens et al. 2006; Bammann et al. 2006), are filling this gap.

The HELENA project included four different sub-studies. The most relevant in relation with adolescent obesity were (a) a cross-sectional assessment of risk factors and (b) the pilot of a web-based computer tailored lifestyle intervention study. In the cross-sectional study, more than 3,000 adolescents were recruited in ten European cities. A comprehensive set of measurements of the nutritional status and lifestyle was applied. Dietary intake was assessed by means of two 24-h recalls obtained for two non-consecutive days, using a computer-based method (Vereecken et al. 2008). Nutrition knowledge and eating attitudes as well as food choices and preferences were also assessed. Body composition was measured using anthropometry and bioelectrical impedance (Nagy et al. 2008). Physical activity was measured using accelerometry and the International Physical Activity Questionnaire (IPAQ), adapted for adolescents (Hagströmer et al. 2008). Different physical fitness dimensions were determined using a fitness test battery (Ortega et al. 2008). Plasma lipids and metabolic profile, vitamin status, inflammation, and immune function were analyzed in centralized laboratories (González-Gross et al. 2008). More than 700 SNPs in more than 70 genes were genotyped. The web-based computer tailored program indicated to be effective in terms of modifying physical activity patterns, when compared with a conventional intervention (De Bourdeaudhuij et al. 2010).

The IDEFICS study is a so-called Integrated Project that pursues two aims. On the one hand, it investigates the etiology of diet- and lifestyle-related diseases and disorders with a strong focus on overweight and obesity in children. On the other hand, it develops, implements and evaluates primary prevention programs to tackle the obesity epidemic. The primary prevention modules of the IDEFICS study dwell on the current evidence-base in this research area and are harmonized across Europe allowing for country-specific modifications in each intervention region that is to be compared with a control region in a longitudinal design (Pigeot et al. 2010). For these purposes, the IDEFICS study has recruited about 16,000 children aged 2–8 years old in eight European countries. These children are examined based on an extensive protocol in a baseline and a follow-up survey. The overall examination program includes standard anthropometric measures, clinical parameters such as blood pressure, ultrasonography of the calcaneus to assess bone stiffness, collection of urine, saliva, blood for further medical parameters and genetic analyses, accelerometry to assess physical activity, tests for physical fitness, assessment of nutritional behavior via a food frequency questionnaire and a computer-based 24-h dietary recall, parental questionnaires to assess medical, behavioral and socio-demographic factors, tests of sensory perception and food preferences, experiments to assess consumer behavior, and characterization of the built environment based on GIS (Geographic Information System) data.

To have a clear idea of the prevalence of obesity, the standardized approach of studies like HELENA and IDEFICS should be adopted by other projects. Especially nationally representative studies with such a standardized protocol are needed. They already exist in some areas, but they need to be developed in the great majority of the world. At the European level, the WHO Regional Office for Europe is establishing a standardized surveillance system. Nationally representative samples of children aged 6–9 years will be considered. The first data collection round was performed during the school year 2007/2008 in more than ten countries. It will be followed by further rounds at 2-year intervals in order to describe temporal trends.

The need for harmonized methods and comparable data in different geographic areas does not only apply to the basic measurements to assess the prevalence of obesity (weight, height and other anthropometric measurements), but also to those addressing environmental and lifestyle factors. From infancy through childhood to adolescence, these methods should be adapted to the different physical and cognitive developmental phases. From this point of view, both the IDEFICS and HELENA study did a considerable effort, and the developed methodologies should be considered for future studies in the field.

There is also the need to close the gaps in our understanding of causal mechanisms. The multiplicity of obesity risk factors should be addressed in large cohort and intervention studies. These studies should focus not only on identifying independent risk factors, but also on prioritizing these factors and assessing their interactions. Obesity is certainly caused by the presence of several risk factors in the same individuals. Therefore, identification of clusters of these risk factors is a promising avenue of further research.

References

Ahrens, W., Bammann, K., De Henauw, S., Halford, J., Palou, A., Pigeot, I., Siani, A., & Sjöström, M., on behalf of the European Consortium of the IDEFICS Project (2006). Understanding and preventing childhood obesity and related disorders - IDEFICS: A European multilevel epidemiological approach. *Nutrition, Metabolism & Cardiovascular Diseases, 16,* 302–308.

Allender, S., & Rayner, M. (2007). The burden of overweight and obesity-related ill health in the UK. *Obesity Reviews, 8(5),* 467–473.

Bammann, K., Peplies, J., Sjöström, M., Lissner, L., De Henauw, S., Galli, C., Iacoviello, L., Krogh, V., Marild, S., Pigeot, I., Pitsiladis, Y., Pohlabeln, H., Reisch, L., Siani, A., & Ahrens, W., on behalf of the IDEFICS Consortium (2006). Assessment of diet, physical activity biological, social and environmental factors in a multi-centre European project on diet- and lifestyle-related disorders in children (IDEFICS). *Journal of Public Health, 14,* 279–289.

De Bourdeaudhuij, I., Maes, L., De Henauw, S., De Vriendt, T., Moreno, L.A., Kersting, M., Sarri, K., Manios, Y., Widhalm, K., Sjöström, M., Ruiz, J.R., & Haerens, L., on behalf of the HELENA Study Group (2010). Evaluation of a computer-tailored physical activity intervention in adolescents in six European countries: The Activ-O-Meter in the HELENA Intervention Study. *Journal of Adolescent Health,* in press.

Eisenmann, J.C., Welk, G.J., Wickel, E.E., Blair, S.N., & Aerobics Center Longitudinal Study (2004). Stability of variables associated with the metabolic syndrome from adolescence to adulthood: the Aerobics Center Longitudinal Study. *American Journal of Human Biology, 16,* 690–696.

Flodmark, C.E., Lissau, I., Moreno, L.A., Pietrobelli, A., & Widhalm, K. (2004). New insights into the field of children and adolescents' obesity: the European perspective. *International Journal of Obesity, 28,* 1189–1196.

Franks, P.W., Hanson, R.L., Knowler, W.C., Sievers, M.L., Bennett, P.H., Looker, H.C. (2010). Childhood obesity, other cardiovascular risk factors, and premature death. *New England Journal of Medicine, 362(6),* 485–493.

Freedman, D.S., Khan, L.K., Serdula, M.K., Dietz, W.H., Srinivasan, S.R., & Berenson, G.S. (2005). Racial differences in the tracking of childhood BMI to adulthood. *Obesity Research, 13,* 928–935.

González-Gross, M., Breidenassel, C., Gómez, S., Ferrari, M., Béghin, L., Spinneker, A., Díaz, L., Maiani, G., Demailly, A., Al-Tahan, J., Albers, U., Wärnberg, J., Stoffel-Wagner, B., Jiménez-Pavón, D., Libersa, C., Pietrzik, K., Marcos, A., & Stehle, P., on behalf of the HELENA study group (2008). Sampling and processing of fresh blood samples within a European multicenter nutritional study: Evaluation of biomarker stability during transport and storage. *International Journal of Obesity (London), 32 (Suppl 5),* S66–S75.

Guh, D.P., Zhang, W., Bansback, N., Amarsi, Z., Birmingham, C.L., & Anis, A.H. (2009). The incidence of co-morbidities related to obesity and overweight: a systematic review and meta-analysis. *BMC Public Health, 9,* 88.

Hagströmer, M., Bergman, P., De Bourdeaudhuij, I., Ortega, F.B., Ruiz, J.R., Manios, Y., Rey-López, J.P., Phillipp, K., von Berlepsch, J., & Sjöström, M., on behalf of the HELENA Study Group (2008). Concurrent validity of a modified version of the International Physical Activity Questionnaire (IPAQ-A) in European adolescents – The HELENA Study. *International Journal of Obesity (London), 32 (Suppl 5),* S42–S48.

Hedley, A.A., Ogden, C.L., Johnson, C.L., Carroll, M.D., Curtin, L.R., & Flegal, K.M. (2004). Prevalence of overweight and obesity among US children, adolescents, and adults, 1999-2002. *Journal of the American Medical Association, 291,* 2847–2850.

Katzmarzyk, P.T., & Janssen, I. (2004). The economic costs associated with physical inactivity and obesity in Canada: an update. *Canadian Journal of Applied Physiology, 29(1),* 90–115.

Martínez Vizcaíno, F., Salcedo Aguilar, F., Rodríguez Artalejo, F., Martínez Vizcaíno, V., Domínguez Contreras, M.L., & Torrijos Regidor, R. (2002). Obesity prevalence and tracking of body mass index after a 6 years follow up study in children and adolescents: the Cuenca Study, Spain. *Medicina Clinica (Barcelona), 119,* 327–330.

McArthur, L.H., Holbert, D., & Peña, M. (2003). Prevalence of overweight among adolescents from six Latin American cities: a multivariable analysis. *Nutrition Research, 23,* 1391–1402.

McKinnon, R.A., Orleans, C.T., Kumanyika, S.K., Haire-Joshu, D., Krebs-Smith, S.M., Finkelstein, E.A., Brownell, K.D., Thompson, J.W., & Ballard-Barbash, R. (2009). Considerations for an obesity policy research agenda. *American Journal of Preventive Medicine, 36(4),* 351–357.

Moreno, L.A., De Henauw, S., González-Gross, M.M., Kersting, M., Molnár, D., Gottrand, F., Barrios, L., Sjöström, M., Manios, Y., Gilbert, C.C., Leclercq, C., Widhalm, K., Kafatos, A., & Marcos, A., on behalf of the HELENA Study Group (2008a). Design and implementation of the Healthy Lifestyle in Europe by Nutrition in Adolescence Cross-Sectional Study. *International Journal of Obesity (London), 32 (Suppl 5),* S4–S11.

Moreno, L.A., González-Gross, M., Kersting, M., Molnár, D., De Henauw, S., Beghin, L., Sjöström, M., Hagstromer, M., Manios, Y., Gilbert, C.C., Ortega, F.B., Dallongeville, J., Arcella, D., Wärnberg, J., Hallberg, M., Fredriksson, H., Maes, L., Widhalm, K., Kafatos, A.G., & Marcos, A., on behalf of the HELENA Study Group (2008b). Assessing, understanding and modifying nutritional status, eating habits and physical activity in European adolescents. The HELENA Study. *Public Health Nutrition, 11,* 288–299.

Morrison, J.A., Friedman, L.A., Harlan, W.R., Harlan, L.C., Barton, B.A., Schreiber, G.B., & Klein, D.J. (2005). Development of the metabolic syndrome in black and white adolescent girls: a longitudinal assessment. *Pediatrics, 116,* 1178–1182.

Müller-Riemenschneider, F., Reinhold, T., Berghöfer, A., & Willich, S.N. (2008). Health-economic burden of obesity in Europe. *European Journal of Epidemiology, 23(8),* 499–509.

Nagy, E., Vicente-Rodríguez, G., Manios, Y., Béghin, L., Iliescu, C., Censi, L., Dietrich, S., Ortega, F.B., De Vriendt, T., Plada, M., Moreno, L.A., & Molnár, D., on behalf of the HELENA Study Group (2008). Harmonization process and reliability assessment of anthropometric measurements in a multicenter study in adolescents. *International Journal of Obesity (London), 32 (Suppl 5),* S58–S65.

Ogden, C.L., Carroll, M.D., & Flegal, K.M. (2008). High body mass index for age among US children and adolescents, 2003-2006. *Journal of the American Medical Association, 299,* 2401–2405.

Olds, T.S., Tomkinson, G.R., Ferrar, K.E., & Maher, C.A. (2009). Trends in the prevalence of childhood overweight and obesity in Australia between 1985 and 2008. *International Journal of Obesity, 34,* 57–66.

Ortega, F.B., García-Artero, E., Ruiz, J.R., Vicente-Rodríguez, G., Bergman, P., Hagströmer, M., Ottevaere, C., Nagy, E., Konsta, O., Rey-López, J.P., Polito, A., Dietrich, S., Plada, M., Béghin, L., Manios, Y., Sjöström, M., & Castillo, M.J., on behalf of the HELENA study group (2008). Reliability of health-related physical fitness tests in European adolescents. The HELENA study. *International Journal of Obesity (London), 32 (Suppl 5)*, S49–S57.

Péneau, S., Salanave, B., Maillard-Teyssier, L., Rolland-Cachera, M.F., Vergnaud, A.C., Méjean, C., Czernichow, S., Vol, S., Tichet, J., Castetbon, K., & Hercberg, S. (2009). Prevalence of overweight in 6- to 15-year-old children in central/western France from 1996 to 2006: trends toward stabilization. *International Journal of Obesity (London), 33*, 401–407.

Pigeot, I., De Henauw, S., Foraita, R., Jahn, I., & Ahrens, W. (2010). Primary prevention from the epidemiology perspective: three examples from the practice. *BMC Medical Research Methodology, 10*, 10.

Pratt, C.A., Stevens, J., Daniels, S. (2008). Childhood obesity prevention and treatment: recommendations for future research. *American Journal of Preventive Medicine, 35(3)*, 249–252.

Stamatakis, E., Wardle, J., & Cole, T.J. (2009). Childhood obesity and overweight prevalence trends in England: evidence for growing socioeconomic disparities. *International Journal of Obesity, 34*, 41–47.

Sundblom, E., Petzold, M., Rasmussen, F., Callmer, E., & Lissner L. (2008). Childhood overweight and obesity prevalences levelling off in Stockholm but socioeconomic differences persist. *International Journal of Obesity (London), 32*, 1525–1530.

Vereecken, C.A., Covents, M., Sichert-Hellert, W., Fernández-Alvira, J.M., Le Donne, C., De Henauw, S., De Vriendt, T., Phillipp, K., Béghin, L., Manios, Y., Hallström, L., Poortvliet, E., Matthys, C., Plada, M., Nagy, E., & Moreno, L.A., on behalf of the HELENA Study Group (2008). Development and evaluation of a self-administered computerized 24-hour dietary recall method for adolescents in Europe. *International Journal of Obesity (London), 32 (Suppl 5)*, S26–S36.

Vogels, N., Posthumus, D.L., Mariman, E.C., Bouwman, F., Kester, A.D., Rump, P., Hornstra, G., & Westerterp-Plantenga, M.S. (2006). Determinants of overweight in a cohort of Dutch children. *American Journal of Clinical Nutrition, 84*, 717–724.

Wang, G., & Dietz, W.H. (2002). Economic burden of obesity in youths aged 6 to 17 years: 1979-1999. *Pediatrics, 109(5)*, E81.

Wang, Y., Beydoun, M.A., Liang, L., Caballero, B., & Kumanyika, S.K. (2008). Will all Americans become overweight or obese? Estimating the progression and cost of the US obesity epidemic. *Obesity (Silver Spring), 16(10)*, 2323–2330.

Wolf, A.M., & Colditz, G.A. (1998). Current estimates of the economic cost of obesity in the United States. *Obesity Research, 6(2)*, 97–106.

World Health Organization (WHO) (2009). *Global database on child growth and malnutrition*. Retrieved March 2009, http://www.who.int/nutgrowthdb/database/en/.

Chapter 2
Ethics and Public Policy

Dita Wickins-Drazilova and Garrath Williams

Introduction

Ethical reflections help us decide what are the best actions to pursue in difficult and controversial situations. Reflections on public policy consider how to alter patterns of individual activity and institutional policies or frameworks for the better. The rising prevalence of childhood and adolescent obesity may pose serious health issues. As such, it is related to ethical and public policy questions including responsibility for health, food production and consumption, patterns of physical activity, the role of the state, and the rights and duties of parenthood.

The problem of rising prevalence of obesity is mainly an issue in the Western world. Many developing countries going through rapid economic growth now face or might soon face similar problems. However, in this chapter we will offer only a Western perspective on the current problem of rising childhood and adolescent obesity, drawing many of our examples from the British context.

What are Childhood and Adolescence?

Every society constantly receives an influx of strangers into its midst – children. The concept of childhood has been long discussed by ethicists and philosophers. However, only recently has the philosophy of childhood been recognized as a specific area of philosophy concerned with what childhood is, what are children's rights and interests, societies' attitudes toward children, and the role of children in society (Matthews 2005). While philosophers don't often agree on how to best describe childhood and what is the role of children in society, they do agree that children have limited responsibility for their actions and that adults owe them a strong duty of care. Together with cognitive development and increasing experience, a child's moral development is a gradual progress towards adulthood. This means that crucial decisions in children's interests have to be made by parents, responsible guardians, schools, other public institutions and state bodies until the individual reaches a level of moral development, or attains an age that his/her society accepts as indicating adulthood. This may be general, or situation-specific.

How should we decide the ages when a child becomes an adolescent and an adolescent an adult? Both transitions relate to social and legal norms that have altered considerably in the recent history of Western societies. Since childhood, adolescence and adulthood represent a gradual and continuous

D. Wickins-Drazilova (✉) and G. Williams
Department of Philosophy, Furness College, Lancaster LA1 4YL, UK
e-mail: g.d.williams@lancester.ac.uk

L.A. Moreno et al. (eds.), *Epidemiology of Obesity in Children and Adolescents*,
Springer Series on Epidemiology and Public Health 2, DOI 10.1007/978-1-4419-6039-9_2,
© Springer Science+Business Media, LLC 2011

personal and social development, it is impossible to exactly mark the age of transition into a fully responsible member of a society. Moreover, this development clearly varies considerably between individuals. David Archard writes: "Adulthood is to be thought of as a state of mind rather than a question of age" (Archard 1995, p. 6). However, adulthood is also a status, involving increased rights and responsibilities. As such, it depends on others recognizing a person as an adult. The law necessarily draws some clear lines marking such a status, for instance, ages for criminal and civil responsibility. At the same time, parents and institutions that deal with children are under a clear duty to recognize – and foster – the child's increasing independence and responsibility for self and others as it enters adolescence and adulthood.

Just as the concept of childhood varies culturally, so do the rights accorded to parents. This can be seen in the thought of Aristotle, the Greek philosopher from the fourth century B.C. He claimed that what happens inside families are private matters that are regulated by the head of the family, and not regulated by laws as are public relations between citizens: "What is just for a master and for a father are not the same as [political justice], though they are similar. For there is no unqualified injustice in relation to what is one's own, and a man's property, as well as his child until it reaches a certain age, are, as it were, a part of him; and no one rationally chooses to harm himself, which is why there is no injustice in relation to oneself. So nothing politically just or unjust is possible here" (Aristotle 2000, p. 1134b). Aristotle's idea is that a father's children are, just like slaves, "part of him," and as no one chooses to hurt himself, there can be no injustice done to children by parents. This is similar to the concept of childhood that appeared in Roman law where parents had absolute power over their children (Archard 1995, p. 9). There is no doubt that the idea that children fully "belong" to their father was long accepted and practiced in European history. However, in recent centuries, we have moved far from the idea of parent's absolute power over the child. Cases of domestic abuse especially have changed public attitudes, and societies – in particular state-sponsored institutions – intervene far more in the name of children's interests. Nowadays, while parents or legal guardians have direct responsibility for their children, it is essentially the state that has the last word in protecting child's interests. This doctrine involves an immense extension of state power into what Aristotle saw as the "private sphere" – although, at the societal level, it may also be related to adults taking a lower degree of responsibility for children who are not their own (Furedi 2001).

Obesity and Individual Choice

Without entering into the debate as to whether it is a disease or not, obesity is defined by the World Health Organization as a body mass index (BMI) over 30. It is widely held that obesity carries significant health risks to individuals; it therefore has implications for national health systems, and as such imposes costs on others. It is more controversial – and in any case a distinct claim – to maintain that increased body weight below this high threshold also poses health risks. (The frequently used term "overweight" seems to assume that it does; we will generally avoid this term because this assumption is dubious. Further, although it might be argued that overweight is a stage "on the way" to obesity, most "overweight" children and adults never become obese.) The majority of authors accept that it is in each individual's best interest not to be obese, and that having non-obese citizens is also a good for the whole society. Questions for ethics and public policy arise when we ask what these interests imply for people's individual responsibilities and the responsibilities of a whole series of institutions – from schools to companies to local councils to state bodies.

Many of the questions that arise around obesity in adults can be set aside when we consider the situation of children. For instance, some argue that adults who engage in unhealthy behaviors impose costs upon other members of society, and that it is unfair to allow people to impose this responsibility on others. (A parallel argument could be offered that parents who "allow" their children to become obese should be judged responsible for imposing costs on society. We consider arguments concerning the responsibilities of parents in the next section.) Whether or not people who become obese should be considered responsible or as imposing costs on others, it is clear that children should not be. An opposing argument – usually based on a liberal notion of autonomy – contends that neither state nor society have a right to impose "paternalistic" policies on adults. For example, governmental policies advising us to eat "five [fruit and vegetables] a day" are often derided as the voice of a "nanny state." Paternalism, however, is precisely the course of action that parents, or those helping to fulfill duties of care to children, ought to adopt. Children need nannies, so to speak – although they also need to be equipped with the education and skills that will enable them to act independently, and to be granted an increasing freedom (especially in adolescence) so that they can meaningfully practise those skills.

However, it is worth observing some important difficulties in the common line of thought that adults make their own choices – whether it is held that they are responsible for those choices, or ought to be allowed to make those choices free of state interference. These difficulties have important implications for how we think about children's upbringing and parental duties.

In the first place, the choices we make depend very much on the range of opportunities open to us and the costs of those choices, not to mention a whole range of social pressures, many magnified through the mass media or by the advertising of commercial bodies. All sorts of organizations are continually acting to alter and structure the opportunities open to us. Market forces promise to promote choice but also channel and stimulate it in particular ways. State and other bodies continually influence our field of opportunities – sometimes in obvious ways, but sometimes in important ways that we may not notice.

In other words, although most authors reject the use of state coercion against, for example, adults who are acting to damage their own health, there are many social, economic and state activities that affect the opportunities available to people and the choices that they make. While some of these measures make unhealthy behaviors more costly or less attractive, others may create pressures toward unhealthy behaviors. Simple examples of the first sort would be the taxation of tobacco and the ban on smoking in public areas. But it is easy to cite examples where collective actions undermine healthier choices. For instance, European Union subsidies of meat, animal fats, grains and sugar contribute toward an "obesogenic" environment – one that makes energy-dense and processed foods cheaper as compared to, say, fresh fruits and vegetables. Or again: many media representations simplistically equate health and thinness, as well as promoting unrealistic and unhealthy ideals of body shape. They therefore play a role in encouraging widespread, harmful "yo-yo" dieting, as well as more extreme eating disorders.

Moreover, people's ability to navigate such opportunities, constraints, and pressures in their own interests is related to their socio-economic status (SES, in which we may include social advantages or disadvantages linked to race and ethnicity). Complex and contested as the connections involved are, it is clear that both subjective factors (such as education or locus of control) and objective factors (actual opportunities and costs) will tend to vary with SES. More simply, "choice" is generally more real and meaningful for higher social classes. One implication of this is that discourses emphasizing individual responsibility may have invidious effects from the point of view of social justice.

While many adults have only a partial awareness of the complex forces that structure and constrain their choices, young children have none, while adolescents obviously vary greatly in this regard. Likewise, children have very restricted choices. This suggests two different routes for interventions at a public policy level. On the one hand, we might try to limit the sorts of opportunities and choices that we extend to children, or the sorts of pressures we expose them to. (For instance, we might try to limit the power of companies to promote their products to children.) But as they grow up, those children will eventually be expected to make their own choices in a very complex environment. This suggests a second priority. We need to foster children's abilities to handle the freedom of choice they will eventually be granted – which means that we must also equip them with some ability to recognize the ways in which others may be affecting their choices, or making choices on their behalf. In this regard, it may even be counter-productive to shelter children from the sorts of choices, risks and pressures that they will later encounter. As most parents find out, at some point our natural desire to protect children actually becomes risky for them. For example keeping children in a "safe" home environment where they spend much of their leisure time watching television and playing video games increases their risk of becoming obese (Hancox and Poulton 2006). Letting children play outside or cycle on the road involves risks, to be sure. One might argue, however, that the long-term risks of bringing up "cotton-wool kids" are far greater. In general, allowing children to be active in their own right, and to socialize with their peers, is essential to their development into adults capable of dealing with a wider world. To some extent, this point must also extend to their food choices.

Finally, there is an obvious difficulty with the common liberal idea that adults may do as they please, as long as they do not harm others (and so long as they respect the contractual undertakings they have made – for instance, in employment). Adults who become parents have responsibilities to care for children. Although the points at which state intervention may be legitimate are difficult to judge, no one any longer holds – as Aristotle seemed to claim – that it is enough for parents to avoid harming their children. Many authors and some laws pronounce that parents are obliged to act in a child's "best interests" – a very demanding standard. Certainly, parents must show active care and concern for their children, as must some institutions, schools and health services for instance. States, as noted already, are charged with ensuring that parents do this, and with taking that responsibility over where parents fail.

Parental Responsibility

The previous section has suggested that many organizations, including the state, are constantly influencing the choices we make and altering the opportunities that are open to us. We may desire to protect children from the responsibilities of individual choice and the pressures to unhealthy behaviors of our "obesogenic" environment. However, we have pointed out that protecting children may come at a price, insofar as children also need to learn how they can handle the choices, pressures and responsibilities that they will soon be exposed to.

In the first instance, children learn from their parents what are acceptable and desirable behaviors. It is in the family that children pick up elementary dietary and lifestyle habits and receive the first guidance that influences their health, fitness and wellbeing. Parents (or legal guardians) decide what a child eats, drinks, what sorts of activity are open to them, and what environment they live in. Parental influence plays a strong role in children's future health from the day a child is born. For example, research on breastfeeding suggests that it has not only positive effects on child's health but also on reducing the risk of childhood obesity (Armstrong et al. 2002).

Indeed, parents affect the health of their children even before they are born. The effect that a pregnant mother's alcoholism and drug addiction has on health of the fetus has been long recognized. Latest research results suggest that the food mothers eat during pregnancy may be important; research conducted on animals has showed that BMI of their young increases significantly after the mothers were fed on junk food during pregnancy and lactation (Bayol et al. 2007). Mothers' dietary and lifestyle habits during pregnancy may even affect future food and taste choices of their children. In one study a group of pregnant mothers was given carrot juice to drink during pregnancy. As a result, their children later showed less distasteful faces when they first tasted carrots compared to children whose mothers didn't drink carrot juice during pregnancy (Mennella et al. 2001).

However, the responsibility of parents for their children becoming overweight or obese is often overestimated (Food Ethics Council 2005, pp. 21–29). Much media coverage and a good deal of political discussion assume that the parents of obese children and adolescents should shoulder most of the responsibility – or blame – for the weight of their children. We see this in extreme form in many television "reality shows." Obese children and their parents receive not only public, and often insensitive, criticisms of their lifestyle habits, but are also inducted into radical lifestyle changes by supposed "experts." We now consider four reasons why parents should not be expected to shoulder such a heavy responsibility.

1. Firstly, parents may not be responsible for their child's obesity as they often don't know what to do. Today's parents may not have received much dietary education in school (if any at all) – nor, perhaps, much guidance from their parents in planning and preparing meals. Even if parents are resolved to make the best health choices for their children, they may be discouraged by the fact that it is difficult to find clear and helpful advice.

   Parents get conflicting messages on what is best for children from their GPs, available literature, media, scientists and government. This is often because scientific results with regard to nutrition and obesity are uncertain, and the way this research is reported in the media and translated into medical advice is confusing or contradictory. (We should not forget that there are many commercial interests that sponsor and influence research in nutrition and related areas.) For example, a woman seeking advice on whether it is harmful to have an occasional glass of wine during pregnancy might end up utterly confused. If she looked at the scientific evidence, she would realize that there is no clear evidence whether a small amount of alcohol (1–2 units once or twice a week) causes any harm to the fetus. As a result, in some countries one or two glasses of wine or beer a week during pregnancy is allowed or even recommended, while in other countries mothers-to-be are strictly discouraged from any alcohol whatsoever. In Britain a small amount of alcohol wasn't regarded as harmful until the British Medical Association recently changed their recommendations to zero tolerance. The reason the recommendations changed wasn't due to new research; rather, the judgment that it is better to recommend zero tolerance as it is – somewhat patronizingly – deemed difficult for women to tell how many units they are consuming (British Medical Association 2008).

   Of course, there are some clear, simple and useful messages such as the benefits of eating more fruit and vegetables, currently promoted by the "five-a-day" campaign. Although regarded as an overall success across Europe, even this campaign has been criticized. A recent survey showed that while most adults are aware of the "five-a-day" message, most of them eat only two or three portions daily. Moreover, there is a wide-spread confusion about what counts as a portion, with 25% believing that a glass of squash counts and 3% that potato chips (fries) count too. Also, some 60% of people believed five pieces of fruit alone ticked the "five-a-day" box, while there should be a mix of portions (Hickman 2008).

   These confusions point to a broad issue with any general formula such as improving diet, increasing physical activity, or decreasing the amount of time children watch TV. While easy to understand in the abstract, they are not always easy to translate into action in particular circumstances. One reason is that in many cases individual factors may be at work and might affect possible courses of action. The primary causes of a child's becoming obese may not be dietary and lifestyle habits themselves. For example, a child being bullied at school or abused at home might find overeating as a solution (comfort food) or even a way of calling for help (attention seeking). Trying to change the child's diet or exercise regime might work in the short term, but will not address the root problem.

2. This leads us to a second difficulty with the argument that parents bear primary responsibility for their child's obesity, which is that so many other social factors make it difficult to put advice about healthy living into practice. The "obesogenic" society can be described as an environment where there is an abundance of cheap and easily accessible high-calorie food, cars are used even for small distances instead of walking and cycling, and sedentary activities predominate over

manual labor and physical exercise. For children, opportunities for play and activity depend especially heavily upon the environment and social structures. Similarly, many organizations – especially companies selling confectionary, other processed foods, fast food and games – seek to influence children's choices and opportunities.

3. Although all parents act in an environment that can make it difficult to institute healthier behaviors and eating in their children's lives, these factors do not impact equally on all families. A third factor that undermines parental responsibility concerns the effects of low socio-economic status (SES). Most studies show that low SES is related to higher prevalence of obesity in both children and adults. For example a study done across the US, Canada and Norway on 6–10 year olds proved that children from poor families are more likely to be obese (Phipps et al. 2006). While it remains controversial just what causal factors underlie such associations, it is surely true that parents from lower SES groups have relatively less power to alter their lifestyles and those of their children. That is, after all, part of what it means to be socially disadvantaged. And it would surely be wrong to blame parents for being poor!

   It should be added that correlations between low SES and exposure to factors conducing to obesity are no simple matter. For example, one study of levels of overweight and obesity in various socio-economically deprived areas of the city of Liverpool asked why it is that some areas have higher levels of childhood obesity, while other even more impoverished areas (among the most deprived areas of England) have almost the lowest prevalence of childhood obesity in Liverpool. In looking at the differences between these areas, what became apparent was that the areas with high prevalence of overweight and obesity are heavily built on with Victorian terraces, narrow streets and parks too dangerous to play in. On the other hand, the other areas are estates built in the 1970s with wide streets, many green areas around houses and plenty of other grass areas to play on. The team concluded that rather than socio-economic status as such, the prevalence of obesity depends on whether the built environment that children live in encourages or discourages physical activity (Dummer et al. 2005; see also Public Health Information for Scotland 2008, for some further complexities in the relation between SES and obesity rates). Naturally, however, it will often be the case that lower SES families live in environments that are less conducive to safe outdoor activities than wealthier families.

4. A last and major reason why parents cannot be expected to bear sole responsibility for their child's diet and health is that every child's development is also in the hands of public institutions (such as kindergartens and schools) as well as the state. Although there is no doubt that parents are in charge of everyday active care for their children, then, their efforts need to be supported by state and other institutions – and are sometimes undermined by those bodies. So it is also necessary to discuss the role that public policy measures may play with regard to the prevalence of childhood obesity. We turn, first, to the possibility of intervening via schools and kindergartens.

Interventions Through Schools and Kindergartens

The range of possible anti-obesity interventions is very broad, from small initiatives on local levels (such as a community's joint effort to build a new playground) to large-scale interventions and policy changes at national and international level. In this section we focus on interventions aimed at tackling childhood obesity happening in or through schools and kindergartens, with or without the involvement of parents. The next section will consider some proposals for changes at the public policy level.

Interventions in schools and kindergartens can be very influential as that is where children spend much of their time and receive much of their education. Introducing lessons on dietary education as well as cooking classes have been one of the main initiatives in recent years. Schools can tackle childhood obesity by offering healthy lunches, snack options and low-sugar drinks. There has also been a call to increase weekly hours of physical education, to improve sports facilities and playgrounds. The role, amount and quality of physical education have been under threat in many countries (Marshall and Hardman 2000). School based interventions may also be attractive because they have the potential to be specifically targeted at areas of relative economic deprivation.

There are other intervention programs that contact children through schools but go beyond school settings. For example, the MEND program that started in Britain in 2002 offers free after-school courses that include teaching children how to play physically active games or showing them how to eat healthily by offering cooking lessons, food tasting and visits to supermarkets. MEND can be regarded as a success so far as it started as a small-scale trial; after continuous evaluation it currently operates in over 230 locations in Britain and is even expanding to other countries (MEND 2008).

Without denying the importance and advantages of school- and kindergarten-based interventions, however, we should note some significant problems and limitations that they face.

Firstly, many interventions don't get evaluated. We will only know what interventions are truly effective by checking their effects. This evaluation cannot be done on short-term basis, but needs to be monitored for many years since a truly effective intervention is meant to have long-lasting impacts. Therefore it is useful to have intervention studies such as IDEFICS that include school- and kindergarten-based interventions that will be evaluated over 2 years with an option for future follow-up (IDEFICS 2008). One might argue, of course, that even 2 years is rather short: we are hoping, after all, that the interventions will have lasting effect on *adult* health.

A related difficulty is that most interventions include many different actions and are done on many levels, so it is difficult later to identify which parts worked and which didn't. For example an evaluation of a school-based intervention including lunch meals, regular dietary lessons and increased physical activities can hardly identify which parts of the intervention had positive, negative or no effect on the health and weight of children. It cannot be doubted that there are very good reasons for intervening in this way, since a multiplicity of factors are undoubtedly at work here, but there is a price in terms of evaluation. Although it is possible to compare an intervention region with a control region, and hence to gain some sense as to whether an intervention program has significant effects, there are many difficulties in assessing which aspects of the intervention were most important, or whether any aspects were, perhaps, counter-productive.

A third difficulty with childhood-obesity interventions done in school or kindergarten settings is that it might be too late as some children enter these institutions already overweight or obese. Furthermore, by the time children enter a kindergarten or school, they have tasted thousands of foods and have very clear taste preferences as well as other habits (such as how much or when they eat, or how much they like to exercise). It is very difficult to change such behaviors without the involvement of their families.

This relates to a fourth problem. Many school- and kindergarten interventions are done without the involvement of parents and families. Even the best school taking the most comprehensive anti-obesity measures has a limited impact on what children do and eat outside of school hours, when children may well not do, or be unable to do, what their teachers tell them. Children spend most of their time outside of school, where they follow eating and lifestyle habits of parents (the more so, the more parents supervise their children's activity, perhaps fearing that it would be irresponsible to allow their children to play independently). So a truly effective intervention has to have impact on both children and their families. For example the MEND Program agrees to enroll only children who come with at least one parent. That way parents learn together with their children, and the courses have a chance to have long-lasting effects on the whole family's lifestyle. It should be added, however, that a well-known problem in addressing lower socio-economic status groups is the greater difficulty of involving parents. While the MEND policy is well-founded from the point of view of effectiveness for individual children, it may have an unwanted effect in terms of reaching children from lower SES backgrounds.

A final problem that we need to be aware of is that most interventions aren't aimed at individual children, but are implemented on whole groups. As a result, children who are of a perfectly healthy weight – or even underweight – may come to think of themselves as "overweight." Teenage girls especially have a tendency to overestimate their body weight, and this is also a group where acutely dangerous eating disorders such as bulimia and anorexia are real problems. On the other hand, many obese children, or children who may be deemed "overweight" by those conducting the intervention, think that they have a reasonable body weight. Weighing and measuring children and informing them and their parents that they are obese – or "overweight" – is therefore a sensitive activity. For example, schools in several U.S. states have sent parents report cards on their child's risk of becoming obese. While some parents thought the report card a great idea, many complained "the notices are stigmatizing and damaging to a child's self-esteem" (Wadas-Willingham 2008). For this and other reasons, we would strongly argue that interventions should be focused on promoting healthy lifestyles rather than weight loss per se. Nonetheless, there remains a clear danger that children and parents will still perceive thinness itself as a healthy goal, and treat it as a measure of their individual or family success.

Possible Public Policy Measures

Policy changes on national and international level aim to affect whole groups of citizens. One problem with large-scale interventions is that they require significant political will, over an extended period of time. As a result, they are very difficult to administer, never mind to guarantee success. Apart from the difficulties of pursuing any policy or political reform, the biggest challenge is to decide which policies will bring the most benefit and involve a proper division of responsibilities between state, organizations and families. While we know that the prevalence of obesity is rising in the developed world, we don't know exactly what factors are causing and affecting it. The idea that changes in BMI correspond to imbalances between energy intake and energy expenditure may be strictly correct (for a person who is not growing), but it is not very informative, practically speaking.* That is, it points to no obvious policy changes needed to halt the trend towards increasing obesity in our societies. In this section we briefly review three possible policy measures. The first is higher taxation of foods contributing to obesity, or the subsidy of healthier options such as fruit and vegetables. The second one is the proposal to ban or restrict advertising of "unhealthy" foods on one hand, and/or to promote healthier eating by advertising on the other. A third possible intervention concerns changes in transport infrastructures. These three types of interventions are amongst the most prominent measures suggested in the policy literature (Millstone et al. 2006).

---

*There is much scope for simplification on both sides of this equation. On the one hand, food eaten does not simply correspond to energy uptake by the body. (For example, the calorie value of foodstuffs corresponds to the energy uptake expected in a normal digestive tract. But this will clearly differ between individuals and in the same individual over time.) On the other, energy expenditure is not directly proportionate to the amount of "exercise" that a person undertakes. Even an intervention that is simply aimed at reducing BMI – as we argue above, not a goal that we think is helpful for policy purposes – might therefore intervene at numerous points that have no obvious relation to calorie intake or amount of physical activity. For some indication of the range of such factors, including the impact of ambient temperature control, pollution, smoking, medications and amount of sleep, see Keith et al. (2006).

One intervention that has often been aired to tackle obesity is the idea of altering food prices in line with their supposed effects on health or body weight. This might include higher taxation of high-fat, high-sugar and high-salt food products, or the subsidy of healthy foods such as fruit and vegetables, or both (Garson and Engelhard 2007). Some people argue that prices of food should be higher in general as people are overeating as a result of cheap food (Pollan 2008, p. 187). (A complementary suggestion might be that people are eating too much of the wrong sorts of food – meats from animals fed and reared in damaging ways, for instance.) In Britain the proportion of family income that is spent on buying food has been dropping for the last half of century. Statistics show that both in Britain as well as in the US the percentage of the average family budget spent on food and non-alcoholic drinks has decreased by approximately half in last 50 years (National Statistics 2008). This trend may be slightly changing with recent worldwide rises in food prices (Department of Agriculture and Economic Research Service 2008). In general, however, it can be said that the percentage of average income spent on food decreases with a country's economic development. This can be clearly seen in Europe, where the average citizen of the European Union spent 17.4% of their income on food in 2004, while people spent almost half of their income on food in the EU accession countries (FAO 2004).

Most commentators, however, oppose such direct state interventions. One objection is that any such system would inevitably create somewhat arbitrary food groups; another that it would be difficult to implement. The EU-funded PorGrow project interviewed stakeholders on their opinions of anti-obesity interventions, and found many doubts over strategies based on taxation of certain types of food. Overall, stakeholders representing food industry, non-governmental public sector as well as policy makers rated the idea of taxing of high-fat and high-sugar foods very negatively. One of many concerns raised was that the taxation option would impact most on lower socio-economic groups (Millstone et al. 2006, pp. 120–123). It might be argued that this should not be of concern, since a similar effect arises with regard to the high taxation of tobacco, which affects lower socio-economic groups most since they smoke more than other groups. On the other hand, many have contended that healthier foods are less easily available in poorer neighborhoods; if true, that should surely count against the justice of such a policy (unless, perhaps, it were accompanied by additional interventions with regard to food availability).

In addition, we should not ignore the fact that governments already intervene extensively in the price of food. In the European Union this is principally via the Common Agricultural Policy. This policy may have made sense in a time of food shortages. Now, however, it is perverse in terms of food and health, as well as damaging to food production in developing countries (Oxfam 2002a, b, 2004a, b). The EU system of subsidizing and supporting agriculture artificially lowers the prices of foods (especially those high in sugar or fat, including meat and dairy products) and rewards large-scale industrial agriculture (often to the detriment of the (micro-)nutritional value of the resulting foodstuffs) (Pollan 2008, p. 108). From the point of view of obesity – or of healthy eating in general – there is little doubt that this policy is counter-productive (Schafer Elinder 2005).

A second example of a possible policy intervention is the proposal to ban or restrict advertising of "unhealthy" foods or to advertise healthier eating, or both. Some of these interventions are already taking place. For example, the United Kingdom has a ban on advertising "junk" foods before, during and after educational TV programs aimed at children. There is also a call to restrict advertising of high-fat and high-sugar food in all media in the same way as tobacco and alcohol advertising. In the last few years the British government has been regularly warning the food industry as well as the media that if they don't start acting "responsibly," strict restrictions on food advertising will be introduced (BBC 2006). On the face of it, this seems like an eminently sensible policy measure, and there is certainly something deeply unattractive about large companies exercising finely-honed marketing skills on young children to the likely detriment of their health. Despite the gut-appeal of such a policy, however, it may still leave important questions unaddressed.

In the first place, there are some doubts as to whether restricted advertising would have a significant effect, given how pervasive is children's exposure to the full panoply of marketing techniques –

from supermarkets through bill-boards to the internet and disguised advertising in the form of "product placement" in many films and television shows. Whatever restrictions are imposed, children are bound to see or watch thousands of adverts and brand messages. Moreover, they often watch a great deal of adult television, or will soon do so. Second, observe that there is an important connection to socio-economic status here. It might, indeed, be argued that restrictions on advertising might benefit lower SES children more, because they are more susceptible to advertising messages (cf. respondent quoted in Millstone et al. 2006, p. 107). It seems to be true that subjective abilities to deal with consumer choices tend to vary with SES, and are to some extent independent from the restrictions on choice imposed by lower income. To the extent that advertising restrictions were effective, then, they might "protect" children in the short-term. However, those children will still be exposed to some advertising and will soon be adolescents who must develop sophisticated consumer skills to navigate the full gamut of marketing techniques. One may argue, therefore, that we should be more concerned with developing children's ability to respond to advertising intelligently, than with the (probably vain) attempt to prevent their being exposed to it.

In this context it is also worth emphasizing how much is involved in educating future consumers. Children need to learn how to enter the market place and make choices that relate to their own interests, as opposed to the interests of those who are selling. They need to learn how to see past all manner of largely irrelevant or misleading factors, such as branding, advertising, one-sided health claims, not to mention the latest dietary fads and health-related panics being aired in the media. This sort of education is not only a matter of providing people with information. The skills involved are primarily practical, and are developed through actual experience of navigating consumer and life-style choices. This is not, of course, a reason to reject information-based measures, such as education about healthier lifestyles or better nutrition labeling of food. Nonetheless, the importance of these practical consumer skills does suggest a critical channel that interventions – not least school-based interventions – might also seek to address.

A third possible intervention concerns transport systems and infrastructure, given our societies' over-reliance on the private car. (This is also a major issue for developing countries, as many are rapidly moving to car-based economies). There is no doubt that many measures to improve transport infrastructures and public transport, or to alter urban planning, would be very expensive and would take a lot of time (Millstone et al. 2006). However, states have easier and cheaper options such as building safe footpaths and cycle-paths to promote walking and cycling to school. That could reduce how often children are driven to school, and regular exercise before and after school would obviously increase the amount of time children are physically active. There are currently many new initiatives of local councils, governments and independent groups to promote healthy walking and cycling to school as a way of tackling childhood obesity (Surrey County Council 2008; Walk to School Campaign 2008).

However, many parents are reluctant to allow children to go far from the house due to perceived dangers from road traffic. According to a survey conducted by the government-backed "Cycling England" initiative, although the number of children involved in cycling accidents has been dropping in recent years, eight out of ten parents don't allow their children to cycle to school for safety reasons. While most parents admit they used their bike as regular transport when they were school age, most of them ban their children from enjoying the same freedoms (Taylor 2008).. But as a separate survey for sustainable transport charity "Sustrans" found, nearly half of all pupils answered that they want to cycle to school, yet only 2% of British schoolchildren actually do (BBC 2008).

Street crime and violence – or rather, the fear of these – may also play a role in parents' decisions whether to allow their children to walk and cycle to school, or to play independently. Although the statistics remain more or less static, perceptions of risk and danger seem to have increased considerably, which may have something to do with increasing media coverage of (for example) pedophilia or the place of crime on politicians' agendas (Gill 2007). They also relate to parents' increasing tendency not to expect other adults to take responsibility for their children (Furedi 2001).

Such concerns affect how many children are allowed to play outside, if they are allowed to use a bicycle, and account for the increasing tendency to drive children to school.

There are many stereotypes about children and childhood that are related to the current preoccupation with safety concerns. For example, media representations in the UK often see-saw between picturing children as either powerless victims or dangerous and potentially criminal. This schizophrenic attitude reflects a more realistic concern that our societies are overly protective of (most) children, and as a result are not bringing up a generation of responsible and independent adults. As discussed above with regard to children's walking and biking to school, many are concerned about the effect these overprotective attitudes have on children. Terms such as "cotton-wool kids," "cul-de sac generation" and (on the other hand) "free-range" children have recently appeared in the media. American journalist Lenore Skenazy published an article about her 9-year old son traveling on his own on public transport across New York. She subsequently described how this sparked more negative responses than anything she had written in her 28-years career as a political and war journalist. Major TV channels labeled her as "America's Worst Mom"; yet in her words, "My son got home, ecstatic with independence" (McDermott 2008). Only a generation ago, it was common for children to play together unsupervised, and to make their own way to and from school. As many commentators have emphasized, letting children take risks is part of their development. As Penny Nicholls, strategy director at the Children's Society, recently pointed out: "Over-protecting children carries different risks to under-protecting them, but can still cause long-term damage to their well-being" (BBC 2007). A society that is overprotective of its children may soon find out that they are not learning how to become responsible adults.

Concluding Reflections

We have discussed Western perspectives on childhood and adolescence, the responsibilities that their parents or guardians have for their development, interventions in schools, as well as the possible role of the state. We have presented many doubts as to why parents cannot be fully responsible for their children. It is not only that there is much confusion over what is best for children, but also developed societies constitute an "obesogenic" environment, so that our social structures and environments often contradict the clearest and most general aspects of the advice that is given. At the same time, it is difficult to say exactly what changes would render that environment healthier for children and adults, or how they might be brought about. What is certain is that parental efforts need to be supported by public institutions, and that commercial interests often run counter to the efforts of both. We have therefore discussed some ways in which states and local authorities can alter the opportunities available to children, and suggested that schools and health campaigns need to support the development of children's abilities to respond intelligently to widespread social pressures for all sort of unhealthy behaviors. We have also discussed three possible policy measures that could counter the rise of childhood obesity: altering food prices, banning or restricting food advertising to children, and altering children's use of different modes of transport. While all of these point to useful areas for change at community, social or policy levels, however, none of them promises a simple or direct remedy. This is because in each case we are pointed to more complex surrounding factors. Proposals to tax unhealthy foods really point us back to our system of food production, already subject to extensive state intervention and enormous commercial forces. Measures to do with advertising point us to children's – and adults' – abilities to act as intelligent, independent consumers in a complex market-place. Measures relating to transport point us to many factors, not least to children's freedom of movement and safety in societies of strangers – societies that increasingly see adult strangers as a threat to children, rather than a source of guidance and oversight.

Rather than offering particular prescriptions, then, we conclude by emphasizing how great are the challenges involved here, both culturally and institutionally. Culturally speaking, a number of popular stereotypes may get in the way of sensible responses to the issues. We have already noted that contemporary ideas about childhood often over-emphasize children's vulnerability and inability to act independently – increasing pressures upon parents while limiting children's freedom to socialize and be active. Furthermore, we have only touched on other stereotypes that affect how we think about food and health. While we clearly need to develop children's abilities to navigate an environment which favors low levels of physical activity, unhealthy food choices, and so on, we also need to avoid playing into the stigma and prejudices surrounding "fat."

There can be little doubt that Western societies entertain many dubious stereotypes about body image, and there is emerging opposition to our recent obsession with "overweight" and obesity. Feminists have long argued that women are oppressed by developed societies' very slim, indeed boyish, body ideals, while pro-fat activists argue more broadly that our society has cultivated a "fat phobia" (NAAFA 2008). Anorectic supermodels are presented in the popular media as examples of desirable body shape, or even as images of health, while fatness is popularly associated with laziness, incompetence and stupidity. "Letting yourself" become obese is seen as a moral and social failure. Given this background, there is a real danger that anti-obesity interventions might contribute – in effect, though not of course in intention – to increased stigma upon "overweight" or obese children. There is also a danger that anti-obesity interventions may play into social tendencies to demonize (some) foods, to regard food merely in terms of its (supposed) health effects, and to ignore or even spoil the pleasures and sociability that most people and cultures have traditionally found in eating.

Institutionally, it is also worth bearing in mind how powerful are the commercial interests at stake here. Many argue that the food industry is irresponsibly contributing to obesity and indeed profiting from it, a point that we have only touched on in this chapter. Processed foods, which are certainly a major factor in the rise of obesity and dietary problems, generate much more profit than whole foods; they can be branded, and are easier to store and transport. The food industry has also played into confusion among the general public as to what constitutes a healthy diet. Consider the manifold ways in which packaging makes or implies health claims for all sorts of foods, or the ways in which images of forbidden indulgence are attached to all sorts of allegedly unhealthy foods. It might also be argued that we rely too much on – at any rate, are often confused by – what the latest research claims is beneficial to our health, forgetting that powerful food companies often fund research. Other industries profit from obesity too, such as the pharmaceutical and dieting industries. Think not only of the thousands of books available on the topic of dieting, but also the enormous number of "low fat," "low carb" and "diet" foods available for sale, and the various commercial weight-loss programs. Insofar as institutional changes are unlikely, this again highlights the importance of equipping children – and adults – with the skills and independence to make consumer-choices that serve their own interests, rather than those of private companies.

The need to equip children with the personal and social resources to make such choices points us back to one of the most difficult questions for all health-oriented social policies. This is the undoubted link between social class and poorer health, which in developed countries is now manifesting itself in problems of overweight rather than underweight. Immensely complex as this link is, it certainly relates to the greater difficulty people with fewer opportunities and lower education will always face in negotiating social life to their lasting advantage. None of the measures we have discussed provides any straightforward answers to this problem, nor could it, for it relates to the most fundamental problems of social justice.

In sum, simple interventions to tackle the rise of childhood obesity are not available, and all the measures we have touched on face considerable challenges. They must tackle the opportunities we extend to children, the ways we have come to think and feel about food, powerful institutional and commercial pressures, and deep social inequalities. At the same time, we might take heart from the thought that developing children's abilities to be active, independent and informed promises social benefits much beyond a reduced incidence of obesity and improved health.

References

Archard, D. (1995). *Children, rights and childhood*. London: Routledge.

Aristotle (2000). *Nicomachean ethics*. translated by Roger Crisp. Cambridge: Cambridge University Press.

Armstrong, J., Reilly, J.J., & Child Health Information Team (2002). Breastfeeding and lowering the risk of childhood obesity. *Lancet, 359*, 2003–2004.

Bayol, S.A., Farrington, S.J., & Stickland, N.C. (2007). A maternal 'junk food' diet in pregnancy and lactation promotes an exacerbated taste for 'junk food' and a greater propensity for obesity in rat offspring. *British Journal of Nutrition, 98*, 843–851.

BBC (2006, July 25). Blair threatens junk food ad ban. (October 21, 2010); www.bbc.co.uk/1/hi/uk_politics/5215288.stm.

BBC (2007, October 28). Fear stops child development. (October 21, 2010); www.bbc.co.uk/1/hi/education/7062545.stm.

BBC (2008, May 5). Parents 'stop children cycling'. (October 21, 2010); news.bbc.co.uk/1/hi/education/7380691.stm.

British Medical Association (2008). Fetal alcohol spectrum disorders: a guide for healthcare professionals. (October 21, 2010); www.bma.org.uk/health_promotion_ethics/alcohol/Fetalalcohol.jsp.

Department of Agriculture Economic Research Service (2008). Food CPI, prices and expenditures: food expenditure tables. Washington (October 21, 2010); www.ers.usda.gov/briefing/CPIFoodAndExpenditures/Data/.

Dummer, T.J.B., Gibbon, M.A, Hackett, A.F., Stratton, G., & Taylor, S.R. (2005). Is overweight and obesity in 9-10-year-old children in Liverpool related to deprivation and/or electoral ward when based on school attended? *Public Health Nutrition, 8*, 636–641.

FAO (2004). Twenty-fourth FAO regional conference for Europe, food safety and quality in Europe, Montpellier, France. (October 21, 2010); ftp://ftp.fao.org/unfao/bodies/erc/erc24/J1876e.doc.

Food Ethics Council (2005). Getting personal: shifting responsibilities for dietary health. London (October 21, 2010); www.foodethicscouncil.org/node/115.

Furedi, F. (2001). *Paranoid parenting*. London: Allen Lane.

Garson, A. Jr., & Engelhard, C.L. (2007). Attacking obesity: lessons from smoking. *Journal of the American College of Cardiology, 49*, 1673–1675.

Gill, T. (2007). *No fear: growing up in a risk averse society*. London: Calouste Gulbenkian Foundation.

Hancox, R.J., & Poulton, R. (2006). Watching television is associated with childhood obesity: but is it clinically important? *International Journal of Obesity, 30*, 171–175.

Hickman, M. (2008, May 8). Confusion over official advice on healthy diet. *The Independent* (October 21, 2010); www.independent.co.uk/life-style/health-and-wellbeing/health-news/confusion-over-official-advice-on-healthy-diet-822823.html.

IDEFICS (2008). Identification and prevention of dietary- and lifestyle-induced health effects in children and infants. (October 21, 2010); www.ideficsstudy.eu.

Keith, S.W, Redden, D.T., Katzmarzyk, P.T., Boggiano, M.M., Hanlon, E.C., Benca, R.M., Ruden, D., Pietrobelli, A., Barger, J.L., Fontaine, K.R., Wang, C., Aronne, L.J., Wright, S.M., Baskin, M., Dhurandhar, N.V., Lijoi, M.C., Grilo, C.M., DeLuca, M., Westfall, A.O., & Allison, D.B. (2006). Putative contributors to the secular increase in obesity: exploring the roads less traveled. *International Journal of Obesity, 30*, 1585–1594.

Marshall, J., & Hardman, K. (2000). The state and status of physical education in schools in international context. *European Physical Education Review, 6*, 203–229.

Matthews, G. (2005). Philosophy of childhood. Stanford Encyclopedia of Philosophy. (October 21, 2010); plato.stanford.edu/entries/childhood.

McDermott, N. (2008, April 30). I've been labelled the world's worst mom. *Spiked*. (October 21, 2010); www.spiked-online.com/index.php?/site/earticle/5043/.

MEND Programme (2008). Mind, Exercise, Nutrition... Do It! London (October 21, 2010); www.mendprogramme.org.

Mennella, J.A., Jagnow, C.P., & Beauchamp, G.K. (2001). Prenatal and postnatal flavor learning by human infants. *Pediatrics, 107*, 88.

Millstone, T., & Lobstein, T. (2006). Policy options for responding to obesity: evaluating the options. Summary report of the EC-funded project to map the views of stakeholders involved in tackling obesity - the PorGrow project. University of Sussex.

NAAFA (2008). National Association to Advance Fat Acceptance. Oakland, California (October 21, 2010); www.naafa.org.

National Statistics (2008). Family spending. (October 21, 2010); www.statistics.gov.uk/cci/nugget.asp?id=1921.

Oxfam (2002a). Stop the dumping! How EU agricultural subsidies are damaging livelihoods in the developing world, 31, Oxford (October 21, 2010); www.oxfam.org.uk/resources/policy/index.html.

Oxfam (2002b). Milking the CAP: How Europe's dairy regime is devastating livelihoods in the developing world, 34, Oxford (October 21, 2010); www.oxfam.org.uk/resources/policy/index.html.

Oxfam (2004a). Spotlight on subsidies: cereal injustice under the CAP in Britain, 55, Oxford (October 21, 2010); www.oxfam.org.uk/resources/policy/index.html.

Oxfam (2004b). Dumping on the world how EU sugar policies hurt poor countries, 61, Oxford (October 21, 2010); www.oxfam.org.uk/resources/policy/index.html.

Phipps, S.A., Burton, P.S., Osberg, L.S., & Lethbridge, L.N. (2006). Poverty and the extent of childhood obesity in Canada, Norway and the United States. *Obesity Reviews, 7*, 5–12.

Public Health Information for Scotland (2008). Obesity by class. (October 21, 2010); www.scotpho.org.uk/home/Clinicalriskfactors/Obesity/obesity_data/obesity_deprivation.asp.

Schafer Elinder, L. (2005). Obesity, hunger, and agriculture: the damaging role of subsidies. *British Medical Journal, 331*, 1333–1336.

Surrey County Council (2008). Safe routes to schools' initiative. Surrey (October 21, 2010); www.saferoutesto-schools.com.

Taylor, M. (2008, May 6). Parents afraid to allow their children to cycle on roads. *The Guardian*. (October 21, 2010); www.guardian.co.uk/uk/2008/may/06/transport.children.

Wadas-Willingham, V. (2008, May 25). Six states get an 'A' for work against kids' obesity. *CNN News: Health*; www.cnn.com/2007/HEALTH/diet.fitness/01/30/obesity.report/index.html.

Walk to School Campaign (2008). London (October 21, 2010); www.walktoschool.org.uk.

Chapter 3
Methodological Aspects for Childhood and Adolescence Obesity Epidemiology

Gerardo Rodríguez, Angelo Pietrobelli, Youfa Wang, and Luis A. Moreno

Introduction

Body composition assessment methods are useful for the screening of excess body fat and its related metabolic complications. Reliable and practical measurements of body fatness and its distribution pattern are necessary in epidemiological, clinical and population studies for monitoring overweight and obesity and its outcomes or consequences. Childhood and adolescence are critical periods in human life due to the multiple changes that take place between birth and adulthood. The global acceleration of both growth and maturation, especially during the first 2 years of life and adolescence, imply that parameters to assess nutritional status differ considerably in every stage.

While body mass and body compartments constantly increase until adulthood, annual growth velocity and proportional weight gain decrease progressively, except during puberty. A characteristic sexual dimorphism of body composition patterns is present at the end of childhood and during adolescence. Sex differences in total fat mass and its body distribution are apparent even long before puberty starts (Daniels et al. 1997). The amount of fat mass in girls is usually higher than in boys at all ages (Daniels et al. 1997; Rodríguez et al. 2004b). These body composition differences related to sex support the concept that population standard growth curves must be constructed separately for both sexes. Furthermore, sexual maturation is related to adiposity measures and the association varies by sex (Wang 2002), and it has been argued that sexual maturation status should be considered when assessing young people's nutritional status including obesity (Wang and Adair 2001; WHO 1995).

The body mass index (BMI: kg/m^2), frequently used as an adiposity index, also varies in a characteristic way during growth. It decreases during childhood until the so-called "adiposity rebound" which is a rise in BMI measure that occurs normally between 3 and 7 years. After the "adiposity

G. Rodríguez
Growth, Exercise, Nutrition and Development (GENUD) Research Group, Departamento de Pediatría,
Universidad de Zaragoza, Instituto Aragonés de Ciencias de la Salud, Zaragoza, Spain

A. Pietrobelli
Pediatric Unit, Verona University Medical School, and Applied Dietetic Technical Sciences Chair,
Modena and Reggio Emilia University, Verona, Italy

Y. Wang
Center for Human Nutrition, Department of International Health, Bloomberg School of Public Health,
Johns Hopkins University, 615 North Wolf Street, Baltimore, MD 21205, USA

L.A. Moreno (✉)
(Growth, Exercise, Nutrition and Development) GENUD Research Group,
E. U. Ciencias de la Salud, Universidad de Zaragoza, Zaragoza, Spain
e-mail: lmoreno@unizar.es

L.A. Moreno et al. (eds.), *Epidemiology of Obesity in Children and Adolescents*,
Springer Series on Epidemiology and Public Health 2, DOI 10.1007/978-1-4419-6039-9_3,
© Springer Science+Business Media, LLC 2011

rebound," BMI increases again until the adulthood. It has been observed that changes in BMI during adiposity rebound are due to changes in body fat and not to variations in lean mass or height. At the individual level, an early "adiposity rebound" is known to be a risk factor for later obesity (Cole 2004; Rolland-Cachera et al. 1984).

Chronological and biological factors significantly affect growth patterns in children and adolescents. Growth, maturation and development are dynamic processes which influence anthropometric proportions and body composition along these life periods. Therefore, epidemiological assessment of obesity in children and adolescents should consider all these factors. This chapter reviews concepts and methods, specific body composition assessment techniques, and epidemiological aspects that should be considered for obesity assessment during childhood and adolescence.

Definition and Diagnosis of Obesity

Obesity is defined as an excess of body fat (WHO 2000). However, the obesity concept means more than body fat deposition because adiposity is associated with short- and long-term adverse metabolic complications, as well as with significant physical and psychosocial problems, that must be all included in the same concept (Fisberg et al. 2004; Koletzko et al. 2002). In order to manage obesity and its consequences (definitions, diagnosis, quantification and classification), objective and standard parameters of body fatness are required.

In children and adolescents, as they grow, anthropometric and body composition measures change considerably over the years. Especially during adolescence, a global acceleration of growth and maturation occurs, with differential changes between both sexes. Annual gain of height, weight and fat-free mass continuously increase during childhood and adolescence. Among other sex differences, the amount of fat mass is usually higher in girls than in boys and, independently of the chronological age (CA), pubertal development is associated with an increase of body fat in girls. However, the characteristic body composition pattern that appears in adolescent boys is a decrease of body fat (Rodríguez et al. 2004a; Taylor et al. 1997). Body composition and body mass distribution are sex and age related in both children and adolescents and, therefore, growth charts and population references are necessary to define obesity.

Screening for Excess Body Fat

Population-based cut-off values for body fat determined by body composition reference methods are theoretically the best criterion for the definition of overweight and obesity. However, the definition of excess body fat is somewhat arbitrary even when total body fat mass or body fat mass percentage (%FM) are accurately measured. Nowadays, there is no consensus about %FM cut-offs for obesity in children and adolescents. Especially during adolescence, the level of adiposity may vary widely by age, sex and pubertal development. In the absence of clear cut-off points, usually accepted %FM values for the definition of excess body fat range between 30–35% in female adolescents and 20–25% in males aged 4–6 years and 15–18 years (Sardinha et al. 1999; Taylor et al. 2002; Taylor et al. 2003.

During recent years, BMI is the parameter most frequently used for the screening of excess body fat in children and adolescents for a number of reasons, such as that it is easy to determine, it tends to correlate well with body fat, and it has been widely used in adults to define obesity. In a 1995 report, a WHO expert committee ever suggested using the sex-age-specific 85th BMI percentile based on data collected in the United States to classify overweight in ado-

Table 3.1 International cut-off points for body mass index for overweight and obesity by sex between 2 and 18 years, defined to pass through body mass index of 25 and 30 kg/m² at age 18 (Cole et al. 2000)

Age	Body mass index 25 kg/m²		Body mass index 30 kg/m²	
	Males	Females	Males	Females
2	18.41	18.02	20.09	19.81
2.5	18.13	17.76	19.80	19.55
3	17.89	17.56	19.57	19.36
3.5	17.69	17.40	19.39	19.23
4	17.55	17.28	19.29	19.15
4.5	17.47	17.19	19.26	19.12
5	17.42	17.15	19.30	19.17
5.5	17.45	17.20	19.47	19.34
6	17.55	17.34	19.78	19.65
6.5	17.71	17.53	20.23	20.08
7	17.92	17.75	20.63	20.51
7.5	18.16	18.03	21.09	21.01
8	18.44	18.35	21.60	21.57
8.5	18.76	18.69	22.17	22.18
9	19.10	19.07	22.77	22.81
9.5	19.46	19.45	23.39	23.46
10	19.84	19.86	24.00	24.11
10.5	20.20	20.29	24.57	24.77
11	20.55	20.74	25.10	25.42
11.5	20.89	21.20	25.58	26.05
12	21.22	21.68	26.02	26.67
12.5	21.56	22.14	26.43	27.24
13	21.91	22.58	26.84	27.76
13.5	22.27	22.98	27.25	28.20
14	22.62	23.34	27.63	28.57
14.5	22.96	23.66	27.98	28.87
15	23.29	23.94	28.30	29.11
15.5	23.60	24.17	28.60	29.29
16	23.90	24.37	28.88	29.43
16.5	24.19	24.54	29.14	29.56
17	24.46	24.70	29.41	29.69
17.5	24.73	24.85	29.70	29.84
18	25	25	30	30

lescents (WHO 1995). In 2000, the International Obesity Task Force (IOTF) proposed BMI cut-off points for overweight and obesity screening, for each half-year of age both in males and females, which correspond to BMI values of 25 and 30 kg/m² at the age of 18 years (Cole et al. 2000) (Table 3.1). Other studies have used the BMI for the screening of excess body fat in children and adolescents based on BMI-for-age percentiles derived from international and national population data. Among these studies, the most frequent criterion for obesity definition has been a BMI higher than the 95th percentile for a specific age and sex subgroup, and for overweight a BMI between the 85th and 95th percentile (Moreno et al. 2000; Must et al. 1991; Power et al. 1997; Serra et al. 2001). The IOTF BMI values represent standard international references that allow the screening of adiposity in children and adolescents worldwide under the same criterion, without variations depending on geographic, social and secular trends (Cole et al. 2000). The IOTF approach is questionable at the individual level but is useful in epidemiological studies when obesity prevalence is estimated and then compared with results from other populations.

Reference Population Standards

Body composition and BMI-for-age sex-specific charts are graphic tools that contain a series of curved lines indicating specific percentiles. The percentile curves show the pattern of growth according to anthropometric, compartment measurement or derived index values. Healthcare professionals use the established percentile cut-off points to identify nutritional risk status in children and adolescents. The meaning and interpretation of the percentiles is a matter of great importance. For instance, if a child's BMI equals the 75th percentile, it means that 75% of children with the same sex and age from reference population considered for this specific chart have a lower BMI than the measured subject. As an index of adiposity, a BMI value ≥95th percentile defines the cut-off for obesity; a BMI between the 85th and 95th percentile defines the range for overweight; a BMI < 5th percentile indicates underweight; and a BMI from the 5th percentile to <85th percentile means normal weight. Besides providing an isolated point of reference for the definition of overweight, BMI percentile curves are very useful in growing children and adolescents, to assess sequential long term changes of nutritional status in individuals and groups, and to compare BMI percentile values between subjects of different age and sex subgroups (Rodríguez and Moreno 2006).

Many other national and international reference standards for children and adolescents have been proposed for the assessment of adiposity. Their different methodological possibilities are reviewed in this chapter. It is accepted that anthropometric or body composition measurements over the 95th percentiles, or +2 standard deviations (SD) over mean population values, are considered excessive or abnormally high. To know the number of SDs that a measurement moves away from the mean value of the reference population, a "z-score" can be calculated by the formula: $z\text{-}score = (measurement - mean)/SD$.

Methodological Aspects Depending on the Aims

Depending on the aims of each study, population standards and methods used must be in agreement with its purpose. We should consider the reliability of the methods for each pediatric age group, the use of up-to-date reference data and an appropriate measurement method for each aim. Some practical examples of method selection are given below:

1. When aiming to measure the total amount of body fat or its regional distribution and, at the same time, to test the agreement with population means, up-to-date reference charts must be appropriately selected among all that already exist for the corresponding method, sex and age group. In the case of population samples with a large number of subjects, when fast and easy population mean measurements are required, "field methods" such as anthropometry or bioelectrical impedance are appropriate to have a global epidemiological view of the sample characteristics.
2. When accuracy and precision are required to assess total or regional body fat (e.g., intra-abdominal fat), aiming to correlate body measurements with associated co-morbidities at the individual level or in a reduced sample, reference methods must be selected such as "air displacement plethysmography," magnetic resonance imaging or dual-energy X-ray absorptiometry (Pietrobelli et al. 2001; Rodríguez et al. 2004a).
3. If the aim is to monitor changes of body fat or abdominal circumference, after individual or population interventions, regional or national body composition charts are adequate enough to control longitudinal variations.
4. When overweight prevalence needs to be assessed, the IOTF BMI reference standards represent the best option (Cole et al. 2000). Although the classification of subjects by these BMI criteria does not have enough accuracy and precision at the individual level, standard and global international reference criteria allow to assess obesity prevalence in epidemiological studies in children and adolescents with the same pre-fixed cut-offs in a comparable way over the world and over the time.

Assessment of Body Composition

Significant physical changes occur during the years spanning infancy through young adulthood. These changes are apparent both externally and internally. External changes such as body proportions, height, weight, and pubertal status changes are easily measured by physical examination and by simple anthropometric measurements; however, internal changes such as body composition and hormonal status require specialized testing (Pietrobelli et al. 2001).

The physical changes that occur throughout childhood are generally related to growth and maturation. Growth and maturation are complex biological processes influenced by multiple factors including genes, environment (e.g., diet and physical activity), demography (age, sex, and race), hormones, and health status. Clinical assessment of growth and maturation may be enhanced by accurate measurement of body composition (Pietrobelli et al. 2007).

Over the past several decades body composition methods have been gaining acceptance in both research and clinical medicine; however, studies have demonstrated that adult body composition measurement methods and data may not be directly applicable to pediatric populations. The value of understanding pediatric body composition methods and applications is manifold. Body composition analysis in children provides a window into the complex changes that occur throughout childhood and provides the opportunity to assess metabolic and physiological correlates. Once body composition is determined in large groups of healthy children, it will be possible to understand the normal compartmental changes that occur with growth and development and to attain a greater understanding of the effect of disease and medications on body composition. Additionally, longitudinal body composition studies will clarify the relationship between body composition measurements during childhood and during adulthood.

Body Composition Changes Throughout Childhood and Adolescence

Body composition measurements at the molecular level are most simply divided into fat mass (FM) and fat-free mass (FFM), representing a two-compartment model of the body. Features of the two-compartment model are influenced by age and maturation (Butte et al. 2000). It has been demonstrated that the proportion of FM to FFM changes throughout childhood and adolescence, and the changes in boys are different from those in girls (Maynard et al. 2001).

Early growth is a consequence of cellular hypertrophy and hyperplasia. Throughout infancy, childhood and adolescence, there is a change in the chemical composition of FFM as defined in terms of total body water (TBW), extracellular water, cellular water, osseous minerals, non-osseous minerals, carbohydrates and total body potassium (TBK). The use of age-specific and sex-specific constants for converting chemical components such as total body water (TBW), total body potassium (TBK), and body density into FFM can eliminate systematic errors in two-compartment pediatric molecular body composition methods (Forbes 1987). The components of FFM include protein, mineral mass, lipid, and water. These FFM components also change as absolute and relative mass with age (Fomon and Nelson 2002; Fomon et al. 1982).

The following section reviews available pediatric body composition methodologies used to monitor the changes during growth and development and to classify the level of these changes.

Anthropometry

Anthropometry represents a group of inexpensive and non-invasive methods to assess the size, shape and composition of the human body. Anthropometric measurements include weight, height, circumferences, and skinfold thicknesses. Relative measures such as weight-for-height (kg/m) and BMI (kg/m^2) are derived from weight and height measurements (WHO 1995). Circumferences and skinfold thicknesses may be used to assess the size and proportion of body segments (Cameron 1986).

Anthropometric measurements may be used as indirect markers of adiposity (e.g., BMI, waist circumference) or as markers of fat distribution (e.g., waist circumference, adiposity index).

Length/Height

The ability to accurately measure length in infancy and height in childhood contributes to the ability to assess the presence of normal growth and growth velocity. Poor growth in children can represent a wide array of disorders including poor nutrition, hypothyroidism, growth hormone deficiency, chronic infection, inflammatory bowel disease, celiac disease, and malignancy. Although this measurement is relatively easy to perform, it requires a certain degree of technical knowledge.

Length is measured from birth to age two using an infant stadiometer. Optimally two observers should measure length. One observer stands behind the headboard and positions the child's head with the Frankfort Plane with the shoulders and hips flat against the board plane; the Frankfort Plane is perpendicular to the board plane. The second observer stands at the child's feet and reads the measurement.

Stature or standing height is measured in the standard upright posture starting at age two. It is important to note that stature is shorter than length; this discrepancy is accounted for on the National Center for Health Statistics growth curves when the child's data are transitioned between the 0–36 month and the 2–20 year curves. A stadiometer with a fixed or movable rod is used to measure height. During the measurement the child should stand straight with arms by the sides, palms facing the thighs, heels together touching the vertical board of the stadiometer with the feet positioned at a $60°$ angle to each other, and the weight distributed equally between both feet (Heyward and Stolarczyk 1996).

Weight

Infants (0–2 years) should be weighed unclothed on a leveled pan scale. The pan should be 100 cm long in order to support a 2-year-old child. Children should be weighed in their underwear with a digital or balance scale. Weight is recorded to the nearest 100 g. This measurement should be repeated three times and averaged.

Weight-for-Stature Indices

Weight-for-stature indices are expressed as a percentage of the median reference values, as a percentile and as a z-score. The percentage of the median is one hundred times the measurement divided by the median or mean reference value for the child's age. To determine the percentile the measurement is plotted on a growth percentile chart (growth curve). The z-score indicates the number of standard deviations the measurement is above or below the mean or median reference value (Cole 1993).

Body Mass Index (BMI)

BMI is an anthropometry-based index of weight-for-height that is safe, non-invasive, simple, and inexpensive to obtain. The equation for BMI is W/H^2, where weight (W) is expressed in kilograms and height (H) in meters (Quetelet 1869). Several studies suggest that BMI is a useful measure of growth and development in children (Cole et al. 2000; Dietz and Bellizzi 1999); additionally, BMI is widely used to characterize childhood fatness in epidemiological studies (Moreno et al. 2006; Pietrobelli et al. 1998; Rodríguez and Moreno 2006).

Longitudinal studies have aided in the characterization of the BMI curve in childhood. BMI increases during infancy, peaks at approximately 9 months of age, decreases until approximately 6 years of age, and thereafter increases until adulthood. The earliest published pediatric BMI curves were based on data obtained from French children (Pietrobelli et al. 1998). Currently, BMI curves are available for American (Kuczmarski et al. 2000), British (Cole et al. 1995), Swedish (He et al. 2000), Hong Kong (Leung et al. 1998), Dutch (Cole and Roede 1999) and Italian (Cacciari et al. 2002) pediatric populations.

In the United States, BMI values are used to classify children as either underweight, normal weight (<85th), at risk for overweight (85th–95th), and overweight (>95th) (Dietz and Bellizzi 1999; Himes and Dietz 1994). In an international context, the IOTF reference standards (Cole et al. 2000) are strongly recommended in order to allow adequate comparisons.

Skinfold Thickness

Skinfold thickness measurement is another anthropometry-based body composition method. A skinfold consists of a double fold of skin and subcutaneous adipose tissue. To obtain a skinfold thickness measurement the skinfold is held by the investigator's non-dominant hand between finger 1 and fingers 2 and 3, and a caliper, held in the dominant hand, provides a measurement of the skinfold in millimeters (Lohman 1989) (Fig. 3.1). A high quality skinfold caliper is necessary to accurately measure the skinfold. A flexible measuring tape is necessary to determine the exact point of measurement for certain skinfold thickness measurements. Skinfold thickness measurements can be used to estimate body density, FFM, FM, and %BF in conjunction with appropriate and validated prediction equations (Brambilla et al. 2006; Rodríguez et al. 2005). Assumptions of the skinfold thickness-based equations are that skinfold thickness measurements quantify subcutaneous fat

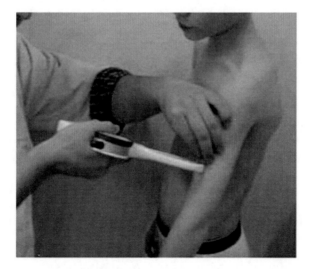

Fig. 3.1 To obtain a skinfold thickness measurement the skinfold is held by the investigator's non-dominant hand between finger 1 and fingers 2 and 3, and a caliper, held in the dominant hand, provides a measurement of the skinfold in millimeters

mass, and that subcutaneous fat mass is a constant fraction of total body fat. These equations may be used when a relative index of fatness is required in field or clinical studies but their accuracy for the assessment of %BF at the individual level is poor (Rodríguez et al. 2005).

The most useful skinfold thickness measurements in the pediatric age group are the triceps and subscapular skinfolds. The biceps, suprailiac, thigh and calf skinfolds are also frequently used. Triceps is a good indicator of energy reserves, it correlates well with percent body fat and reference data for triceps from children 1 year of age through adulthood is available. The anatomical reference point of the triceps skinfold is the acromial process of the scapula and the olecranon process of the ulna. A tape measure is used to measure the distance between the lateral projection of the acromial process and the inferior margin of the olecranon process on the lateral aspect of the arm while the elbow is flexed 90°; the midpoint is then marked on the lateral side of the arm. The triceps skinfold is subsequently measured with a caliper one centimeter above the measured midpoint on the posterior aspect of the arm.

Subscapular skinfold correlates highly with total body fat and is a good measure of fat stores on the trunk and is less sensitive to short term fluctuation in nutritional status. The anatomical reference point for the subscapular skinfold thickness is the inferior angle of the scapula, and the skinfold is located along the natural cleavage line of skin inferior to this landmark. The measurement is taken with a caliper applied one centimeter below the grasping fingers. Standard error of the estimate for %BF ranges from 3.6 to 3.9% of body fat. Percent body fat determined by equations that use two or more skinfolds correlates well with %BF determined by underwater weighing (Pearson´s correlation coefficient $r=0.65$ to 0.90) (Harsha et al. 1978).

Circumferences and Diameters

Body size and body proportions are important components of pediatric body composition measurement. Circumferences and skeletal breadth are anthropometric measurements that are useful in determining body size and body proportions. The principles for the use of these anthropometric-based measurement methods are that circumferences reflect FM and FFM and that skeletal size reflect FFM (Wagner and Heyward 1999). Waist, hip and thigh circumferences are used to predict body fat distribution in children, and waist and hip circumferences are both good predictors of intra-abdominal adipose tissue (Brambilla et al. 2006; Goran et al. 1998). A flexible plastic tape measure with a spring-loaded handle is used for the measurement. The measurements should not be made over clothing. The subject stands erect with the abdomen relaxed, the arms at the sides and the feet together.

There have been many different recommendations about where is the correct anatomic place to measure the waist circumference: at the level of umbilicus, around the most prominent part of abdomen, around the narrowest abdominal perimeter, etc. The most recent recommendation is that the examiner faces the children and places an inelastic tape around, in a horizontal plane, at the level of the natural waist, which is the narrowest part of the torso in the area between the spina iliaca superior and the costal edge in the midaxillary line. The waist measurement should be taken at the end of a normal expiration, without the tape compressing the skin.

For the hip circumference, the examiner squats at the side of the subject so that the level of maximum extension of the buttocks can be seen. The tape is placed around the buttocks in a horizontal plane at this level without compressing the skin. The tape is in contact with the skin but it should not indent the soft tissues.

Among others, waist circumference curves are available for American children providing data from 2 to 18 years at the 10th, 25th, 50th and 90th percentiles in a nationally representative sample of African-American, Hispanic and Caucasian children (Fernandez et al. 2004); and in Spanish children (Moreno et al. 1999) and adolescents (Moreno et al. 2007).

Non-Anthropometric Methods

Bioimpedance Analysis

The bioimpedance (BIA) method is based on the concept that tissues rich in water and electrolytes conduct better the flow of an electrical current than adipose tissue. Bioimpedance systems measure the impedance of a low energy electrical signal as it flows through body tissues; impedance is proportional to the conductor length (i.e., height) and inversely proportional to the conductor cross-sectional area. Four electrodes are usually attached to the individual during measurement: one each to the ankle and foot, and one each to the wrist and back of the hand. Measurements are also taken from hand to hand or from foot to foot with the subject standing. Conduction of the electrical current through body tissues is related to the water and electrolyte content of the tissue.

The BIA method provides an estimate of total body water, which is then transformed into FFM. Systems may also be calibrated directly to FFM. While hydration in adults is reasonably stable at ~73%, the hydration of FFM is 77% in 5–6 year old boys and 78% in girls; at age 7–8 years is 76.8% in boys and 77.6% in girls; and at 8–9 years is 76.2% in boys and 77.0% in girls. A pediatric FFM BIA prediction equation must therefore be developed using a reference method for FFM rather than relying on an assumed adult hydration value.

Several population-specific BIA prediction equations have been developed for use in children (Yanovski et al. 1996). Houtkooper et al. (1992), using a three-component model, developed a BIA equation for estimating FFM and cross-validated the equation in subjects 10–19 years of age. An equation developed for subjects younger than 10 years of age and validated by deuterium dilution method was used to obtain reference values for TBW (the prediction error for this equation was 1.411 kg) (Kushner et al. 1992). Lohman's age and sex constants for hydration of FFM are then used to convert TBW estimates to FFM (Lohman 1989). Race-specific BIA FFM equations have been also developed and cross-validated with prediction errors ranging from 1.3 to 2.0 kg (Ellis 1996).

Finally, it is important to note that measurement conditions are fundamental for obtaining accurate BIA body composition estimates. The BIA model, the equation used for body composition estimation, room and subject temperature, body position, electrode placement and several other factors (e.g., eating or drinking, dehydration, exercise) can all influence measurements and should be standardized during measurement (Pietrobelli et al. 2001). The subject must be laying horizontal at least 5 min or more before measurement, to allow an even distribution of all the body fluids. In presence of fever BIA data are not valid. Since the volume to be assessed is the entire length between the foot and the arm it is important to avoid any contact that short circuits such pathway. If the subject is not dressed, arms and legs must be separated from each other, or insulated. To avoid acute fluid shifts, subjects will be instructed to refrain from strenuous exercise for 12 h before the measurement. The examination must be done after an overnight fasting. Room temperature must be kept between 20 and 24°C to prevent undesired effects on cutaneous blood flow or compartmental changes in water. Subjects will be measured while lying supine on a non-conductive surface.

Hydrodensitometry

Hydrodensitometry or underwater weighing is a method based on Archimedes' principle that measures body volume by subtracting submerged weight from land weight and dividing by the density of water. Body density (BD) may be calculated from the body volume measurement, %BF may then be determined using the Siri equation:

$$\%BF = (4.95/BD - 4.5) \times 100.$$

Traditionally, this method has been considered as the gold standard but nowadays it is less widely used because of its technical limitations and it has been replaced by other methods such as dual-energy X-ray absorptiometry or air displacement plethysmography.

Air Displacement Plethysmography (ADP)

ADP by BOD POD is a body composition method that measures body volume and calculates body density. The BOD POD software calculates BF from body density using the Siri equation. ADP is an attractive body composition method for children because of its ease of use and safety (Fields et al. 2002).

During the volume measurement, small changes in volume are produced inside the ADP chamber and the pressure response to these small volume changes is measured. This is done by measuring the interior volume of the empty chamber, then testing it again when the subject is inside. Test conditions are extremely important for accurate ADP results. ADP by BOD POD is performed under adiabatic conditions (it means that there is no heat transfer out of the system) and is based on Poisson's law: $P_1/P_2 = (V_2/V_1)^\gamma$ where γ is the ratio of specific heat of the gas at constant pressure (P) to that of constant volume (V) and is equal to 1.4 for air (Fields et al. 2002). Adiabatic conditions allow for free gain and loss of heat during compression and expansion of air (Fields et al. 2002); however clothing, body hair, and skin surface may create partially isothermal conditions, and isothermal air is 40% more compressible than adiabatic air. The surface area artifact accounts for the isothermal conditions introduced by the skin surface. This small artifact (an apparent reduction in the subject's body volume) is automatically calculated by the BOD POD and used to correct subject body volume. The manufacturer recommends that a swim cap is worn on the head to minimize the effect of hair on creating isothermal conditions. Additionally, the manufacturer recommends that skintight clothing, such as Lycra or spandex, be worn to minimize air trapping in lose clothing. Excess and lose clothing cause underestimation in BF measurement by BOD POD (Fields et al. 2002).

Dual-Energy X-Ray Absorptiometry (DXA)

Recent advances in techniques to measure body composition have provided DXA for assessment of whole-body, as well as regional measurements of bone mass, lean mass and fat mass (Pietrobelli et al. 1996). DXA quantifies relative attenuation of the two main photon peaks as they pass through the body. They resolve body weight into bone mineral and lean tissue mass and subsequently fat tissue mass. Reproducibility for DXA is approximately 0.8% for bone, 1.7% for fat, and 2% of body weight.

DXA scans are increasingly available and easily performed for children of all ages making this method attractive for pediatric body composition measurement. The two major manufacturers of DXA are GE Lunar Corp. and Hologic, Inc, and each has its own measurement algorithm. Each manufacturer produces several different models of DXA. If each DXA system's specific character-istics are taken into account, they all have great potential as pediatric research and clinical tools. An example of a research use of DXA that may lead to clinical application is the prediction of the risk of comorbidities in obese children and adolescents (Higgins et al. 2001). The radiation dose of a whole body DXA scan is low, it accounts only for 0.001 millisieverts which is the hundredth part of a chest radiography dose.

Recognition that DXA measures may differ from results obtained by other methods, and that not all DXA systems are the same, will lead to better interpretation of research and clinical results. Future areas of investigation include pediatric DXA precision studies and comparisons between DXA systems. Results from these will enhance the use of DXA for defining the relationship between body composition and health outcomes.

Imaging Methods

Computerized axial tomography (CT) and magnetic resonance imaging (MRI) provide investigators the opportunity to evaluate tissue organ level components in pediatric subjects in vivo (Heymsfield et al. 1997). CT and MRI produce cross-sectional high-resolution images and multiple cross-sectional images can be used to reconstruct tissue volumes in pediatric subjects including total, subcutaneous and visceral adipose tissue, skeletal muscle, brain, heart, kidney, liver, skin, and bone. Imaging techniques offer new insights into the associations between intra-abdominal adipose tissue and metabolic factors (Goran 1998). None of the currently available methods can assess tissue-system level body composition components with the same accuracy as CT and MRI.

The accumulation of visceral adipose tissue (VAT) in childhood is clinically relevant as there are significant relationships between VAT and adverse health, including dyslipidemia and glucose intolerance, in obese children (Brambilla et al. 2006; Caprio et al. 1996). The accuracy of the measurements that we have with CT and MRI should help to understand ethnic differences in fat distribution as well as sex differences (Goran 1998).

CT and MRI are accurate imaging techniques for assessing body fat distribution, but the disadvantages are cost and radiation exposure (i.e., CT; radiation dose of an abdominal CT accounts for 10 millisieverts), and limited use to a research setting.

Epidemiological Aspects

The current prevalence and trends of obesity among children and adolescents vary considerably worldwide (see also Part I of this book). North America and some European countries have the highest prevalence of overweight (approximately 20 to 30%) and obesity (about 5 to 15%), as well as the highest rate of increase (e.g., 0.5% annually in the USA) (Lobstein et al. 2004; Wang and Lobstein 2006). The prevalence remains very low in most developing countries, especially those in Asia and Africa (overweight <5%, obesity <2%) based on available data, where undernutrition is still the major nutrition problem (Wang and Lobstein 2006). However, in some developing countries, in particular, those that have enjoyed rapid socio-economic growth such as China and Brazil have seen a fast increase in the obesity problem in both their adult and child populations (Wang et al. 2002; Wang et al. 2007).

Different regions (geographic and rural/urban areas), socio-economic status (SES), ethnic/racial groups, age groups, and sex groups are affected differently (Wang and Lobstein 2006; Wang and Wang 2002; Wang and Zhang 2006; Wang et al. 2002; Zhang and Wang 2007). This fact is due to the considerable socio-economic and lifestyles differences between populations. Another reason for prevalence variations is the different composition of the study samples and the different definition of obesity and overweight (e.g., various BMI cut points). Several factors that may affect the findings of descriptive epidemiological studies are addressed in this section of the chapter.

Various studies have provided different estimates of the scope of the obesity problem in the same population or country due to a combination of multiple factors. Policy makers, researchers and the general public should pay close attention to this fact when they interpret such obesity related findings. Table 3.2 shows an example of the differences in the estimated prevalence of overweight and obesity in a large representative sample of children and adolescents in Beijing, China according to various recommended BMI cut points (Mi et al. 2006). For example, the prevalence of obesity in girls aged 10–12 years old ranged from 4.0% based on the IOTF reference to 9.5% if the local Chinese reference is used.

Table 3.2 Comparisons of estimated prevalence (%) of overweight and obesity among children and adolescents in Beijing according to the Chinese, US CDC (Centers for Disease Control and Prevention), and IOTF references

Age (years)	Total Overweight or obesity	Obesity	Boys Overweight or obesity	Obesity	Girls Overweight or obesity	Obesity
Chinese ref						
7–9	20.9	11.4	25.2	14.5	16.6	8.3
10–12	25.1	11.9	31.2	14.2	18.6	9.5
13–15	20.4	8.7	25.2	11.4	15.7	6.0
16–18	18.7	5.9	23.2	8.3	14.8	3.9
7–18	21.6	9.8	26.7	12.4	16.5	7.1
US CDC ref						
7–9	20.7	10.5	26.1	15.2	15.1	5.7
10–12	25.8	12.0	31.8	16.3	19.3	7.4
13–15	19.7	8.1	24.9	12.3	14.5	4.0
16–18	14.2	4.9	18.9	7.8	10.0	2.4
6–18	20.6	9.2	26.1	13.3	15.1	5.1
IOTF ref						
7–9	18.0	6.4	21.9	9.1	18.4	3.6
10–12	23.9	7.2	29.1	10.3	18.4	4.0
13–15	18.9	5.3	24.3	7.8	13.6	2.8
16–18	15.4	3.6	20.3	5.2	11.2	2.3
6–18	19.3	5.8	24.2	8.3	14.5	3.1

Based on data collected from a representative sample of 21,198 subjects in Beijing in 2004. The Chinese reference only covers children aged 7 and older (adapted from Mi et al. 2006)

Strengths and Limitations of Using BMI in Assessing Childhood Obesity

It is recommended that an ideal measure of body fatness should meet several requirements (Power et al. 1997; Wang 2004), including: a) It should be accurate in assessing the amount of body fat; b) It needs to be precise with small measurement error; c) The measure can predict risks of health consequences; d) It should be possible to develop cut-offs to separate individuals according to their adiposity-related health risks; and e) It needs to be feasible in terms of simplicity, cost and ease of use, and acceptability to the subjects.

Although none of the existing measures satisfies all these criteria, the current consensus is that BMI is probably the best choice among available measures including weight-for-height, which can be easily assessed at low cost and has a strong association with body fat and health risks. BMI has been recommended for use in children, adolescents, and adults to assess body weight status (WHO 1995, 2000). BMI is widely recommended because it is a weight-for-height index that is independent from height in adults. However, BMI also has a number of limitations as an indirect measure of fatness in children (Prentice and Jebb 2001; Wang 2004), in particular its association with height. BMI variability throughout childhood strongly depends on height variation instead of fatness deposition (Fig. 3.2). Ideally, cut-offs should be established based on related health risk. The selection of appropriate cut points for assessing "high risk" individuals should be based on evidence of increased risk for morbidity, mortality, or/and impaired function (Power et al. 1997). The relationship between different indicators or cut-offs and health outcomes is more difficult to assess in children than it is in adults. In children, two different types of health outcomes may need to be considered: short- and intermediate-term health outcomes during childhood and adolescence, and long-term health outcomes in adulthood. For this reason, well-designed long-term longitudinal studies examining the long-term health consequences of childhood obesity are needed.

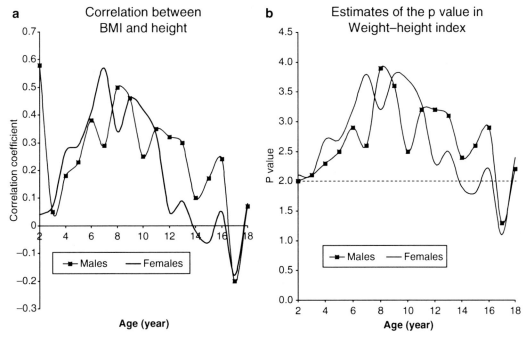

* p value, to calculate the weight-height index using height to the power of p, e.g., it is 2 for body mass index (=weight (kg)/height (m)^2)

Fig. 3.2 The correlation coefficients between BMI and height and estimates of the *p* value* in weight–height^p index in American boys and girls, by age. *Source a*: NHANES III (1988–94); *Source b*: adapted from Wang (2004)

Secular Changes in Growth, Body Composition, and Sexual Maturation and Differences Within and Between Populations

(a) *Secular changes:* Secular changes in growth and body composition, and related between-population differences in these measures (e.g., Table 3.3) may complicate the interpretation of anthropometric measures such as weight-for-height and BMI, and thus affect the appropriate assessment of adiposity and obesity prevalence throughout childhood and adolescence both at individual and population levels (Wang 2004; Wang et al. 2006). Height, weight, BMI and fatness have increased nowadays in children compared with preexisting reference data which are no longer representative of the current population. In addition, this also poses a challenge for the development of anthropometric references, both local and international ones. For example, contemporary Cambridge children had more fat mass and less lean mass than the British reference child for a given BMI value (Wells et al. 2002). These findings suggest that BMI-based assessments have underestimated the secular increase in children's fatness. Changes over time in the relationship between BMI and body composition will give a misleading prediction of adult illness. Such changes may make it hard to justify using fixed age-sex-specific BMI cut-offs developed from another country such as the United States to assess obesity, particularly in societies that have been experiencing dramatic socio-environmental transitions. Thus, there are two key decisions being involved when BMI is going to be used as a body fat index, one is the selection of the population reference (local data vs. data from other places) and the other is the choice of appropriate cut-offs (e.g., 85th or 90th percentile). However, a reality is that unless each country develops its own reference, we have to use references from other countries (Reilly 2002; Wang et al. 2006).

Table 3.3 Comparison of height medians in different populations and growth references, for 10 and 12 years old boys and girls (adapted from Wang et al. 2006)

Country	Boys		Girls		References
	10 year	12 year	10 year	12 year	
WHO/NCHS	137.5	149.7	138.3	151.5	Hamill et al. (1979)
US 2000 CDC	140.1	150.9	139.8	153.4	Kuczmarski et al. (2000)
UK 1990	138.4	148.4	138.4	149.8	Freeman et al. (1995)
China					Ge (1995)
National average	132.5	142.5	132.1	143.6	
High-income group	136.2	146.2	136.3	148.5	
France	135.6	145.9	134.7	147.7	Sempé et al. (1979)
Italy (Central and North)	139.5	151.3	139.6	152.6	Cacciari et al. (2002)
Italy (South)	137.9	149.1	138.6	150.9	Cacciari et al. (2002)
Netherlands	143.2	154.0	143.3	155.3	Fredriks et al. (2000)
Spain	136.5	146.7	136.7	148.4	Hernández et al. (1988)
Swedish 1995	140.1	150.5	140.1	153.0	Lindgren et al. (1995)
Swedish 2002	141.1	152.1	141.1	153.9	Wikland et al. (2002)

(b) *Sexual maturation:* Studies show that sexual maturation (SM) is associated with adiposity in female and male adolescents and the prevalence of obesity in older children and adolescents varies depending on sex (e.g., Wang 2002). Pubertal development is associated with an increase of body fat in girls and with a decrease of body fat in boys. Sex differences in fat mass are apparent even long before puberty tends to start. There are large intra- and inter-population variations in the patterns of sexual maturation (Eveleth and Tanner 1990; Morabia and Costanza 1998). Although the relation between SM and fatness remains controversial, a growing body of evidence suggests that SM has a more important effect on levels of fatness than fatness does on the timing of SM. Fatness and BMI correlate more closely with the maturation stage (or developmental age (MA)) than with chronological age (CA). The secular trends towards early SM continue in both industrialized and developing countries. Using national representative cross-sectional survey data, we found that compared to non early maturers early SM was positively associated with obesity in American adolescent girls (odds ratio (OR) = 2.0 and 95% confidence interval (CI) = (1.1, 3.5)), but the association between early SM and obesity was reverse for adolescent boys (OR = 0.4; 95% CI = (0.2, 0.8)). Furthermore, we found that most of the significant ethnic differences in measures of overweight, obesity, and body fatness disappeared after controlling for SM (Wang 2002).

However, to our knowledge, none of the current widely used obesity references have provided a practical approach to address this issue. Previously we have proposed a population-based approach for adjusting maturity difference between the study and reference populations (Wang and Adair 2001). We illustrated the approach using the WHO/NCHS (National Center for Health Statistics) reference and data collected in three populations. The adjustment increased the estimates of overweight prevalence by about one-quarter to one-third (in relative terms) in Chinese and Russian adolescent girls, where children matured later than the reference populations, but decreased it in the US where children matured earlier (Fig. 3.3). The adjustment had a greater effect in girls at ages around puberty (10–13 years) than in older girls (14–18 years).

(c) *Adiposity rebound (AR):* It is of concern that considerable difference may exist in the timing and patterns of adiposity rebound between populations – in particular, between populations in

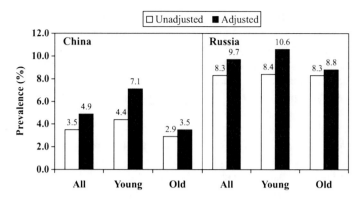

*Young (10-13 y), old (14-18 y). Adjusted prevalence was calculated using MA-matched BMI cut-offs (MA=CA-0.9 for China, and MA=CA-0.4 for Russia); unadjusted prevalence was calculated using CA-matched BMI cutoffs. Total sample size was 1,316 for China and 744 for Russia

Fig. 3.3 Unadjusted and maturation-adjusted overweight prevalence (%) in Chinese and Russian girls (adapted from Wang and Adair 2001)

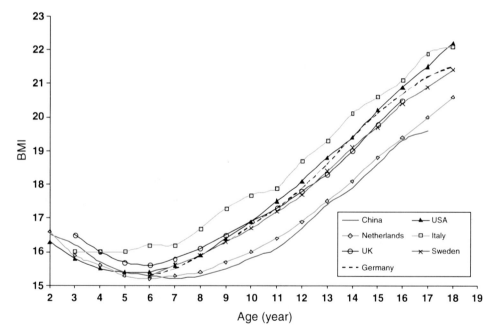

Fig. 3.4 BMI (median) by age and adiposity rebound among boys in China, Germany, Italy, Netherlands, Sweden, UK, and USA (adapted from Wang et al. 2006)

industrialized and in developing countries. This may affect the estimate of obesity prevalence for children from developing countries at around the age of adiposity rebound when using the so-called international references developed based upon data collected in wealthy societies (Wang 2004). Considerable differences in the timing of AR onset exist and there are secular trends towards an earlier onset of AR (Fig. 3.4). For example, national representative survey data show that the onset of AR happens around 6 years of age among children in France, the Netherlands, and UK, 5.5 years in the US, and about 5 years in Italy, but much later among Chinese children at around age 7 years (Wang 2004). It seems that the timing of AR might change over time in some populations, and can vary between groups even within the same country. For example, recent data collected in Shanghai, the largest and most prosperous city in China where people's living standards are comparable to that in many industrialized countries, showed that the onset of AR advanced to around 5 years compared to the national Chinese average of 7 years.

(d) *Other important factors:* Furthermore, the following factors could also greatly affect the findings from individual studies, and should be taken into consideration when researchers design their studies and read published data: (1) *Large within-country variations:* For many countries there are large differences in the prevalence of obesity as well as in secular trends between regions, racial/ ethnic groups, age cohorts, and socio-economic groups. Therefore, ideally representative samples should be drawn when one aims to estimate the national situation regarding obesity. (2) *Sampling problems and lack of representativeness:* To obtain representative samples is too costly or imprac- tical in many countries, especially in developing countries. Some of the results presented in the current literature may be based upon national, representative data, while others are based on small, non-representative data. (3) *Measurement errors:* Data collected in different studies, different countries, and different time periods may not have the same quality. Different studies may have adopted different protocols for quality control and the standard for data accuracy. For example, in some large scale studies or monitoring programs (including some from developed countries such as the United States), often children are measured regarding their height and weight with clothes and the reading may rounded to pound or ¼ pound. To accurately measure height can be more challenging than that of weight due to the inherent inter- and intra-observer variability of height measures which decreases measurement precision. Compared to data measured directly, subjects' self-reported data suffer misreporting leading to systematical errors such as overreporting of height and under-reporting of weight. The potential influence of measurement errors should not be ignored both in study design, data collection, and for data interpretation.

Conclusions

Current prevalence and trends of obesity among children and adolescents vary considerably world- wide even within countries. Different regions (geographic and rural/urban areas), SES, ethnic/racial groups, age groups, and sex groups are affected differently. The key reason for the variations is due to the considerable socio-economic and lifestyle differences between them. In addition, they are also exaggerated by differences in sampling and differing reference criteria for obesity and over- weight. Nowadays, there is still no international consensus for excess body fat definition, and clear %FM or BMI cut-offs for obesity/overweight classification in children and adolescents. Charts for BMI and body composition that are stratified by age and sex are needed by healthcare professionals to identify individual adiposity. In this context, depending on the concrete purpose of each study and sample characteristics, careful selection of methods and references must be done.

Body composition techniques measure components of the body on the basis of their differing physical characteristics, and body composition can be described by models of varying complexity that use one or more measurement techniques. Body composition analysis has been used to study physiologic processes such as growth, development and exercise physiology and is increasingly being applied to the study and clinical management of pediatric pathologic conditions. It is crucial to understand exactly what is being measured and how estimates of body composition are derived (Battistini et al. 2006). Whatever the reason for assessing body composition, nutritionists and clini- cians in health-related fields should have a general understanding of the most commonly used techniques for assessing body composition in pediatric subjects.

BMI may be used in population-based epidemiological studies for the screening of excess body fat in children and adolescents because it is easy to determine and it correlates well with body fat. IOTF BMI cut-offs have good sensitivity and specificity but a considerable number of subjects may be erroneously classified as overweight or obese by this criterion. So, the IOTF approach may be questionable at the individual level but it is useful in large scale studies and as a relative index of excess body fat in clinical practice. When aiming to measure the total amount of body fat or its regional distribution in large scale studies fast and easy methods are required. Anthropometry or bioelectrical impedance are both appropriate methods to have a global epidemiological view of the sample characteristics and represents a group of inexpensive and non-invasive methods to assess the size, shape and composition of the human body. Waist circumference is the best simple anthropometric predictor of body fat distribution (intra-abdominal adipose tissue) and risk of metabolic syndrome in children and adolescents.

When accurate measures of total or regional body fat (e.g., intra-abdominal fat) are required at the individual level or in a reduced sample, methods such as ADP, MRI or DXA must be used. ADP is a good option if the aim is to assess %BF, DXA is able to assess three body compartments (bone mineral content, BF and FFM) in the whole body and in several body regions and MRI is the "gold standard" when accurate measures of intra-abdominal fat are required. It would be desirable that these accurate methods of body composition assessment used as "laboratory methods" in current research and applied clinical studies could all be finally incorporated in large scale epidemiological studies. If subjects are commonly admitted to a "body composition laboratory" these methods will be more economically acceptable also for field studies.

References

Battistini, N.C., Poli, M., Malavolti, M., Dugoni, M., & Pietrobelli, A. (2006). Healthy status and energy balance in pediatrics. *Acta Biomedica, 77*, 7–13.

Brambilla, P., Bedogni, G., Moreno, L.A., Goran, M.I., Gutin, B., Fox, K.R., Peters, D.M., Barbeau, P., De Simone, M., & Pietrobelli, A. (2006). Crossvalidation of anthropometry against magnetic resonance imaging for the assessment of visceral and subcutaneous adipose tissue in children. *International Journal of Obesity (London), 30*, 23–30.

Butte, N.F., Hopkinson, J.M., Wong, W.W., O'Brian Smith, E., & Ellis, K.J. (2000). Body composition during the first 2 years of life: an updated reference. *Pediatric Research, 47*, 578–585.

Cacciari, E., Dilani, S., Balsamo, A., Dammacco, F., De Luca, F., Chiarelli, F., Pasquino, A.M., Tonini, G., & Vanelli, M. (2002). Italian cross-sectional growth charts for height, weight and BMI (6-20). *European Journal of Clinical Nutrition, 56*, 171–180.

Cameron, N. (1986). The methods of auxological anthropometry. In F. Falkner & J.M. Tanner (Eds.), *Human growth: a comprehensive treatise* (pp 3–46). New York: Plenum.

Caprio, S., Hyman, L.D., McCarthy, S., Lange, R., Bronson, M., & Tamborlane, W.V. (1996). Fat distribution and cardiovascular risk factors in obese adolescent girls: importance of the intra-abdominal fat depot. *American Journal of Clinical Nutrition, 64*, 12–17.

Cole, T.J. (1993). The use and construction of anthropometric growth reference standards. *Nutrition Research Review, 6*, 19–50.

Cole, T.J. (2004). Children grow and horses race: is the adiposity rebound a critical period for later obesity? *BioMed Central Pediatrics, 4*, 6.

Cole, T.J., & Roede, M.J. (1999). Centiles of body mass index for Dutch children aged 0-20 years in 1980 – a baseline to assess recent trends in obesity. *Annals of Human Biology, 26*, 303–308.

Cole, T.J., Freeman, J.V., & Preece, M.A. (1995). Body mass index reference curves for the UK, 1990. *Archives of Disease in Childhood, 73*, 25–29.

Cole, T.J., Bellizzi, M.C., Flegal, M., & Dietz, W.H. (2000). Establishing a standard definition for child overweight and obesity worldwide: international survey. *British Medical Journal, 320*, 1240–1243.

Daniels, S.R., Khoury, P.R., & Morrison, J.A. (1997). The utility of body mass index as a measure of body fatness in children and adolescents: Differences by race and gender. *Pediatrics, 99*, 804–807.

Dietz, W.H., & Bellizzi, M.C. (1999). Assessment of childhood and adolescent obesity. *American Journal of Clinical Nutrition, 70(1 part2)*, S117–S175.

Ellis, K.J. (1996). Measuring body fatness in children and young adults: comparison of bioelectrical impedance analysis, total body electrical conductivity, and dual energy X-ray absorptiometry. *International Journal of Obesity, 20*, 866–873.

Eveleth, P.B., & Tanner, J.M. (1990). *Worldwide variation in human growth*. New York: Cambridge University Press.

Fernandez, J.R., Pietrobelli, A., Redden, T.D., & Allison, D.B. (2004). Waist circumference percentile in nationally representative samples of black, white, and Hispanic children. *The Journal of Pediatrics, 145*, 439–444.

Fields, D.A., Goran, M.I., & McCrory, M.A. (2002). Body-composition assessment via air-displacement plethysmography in adults and children: a review. *American Journal of Clinical Nutrition, 75*, 453–467.

Fisberg, M., Baur, L., Chen, W., Hoppin, A., Koletzko, B., Lau, D., Moreno, L.A., Nelson, T., Strauss, R., & Uauy, R. (2004). Obesity in children and adolescents: Working Group Report of the Second World Congress of Pediatric Gastroenterology, Hepatology, and Nutrition. *Journal of Pediatric Gastroenterology and Nutrition, 39*, S678–S687.

Fomon, S.J., & Nelson, S.E. (2002). Body composition of the male and *female* reference infants. *Annual Review Nutrition, 22*, 1–17.

Fomon, S.J., Haschke, F., Ziegler, E.E., & Nelson, S.E. (1982). Body composition of reference children from birth to age 10 years. *American Journal of Clinical Nutrition, 35*, 1169–1175.

Freeman, J.V., Cole, T.J., Chinn, S., Jones, P.R., White, E.M., & Preece, M.A. (1995). Cross sectional stature and weight reference curves for the UK, 1990. *Archives of Disease in Childhood, 73*, 17–24.

Fredriks, A.M., van Buuren, S., Burgmeijer, R.J., Meulmeester, J.F., Beuker, R.J., Brugman, E., Roede, M.J., Verloove-Vanhorick, S.P., & Wit, J.M. (2000). Continuing positive secular growth change in The Netherlands 1955-1997. *Pediatric Research, 47*, 316–323.

Ge, K. (1995). *The dietary and nutritional status of Chinese population (1992 national nutrition survey).* Beijing: Institute of Nutrition and Food Hygiene (and additional analysis).

Goran, M.I. (1998). Measurement issue related to studies of childhood obesity: assessment of body composition, body fat distribution, physical activity and food intake. *Pediatrics, 101*, 505–518.

Goran, M.I., Gower, B.A., Treuth, M., & Nagy, T.R. (1998). Prediction of intra-abdominal and subcutaneous abdominal adipose tissue in healthy pre-pubertal children. *International Journal of Obesity, 22*, 549–558.

Hamill, P.V., Drizd, T.A., Johnson, C.L., Reed, R.B., Roche, A.F., & Moore, W.M. (1979). Physical growth: National Center for Health Statistics percentiles. *American Journal of Clinical Nutrition, 32*, 607–629.

Harsha, D.W., Frerichs, R.R., & Berenson, G.S. (1978). Densitometry and anthropometry of black and white children. *Human Biology, 50*, 261–280.

He, Q., Albertsson-Wikland, K., & Karlberg, J. (2000). Population bases body mass index reference values from Goteborg, Sweden: birth to 18 years of age. *Acta Pediatrica, 89*, 582–592.

Hernández, M., Castellet, J., Narvaíza, J.L., Rincón, J.M., Ruiz, I., Sánchez, E., Sobradillo, B., & Zurimendi, A. (1988). *Curvas y tablas de crecimiento. Instituto de Investigación sobre Crecimiento y Desarrollo. Fundación Faustino Orbegozo.* Madrid: Garsi Editorial.

Heymsfield, S.B., Ross, R., Wang, Z.M., & Frager, D. (1997). Imaging techniques of body composition: advantages of measurement and new uses. In S.J. Carlson-Newbarry & R.B. Costello (Eds.), *Emerging technologies for nutrition research* (pp 127–150). New York: New York Academic Press.

Heyward, V.H., & Stolarczyk, L.M. (1996). *Applied body composition assessment.* Champaign, IL: Human Kinetics.

Higgins, P.B., Gower, B.A., Hunter, G.R., & Goran, M.I. (2001). Defining health related obesity in prepubertal children. *Obesity Research, 9*, 233–240.

Himes, J.H., & Dietz, W.H. (1994). Guidelines for overweight in adolescent preventive services: recommendations from an expert committee. *American Journal of Clinical Nutrition, 59*, 307–316.

Houtkooper, L.B., Going, S.B., Lohman, T.G., Roche, A.F., & Van Loan, M. (1992). Bioelectrical impedance estimation of fat free body mass in children and youth: a cross validation study. *Journal of Applied Physiology, 72*, 366–373.

Koletzko, B., Girardet, J.P., Klish, W., & Tabacco, O. (2002). Obesity in children and adolescents worldwide: current views and future directions. *Journal of Pediatric Gastroenterology and Nutrition, 35*, S205–S212.

Kuczmarski, R.J., Ogden, C.L., Grummer-Strawn, L.M., Flegal, K., Guo, S.S., Wei, R., Mei, Z., Curtin, L.R., Roche, A.F., & Johnson, C.L. (2000). *CDC growth chart: United States. Advance data from Vital and Health Statistics: n. 314.* Hyattsville, Maryland: National Center for Health Statistics.

Kushner, R.F., Schoeller, D.A., Fjeld, C.R., & Danford, L. (1992). Is the impedance index (ht2/R) significant in predicting total body water? *American Journal of Clinical Nutrition, 56*, 835–839.

Leung, S.S.F., Cole, T.J., Tse, L.Y., & Lau, J.T.F. (1998). Body mass index reference curves for Chinese children. *Annals of Human Biology, 25*, 169-174.

Lindgren, G., Strandell, A., Cole, T., Healy, M., & Tanner, J. (1995). Swedish population reference standards for height, weight and body mass index attained at 6 to 16 years (girls) or 19 years (boys). *Acta Paediatrica, 84*, 1019–1028.

Lobstein, T., Baur, L., Uauy, R.; for the IOTF Childhood Obesity Working Group (2004). Obesity in children and young people: A crisis in public health. *Obesity Reviews, 5(Suppl 1)*, 4–85.

Lohman, T.G. (1989). Assessment of body composition in children. *Pediatric Exercise Science, 1*, 19–30.

Maynard, L.M., Wisemandle, M.A., Roche, A.F., Chumlea, W.C., Guo, S.S., & Siervogel, R.M. (2001). Childhood body composition in relation to body mass index. *Pediatrics, 107*, 344–350.

Mi, J., Cheng, H., Hou, D.Q., Duan, J.L., Teng, T.T., & Wang, Y. (2006). Prevalence of overweight and obesity among children and adolescents in Beijing in 2004. *Chinese Journal of Epidemiology, 27*, 474–479.

Morabia, A., & Costanza, M.C. (1998). International variability in ages at menarche, first live birth, and menopause. *American Journal of Epidemiology, 148*, 1195–1205.

Moreno, L.A., Fleta, J., Mur, L., Rodríguez, G., Sarría, A., & Bueno, M. (1999). Waist circumference values in Spanish children. Gender related differences. *European Journal of Clinical Nutrition, 53*, 429–433.

Moreno, L.A., Sarría, A., Fleta, J., Rodríguez, G., & Bueno, M. (2000). Trends in body mass index and overweight prevalence among children and adolescents in the region of Aragón (Spain) from 1985 to 1995. *International Journal of Obesity, 24*, 925–931.

Moreno, L.A., Blay, M.G., Rodríguez, G., Blay, V.A., Mesana, M.I., Olivares, J.L., Fleta, J., Sarría, A., Bueno, M., & the AVENA-Zaragoza Study Group (2006). Screening performances of the International Obesity Task Force body mass index cut-off values in adolescents. *Journal of American College of Nutrition, 25*, 403–408.

Moreno, L.A., Mesana, M.I., González-Gross, M., Gil, C.M., Ortega, F.B., Fleta, J., Wärnberg, J., León, J., Marcos, A., & Bueno, M. (2007). Body fat distribution reference standards in Spanish adolescents: the AVENA Study. *International Journal of Obesity (London), 31*, 1798–1805.

Must, A., Dallal, G.E., & Dietz, W.H. (1991). Reference data for obesity: 85th and 95th percentiles of body mass index (wt/ht^2) and triceps skinfold thickness. *American Journal of Clinical Nutrition, 53*, 839–846.

Pietrobelli, A., Formica, C., Wang, Z., & Heymsfield, S.B. (1996). Dual-energy X-ray absorptiometry body composition model: review of physical concepts. *American Journal of Physiology, 271*, E941–E951.

Pietrobelli, A., Faith, M.S., Allison, D.B., Gallagher, D., Chiumello, G., & Heymsfield, S.B. (1998). Body mass index as a measure of adiposity among children and adolescent: a validation study. *Journal of Pediatrics, 132*, 204–210.

Pietrobelli, A., Heo, M., & Faith, M.S. (2001). Assessment of childhood and adolescents body composition: a practical guide. In P. Dasgupta & R. Hauspie (Eds.), *Perspectives in human growth, development and nutrition* (pp 67–76). London: Kluwer.

Pietrobelli, A., Malavolti, M., Fuiano, N., & Faith, M.S. (2007). The invisible fat. *Acta Paediatrica, 96*, 35–38.

Power, C., Lake, J.K., & Cole, T.J. (1997). Body mass index and height from childhood to adulthood in the 1985 British birth cohort. *American Journal of Clinical Nutrition, 66*, 1094–1101.

Prentice, A.M., & Jebb, S.A. (2001). Beyond body mass index. *Obesity Reviews, 2*, 141–147.

Quetelet, L.A.J. (1869). *Physique sociale, Vol 2*. Brussels: C. Muquardt.

Reilly, J.J. (2002). Assessment of childhood obesity: national reference data or international approach? *Obesity Research, 10*, 838–840.

Rodríguez, G., & Moreno, L.A. (2006). Body mass index and body fat composition in children and adolescents. In L.A. Ferrera (Ed). *Focus on body mass index and health research* (pp 79–95). New York: Nova Science.

Rodríguez, G., Moreno, L.A., Blay, M.G., Blay, V.A., Garagorri, J.M., Sarría, A., Bueno, M, & AVENA Zaragoza Study Group (2004a). Body composition in adolescents: measurements and metabolic aspects. *International Journal of Obesity, 28(Suppl 3)*, S54–S58.

Rodríguez, G., Samper, M.P., Ventura, P., Moreno, L.A., Olivares, J.L., & Pérez-González, J.M. (2004b). Gender differences in newborn subcutaneous fat distribution. *European Journal of Pediatrics, 163*, 457–461.

Rodríguez, G., Moreno, L.A., Blay, M.G., Blay, V.A., Fleta, J., Sarría, A., Bueno, M, & AVENA Zaragoza Study Group (2005). Body fat measurement in adolescents: Comparison of skinfold thickness equations with dual-energy X-ray absorptiometry. *European Journal of Clinical Nutrition, 59*, 1158–1166.

Rolland-Cachera, M.F., Deheeger, M., Bellisle, F., Sempe, M., Guilloud-Bataille, M., & Patois, E. (1984). Adiposity rebound in children: a simple indicator for predicting obesity. *American Journal of Clinical Nutrition, 39*, 129–135.

Sardinha, L.B., Going, S.B., Teixeira, P.J., & Lohman, T.G. (1999). Receiver operating characteristic analysis of body mass index, triceps skinfold thickness, and arm girth for obesity screening in children and adolescents. *American Journal of Clinical Nutrition, 70*, 1090–1095.

Sempé, M., Pédron, G., & Roy-Pernot, M.P. (1979). *Auxologie: méthode et séquences*. Paris: Laboratoire Theraplix.

Serra, L.L., Ribas, L., Aranceta, J., Pérez, C., & Saavedra, P. (2001). Epidemiología de la obesidad infantil y juvenil en España. Resultados del studio enKid (1998-2000). In L.L. Serra & J. Aranceta (Eds.), *Obesidad infantil y juvenil. Estudio enKid* (pp 821–108). Barcelona: Masson.

Taylor, R.W., Gold, E., Manning, P., & Goulding, A. (1997). Gender differences in body fat content are present well before puberty. *International Journal of Obesity, 21*, 1082–1084.

Taylor, R.W., Jones, I.E., Williams, S.M., & Goulding, A. (2002). Body fat percentages measured by dual-energy X-ray absorptiometry corresponding to recently recommended body mass index cutoffs for overweight and obesity in children and adolescents aged 3-18 y. *American Journal of Clinical Nutrition, 76*, 1416–1421.

Taylor, R.W., Falorni, A., Jones, I.E., & Goulding, A. (2003). Identifying adolescents with high percentage body fat: a comparison of BMI cutoffs using age and stage of pubertal development compared with BMI cutoffs using age alone. *European Journal of Clinical Nutrition, 57*, 764–769.

Wagner, D.R., & Heyward, V.H. (1999). Techniques of body composition assessment: a review of laboratory and fields methods. *Research Quarterly for Exercise and Sport, 70*, 135–149.

Wang, Y. (2002). Is obesity associated with early sexual maturation? A comparison of the association in American boys versus girls. *Pediatrics, 110*, 903–910.

Wang, Y. (2004). Epidemiology of childhood obesity–methodological aspects and guidelines: What's new? *International Journal of Obesity, 28*, S21–S28.

Wang, Y., & Adair, L. (2001). How does maturity adjustment influence the estimates of obesity prevalence in adolescents from different populations using an international reference? *International Journal of Obesity, 25*, 550–558.

Wang, Y., & Lobstein, T. (2006). Worldwide trends in childhood obesity. *International Journal of Pediatric Obesity, 1*, 11–25.

Wang, Y., & Wang, J.Q. (2002). A comparison of international references for the assessment of child and adolescent overweight and obesity in different populations. *European Journal of Clinical Nutrition, 56*, 973–982.

Wang, Y., & Zhang, Q. (2006). Are American children and adolescents of low socioeconomic status at increased risk of obesity? Changes in the association between overweight and family income between 1971 and 2002. *American Journal of Clinical Nutrition, 84*, 707–716.

Wang, Y., Monteiro, C., & Popkin, B.M. (2002). Trends of obesity and underweight in older children and adolescents in the United States, Brazil, China and Russia. *American Journal of Clinical Nutrition, 75*, 971–977.

Wang, Y., Moreno, L.A., Caballero, B., & Cole, T.J. (2006). Limitations of the current World Health Organization growth references for children and adolescents. *Food and Nutrition Bulletin, 27*, s175–s188.

Wang, Y., Mi, J., Shan, X., Wang, Q.J., & Ge, K. (2007). Is China facing an obesity epidemic and the consequences? The trends in obesity and chronic disease in China. *International Journal of Obesity, 31*, 177–188.

Wells, J.C., Coward, W.A., Cole, T.J., & Davies, P.S. (2002). The contribution of fat and fat-free tissue to body mass index in contemporary children and the reference child. *International Journal of Obesity and Related Metabolic Disorders, 26*, 1323–1328.

WHO (1995). *Expert Committee. Physical status, the use and interpretation of anthropometry.* WHO Technical Report Series 854. Geneva: World Health Organization.

WHO (2000). *Obesity: preventing and managing the global epidemic. Report of a WHO consultation.* WHO Technical Report Series 894. Geneva: World Health Organization.

Wikland, K.A., Luo, Z.C., Niklasson, A., & Karlberg, J. (2002). Swedish population-based longitudinal reference values from birth to 18 years of age for height, weight and head circumference. *Acta Paediatrica, 91*, 739–754.

Yanovski, S.Z., Van Hubbard, S., Heymsfield, S.B., & Lukaski, H.C. (1996). Bioelectrical impedance analysis. *American Journal of Clinical Nutrition, 64(S3)*, S387–S531.

Zhang, Q., & Wang, Y. (2007). Using concentration index to study changes in socio-economic inequality of overweight among US adolescents between 1971 and 2002. *International Journal of Epidemiology, 36*, 916–925.

Part I
Descriptive Epidemiology

Chapter 4
Childhood Obesity in the WHO European Region

Yannis Manios and Vassiliki Costarelli

Introduction

Overweight and obesity in most countries of Europe show rising secular trends and are predicted to continue rising if counteracting measures are not taken (Wan et al. 2007). In the European Union, the number of children who are overweight is expected to rise by 1.3 million children per year, with more than 300,000 of them becoming obese each year (Kosti and Panagiotakos 2006). Obesity is a multifactorial disease with a complex etiology.

Changes in social settings and lifestyle in Europe during the last decades have impacted on children's behavior, with unhealthy dietary habits and sedentary lifestyle becoming the norm (Lasserre et al. 2007; Manios et al. 2004; Moreno et al. 2001c). It is well documented that overweight and obesity in childhood can lead to a wide array of health and social consequences (Tounian 2007). Conditions such as type 2 diabetes mellitus, hypercholesterolemia and hypertension, which were previously seen mainly in adults, are becoming more common among children as the prevalence of obesity increases (Angelopoulos et al. 2006; Franks et al. 2007; Manios et al. 2005; Pastucha et al. 2007; Tounian 2007). Most importantly, the psychological well-being and the quality of life of the obese children can also be affected (de Beer et al. 2007; Janicke et al. 2007). In addition, a number of recent studies have suggested that childhood obesity in most cases tracks into adulthood (Freedman et al. 2004; Wright et al. 2001) and increases the risk of degenerative diseases later in life (DiPietro et al. 1994; Nieto et al. 1992; O'Neill et al. 2007).

Recording and understanding the prevalence of obesity in children and the social, geographic and cultural parameters related to the phenomenon can facilitate the formation of effective public health intervention policies in counteracting childhood obesity. It is known that early prevention is more effective in managing the epidemic of obesity (O'Neill et al. 2007) in comparison to treating obesity later in life.

In spite of the fact that currently there are several initiatives by the WHO Regional Office for Europe to assemble comparable data on overweight and obesity, there is a distinctive lack of harmonized cross-national surveys of overweight and obesity prevalence levels in children (Lobstein

Y. Manios (✉)
Department of Nutrition and Dietetics, Harokopio University of Athens,
70, E.Venizelou Avenue, Kallithea, Athens 17671, Greece
e-mail: manios@hua.gr

V. Costarelli
Department of Home Economics & Ecology, Harokopio University of Athens,
70, E.Venizelou Avenue, Kallithea, Athens, 17671, Greece

L.A. Moreno et al. (eds.), *Epidemiology of Obesity in Children and Adolescents*,
Springer Series on Epidemiology and Public Health 2, DOI 10.1007/978-1-4419-6039-9_4,
© Springer Science+Business Media, LLC 2011

and Millstone 2006). The International Obesity Task Force (IOTF) has previously collected data based on surveys of national and sub-national samples collected as part of national monitoring activities (IASO/IOTF 2007). However, the data on many occasions reflect surveys undertaken in different years, covering different age groups, using varying criteria for defining obesity and in some cases relying on self-reported measures of weight and height.

The literature on childhood and adolescent obesity in the European region is vast, however, there is an apparent lack of properly conducted descriptive epidemiological surveys, which make the prevalence comparison among the different countries and regions very difficult to achieve. Efforts should be made from research groups of different countries to measure prevalence of obesity in children and adolescents using nationally representative samples of children and adopt methodologies and cut-off points which render their data useful for cross country comparisons.

There is evidence for associations between increased children's body mass index (BMI) and short- and long-term health outcomes (Mutunga et al. 2006), but this is currently insufficient to establish appropriate cut-off points of BMI. The definition for excess body weight and obesity is based on the percentile values of BMI adjusted for age and sex corresponding to BMI of 25 and 30 kg/m^2 at age 18 years, however, this causes a problem when used in children and adolescents, since they are in a phase when it is natural to grow and gain weight. A number of different cut-off points based on percentiles of BMI have been used (Cole et al. 2000; de Onis et al. 2006; Kuczmarski et al. 2002; Wright et al. 2008). It is important to underline that appropriate cut-off points are very important in order that trends over time can be monitored and comparisons made between populations. Currently, our understanding of the prevalence and etiology of obesity in children is relatively limited due to lack of comparable representative data from different countries, and the varying criteria for defining obesity (Lasserre et al. 2007; Popkin et al. 2006).

The purpose of the current chapter is to thoroughly describe the geographic variation in prevalence of obesity in children and adolescents in WHO European Region, by age, sex, time trends, socio-economic status and ethnic origin and to concurrently identify the key postulated risk factors for the above variation in prevalence of obesity.

Geographic Area

Definition

In the current chapter, prevalence of childhood and adolescent overweight and obesity is presented for 29 countries of the WHO Region, where it was possible to find adequately reliable and recent prevalence data: Austria, Belgium, Bulgaria, Cyprus, Czech Republic, Demark, Estonia, Finland, France, Germany, Greece, Hungary, Iceland, Ireland, Israel, Italy, Lithuania, Malta Netherlands, Norway, Poland, Portugal, Russian Federation, Slovakia, Spain, Sweden, Switzerland, Turkey and the United Kingdom.

Socio-Demographic and Economic Characteristics

Prior to tabulating and discussing the prevalence of obesity in children and adolescents in Europe and Russia, it is important to present some key socio-demographic and economic characteristics of the countries whose prevalence data were used. The socio-demographic and economic characteristics presented in Table 4.1 were taken from the WHO Statistical Information System (World Health

Table 4.1 Socio-demographic and economic characteristics in countries of the WHO European Region – WHO Statistical Information System, WorldBank database, Wikipedia

Country	Area km²	Population in thousands (N)	Population below the age of 20 years (%)	GDP per capita $	Population below poverty line (% living on <US$1 per day)	Life expectancy at birth (years, men–women)	Human Development Index (rank order)	Crude birth rate in ‰	Crude death rates in ‰ men–women	Infant mortality‰
Austria	83,858	8,189	22.05	38,961	–	77–82	14	9.2	114–55	4
Belgium	30,528	10,419	23.32	37,214	–	76–82	13	10.4	122–65	4
Bulgaria	110,912	7,726	17.66	3,995	<2	69–76	54	8.9	217–92	12
Cyprus	9,251	835	23.61	23,676	–	77–82	29	12.2	94–47	4
Czech Republic	78,866	10,220	21.22	13,848	–	73–79	30	9.2	161–69	3
Denmark	43,094	5,431	23.55	50,965	–	76–80	15	11.2	117–72	4
Estonia	45,100	1,330	23.45	12,203	<2	67–78	40	10.8	301–108	6
Finland	338,145	5,249	23.43	40,197	–	76–82	11	11.2	137–62	3
France	551,500	60,496	25.02	35,404	–	77–84	16	12.2	132–60	4
Germany	357,022	82,689	20.32	35,204	–	76–82	21	8.2	112–58	4
Greece	131,957	11,120	19.78	27,610	–	77–82	24	9.3	110–46	4
Hungary	93,032	10,098	21.76	11,340	<2	69–77	35	9.3	249–108	6
Iceland	103,000	295	29.55	54,858	–	79–83	2	14.3	79–52	2
Ireland	70,273	4,148	27.70	44,500	–	77–81	4	15.5	105–60	4
Israel	20,770	6,725	36.63	20,399	–	78–82	23	19.7	91–48	4
Italy	301,318	58,093	19.02	31,791	–	78–84	17	9.2	91–47	4
Lithuania	65,300	3,431	24.63	8,610	<2	65–77	41	9.1	304–102	7
Malta	316	402	24.55	15,293	–	77–81	32	9.8	82–48	5
Netherlands	41,528	16,299	24.46	40,571	–	77–81	10	12.5	89–63	4
Norway	385,155	4,620	25.85	72,306	–	77–82	1	11.1	93–57	3
Poland	312,685	38,530	23.90	8,890	<2	71–79	37	9.5	198–79	6
Portugal	91,982	10,495	21.49	18,465	–	75–81	28	10.5	144–61	4
Russian Federation	17,098,242	143,202	23.45	6,856	<2	59–72	65	10.7	485–180	11
Slovakia	49,033	5,401	24.11	10,158	–	70–78	42	10.0	203–76	7
Spain	505,992	43,064	19.83	27,767	–	77–84	19	10.8	113–45	4
Sweden	449,964	9,041	23.84	42,383	–	79–84	5	11.3	82–51	3
Switzerland	41,284	7,252	22.62	51,771	–	79–84	9	9.2	87–49	4
Turkey	783,562	73,193	32.74	5,408	3.4	69–74	92	18.4	180–112	26
United Kingdom	242,900	59,668	24.78	39,213	–	77–81	18	12.0	102–63	5

Organization 2005) apart from the Gross Domestic Product (GDP) per capita in $ for each country, which was obtained from the WorldBank database (http://www.worldbank.org) and the Human Development Index (rank order) from Wikipaedia (http://en.wikipedia.org/wiki/Human_Development_Index).

Methods

Prevalence data of overweight and obesity among children and adolescents have been compiled from published literature, personal communication with expert scientists, health agencies and existing databases. A search was performed on relevant papers on "Prevalence of Obesity and Overweight" using MEDLINE and the ISI Web of Science. The search was limited to the age range 0–18 years, to the countries of the WHO European Region and to publications in English and French. The key words used were "Obesity", "Overweight", "Children", "Childhood", "Adolescents", "Adolescence" and "Europe". A total of 3,594 hits were found. Emphasis was given on the most recent work available and in particular on cross-sectional and school-based studies with large and nationally representative samples, where body weight was measured and not self-reported and the IOFT cut-off points have been used. It was decided to present the prevalence data in three separate tables according to the age group of the children: pre-school children (0–6 years), school children (6–12 years) and adolescents (12–18 years). It is important to note that unfortunately, for a number of countries, it was not possible to find a published study meeting all the above criteria and as a result, occasionally, studies with self-reported data and with smaller sample sizes have been used in the tables (Tables 4.2–4.4). The very few studies that used self-reported anthropometric data are indicated in the relevant tables. Finally, online databases for obesity prevalence from the WHO and the International Association of the Study of Obesity (IASO/IOTF 2007) where used, together with the World Bank (http://www.worldbank.org) and the WHO Statistical Information System (World Health Organization 2005), for data on the socio-demographic and economic characteristics of the region.

In order to make the findings presented in this chapter most useful for comparison, the vast majority of the studies that are described here have applied the International Obesity Task Force (IOTF) cut-off points (Cole et al. 2000). However, when this was not possible, prevalence data from studies using either the Kromeyer-Hauschild reference system for Central Europe (Kromeyer-Hauschild and Zellner 2007) or the Centres for Disease Control (CDC) cut-off points (Ogden et al. 2002) have been used. Finally, a very small number of studies presenting obesity prevalence data in adolescents using Internal Study Reference Standards for obesity classification, have also been used (Table 4.4).

The IOTF cut-off points for overweight and obesity were developed based on an international survey of six large nationally representative cross-sectional growth studies from Brazil, Great Britain, Hong Kong, the Netherlands, Singapore, and the United States. For each of the surveys, percentile curves were drawn such that at age 18 years they passed through the widely used cut-off points of 25 and 30 kg/m^2 for adult overweight and obesity. The resulting curves were averaged to provide age and sex specific cut-off points from 2–18 years (Cole et al. 2000).

According to the Kromeyer-Hauschild reference system the terms "overweight" and "obese" are defined based on percentiles of the BMI (exceeding the 90th and 97th percentile for overweight and obesity respectively) (Kromeyer-Hauschild and Zellner 2007; Kromeyer-Hauschild et al. 2001). The main advantage of the Kromeyer-Hauschild reference system is that it has been specifically designed for children living in Central Europe.

Finally the CDC 2000 Growth Charts for the United States (CDC criteria) were based on the US National data collected in a series of five surveys between 1963 and 1994 for children and adolescents aged 2–20 years. Overweight and obesity were defined as BMI-for-age ≥85th and ≥95th percentiles, respectively (Ogden et al. 2002).

Table 4.2 Prevalence (%) of overweight and obesity in children 0–6 years old, WHO European Region

Country	Survey	Year of survey	Number of children	Age (years)	Total Overweight (including obese)	Total Obese	Boys Overweight (including obese)	Girls Overweight (including obese)	Boys Obese	Girls Obese	Cut-off points
Austria	Kirchengast and Schober (2006b)	Longitudinal study	794 (455 boys/339 girls)	6	17.8	8.6	17.8	17.9	9.4	7.6	Kromeyer-Hauschild
Cyprus	Savva et al. (2005)	Cross-sectional study, 2004	1,414	2–5	13.5	2.9	11.1	15.9	2.7	3.1	CDC
France	Lioret et al. (2007) (personal communication)	Cross-sectional study, 1998–1999	242 (self reported weight and height)	3–5	17.9	7.7					IOTF
Germany	Kurth and Schaffrath Rosario (2007)	Cross-sectional study, 2003–2006	17,641; 0–17 years 8,985 boys/8,656 girls	3–6	11.9	2.9	11.9	2.9	11.9	2.9	Kromeyer-Hauschild
Greece	Manios et al. (2007)	Retrospective cohort study, 2003–2004	2,374 (1,218 boys/1,156 girls)	1–5	21.3	7.1	19.1	23.6	6.2	8.1	IOTF
Hungary	Kern (2007)	Cross-sectional study, 2003–2006	1,135 (582 boys/553 girls)	5	12.6	4.5	10.1	15.3	3.4	5.7	IOTF
Ireland (ROI)	Whelton et al. (2007)	Cross-sectional study, 2001–2002	1,352 (630 boys/722 girls)	4	27.7	7	26	29	7	7	IOTF
Italy	Luciano et al. (2003) north/south	Cross-sectional study, 2002	2,150 (1,137 boys/1,013 girls)	2–6	20.2/31.5	5.7/11.6	17/30.1	23.7/33.1	5.7/12.3	5.8/10.7	IOTF
Lithuania	Jakimaviciene and Tutkuviene (2007)	Cross-sectional study, 2003–2006	205 (90 boys/115 girls)	4	9.6	0.8	7.3	11.48	0.8	0.82	IOTF
Netherlands	van den Hurk et al. (2007)	Cross-sectional study, 2002–2004	1,781	4			12.3	16.2	2.3	3.4	IOTF

(continued)

Table 4.2 (continued)

Country	Survey	Year of survey	Number of children	Age (years)	Total Overweight (including obese)	Total Obese	Boys Overweight (including obese)	Girls Overweight (including obese)	Boys Obese	Girls Obese	Cut-off points
Norway	Juliusson et al. (2007)	Cross-sectional study, 2003–2006	4,115; 4–17 years (2,086 boys/ 2,029 girls)	6			8.2	19.2	1.76	7.14	IOTF
United Kingdom	Crowther et al. (2007)	Cross-sectional study, 2003–2006	297,600 (152,400 boys/ 145,200 girls)	4–5	22.8	10	24.1	21.4	10.7	9.2	IOTF
Spain	Larranaga et al. (2007)	Cross-sectional study, 2004–2005	161 (76 boys/ 85 girls)	4–6	29.4	9.3					IOTF
Sweden	Holmback et al. (2007)	Retrospective cohort study, 2002	183 (88 boys/ 95 girls)	4	20	4	18	22	2	6	IOTF
Turkey	Ozer (2007)	Cross-sectional study	68 (34 boys/ 34 girls)	6	25	4.7	31.2	18.7	6.2	3.1	IOTF

Table 4.3 Prevalence of overweight and obesity in children 6–12 years old, WHO European Region

Country	Survey	Year of survey	Number of children	Age (years)	Total Overweight (including obese)	Total Obese	Boys Overweight (including obese)	Girls Overweight (including obese)	Boys Obese	Girls Obese	Cut-off points
Austria	Kirchengast and Schober (2006b)	Longitudinal study, 2006	794 (455 boys/339 girls)	10	26.8	10.6	28.3	24.8	11.6	9.4	Kromeyer-Hauschild
Belgium	Yngve and Sjostrom (2001) reported by parents	Cross-sectional study, 2003	965 (496 boys/469 girls)	11	8.9	1.3	9.5	8.4	0.6	2.1	IOTF
Bulgaria	Lobstein and Frelut (2003)	Cross-sectional study, 1998	6,655; 7–17 years	7–11	18						IOTF
Cyprus	Savva et al. (2002)	Cross-sectional study, 1999–2000	221 (221 boys/120 girls)	10	32.1	12.2	31.7	32.5	11.9	12.5	IOTF
Czech Republic	Lobstein and Frelut (2003)	Cross-sectional study, 2001	32,453; 7–18 years	7–11	17						IOTF
Denmark	Yngve and Sjostrom (2001) reported by parents	Cross-sectional study, 2003	1,066 (528 boys/538 girls)	11	10	1.0	12.7	7.3	1.6	0.4	IOTF
Estonia	Villa et al. (2007)	Cross-sectional study, 1998–1999	542 (258 boys/284 girls)	9	10	0.7	11.2	8.9	0.4	1	IOTF
Finland	Hakanen et al. (2006)	Prospective randomized trial, 2000–2002	585	10			23.6	19.1			IOTF
France	Lioret et al. (2007) (personal communication, self reported)	Cross-sectional study, 1998–1999	578	6–12	15.7	2.4					IOTF
East Germany	Frye and Heinrich (2003)	Cross-sectional study, 1998–1999	732 (377 boys/355 girls)	8–10	26.6	5.6	26.8	26.5	6.9	4.2	IOTF
Germany	Kurth and Schaffrath Rosario (2007)	Cross-sectional study, 2003–2006	17,641; 0–17 years (8,985 boys/8,656 girls)	7–10	21.4	6.4	21.4	6.4	21.4	6.4	Kromeyer-Hauschild

(continued)

Table 4.3 (continued)

Country	Survey	Year of survey	Number of children	Age (years)	Total Overweight (including obese)	Total Obese	Boys Overweight (including obese)	Girls Overweight (including obese)	Boys Obese	Girls Obese	Cut-off points
Greece	Moschonis et al. (2008)	Cross-sectional study, 2007–2008	1,192 (626 boys/566 girls)	10–12	38.9	10.9	43.0	34.5	13.9	7.6	IOTF
Hungary	Kern (2007)	Cross-sectional study, 2003–2006	1,661 (823 boys/838 girls)	10	21.3	5.7	18.9	23.5	4.7	6.7	IOTF
Iceland	Jackson-Leach and Lobstein (2006)	Cross-sectional study, 1998		9			22	25.5	5.8	4.2	IOTF
Ireland	Whelton et al. (2007)	Cross-sectional study, 2001–2002	2,699 (1,372 boys/1,327 girls)	8	27	7.5	24	30	7	8	IOTF
Israel	Huerta et al. (2006)	Cross-sectional study, 2000	1,042 (445 boys/596 girls)	7–8		6.8			8.6	5.5	CDC
Italy	Bertoncello et al. (2008)	Cross-sectional study, 2001	6,508 (3,325 boys/3,183 girls)	9	29.3	5.8	31.1	27.4	6	5.6	IOTF
Lithuania	Tutkuviene (2007)	Cross-sectional study, 2000–2002	1,240 (618 boys/622 girls)	7–13	8.7	1.42	8.94	8.46	1.71	1.13	IOTF
Malta	Lobstein and Frelut (2003)	Cross-sectional study, 1992	519	7–11	35						IOTF
Netherlands	van den Hurk et al. (2007)	Cross-sectional study, 2002–2004	12,610	10			13.4	15.9	2.7	2.8	IOTF
Norway	Juliusson et al. (2007)	Cross-sectional study, 2003–2006	4,115; 4–17 years (2,086 boys/2,029 girls)	10			16.7	17.8	2.85	2.8	IOTF
Poland	Matusik et al. (2007)	Cross-sectional study	2,916 (1,471 boys/1,445 girls)	7–9	15.4	3.6	15	15.8	3.6	3.7	IOTF
Portugal	Padez et al. (2004)	Cross-sectional study, 2002–2003	4,508 (2,234 boys/2,274 girls)	8	31.3	11.3	29.5	33.2	10.9	11.8	IOTF
Russian Federation	Lobstein and Frelut (2003)	Cross-sectional study, 1998	2,688; 6–18 years	7–11	10						IOTF
United Kingdom	Crowther et al. (2007)	Cross-sectional study, 2005–2006	240,800 (125,400 boys/115,400 girls)	10–11	31.1	17.3	32.7	29.2	18.9	15.4	IOTF

Country	Reference	Study	Sample	Age							Criteria
Slovakia	Lobstein and Frelut (2003)	Cross-sectional study, 1995–1999	5.514	7–11	12						IOTF
Spain	Larranaga et al. (2007)	Cross-sectional study, 2004–2005	327 (185 boys/175 girls)	7–10	32.6	4.5					IOTF
Sweden	Villa et al. (2007)	Cross-sectional study, 1998–1999	544 (259 boys/285 girls)	9	14.7	2.5	12.3	17	3.7	1.4	IOTF
Switzerland	Zimmermann et al. (2000)	Cross-sectional study	595	6–12	21.7	9.7	22.9	20.4	10.3	9.1	IOTF
Turkey	Ozer (2007)	Cross-sectional study	139 (77 boys/62 girls)	9	18.5	3.5	17.3	20	2.3	5	IOTF

Table 4.4 Prevalence of overweight and obesity in children 12–18 years old, WHO European Region

Country	Survey	Year of the survey	Number of children	Age (years)	Total Overweight (including obese)	Total Obese	Boys Overweight (including obese)	Girls Overweight (including obese)	Boys Obese	Girls Obese	Cut-off points
Austria	Kirchengast and Schober (2006b)	Longitudinal study, 2006	794 (455 boys/339 girls)	15	23.6	10	23.1	24.2	11.3	8.4	Kromeyer-Hauschild
Belgium (Flemish)	Lissau et al. (2004)	Cross-sectional study, 1997–1998	2,643; 13 and 15 year old children (self-reported)	15			13.1	15.4	5.2	5.8	Internal Study Reference Standard
Bulgaria	Lobstein and Frelut (2003)	Cross-sectional study, 1998	6,655; 7–17 years	14–17	17						IOTF
Cyprus	Savva et al. (2002)	Cross-sectional study, 1999–2000	206 (105 boys/101 girls)	15	17.9	4.8	20.0	15.8	5.7	4	IOTF
Czech Republic	Lobstein and Frelut (2003)	Cross-sectional study, 1998	32,453, 7–18 years	14–17	9						IOTF
Estonia	Villa et al. (2007)	Cross-sectional study, 1998–1999	556 (249 boys/307 girls)	15	8.3		8.9	7.8			IOTF
Finland (self-reported)	Kautiainen et al. (2005) (unpublished data, personal communication)	Cross-sectional study, 2005	57,407; 14–18 years	16			20.3	13.1	4.2	3.5	IOTF
France	Lissau et al. (2004)	Cross-sectional study, 1997–1998	2,243 (self reported weight and height)	15			9.8	12.8	2.7	4	Internal Study Reference Standard
Germany	Kurth and Schaffrath Rosario (2007)	Cross-sectional study, 2003–2006	17,641; 0–17 years 8,985 boys /8,656 girls	14–17	25.5	8.5	25.5	8.5	25.5	8.5	Kromeyer-Hauschild

Country	Reference	Study type	Sample	Age							Reference standard
Greece/Thes.	Hassapidou et al. (2006)	School based study	502 (268 boys/234 girls)	12–14	26.3		31	21			IOTF
Greece/Crete	Magkos et al. (2006)	Cross-sectional study, 2002	240 boys	15					12.1		IOTF
Hungary	Kern (2007)	Cross-sectional study, 2003–2006	1,741 (920 boys/821 girls)	15	14.8	3.9	17	12.5	4.4	3.4	IOTF
Ireland	Whelton et al. (2007)	Cross-sectional study, 2001–2002	1,986 (1,051 boys/935 girls)	15	22	5	22	22	5	5	IOTF
Israel	Lissau et al. (2004)	Cross-sectional study, 1997–1998	991 (self reported)	15			20.1	16.4	6.8	6.2	Internal Study Reference Standard
Italy	Velluzzi et al. (2007) Sardinia	Cross-sectional study	3,946 (2,011 boys/1,935 girls)	11–15	17.6	3.7					IOTF
Lithuania	Tutkuviene (2007)	Cross-sectional study, 2000–2002	1,001 (498 boys/503 girls)	14–18	5.06	0.4	6.77	3.35	0.80	0.00	IOFT
Netherlands	van den Hurk et al. (2007)	Cross-sectional study, 2002–2004	1,521	15			15.4	17.2	3	2.8	IOTF
Norway	Juliusson et al. (2007)	Cross-sectional study, 2003–2006	4,115; 4–17 years (2,086 boys/2,029 girls)	15			9.75	8.35	3.5	1.11	IOTF
Poland	Chrzanowska et al. (2007)	Cross-sectional study, 2000	584 (294 boys/290 girls)	16	8.0	1.0	10.73	5.3	2.15	0.00	IOTF
Portugal	Ramos and Barros (2007)	Cross-sectional study	2,161 (1,045 boys/1,116 girls)	13	25.9	6.1	27.4	24.5	6.6	5.7	CDC
Russian Federation	Wan et al. (2007)	Cross-sectional study, 1992	6,883	10–18	10.6	3.5	11.5	9.7	4.5	2	IOTF
United Kingdom	Jebb et al. (2004)	Cross-sectional study, 1997	1,667 (859 boys/808 girls)	15–17	36.1	7.5	39	33	7	8	IOTF
Slovakia	Lissau et al. (2004)	Cross-sectional study, 1997–1998	2,233; 13 and 15 years (self reported)	15			16.5	11.3	4.4	1.1	Internal Study Reference Standard

(continued)

Table 4.4 (continued)

Country	Survey	Year of the survey	Number of children	Age(years)	Total Overweight (including obese)	Total Obese	Boys Overweight (including obese)	Girls Overweight (including obese)	Boys Obese	Girls Obese	Cut-off points
Spain	Moreno et al. (2005a)	Cross-sectional study, 2000–2002	2,320 (1,192 boys/ 1,128 girls)	13–18	22.5	4.4	25.7	19.1	5.7	3.1	IOTF
Sweden	Villa et al. (2007)	Cross-sectional study, 1998–1999	540 (248 boys/ 292 girls)	15	10.1	1.54	9	11	1	2	IOTF
Turkey	Sur et al. (2005)	Cross-sectional study, 2001–2002	1,044 (516 boys/ 528 girls)	12–13	13.9	2	14.9	12.9	1.7	2.3	IOTF

Prevalence of Overweight and Obesity

Time Trends by Country

Studies from several countries provide strong evidence of the increasing trends in the prevalence of childhood obesity worldwide (Jakimaviciene and Tutkuviene 2007; Kautiainen et al. 2002; Kosti and Panagiotakos 2006; Kromeyer-Hauschild and Zellner 2007; Moreno et al. 2000; Moreno et al. 2005b). The annual rate of increase in the prevalence of childhood obesity has been growing steadily, and the current prevalence is ten times higher than it was in the 1970s (WHO, ENHIS 2007). Overweight and obesity in most countries of Europe show rising secular trends and are predicted to continue rising if not addressed.

In the United Kingdom the prevalence of overweight and obesity among school children has tripled over the past 30 years. More specifically, overweight and obesity among school children has increased from 9.4% and 12.1% for boys and girls respectively in 1974 and 22.8% and 26.3% in 1998 to a 32.7% and 29.2% in 2007 (Crowther et al. 2007). In various regions of Spain, the prevalence of excess body weight has doubled from 1985 to 2002 and is now reaching 32.6% among children 7–10 years old (Larranaga et al. 2007). Most importantly, Moreno et al. (2001a, b) have observed increasing trends of central adiposity, especially in males and at the youngest ages studied (6–11 years in males, and 6–7 years in females), independent of trends in BMI.

According to another study, contemporary Greek boys were found to be heavier and had higher BMI values than their peers in 1982 (Magkos et al. 2006).

In the case of Germany, in comparison to former German reference data for the period 1985–1997 the prevalence of overweight in children has risen by 50% and the obesity rate has doubled within the last 3 years (2003–2006) (KIGGS 2006; Kurth and Schaffrath Rosario 2007). The overweight and obesity prevalence in Polish school boys has increased from 6.5% in 1971 to 15.5% in 2000, a trend that has been followed by other Eastern European countries (Matusik et al. 2007). The only observed decrease in prevalence was in the Russian Federation during the economic crisis that followed the dissolution of the USSR, however, obesity prevalence in Russia Federation is now on the increase (Wan et al. 2007).

It has to be noted that the above reported increase in obesity trends in most European countries is not only seen in school children and adolescents but also in very young children, 0–6 years old (Figs. 4.1–4.4).

Geographic Distribution by Country

From infancy through adolescence, more and more children are becoming overweight (Tables 4.2–4.4). Data from reported prevalence of childhood overweight and obesity in Europe suggest that children and adolescents residing in countries surrounding the Mediterranean Sea show the highest rates ranging from 20 to 40%, while those in northern areas of Europe show rates in the range 10–20%. Scandinavian countries have among the lowest prevalence of obesity in all age groups in comparison to other regions (Table 4.2–4.4), with the exception of Finland where a recent study has reported that the prevalence of overweight and obesity in school children in Finland is 23.6 and 19.1% for boys and girls, respectively (Hakanen et al. 2006). The very high prevalence of childhood obesity in Mediterranean countries such as Spain, Italy, Malta and Greece (Tables 4.2–4.4) could be partly attributed to the gradual shift from the healthy Mediterranean diet to a more Western type of diet. In a recent study conducted in Greece, only 11.3% of children and 8.3% of adolescents were found to follow the traditional Mediterranean diet (Kontogianni et al. 2008). In addition, lower physical activity levels

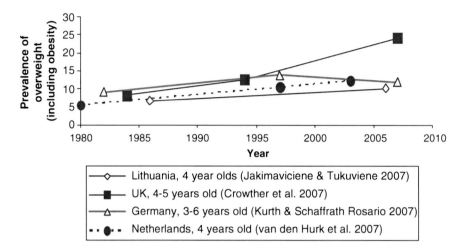

Fig. 4.1 Time trends in overweight prevalence in pre-school children in selected European countries/boys. WHO Statistical Information System (Core Health Indicators in the WHO European Region 2005), WorldBank database and Wikipedia

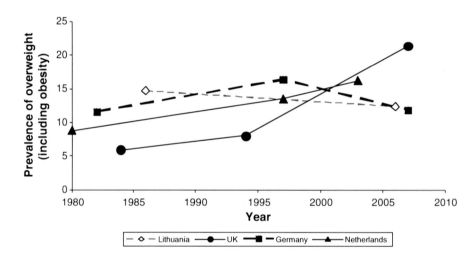

Fig. 4.2 Time trends in overweight prevalence in pre-school children in selected European countries/girls. WHO Statistical Information System (Core Health Indicators in the WHO European Region 2005), WorldBank database and Wikipedia. *Source*: See legend Figure 4.1

have been reported in children and adolescents living in the Mediterranean countries in comparison to children in northern countries of Europe (Rey-Lopez et al. 2008; Samdal et al. 2007).

In the case of central and Eastern Europe, lower levels of overweight have been reported in comparison to children from other parts of Europe, especially from Southern Europe (Tables 4.2–4.4). It is important to note however, that recent studies show a considerable increase in overweight (including obesity) prevalence in children of all ages, in countries such as the United Kingdom (22.8 and 31.1% for pre-school children and school children, respectively) and Austria (26.8 and 17.8% for pre-school children and school children, respectively) (Tables 4.2–4.3) (Crowther et al. 2007; Kirchengast and Schober 2006a). High prevalence rates have also been reported for adolescents, however, they seem to be lower than the prevalence rates for younger children (Table 4.4).

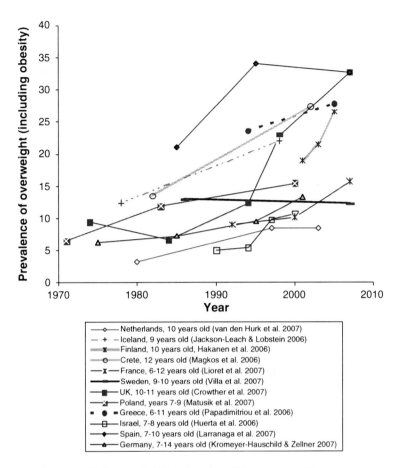

Fig. 4.3 Time trends in overweight in school children in selected European countries/boys

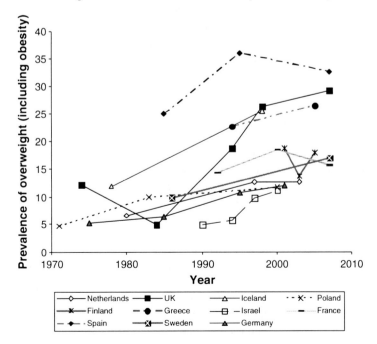

Fig. 4.4 Time trends in overweight in school children in selected European countries/girls.
Source: See legend Figure 4.3

In Lithuania, the Russian Federation, Slovakia and Poland, the overweight and obesity prevalence range from 8.46 to 15.8% among children aged 6–12 years, whereas in countries like Greece,
Spain, Israel and Malta the reported values are from around 26.5 to 35% (Table 4.3). It is likely that
the huge economic burden and the associated poverty following the political transition in the 1990s
may have contributed to the relatively low obesity prevalence in Eastern Europe. However, even
though there is as yet limited available trend data, it is likely that overweight and obesity are
becoming increasingly prevalent throughout the Eastern European Region (Knai et al. 2007).

It is important to note that among pre-school children (Table 4.2), the highest prevalence rates of
overweight and obesity were in Southern Italy (30.1 and 33.1% for boys and girls, respectively) and
Spain (29.4%, both sexes), followed by Ireland (26 and 29% for boys and girls, respectively), the United
Kingdom (24.1 and 21.4% for boys and girls, respectively) and Greece (19.1 and 23.6% for boys and
girls, respectively). The lowest rates were in Lithuania (7.3 and 11.5% for boys and girls, respectively),
Norway (8.2 and 19.2% for boys and girls, respectively) and Germany (11.9%, both sexes).

Recent data revealed that 16.5% of boys and 11.4% of girls between 1 and 2 years old were
classified as "overweight" (based on CDC cut-off points, since IOTF are only valid after the age of
2 years old) (Manios et al. 2007). It is important to note that the reported high prevalence of obesity
in very young children is indicating an increased risk for even higher rates of obesity in adolescence
and adulthood, in the near future, exceeding those currently reported.

Prevalence of Obesity by Ethnicity and Socio-Economic Status

In developed countries worldwide, an inverse relationship has been demonstrated between levels of
socio-economic status and prevalence of obesity in adults. In children, results are less consistent,
however, an increasing number of studies suggest that children in lower-income families in developed countries are particularly vulnerable to becoming obese possibly due to poor dietary habits and
limited opportunities for physical activity (Kumanyika 2008; Wardle et al. 2006).

In Europe, a number of recent studies have attempted to investigate the role of ethnicity and SES
on childhood obesity (Kirchengast and Schober 2006b; Will et al. 2005). In the United Kingdom,
children from lower social classes had marginally higher odds to be obese than their peers from
higher income households (Stamatakis et al. 2005). In the case of Spain, a significant inverse
relationship between socio-economic status and obesity has been reported in boys but not in girls
(Moreno et al. 2005a). According to a recent study from Sweden on obesity prevalence in
10 year-old-children, strong gradients, with more obesity and overweight in socio-economically
disadvantaged areas, were observed in both sexes in 2003 (Sundblom et al. 2008). Similar findings
have been reported in other European countries such as France and Germany (Table 4.6) (Lioret et al. 2007;
Will et al. 2005). Very few studies have examined the possible impact of socio-economic characteristics on the risk of being overweight or obese for children under the age of 6 (Savva et al. 2005;
Whitaker and Orzol 2006). In a recent study in Greece on obesity prevalence in children 1–5 years
old, maternal and paternal educational level, as an indicator of SES, was not found to influence the
risk of overweight (Manios et al. 2007). It is likely that parental education is not related to the presence of overweight and obesity in very young children and only becomes a causative factor in later
years. It can also be postulated that in the case of very young children, there is not enough time for
the social and physical environment to have a significant impact on the prevalence of obesity.

Available evidence also indicates that being an immigrant may affect the risk of obesity development during infancy, childhood and adolescence (Kumanyika 2008). In the UK, the prevalence of
overweight and obesity combined in 11–12 years old children was 25%, with higher rates in girls
(29%) and students from lower socio-economic backgrounds (31%) and the highest rates in black
girls (38%) (Wardle et al. 2006). Similar higher rates in migrant children have been reported in the

Netherlands, where the mean prevalence for Turkish boys and girls was 23.4 and 30.2%, for Moroccans 15.8 and 24.5%, for Dutch youths in large cities 12.6 and 16.5%, and for other Dutch participants 8.7 and 11.3%, respectively (Table 4.5) (Kirchengast and Schober 2006b).

In adults, it has been shown that socio-cultural factors drive the standards of desirable body weight within cultures, which in turn influence certain eating behaviors and physical activity patterns (Flynn and Fitzgibbon 1998). Evidence for example suggests that black women are generally less concerned about their body weight and they tend to report less pressure to be slim, less dissatisfaction with their weight, and greater acceptance of being overweight than white women (Kemper et al. 1994; Powell and Kahn 1995). Differences in the perception of ideal body weight together with food security issues seem to play an important role for the above differences in obesity prevalence in migrant children and children with lower SES in developed countries (Mendoza et al. 2006; Monsivais and Drewnowski 2007).

More specifically, Duncan et al. (2006) investigated the relationship among body esteem and body fat in British children in relation to ethnicity and concluded that the association between body dissatisfaction and body fatness differed across ethnic groups. Body esteem and adiposity were negatively related for all children (White, Black, Asian) and for both sexes. Boys (total) and black children (both boys and girls) had significantly higher body esteem than girls (total) and Asian children (both boys and girls), respectively (Duncan et al. 2004, 2006).

Ethnicity and SES also seem to affect levels of physical activity. A recent study which was set to compare physical activity levels between white and South Asian school children in the UK has concluded that South Asian children are significantly less active than their white peers (Duncan et al. 2008). Most importantly, another study was set to assess developmental trends in physical activity and sedentary behavior in British adolescents in relation to ethnicity and socio-economic status. Ethnicity and SES characteristics were found to be significant contributing factors to sedentary behavior in British youth, which are largely established by age 11–12 years, indicating that any potential intervention should start at an earlier age (Brodersen et al. 2007).

Another important issue is the fact that the actual cost of a healthy diet is gradually increasing (Maillot et al. 2007; Monsivais and Drewnowski 2007). A study by Maillot et al. (2007) investigating self-selected diets of French adults has shown that lower energy density and higher nutritional quality were associated with higher energy-adjusted diet costs. Drewnowski et al. (2007) have recently demonstrated that the more energy-dense diets cost less, whereas low-energy-density diets cost considerably more, adjusting for energy intake, sex, and age, which may partially explain the reason behind the highest rates of obesity observed among groups of limited economic means.

In conclusion, socio-economic status is usually associated with obesity in most Western populations. However, different SES groups are at different risk of obesity and the relationship between SES factors and obesity varies across countries (Manios et al. 2007; Wan et al. 2007). This relationship is complex because socio-economic status may influence obesity and vice versa (Stunkard and Sorensen 1993). For children, the relationship among ethnicity, SES and obesity may result from a number of different underlying causes such as unhealthy eating patterns, sedentary lifestyle, cultural attitudes about body weight and the rising cost of a healthy diet.

Discussion of Key Risk Factors

From infancy through adolescence more and more children are becoming obese in Europe; however the prevalence of obesity differs between countries.

In the case of infants and pre-school children a number of perinatal parameters and factors related to parental characteristics have been implicated in the etiology of obesity. More specifically, studies suggest that *bottle-feeding*, duration of *breastfeeding*, *maternal obesity*, *parental feeding*

Table 4.5 Prevalence (%) of overweight and obesity in children and adolescents by ethnicity

Country	Survey	Age (years)	Ethnicity				Cut-off points
			Boys		Girls		
			Overweight (including obese)	Obese	Overweight (including obese)	Obese	
Austria	Kirchengast and Schober (2006b)	6	Austrian18.1, Turkish 20.7, Yugoslavian 23.1		Austrian18.1, Turkish 20.4, Yugoslavian 25.6		Kromeyer-Hauschild
		10	Austrian 27.1, Turkish 21.1, Yugoslavian 36.6		Austrian 27.1, Turkish 27.7, Yugoslavian 30.9		
		15	Austrian 23.7, Turkish 25, Yugoslavian 27.9		Austrian 23.7, Turkish 29.2, Yugoslavian 27.5		
Germany	Will et al. (2005)	6–7	Migrant children[a] 11.7	1.6	24.1	4.7	IOTF
			German children 8.3	0.7	14	3.3	
Greece	Papadimitriou et al. (2006)	6–11	Migrant children[b] 15.9	7.9	15.2	8.7	IOTF
			Greek children 27.8	12.3	26.5	9.9	
Netherlands	Fredriks et al. (2005)	0–21	Dutch (cities) 15 & rural 10	2 & 1	Dutch (cities) 20 & rural 12	3 & 1	IOTF
			Turkish 28	5	Turkish 37	7	
			Morrocan 19	3	Morrocan 30	5	
United Kingdom	Wardle et al. (2006)	11–12 (followed for 5 years, average)	Asian boys were heavier in comparison to White and Black children, but the differences were not statistically significant		Adjusted for SES White 28, Black 38.2, Asian 19.8		IOTF

[a]Migrant children: Turkish (36%), Russian (25%) and Polish (15%)
[b]Migrant children: Albanian (90%), Georgian, Lithuanian, Polish, Serbian, Ukraine, Russian, Moldavian (10%)

practices, *rapid infancy weight gain* and other cultural or familial factors associated with *childhood eating patterns* and *activity levels* are important risk factors for childhood obesity (Manios et al. 2007; Monteiro and Victora 2005; Ong 2006; Parsons et al. 2003; see also the various chapters of Part II of this book). It is plausible that the differences in prevalence of obesity in very young children among European countries could be partly attributed to differences in social and cultural attitudes, practices and believes which influence the above parameters.

Great differences exist in breastfeeding prevalence and duration among European countries. The prevalence and duration of breastfeeding is higher in countries with relatively lower prevalence of childhood obesity such as Sweden, Finland and Austria, in comparison to countries such as Italy, Greece and the UK where prevalence and duration of breastfeeding is less (Yngve and Sjostrom 2001).

There is evidence that breastfed infants are less likely to be obese. A meta-analysis suggests a 10–20% decreased risk of obesity among those who had been breastfed compared with those who were not breastfed (Arenz et al. 2004; Owen et al. 2005) and a 4% reduction for each additional month of breastfeeding duration (Harder et al. 2005). Compared with bottle-feeding, breastfeeding could help infants to better recognize satiety signals and hence to better self-regulate energy intake (Taveras et al. 2004). Another plausible hypothesized pathway is through the biologic activity of certain breast milk components (Weyermann et al. 2007). Rapid growth during infancy, most commonly observed in nonbreastfed infants, has also received a great deal of attention lately as a factor contributing significantly to overweight during infancy and at later ages (Moschonis et al. 2008; Monteiro and Victora 2005; Ong 2006; Weaver 2006).

Parental feeding practices of the child are also very important. The exertion of control during child feeding has been associated with both underweight and overweight during childhood. Restrictive child feeding practices during infancy predicts lower child weight at age 2 years, which may reinforce mothers' use of this strategy in the longer term despite its potential association with disinhibition and greater child weight in later childhood (Farrow and Blissett 2008).

It has to be underlined that the effect of parental obesity on children's risk for increased adiposity is one of the most consistent findings in the controversial field of obesity (Magarey et al. 2003). Evidence suggests that the growing child remains vulnerable to parental influences, but at the same time becomes increasingly susceptible to wider social and environmental factors. Some researchers argue that children adopt their parents' eating habits as a result of environmental exposure rather than the heredity of "food choice genes", although it is unquestionable that some of this resemblance is attributed to genetic similarities (Guillaume et al. 1995; Zeller and Daniels 2004). A recent study in pre-schoolers in Greece has shown that the prevalence of being overweight was significantly greater for children with one or two obese parents (Manios et al. 2007). As children grow older the parental role and the family environment seem to be less influential and other environmental factors affect the risk of becoming obese. The environment of children has drastically changed in Europe during the last decades as reflected in unhealthy dietary habits and sedentary lifestyle. Obesity is no longer a phenomenon confined to wealthier parts of the world such as Western Europe but is increasingly found in the transition countries of the European Region. Available data show that overweight and obesity prevalence levels are rising even in the less developed countries of the WHO European Region (Knai et al. 2007). Substantial foreign investment has been received by many transition countries and although such investment is associated with benefits, it also enables trans-national companies to promote the adoption of western diets including the consumption of processed foods and drinks, often high in saturated fats and added sugars (Hawkes 2005).

Potential environmental obesogenic factors include easy *availability of inexpensive energy-dense food*, *large portions sizes*, increased use of *fast food outlets* and the consumption of *sugary soft*

Table 4.6 Prevalence (%) of overweight and obesity in children and adolescents by SES

Country	Survey	Age (years)	SES Boys Overweight (including obese)	Girls Overweight (including obese)	Cut-off points
France	Lioret et al. (2007)	3–5	Low 19.1, Medium 19.5, High 9.1		IOTF
		6–10	Low 21.7, Medium 13.5, High 6.1		
		11–14	Low 17.3, Medium 7.2, High 2.1		
Germany	Will et al. (2005)	6–7	Boys and Girls *Social class*		IOTF
			Low 17.9 (Migrant) 23.5 (German)		
			Medium 10.5 (Migrant) 7.5 (German)		
			High 27.6 (Migrant) 10.0 (German)		
Greece	Manios et al. (2007)	1–5	SES was not related to obesity prevalence in pre-school children in both sexes		IOTF
Russian Federation	Wan et al. (2007)	6–9	Boys and Girls		IOTF
			Low-income 32.2		
			Middle-income 28.0		
			High-income 33.0		
		10–18	Low-income 12.5		
			Middle-income 9.1		
			High-income 10.8		
United Kingdom	Wardle et al. (2006)	11–12 (followed for 5 years, average)	Most deprived boys were the heaviest but not significantly	Adjusted for ethnicity Most deprived 35.2 Rest of the groups 27.8	IOTF
Turkey (urban)	Manios et al. (2007)	12–13	Middle/High 13.9 Low 8	Middle/High 16.7 Low 9.9	IOTF

drinks (Gibson 2008; Linardakis et al. 2008; Moreno and Rodriguez 2007; Prentice and Jebb 2003). In addition, *motorized transport* together with *the time spent on sedentary activities* (television viewing, use of internet and video games) have increased dramatically (Galcheva et al. 2008; Rey-Lopez et al. 2008).

More specifically, according to a recent study, data from within 20 European Union countries relating to food promotion to children have shown that unhealthy foods such as savory snacks and confectionary were the most commonly marketed and consumed by children across all countries with television being the prime promotional medium (Matthews 2008). Another recent UK study has shown that exposure to food advertisements promotes over-consumption in younger children (Halford et al. 2007). Very importantly, the time spent watching television or playing video games is a period during which the child remains seated and thus his/her energy expenditure is relatively low (Ekelund et al. 2006). Studies have shown that such leisure activities lead to snacking which results in an increase in energy intake (Pardee et al. 2007; Salmon et al. 2008).

It is important to note that food marketing regulation across Europe is inconsistent. In a recent study, an ineffective and incoherent pattern of regulation was observed across the countries, as few governments imposed tough restrictions with most preferring to persuade industry to voluntarily act with responsibly. The strength of regulatory approaches ranged from very tough, as seen in Norway and Sweden where TV advertisements targeting children under 12 are banned, to non-existent in other countries (Matthews 2008).

Finally, *migrant children* and children of *lower SES* (Tables 4.5 and 4.6) seem to be at increased risk of overweight and obesity in comparison to other children (Freedman et al. 2006). Ethnicity is associated with differences in food-related beliefs, preferences, and behaviors and cultural influences may contribute to the higher than average risk of obesity among children and youth in minority populations. Furthermore, in the poorest population groups, the diet is frequently high in calories, very high in fat intake whereas vegetables, fruits, and whole grain cereals, which are generally more expensive, are normally eaten in smaller quantities (Almerich-Silla and Montiel-Company 2007; Branner et al. 2008; Stone et al. 2007).

Conclusions

Childhood obesity is increasing in the WHO European Region. In spite of the fact that there are currently several initiatives to assemble comparable data on overweight and obesity across the WHO European Region (WHO Global Database on body mass index and the database of the WHO Regional Office for Europe; WHO Global Infobase, 2007), there is a distinctive lack of harmonized cross-national surveys of overweight and obesity prevalence levels in children in the European Region (Lobstein and Millstone 2006). Recording and understanding the prevalence of obesity in children and the social, geographic and cultural parameters related to the phenomenon can facilitate the formation of effective public health intervention policies in counteracting childhood obesity. Since early prevention seems to be more effective in managing the epidemic of obesity in comparison to treating obesity later in life, tailored made public health policies should start early in life.

References

Almerich-Silla, J.M., & Montiel-Company J.M. (2007). Influence of immigration and other factors on caries in 12- and 15-yr-old children. *European Journal of Oral Sciences, 115*, 378–383.

Angelopoulos, P.D., Milionis, H.J., Moschonis, G., & Manios, Y. (2006). Relations between obesity and hypertension: preliminary data from a cross-sectional study in primary schoolchildren: the children study. *European Journal of Clinical Nutrition, 60*, 1226–1234.

Arenz, S., Ruckerl, R., Koletzko, B., & von Kries, R. (2004). Breast-feeding and childhood obesity – a systematic review. *International Journal of Obesity Related Metabolic Disorders, 28*, 1247–1256.

Bertoncello, C., Cazzaro, R., Ferraresso, A., Mazzer, R., & Moretti, G. (2008). Prevalence of overweight and obesity among school-aged children in urban, rural and mountain areas of the Veneto Region, Italy. *Public Health Nutrition, 11*, 887–890.

Branner, C.M., Koyama, T., & Jensen, G.L. (2008). Racial and ethnic differences in pediatric obesity-prevention counseling: national prevalence of clinician practices. *Obesity (Silver Spring), 16(3)*, 690–694.

Brodersen, N.H., Steptoe, A., Boniface, D.R., & Wardle, J. (2007). Trends in physical activity and sedentary behaviour in adolescence: ethnic and socioeconomic differences. *British Journal of Sports Medicine, 41*, 140–144.

Chrzanowska, M., Koziel, S., & Ulijaszek, S.J. (2007). Changes in BMI and the prevalence of overweight and obesity in children and adolescents in Cracow, Poland, 1971–2000. *Economic & Human Biology, 5*, 370–378.

Cole, T.J., Bellizzi, M.C., Flegal, K.M., & Dietz, W.H. (2000). Establishing a standard definition for child overweight and obesity worldwide: international survey. *British Medical Journal, 320*, 1240–1243.

Crowther, R., Dinsdale, H., Rutter, H., & Kyffin, R. (2007). Analysis of the National Childhood Obesity Database 2005–06. *A report for the Department of Health by the South East Public Health Observatory on behalf of the Association of Public Health Observatories NHS, January 2007.*

de Beer, M., Hofsteenge, G.H., Koot, H.M., Hirasing, R.A., Delemarre-van de Waal, H.A., & Gemke, R.J. (2007). Health-related-quality-of-life in obese adolescents is decreased and inversely related to BMI. *Acta Pediatrica, 96*, 710–714.

de Onis, M., Onyango, A.W., Borghi, E., Garza, C., & Yang, H. (2006). Comparison of the World Health Organization (WHO) Child Growth Standards and the National Center for Health Statistics/WHO international growth reference: implications for child health programmes. *Public Health Nutrition, 9*, 942–947.

DiPietro, L., Mossberg, H.O., & Stunkard, A.J. (1994). A 40-year history of overweight children in Stockholm: life-time overweight, morbidity, and mortality. *International Journal of Obesity Related Metabolic Disorders, 18*, 585–590.

Drewnowski, A., Monsivais, P., Maillot, M., & Darmon, N. (2007). Low-energy-density diets are associated with higher diet quality and higher diet costs in French adults. *Journal of the American Dietetics Association, 107*, 1028–1032.

Duncan, M.J., Al-Nakeeb Y., & Nevill, A.M. (2004). Body esteem and body fat in British school children from different ethnic groups. *Body Image, 1*, 311–315.

Duncan, M.J., Al-Nakeeb, Y., Nevill, A.M., & Jones, M.V. (2006). Body dissatisfaction, body fat and physical activity in British children. *International Journal of Pediatric Obesity, 1*, 89–95.

Duncan, M.J., Woodfield, L., Al-Nakeeb, Y., & Nevill, A.M. (2008). Differences in physical activity levels between white and South asian children in the United kingdom. *Pediatric Exercise Science, 20*, 285–291.

Ekelund, U., Brage, S., Froberg, K., Harro, M., Anderssen, S.A., Sardinha, L.B., Riddoch, C., & Andersen, L.B. (2006). TV viewing and physical activity are independently associated with metabolic risk in children: the European Youth Heart Study. *PLoS Medicine, 3(12)*, e488.

Farrow, C.V., & Blissett, J. (2008). Controlling feeding practices: cause or consequence of early child weight? *Pediatrics, 121*, e164–e169.

Flynn, K.J., & Fitzgibbon, M. (1998). Body images and obesity risk among black females: a review of the literature. *Annals of Behavioral Medicine, 20*, 13–24.

Franks, P.W., Hanson, R.L., Knowler, W.C., Moffett, C., Enos, G., Infante, A.M., Krakoff, J., & Looker, H.C. (2007). Childhood predictors of young onset type 2 diabetes mellitus. *Diabetes,* DOI: 10.2337/db06-1639.

Fredriks, A.M., Van Buuren, S., Sing, R.A., Wit, J.M., & Verloove-Vanhorick, S.P. (2005). Alarming prevalences of overweight and obesity for children of Turkish, Moroccan and Dutch origin in The Netherlands according to international standards. *Acta Pediatrica, 94*, 496–498.

Freedman, D.S., Khan, L.K., Serdula, M.K., Dietz, W.H., Srinivasan, S.R., & Berenson, G.S. (2004). Inter-relationships among childhood BMI, childhood height, and adult obesity: the Bogalusa Heart Study. *International Journal of Obesity Related Metabolic Disorders, 28*, 10–16.

Freedman, D.S., Khan, L.K., Serdula, M.K., Ogden, C.L., & Dietz, W.H. (2006). Racial and ethnic differences in secular trends for childhood BMI, weight, and height. *Obesity (Silver Spring), 14*, 301–308.

Frye, C., & Heinrich, J. (2003). Trends and predictors of overweight and obesity in East German children. *International Journals of Obesity Related Metabolic Disorders, 27*, 963–969.

Galcheva, S.V., Iotova, V.M., & Stratev, V.K. (2008). Television food advertising directed towards Bulgarian children. *Archives of Disease in Childhood, 93*, 857–861.

Gibson, S. (2008). Sugar-sweetened soft drinks and obesity: a systematic review of the evidence from observational studies and interventions. *Nutrition Research Review, 21*, 134–147.

Guillaume, M., Lapidus, L., Beckers, F., Lambert, A., & Bjorntorp, P. (1995). Familial trends of obesity through three generations: the Belgian-Luxembourg child study. *International Journal of Obesity Related Metabolic Disorders, 19(Suppl 3)*, S5–S9.

Hakanen, M., Lagstrom, H., Kaitosaari, T., Niinikoski, H., Nanto-Salonen K., Jokinen, E., Sillanmaki, L., Viikari, J., Ronnemaa, T., & Simell, O. (2006). Development of overweight in an atherosclerosis prevention trial starting in early childhood. The STRIP study. *International Journal of Obesity (Lond), 30*, 618–626.

Halford, J.C., Boyland, E.J., Hughes, G., Oliveira, L.P., & Dovey, T.M. (2007). Beyond-brand effect of television (TV) food advertisements/commercials on caloric intake and food choice of 5-7-year-old children. *Appetite, 49*, 263–267.

Harder, T., Bergmann, R., Kallischnigg, G., & Plagemann, A. (2005). Duration of breastfeeding and risk of over-weight: a meta-analysis. *American Journal of Epidemiology, 162*, 397–403.

Hassapidou, M., Fotiadou, E., Maglara, E., & Papadopoulou, S.K. (2006). Energy intake, diet composition, energy expenditure, and body fatness of adolescents in northern Greece. *Obesity (Silver Spring), 14*, 855–862.

Hawkes, C. (2005). The role of foreign direct investment in the nutrition transition. *Public Health Nutrition, 8*, 357–365.

Holmback, U., Fridman, J., Gustafsson, J., Proos, L., Sundelin, C., & Forslund, A. (2007). Overweight more prevalent among children than among adolescents. *Acta Paediatrica, 96*, 577–581.

Huerta, M., Gdalevich, M., Haviv, J., Bibi, H., & Scharf, S. (2006). Ten-year trends in obesity among Israeli school-children: 1990-2000. *Acta Paediatrica, 95*, 444–449.

IASO/IOTF (2007). Database on overweight and obesity. International Association for the Study of Obesity (IASO)/ International Obesity Task Force (IOTF), London, http://www.iotf.org/database/index.asp.

Jackson-Leach, R., & Lobstein, T. (2006). Estimated burden of paediatric obesity and co-morbidities in Europe. Part 1. The increase in the prevalence of child obesity in Europe is itself increasing. *International Journal of Pediatric Obesity, 1*, 26–32.

Jakimaviciene, E.M., & Tutkuviene, J. (2007). Trends in body mass index, prevalence of overweight and obesity in preschool Lithuanian children, 1986-2006. *College Antropology, 31*, 79–88.

Janicke, D.M., Marciel, K.K., Ingerski, L.M., Novoa, W., Lowry, K.W., Sallinen, B.J., & Silverstein, J.H. (2007). Impact of psychosocial factors on quality of life in overweight youth. *Obesity (Silver Spring), 15*, 1799–1807.

Jebb, S.A., Rennie, K.L., & Cole, T.J. (2004). Prevalence of overweight and obesity among young people in Great Britain. *Public Health Nutrition, 7*, 461–465.

Juliusson, P.B., Roelants, M., Eide, G.E., Hauspie, R., Waaler, P.E., & Bjerknes, R. (2007). Overweight and obesity in Norwegian children: secular trends in weight-for-height and skinfolds. *Acta Paediatrica, 96*, 1333–1337.

Kautiainen, S., Rimpela, A., Vikat, A., & Virtanen, S.M. (2002). Secular trends in overweight and obesity among Finnish adolescents in 1977-1999. *International Journal of Obesity Related Metabolic Disorders, 26*, 544–552.

Kautiainen, S., Koivusilta, L., Lintonen, T., Virtanen, S.M., & Rimpela, A. (2005). Use of information and communication technology and prevalence of overweight and obesity among adolescents. *International Journal of Obesity (Lond), 29*, 925–933.

Kemper, K.A., Sargent, R.C., Drane, J.W., Valois, R.F., & Hussey, J.R. (1994). Black and white females' perceptions of ideal body size and social norms. *Obesity Research, 2*, 117–126.

Kern, B. (2007). The prevalence of overweight and obesity in Hungarian children. Intensive Course in Biological Anthropology, 1st Summer School of the European Anthropological Association, 16–30 June, 2007, Prague, Czech Republic *EAA Summer School eBook* 1:181–186.

KIGGS (2006). German children and youth health survey 2006. http://www.kiggs.de.

Kirchengast, S., & Schober, E. (2006a). Obesity among female adolescents in Vienna, Austria – the impact of childhood weight status and ethnicity. *British Journal of Obstetrics & Gynaecology, 113*, 1188–1194.

Kirchengast, S., & Schober, E. (2006b). To be an immigrant: a risk factor for developing overweight and obesity during childhood and adolescence? *Journal of Biosocial Science, 38*, 695–705.

Knai, C., Suhrcke, M., & Lobstein, T. (2007). Obesity in Eastern Europe: an overview of its health and economic implications. *Economics of Human Biology, 5*, 392–408.

Kontogianni, M.D., Vidra, N., Farmaki, A.E., Koinaki, S., Belogianni, K., Sofrona, S., Magkanari, F., & Yannakoulia, M. (2008). Adherence rates to the Mediterranean diet are low in a representative sample of Greek children and adolescents. *Journal of Nutrition, 138*, 1951–1956.

Kosti, R.I., & Panagiotakos, D.B. (2006). The epidemic of obesity in children and adolescents in the world. *Central European Journal of Public Health, 14*, 151–159.

Kromeyer-Hauschild, K., & Zellner, K. (2007). Trends in overweight and obesity and changes in the distribution of body mass index in schoolchildren of Jena, East Germany. *European Journal of Clinical Nutrition, 61*, 404–411.

Kromeyer-Hauschild, K., Wabitsch, M., Kunze, D., Geller, F., Geiß, H.C., Hesse, V., von Hippel, A., Jaeger, U., Johnsen, D., Korte, W., Menner, K., Müller, G., Müller, J.M., Niemann-Pilatus, A., Remer, T., Schaefer, F., Wittchen, H.-U., Zabransky, S., Zellner, K., Ziegler, A., & Hebebrand, J. (2001). Perzentile für den Body-Mass-Index für das Kindes- und Jugendalter unter Heranziehung verschiedener deutscher Stichproben. *Monatsschrift für Kinderheilkunde, 149*, 807–818.

Kuczmarski, R.J., Ogden, C.L., Guo, S.S., Grummer-Strawn, L.M., Flegal, K.M., Mei, Z., Wei, R., Curtin, L.R., Roche, A.F., & Johnson, C.L. (2002). 2000 CDC Growth Charts for the United States: methods and development. *Vital Health Statistics, 11*, 1–190.

Kumanyika, S.K. (2008). Environmental influences on childhood obesity: Ethnic and cultural influences in context. *Physiology & Behaviour, 94(1)*, 61–70.

Kurth, B.M., & Schaffrath Rosario, A. (2007). The prevalence of overweight and obese children and adolescents living in Germany. Results of the German Health Interview and Examination Survey for Children and Adolescents (KiGGS). (In German) *Bundesgesundheitsblatt Gesundheitsforschung Gesundheitsschutz, 50*, 736–743.

Larranaga, N., Amiano, P., Arrizabalaga, J., Bidaurrazaga, J. J., & Gorostiza E. (2007). Prevalence of obesity in 4-18-year-old population in the Basque Country, Spain. *Obesity Reviews, 8*, 281–287.

Lasserre, A.M., Chiolero, A., Paccaud, F., & Bovet, P. (2007). Worldwide trends in childhood obesity. *Swiss Medical Weekly, 137*, 157–158.

Linardakis, M., Sarri, K., Pateraki, M.S., Sbokos, M., & Kafatos, A. (2008). Sugar-added beverages consumption among kindergarten children of Crete: effects on nutritional status and risk of obesity. *BMC, Public Health, 8*, 279.

Lioret, S., Maire, B., Volatier, J.L., & Charles, M.A. (2007). Child overweight in France and its relationship with physical activity, sedentary behaviour and socioeconomic status. *European Journal of Clinical Nutrition, 61*, 509–516.

Lissau, I., Overpeck, M.D., Ruan, W.J., Due, P., Holstein, B.E., & Hediger, M.L. (2004). Body mass index and overweight in adolescents in 13 European countries, Israel, and the United States. *Archives of Pediatrics & Adolescent Medicine, 158*, 27–33.

Lobstein, T., & Frelut, M.L. (2003). Prevalence of overweight among children in Europe. *Obesity Reviews, 4*, 195–200.

Lobstein, T., & Millstone, E. (2006). Policy options for responding to obesity: evaluating the options. Summary report of the EC-funded project to map the views of stakeholders involved in tackling obesity – the PorGrow project. *Brighton, University of Sussex, Science and Technology Policy Research (SPRU), NEST (New and emerging science and technology), DG Research, European Commission.*

Luciano, A., Livieri, C., Di Pietro, M.E., Bergamaschi, G., & Maffeis, C. (2003). Definition of obesity in childhood: criteria and limits. *Minerva Pediatrica, 55*, 453–459.

Magarey, A.M., Daniels, L.A., Boulton, T.J., & Cockington, R.A. (2003). Predicting obesity in early adulthood from childhood and parental obesity. *International Journal of Obesity Related Metabolic Disorders, 27*, 505–513.

Magkos, F., Manios, Y., Christakis, G., & Kafatos, A.G. (2006). Age-dependent changes in body size of Greek boys from 1982 to 2002. *Obesity (Silver Spring), 14*, 289–294.

Maillot, M., Darmon, N., Vieux, F., & Drewnowski, A. (2007). Low energy density and high nutritional quality are each associated with higher diet costs in French adults. *American Journal of Clinical Nutrition, 86*, 690–696.

Manios,Y., Yiannakouris, N., Papoutsakis, C., Moschonis, G., Magkos, F., Skenderi, K., & Zampelas, A. (2004). Behavioral and physiological indices related to BMI in a cohort of primary schoolchildren in Greece. *American Journal of Human Biology, 16*, 639–647.

Manios, Y., Magkos, F., Christakis, G., & Kafatos. A.G. (2005). Twenty-year dynamics in adiposity and blood lipids of Greek children: regional differences in Crete persist. *Acta Paediatrica, 94*, 859–865.

Manios, Y., Costarelli, V., Kolotourou, M., Kondakis, K., Tzavara, C., & Moschonis, G. (2007). Prevalence of obesity in preschool Greek children, in relation to parental characteristics and region of residence. *BMC Public Health, 7*, 178.

Matthews, A.E. (2008). Children and obesity: a pan-European project examining the role of food marketing. *European Journal of Public Health, 18*, 7–11.

Matusik, P., Malecka-Tendera, E., & Klimek, K. (2007). Nutritional state of Polish prepubertal children assessed by population-specific and international standards. *Acta Paediatrica, 96*, 276–280.

Mendoza, J.A., Drewnowski, A., Cheadle, A., & Christakis, D.A. (2006). Dietary energy density is associated with selected predictors of obesity in U.S. Children. *Journal of Nutrition, 136*, 1318–1322.

Monsivais, P., & Drewnowski, A. (2007). The rising cost of low-energy-density foods. *Journal of the American Dietetics Association, 107*, 2071–2076.

Monteiro, P.O., & Victora, C.G. (2005). Rapid growth in infancy and childhood and obesity in later life-a systematic review. *Obesity Reviews, 6*, 143–154.

Moreno, L.A., & Rodriguez, G. (2007). Dietary risk factors for development of childhood obesity. *Current Opinion in Clinical Nutrition and Metabolic Care, 10*, 336–341.

Moreno, L.A., Sarria, A., Fleta, J., Rodriguez, G., & Bueno, M. (2000). Trends in body mass index and overweight prevalence among children and adolescents in the region of Aragon (Spain) from 1985 to 1995. *International Journal of Obesity Related Metabolic Disorders, 24*, 925–931.

Moreno, L.A., Fleta, J., Sarria, A., Rodriguez, G., & Bueno, M. (2001a). Secular increases in body fat percentage in male children of Zaragoza, Spain, 1980-1995. *Preventive Medicine, 33*, 357–363.

Moreno, L.A., Fleta, J., Sarria, A., Rodriguez, G., Gil, C., & Bueno M. (2001b). Secular changes in body fat patterning in children and adolescents of Zaragoza (Spain), 1980-1995. *International Journal of Obesity Related Metabolic Disorders, 25*, 1656–1660.

Moreno, L.A., Sarria, A., Fleta, J., Rodriguez, G., Gonzalez, J.M., & Bueno, M. (2001c). Sociodemographic factors and trends on overweight prevalence in children and adolescents in Aragon (Spain) from 1985 to 1995. *Journal of Clinical Epidemiology, 54*, 921–927.

Moreno, L.A., Mesana, M.I., Fleta, J., Ruiz, J.R., Gonzalez-Gross, M., Sarria, A., Marcos, A., & Bueno, M. (2005a). Overweight, obesity and body fat composition in Spanish adolescents. The AVENA Study. *Annals of Nutrition and Metabolism, 49*, 71–76.

Moreno, L.A., Sarria A., Fleta, J., Marcos, A., & Bueno, M. (2005b). Secular trends in waist circumference in Spanish adolescents, 1995 to 2000-02. *Archives of Disease in Childhood, 90*, 818–819.

Moschonis, G., Grammatikaki, E., & Manios, Y. (2008). Perinatal predictors of overweight at infancy and preschool childhood: the GENESIS study. *International Journal of Obesity (Lond), 32*, 39–47.

Mutunga, M., Gallagher, A.M., Boreham, C., Watkins, D.C., Murray, L.J., Cran, G., & Reilly, J.J. (2006). Socioeconomic differences in risk factors for obesity in adolescents in Northern Ireland. *International Journal of Paediatric Obesity, 1*, 114–119.

Nieto, F.J., Szklo, M., & Comstock, G.W. (1992). Childhood weight and growth rate as predictors of adult mortality. *American Journal of Epidemiology, 136*, 201–213.

O'Neill, J.L., McCarthy, S.N., Burke, S.J., Hannon, E.M., Kiely, M., Flynn, A., Flynn, M.A., & Gibney, M.J. (2007). Prevalence of overweight and obesity in Irish school children, using four different definitions. *European Journal of Clinical Nutrition, 61*, 743–751.

Ogden, C.L., Kuczmarski, R.J., Flegal, K.M., Mei, Z., Guo, S., Wei, R., Grummer-Strawn, L.M., Curtin, L.R., Roche, A.F., & Johnson, C.L. (2002). Centers for Disease Control and Prevention 2000 growth charts for the United States: improvements to the 1977 National Center for Health Statistics version. *Pediatrics, 109*, 45–60.

Ong, K.K. (2006). Size at birth, postnatal growth and risk of obesity. *Hormones Research, 65(Suppl 3)*, 65–69.

Owen, C.G., Martin, R.M., Whincup, P.H., Smith, G.D., & Cook, D.G. (2005). Effect of infant feeding on the risk of obesity across the life course: a quantitative review of published evidence. *Paediatrics, 115*, 1367–1377.

Ozer, B.K. (2007). Growth reference centiles and secular changes in Turkish children and adolescents. *Economics & Human Biology, 5*, 280–301.

Padez, C., Fernandes, T., Mourao, I., Moreira, P., & Rosado, V. (2004). Prevalence of overweight and obesity in 7-9-year-old Portuguese children: trends in body mass index from 1970-2002. *American Journal of Human Biology, 16*, 670–678.

Papadimitriou, A., Kounadi, D., Konstantinidou, M., Xepapadaki, P., & Nicolaidou, P. (2006). Prevalence of obesity in elementary schoolchildren living in Northeast Attica, Greece. *Obesity (Silver Spring), 14*, 1113–1117.

Pardee, P.E., Norman, G.J., Lustig, R.H., Preud'homme, D., & Schwimmer, J.B. (2007). Television viewing and hypertension in obese children. *American Journal of Preventive Medicine, 33*, 439–443.

Parsons, T.J., Power, C., & Manor, O. (2003). Infant feeding and obesity through the lifecourse. *Archives of Diseases in Childhood, 88*, 793–794.

Pastucha, D., Malincikova, J., Hyjanek, J., Horakova, D., Cizek, L., Janoutova, G., & Janout, V.G. (2007). Obesity and insulin resistance in childhood. *Central of European Journal of Public Health, 15*, 103–105.

Popkin, B.M., Conde, W., Hou, N., & Monteiro, C. (2006). Is there a lag globally in overweight trends for children compared with adults? *Obesity (Silver Spring), 14*, 1846–1853.

Powell, A.D., & Kahn, A.S. (1995). Racial differences in women's desires to be thin. *International Journal of Eating Disorders, 17*, 191–195.

Prentice, A.M., & Jebb, S.A. (2003). Fast foods, energy density and obesity: a possible mechanistic link. *Obesity Reviews, 4*, 187–194.

Ramos, E., & Barros, H. (2007). Family and school determinants of overweight in 13-year-old Portuguese adolescents. *Acta Paediatrica, 96*, 281–286.

Rey-Lopez, J.P., Vicente-Rodriguez, G., Biosca, M., & Moreno, LA. (2008). Sedentary behaviour and obesity development in children and adolescents. *Nutrition, Metabolism & Cardiovascular Diseases, 18(3)*, 242–251.

Salmon, J., Ball, K., Hume, C., Booth, M., & Crawford, D. (2008). Outcomes of a group-randomized trial to prevent excess weight gain, reduce screen behaviours and promote physical activity in 10-year-old children: Switch-Play. *International Journal of Obesity (Lond), 32*, 601–612.

Samdal, O., Tynjala, J., Roberts, C., Sallis, J. F., Villberg, J., & Wold, B. (2007). Trends in vigorous physical activity and TV watching of adolescents from 1986 to 2002 in seven European Countries. *European Journal of Public Health, 17*, 242–248.

Savva, S.C., Kourides, Y., Tornaritis, M., Epiphaniou-Savva, M., Chadjigeorgiou, C., & Kafatos, A. (2002). Obesity in children and adolescents in Cyprus. Prevalence and predisposing factors. *International Journal of Obesity Related Metabolic Disorders, 26*, 1036–1045.

Savva, S.C., Tornaritis, M., Chadjigeorgiou, C., Kourides, Y.A., Savva, M.E., Panagi, A., Chrictodoulou, E., & Kafatos, A. (2005). Prevalence and socio-demographic associations of undernutrition and obesity among preschool children in Cyprus. *European Journal of Clinical Nutrition, 59*, 1259–1265.

Stamatakis, E., Primatesta, P., Chinn, S., Rona, R., & Falascheti, E. (2005). Overweight and obesity trends from 1974 to 2003 in English children: what is the role of socioeconomic factors? *Archives of Diseases in Childhood, 90*, 999–1004.

Stone, M.A., Bankart, J., Sinfield, P., Talbot, D., Farooqi, A., Davies, M.J., & Khunti, K. (2007). Dietary habits of young people attending secondary schools serving a multiethnic, inner-city community in the UK. *Postgraduate Medical Journal, 83*, 115–119.

Stunkard, A.J., & Sorensen, T.I. (1993). Obesity and socioeconomic status - a complex relation. *New England Journal of Medicine, 329*, 1036–1037.

Sundblom, E., Petzold, M., Rasmussen, F., Callmer, E., & Lissner, L. (2008). Childhood overweight and obesity prevalences levelling off in Stockholm but socioeconomic differences persist. *International Journal of Obesity (Lond), 32*, 1525–1530.

Sur, H., Kolotourou, M., Dimitriou, M., Kocaoglu, B., Keskin, Y., Hayran, O., & Manios, Y. (2005). Biochemical and behavioral indices related to BMI in schoolchildren in urban Turkey. *Preventive Medicine, 41*, 614–621.

Taveras, E.M., Scanlon, K.S., Birch, L., Rifas-Shiman, S.L., Rich-Edwards, J.W., & Gillman, M.W. (2004). Association of breastfeeding with maternal control of infant feeding at age 1 year. *Pediatrics, 114*, e577–e583.

Tounian, P. (2007). Consequences in adulthood of childhood obesity. *Archives in Pediatrics, 14*, 718–720.

Tutkuviene, J. (2007). Body mass index, prevalence of overweight and obesity in Lithuanian children and adolescents, 1985-2002. *College Anthropology, 31*, 109–121.

van den Hurk, K., van Dommelen, P., van Buuren, S., Verkerk, P.H., & Hirasing, R.A. (2007). Prevalence of overweight and obesity in the Netherlands in 2003 compared to 1980 and 1997. *Archives of Diseases in Childhood, 92*, 992–995.

Velluzzi, F., Lai, A., Secci, G., Mastinu, R., Pilleri, A., Cabula, R., Rizzolo, E., Cocco, P.L., Fadda, D., Binaghi, F., Mariotti, S., & Loviselli, A. (2007). Prevalence of overweight and obesity in Sardinian adolescents. *Eat & Weight Disorders, 12*, e44–e50.

Villa, I., Yngve, A., Poortvliet, E., Grjibovski, A., Liiv, K., Sjostrom, M., & Harro, M. (2007). Dietary intake among under-, normal- and overweight 9- and 15-year-old Estonian and Swedish schoolchildren. *Public Health Nutrition, 10*, 311–322.

Wan, N.J., Mi, J., Wang, T.Y., Duan, J.L., Li, M., Gong, C.X., Du, J.B., Zhao, X.Y., Cheng, H., Hou, D.Q., & Wang, L. (2007). Metabolic syndrome in overweight and obese schoolchildren in Beijing. (In Chinese) *Zhonghua Er Ke Za Zhi (Chinese Journal of Pediatrics), 45*, 417–421.

Wardle, J., Brodersen, N.H., Cole, T.J., Jarvis, M.J., & Boniface, D.R. (2006). Development of adiposity in adolescence: five year longitudinal study of an ethnically and socioeconomically diverse sample of young people in Britain. *British Medical Journal, 332*, 1130–1135.

Weaver, L.T. (2006). Rapid growth in infancy: balancing the interests of the child. *Journal of Paediatric Gastroenterology and Nutrition, 43*, 428–432.

Weyermann, M., Brenner, H., & Rothenbacher, D. (2007). Adipokines in human milk and risk of overweight in early childhood: a prospective cohort study. *Epidemiology, 18*, 722–729.

Whelton, H., Harrington, J., Crowley, E., Kelleher, V., Cronin, M., & Perry, I.J. (2007). Prevalence of overweight and obesity on the island of Ireland: results from the North South Survey of Children's Height, Weight and Body Mass Index, 2002. *BMC Public Health, 7*, 187.

Whitaker, R.C., & Orzol, S.M. (2006). Obesity among US urban preschool children: relationships to race, ethnicity, and socioeconomic status. *Archives of Pediatrics Adolescent Medicine, 160*, 578–584.

World Health Organization (2005). Core Health Indicators in the WHO European Region. Regional Office for Europe Scherfigsvej 8DK–2100 Copenhagen, Denmark.

WHO, ENHIS (2007). ENHIS, version 1.8 (21 October 2008); http://www.enhis.org/object_document/o4745n27385.html.

WHO Global InfoBase online [online database] (2007). Geneva, World Health Organization.

Will, B., Zeeb, H., & Baune, B.T. (2005). Overweight and obesity at school entry among migrant and German children: a cross-sectional study. *BMC Public Health, 5*, 45.

Wright, C.M., Parker, L., Lamont, D., & Craft, A.W. (2001). Implications of childhood obesity for adult health: findings from thousand families cohort study. *British Medical Journal, 323*, 1280–1284.

Wright, C., Lakshman, R., Emmett, P., & Ong, K. (2008). Implications of adopting the WHO 2006 Child Growth Standard in the UK: two prospective cohort studies. *Archives of Disease in Childhood, 93(7)*, 566–569.

Yngve, A., & Sjostrom, M. (2001). Breastfeeding in countries of the European Union and EFTA: current and proposed recommendations, rationale, prevalence, duration and trends. *Public Health Nutrition, 4*, 631–645.

Zeller, M., & Daniels, S. (2004). The obesity epidemic: family matters. *Journal of Paediatrics, 145*, 3–4.

Zimmermann, M.B., Hess, S.Y., & Hurrell, R.F. (2000). A national study of the prevalence of overweight and obesity in 6-12 y-old Swiss children: body mass index, body-weight perceptions and goals. *European Journal of Clinical Nutrition, 54*, 568–572.

Chapter 5
The Epidemiology of Childhood Obesity in Canada, Mexico and the United States

Cynthia L. Ogden, Sarah Connor Gorber, Juan A. Rivera Dommarco,
Margaret Carroll, Margot Shields, and Katherine Flegal

Introduction

Published reports based on different definitions indicate that in Canada, Mexico and the United States childhood overweight and obesity have increased dramatically since 1980, with the US leading the way. The prevalence of overweight, using the International Obesity Task Force (IOTF) definitions (Cole et al. 2000) in 7–13 year old girls doubled in Canada between 1981 and 1996 and tripled in boys (Tremblay et al. 2002). In 2004 in Canada, 26% of children and adolescents aged 2–17 were overweight or obese and 8% were obese (Shields 2006). Among children under 5 years of age in Mexico, overweight prevalence (z-score of weight-for-height above +2 of World Health Organization/ National Center for Health Statistics/Centers for Disease Control and Prevention (WHO/NCHS/CDC)

The findings and conclusions in this chapter are those of the authors and not necessarily those of the CDC.

C.L. Ogden(✉)
Division of Health and Nutrition Examination Surveys at National Center for Health Statistics, Centers for Disease Control and Prevention, Epidemiologis, CDC/NCHS, 3311 Toledo Road room 4414, Hyattsville, MD 20782, USA
e-mail: cogden@cdc.gov

S.C. Gorber
Scientific Research Manager, Public Health Agency of Canada/Agence de la santé publique du Canada, 7th Floor, Room 713B, AL 6807B 785 Carling Avenue Ottawa, Ontario K1A 0K9
e-mail: sarah.connor.gorber@phac-aspc.gc.ca

J.A.R. Dommarco
Centro de Investigacion en Nutricion Y Salud, Instituto Nacional de Salud Publica, Av. Universidad 655, Col. Sta. Maria Ahuacatitlan, Cuernavaca, Morelos C.P. 62563, Mexico
e-mail: jrivera@correo.insp.mx

M. Carroll
National Center for Health Statistics, Centers for Disease Control and Prevention, 3311 Toledo Road, Hyattsville, MD 20782
Mcarroll@cdc.gov

M. Shields
Senior Analyst/Analyste Principale, Health Analysis/Analyse de la santé, R.H. Coats Building Immeuble R.-H.-Coats/Floor Étage 24 C, Statistics Canada 100 Tunney's Pasture Driveway, Ottawa ON K1A 0T6, Statistique Canada 100, Promenade Tunney's Pasture, Ottawa ON K1A 0T6,
e-mail: Margot.Shields@statcan.gc.ca

K. Flegal
Senior Research Scientist/Distinguished Consultant, National Center for Health Statistics, Centers for Disease Control and Prevention, 3311 Toledo Road, Hyattsville, MD 20782
e-mail:Kflegal@cdc.gov

L.A. Moreno et al. (eds.), *Epidemiology of Obesity in Children and Adolescents*,
Springer Series on Epidemiology and Public Health 2, DOI 10.1007/978-1-4419-6039-9_5,
© Springer Science+Business Media, LLC 2011

references (Dibley et al. 1987)) increased from 4.2 to 5.3% between 1988 and 1999 (Rivera et al. 2002). In the US, between 1980 and 2006 the prevalence of high body mass index (BMI ≥95th percentile of the sex specific 2000 CDC growth charts) increased from 6 to 16% among children and teens 2 through 19 years of age (Ogden et al. 2002, 2003, 2007, 2008).

This chapter provides an overview of childhood obesity in Canada, Mexico and the United States. Nationally representative surveys contribute comparable information on prevalence, trends, and risk factors related to childhood obesity in each country.

Geographic and Socio-Economic Characteristics

In 2007, the North American continent had a population of almost 440 million people and a surface area of 21,581,100 km^2. The largest country in terms of area and the smallest in terms of population is Canada with a surface area of 9,984,700 km^2 and a population of approximately 33 million people. Mexico has the smallest surface area at 1,964,400 km^2 with a population of over 105 million and the US's area is 9,632,000 km^2 with a population of almost 301 million. The per capita gross domestic product (GDP) in Canada was $43,368 in 2007. In Mexico it was only $8,385 and in the United States it was $45,046. In the same year, life expectancy in Canada was 81 years while in Mexico it was 75 years and in the US it was 78 years. Infant mortality was lowest in Canada at 4.8 deaths per 1,000 live births, followed by the US at 6.3 deaths per 1,000 live births and Mexico at 16.7 deaths per 1,000 live births (UN Statistics 2009; World and Statistics 2009).

Definitions and Measurement of Overweight and Obesity

The definition of excess body fat or adiposity is not clear-cut and body fat is difficult to measure directly. Consequently, obesity is often defined as excess body weight rather than as excess fat. In epidemiologic studies, body mass index (BMI) calculated as weight in kilograms divided by height in meters squared is used to express weight adjusted for height (Dietz and Robinson 1998; Krebs et al. 2007).

Measured weight and height are more accurate than self-reported data. Cost considerations, however, often lead to surveys and epidemiologic studies not being conducted in-person, so that height and weight are self-reported rather than measured. Inaccurate estimates may result because respondents tend to overestimate their heights and underestimate their weights. Or, in the case of children, parents often do not know their child's measurements or under-estimate their child's height (Connor Gorber et al. 2007; Davis and Gergen 1994; Kuczmarski et al. 2001; Perry et al. 1995; Rowland 1990).

In children, the terminology for different levels of weight or BMI varies considerably (Flegal et al. 2006). The terms overweight, obesity and at risk for overweight can be found in the literature. Even when the same term is used (e.g. "overweight") the meaning of that term may not be the same in different countries or across studies. Whatever the terminology used, definitions are generally based on weight and not on adiposity per se. In children, it is unclear what risk-related criteria to use to determine risk-based definitions of overweight or obesity. As a result, statistical definitions based on the 85th and 95th percentiles of sex specific BMI-for-age in a specified reference population are often used in childhood (Barlow and Dietz 1998; Himes and Dietz 1994; Krebs et al. 2007).

Many reference data sets for childhood BMI exist and BMI reference data are used or recommended as part of monitoring of children's growth in many countries (Cole et al. 1998). Reference data are usually based on representative data from a given country, although the World Health Organization charts (for those under 5 years of age) are based on a different approach. They were created from healthy, breastfed children from around the world and are intended to present a standard of physiologic growth and not a descriptive reference (WHO 2006). In this chapter, the CDC 2000 growth charts (Kuczmarski et al. 2002), developed from five US nationally representative surveys (the National Health Examination Surveys II and III in the 1960s, the National Health and Nutrition Examination Surveys (NHANES) I and II in the 1970s, and, for children under 6 years, NHANES III, 1988–1994), were used to define high BMI. These charts represent a revision of the 1977 NCHS growth charts (Hamill et al. 1977).

The choice of cut-off points within the reference population depends upon what assumptions are made. Expert committees in the United States have recommended using a BMI-for-age at or above the 95th percentile of a specified reference population to screen for "overweight" (Barlow and Dietz 1998; Himes and Dietz 1994) and, more recently, have recommended that this cut-off be labeled "obesity" (Krebs et al. 2007) in adolescents and younger children. Similarly, children with BMI values between the 85th and 95th percentiles were considered "at risk for overweight" but, more recently have been labeled "overweight" by expert committees. In this chapter, we focus on one level of high BMI; at or above the 95th percentile on the 2000 CDC growth charts. Throughout the text "high BMI" refers to BMI-for-age ≥95th percentile of the sex specific CDC growth charts consequently, all estimates from Canada, Mexico, and the US in the text are comparable to each other. Some tables and figures do include estimates of the prevalence of BMI-for-age between the 85th and 95th percentiles.

Prevalence and Trends

Prevalence estimates of high BMI-for-age are usually derived from surveys or population studies because systematic data cannot generally be gathered from medical records or vital statistics. Virtually all data on prevalence and trends are based on measurements of weight and height using the classifications described above rather than on body fat due to the logistical difficulties involved in making measurements of body fat in population studies.

In Canada, national survey data with measured heights and weights for children 2–19 years of age are currently available from two surveys: the 1978/1979 Canada Health Survey (CHS) and the 2004 Canadian Community Health Survey (CCHS). The CHS was one of Canada's first national surveys on the health status of its population and collected detailed assessments of physical health (Health and Welfare Canada, Statistics Canada 1981). The CCHS is designed to provide timely cross-sectional estimates of health determinants, health status and health system utilization in Canada and has been conducted on an ongoing basis since 2001. The household survey usually collects only self-reported information, however, in 2004 physical measures of height and weight were collected for all respondents as part of the survey's focus on nutritional status (Statistics Canada 2005). Both surveys were designed to provide nationally representative data using a stratified multistage cluster sampling design. In the CHS, nurses collected the height and weight measurements, while in the CCHS measures were collected by trained interviewers. In both surveys, measurements were collected in the home for children aged 2 years old and over. Recently the Canadian Health Measures Survey, modeled on the US NHANES, was launched to provide nationally representative direct physical measures data including anthropometry as well as blood and urine sampling. Data from this survey will be available in 2010 (Statistics Canada 2005) and will significantly improve Canada's ability to estimate trends in high BMI over time and across population sub-groups.

Table 5.1 shows the prevalence of high BMI in children and adolescents aged 2–19 years in Canada for 1978/1979 and 2004. There have been increases in high BMI in all age groups for girls and for boys aged 6–19 years old. Overall, for children aged 2–19 years, the prevalence of high BMI has more than doubled in Canada, from 6% in 1978/1979 to 12.3% in 2004. Approximately 14% of 2–5 year olds had BMI's greater than or equal to the 95th percentile on the CDC growth charts in 2004, while for 6–11 year olds and teens 12% were at or above this cut-point.

Data on high BMI among Mexican children are available from three national surveys conducted by the Secretary of Health in 1988 and the Mexican National Institute of Public Health in 1999 and 2006 (Olaiz et al. 2006; Resano-Pérez et al. 2003; Sepúlveda et al. 1990). The National Nutrition

Table 5.1 Prevalence and trends of high body mass index (BMI)-for-age[a] among children, aged 2–19 years, Canada excluding territories, 1978/1979[b] and 2004[c]

Survey	2–19 years				2–5 years				6–11 years				12–19 years			
	85th≤BMI <95th		BMI≥95th		85th≤BMI <95th		BMI≥95th		85th≤BMI <95th		BMI≥95th		85th≤BMI <95th		BMI≥95th	
Sex	Percent	SE	Percent	SE	Percent	SE	Percent	SE	Percent	SE	Percent	SE	Percent	SE	Percent	SE
All																
1978/1979[b]	10.9	0.8	6.0	0.7	17.8	1.9	13.3	2.0	11.0	1.5	5.3[d]	1.5	8.1[d]	1.4	3.6[d]	0.8
2004[c]	15.7*	0.7	12.3*	0.5	16.5	1.6	13.7	1.3	15.5*	1.0	12.4*	1.0	15.6*	1.0	11.7*	0.7
Boys																
1978/1979[b]	12.5	1.4	6.9	1.0	21.5	3.4	18.1	2.7	14.1	2.3	3.6[d]	1.2	7.9	1.1	[e]	
2004[c]	15.7	0.9	13.8*	0.9	16.0	2.1	15.0	1.9	15.4	1.4	13.8*	1.6	15.7*	1.3	13.3*	1.2
Girls																
1978/1979[b]	9.2	1.5	5.0[d]	1.1	13.7[d]	4.6			7.9[d]	2.2			8.4[d]	2.3	2.9[d]	0.7
2004[c]	15.8*	0.9	10.8*	0.7	17.0	2.3	12.4[e]	1.7	15.6*	1.4	11.0[e]	1.3	15.5*	1.3	10.0*	1.1

*Significantly different from estimate for 1978/1979

[a]85th percentile ≤ BMI-for-age <95th percentile; BMI-for-age ≥ 95th percentile. BMI (body mass index) is weight in kilogram divided by height and meters squared. The 85th and 95th percentiles are based on the 2000 CDC growth charts and represent the revised version of the 1977 NCHS growth charts

[b]1978/1979 Canada Health Survey

[c]2004 Canadian Community Health Survey: Nutrition

[d]Use with caution (coefficient of variation between 16.6 and 33.3%)

[e]Too unreliable to be published (coefficient of variation greater than 33.3%)

Note: SE standard error

Survey in 1988, the National Nutrition Survey in 1999 and the National Health and Nutrition Survey in 2006 were national, cross-sectional, multi-stage, stratified and representative surveys of the country. The 1988 survey included boys and girls under 5 years of age and teenage girls while the 1999 survey included boys and girls under 12 years of age and teenage girls. In 2006, all children and teens under age 20 years were sampled. The surveys included measurements of weight and height.

Table 5.2 shows the prevalence of high BMI in 1988, 1999 and 2006. Significant increases have occurred for both boys and girls between 1999 and 2006. Among school-age children 6–11 years of age 8.9% were at or above the 95th percentile of BMI-for-age in 1999 while in 2006 15% were at this level. The prevalence among teenage girls rose from 5.6 to 10.1% over the same period.

In the US, the NHANES program provides national estimates of high BMI-for-age for adolescents and children. A series of cross-sectional, nationally representative examination surveys conducted by the National Center for Health Statistics of the CDC, the NHANES surveys were designed using stratified multistage probability samples (CDC 2009). The program began in the 1960s and was periodically conducted until 1999 when it became a continuous survey. Currently, NHANES includes over sampling of Mexican Americans and African Americans, among other groups, in order to improve estimates for these groups. All of the surveys included a standardized physical examination in a mobile examination center with measurement of stature and weight in children 2 years and older (National Center for Health Statistics 1994; McDowell et al. 1981; Miller 1973).

Estimates of the prevalence of high BMI in the US for children and adolescents between the early 1960s and 2006 are shown in Table 5.3. After little change was seen in the 1960s and 1970s there was an increase between NHANES II and NHANES III and a further increase between NHANES III and NHANES 1999–2000. Between 1999–2000 and 2005–2006, however, there was no significant trend (Ogden et al. 2008). As seen in Table 5.3, there was a significant trend ($P < 0.05$) for the entire time period (1960s–2006). In 2005–2006 over 17% of teens (12–19 years of age) were at or above the 95th percentile on the BMI-for-age growth charts while 15.1% of 6–11 and 11.0% of 2–5 year olds were at or above the same cut-point.

Figure 5.1 shows the prevalence of high BMI for Canada, Mexico and the US together. The most recent prevalence of high BMI among girls, but not boys, was significantly higher in the US compared to Mexico although no significant differences were found in the prevalence of high BMI between Canada and the US for the total population, boys or girls.

Distribution of Body Mass Index

Changes in the prevalence of high BMI do not present a complete picture of the trends in BMI. A more complete picture can be seen in the smoothed distributions of BMI between two time periods. In Canada this is depicted with data for adolescents aged 12–19 year olds for 1978/1979 and 2004. The mean BMI rose from 21.0 to 22.6 kg/m^2 between these two time periods resulting in a shift in the BMI distribution toward higher BMIs (Fig. 5.2). This trend was most pronounced for those with BMIs at or higher than 25 or 30 kg/m^2, which corresponds to the cut-points used to classify adults as overweight or obese. For Mexico the picture is shown separately for 12–19 year old teen girls (Fig. 5.3), 6–11 year old children (Fig. 5.4) and 2–5 year old children (Fig. 5.5). A dramatic shift to the right can be seen among teen girls between 1988 and 2006. To a lesser extent a shift occurred among 6–11 year old children while among 2–5 year old children there has been a much smaller change in the distribution. For the US this picture is shown using data in 1976–1980 and 2003–2006 for teens 12–19 years of age. The distribution of BMI between NHANES II (1976–1980) and NHANES 2003–2006 has shifted to the right (Fig. 5.6), but the shift is greater at the upper percentiles of the distribution, indicating that the distribution has become more skewed and the heaviest individuals have gotten even heavier.

Table 5.2 Prevalence and trends of high body mass index (BMI)-for-age[a] among children, aged 2–19 years, Mexico, 1988[b], 1999[c] and 2006[d]

Survey	2–19 years				2–5 years				6–11 years				12–19 years			
	85th ≤ BMI <95th		BMI ≥95th		85th ≤ BMI <95th		BMI ≥95th		85th ≤ BMI <95th		BMI ≥95th		85th ≤ BMI <95th		BMI ≥95th	
Sex	Percent	SE	Percent	SE	Percent	SE	Percent	SE	Percent	SE	Percent	SE	Percent	SE	Percent	SE
All																
1988[e]	–	–	–	–	11.5	0.6	10.4	0.8	–	–	–	–	–	–	–	–
1999	–	–	–	–	16.8	0.6	10.6	0.5	12.5	0.5	8.9	0.4	16.6	0.5	11.5	0.5
2006	15.4	0.3	12.4	0.4	13.6*	0.7	11.0	0.6	15.0*	0.6	14.6*	0.5	14.8	0.7	12.9	0.9
Boys																
1988[e]	–	–	–	–	12.1	0.9	10.9	0.9	–	–	–	–	–	–	–	–
1999	–	–	–	–	16.2	0.8	11.3	0.7	12.6	0.7	9.3	0.6	–	–	–	–
2006	14.4	0.4	14.0	0.5	13.0*	0.8	12.3	0.9	14.8*	0.8	16.6*	0.7	14.8	0.7	12.9	0.9
Girls																
1988[e]	–	–	–	–	10.8	0.8	10.0	1.3	–	–	–	–	6.8	0.4	2.3	0.3
1999	15.6	0.4	7.7	0.3	17.5	0.9	9.9	0.7	12.4	0.7	8.6	0.6	17.2	0.7	5.6	0.5
2006	16.4	0.5	10.9*	0.4	14.2*	1.1	9.6	0.8	15.1*	0.7	12.7*	0.8	18.3	0.7	10.1*	0.6

*Significantly different (P<0.05) from estimate for 1999

[a]85th percentile ≤ BMI-for-age <95th percentile; BMI-for-age ≥95th percentile. BMI (body mass index) is weight in kilogram divided by height and meters squared. The 85th and 95th percentiles are based on the 2000 CDC growth charts and represent the revised version of the 1977 NCHS growth charts

[b]Mexican National Nutrition Survey 1988 (ages <5 years and teenage girls)

[c]Mexican National Nutrition Survey 1999 (ages <12 years and teenage girls)

[d]Mexican National Health and Nutrition Survey 2006 (ages <20 years)

[e]For pre-school children the group is 2–4 years of ages

Note: SE standard error

Table 5.3 Prevalence and trends* of high body mass index (BMI)-for-age[a] among children, age 2–19 years, United States, 1960–2006

Survey[b]	2–19 years				2–5 years				6–11 years				12–19 years			
	85th≤BMI<95th		BMI≥95th		85th≤BMI<95th		BMI≥95th		85th≤BMI<95th		BMI≥95th		85th≤BMI<95th		BMI≥95th	
	Percent	SE	Percent	SE	Percent	SE	Percent	SE	Percent	SE	Percent	SE	Percent	SE	Percent	SE
All																
1963–1965									8.8	0.4	4.3	0.4	9.7	0.4	4.6	0.3
1966–1970[c]																
1971–1974	10.4	0.6	5.1	0.3	10.9	1.1	4.8	0.6	10.0	0.8	4.0	0.5	10.5	0.8	6.1	0.6
1976–1980	9.2	0.4	5.5	0.4	9.2	0.5	5.0	0.6	9.0	0.9	6.5	0.7	9.2	0.6	5.0	0.5
1988–1994	13.0	0.7	10.0	0.5	10.9	0.6	7.2	0.7	13.5	1.0	11.3	1.0	13.8	1.1	10.5	0.9
1999–2000	14.3	0.9	13.9	0.9	11.7	1.2	10.3	1.7	14.7	2.0	15.1	1.4	15.2	1.2	14.8	0.9
2001–2002	14.6	0.6	15.4	0.9	12.8	1.3	10.6	1.8	15.9	1.0	16.3	1.6	14.4	1.0	16.7	1.1
2003–2004	16.5	0.8	17.1	1.3	12.3	1.4	14.0	1.6	18.5	1.4	18.8	1.3	17.0	1.4	17.4	1.7
2005–2006	14.6	0.9	15.5	1.3	11.6	1.7	11.0	1.2	14.3	1.8	15.1	2.1	16.2	1.0	17.8	1.8
Boys																
1963–1965									8.3	0.6	4.0	0.4	9.4	0.6	4.5	0.4
1966–1970[c]																
1971–1974	10.5	0.8	5.2	0.5	12.3	1.3	4.9	0.8	10.6	1.3	4.3	0.8	9.7	1.2	6.0	0.8
1976–1980	9.4	0.6	5.4	0.4	8.2	0.7	4.6	0.6	9.7	1.1	6.7	0.8	9.5	1.0	4.8	0.5
1988–1994	12.6	0.9	10.2	0.7	10.7	1.0	6.2	0.8	13.7	1.5	11.6	1.3	12.7	1.4	11.3	1.3
1999–2000	15.0	1.9	14.0	1.2	12.5	2.2	9.5	2.3	16.2	3.2	15.8	1.8	15.2	1.6	14.8	1.3
2001–2002	14.2	0.6	16.4	1.0	13.5	1.6	10.7	2.4	15.1	1.4	17.5	1.9	13.9	1.7	17.6	1.3
2003–2004	16.6	1.0	18.2	1.5	12.2	2.3	15.1	1.7	16.6	1.8	19.9	2.0	18.5	1.5	18.2	1.9
2005–2006	14.7	1.2	15.9	1.5	13.3	2.6	10.5	1.7	15.2	2.2	16.2	2.5	14.9	1.4	18.2	2.4
Girls																
1963–1965									9.3	0.5	4.5	0.6	10.1	0.6	4.7	0.3
1966–1970[c]																
1971–1974	10.2	0.8	5.0	0.4	9.4	1.2	4.8	0.8	9.3	1.2	3.6	0.6	11.2	1.3	6.2	0.8
1976–1980	9.0	0.6	5.7	0.6	10.3	0.9	5.4	1.0	8.2	1.3	6.4	1.0	9.0	0.8	5.3	0.8
1988–1994	13.4	0.9	9.8	0.8	11.0	0.9	8.2	1.0	13.2	1.5	11.0	1.4	15.0	1.6	9.7	1.1
1999–2000	13.6	0.8	13.8	1.1	11.0	1.8	11.2	2.5	13.1	1.6	14.3	2.1	15.2	1.9	14.8	1.0
2001–2002	15.0	0.9	14.3	1.3	12.3	1.8	10.5	1.8	16.7	1.7	14.9	2.4	14.9	1.2	15.7	1.9

Table 5.3 (continued)

Survey[b]	2–19 years				2–5 years				6–11 years				12–19 years			
	85th ≤ BMI <95th		BMI ≥95th		85th ≤ BMI <95th		BMI ≥95th		85th ≤ BMI <95th		BMI ≥95th		85th ≤ BMI <95th		BMI ≥95th	
	Percent	SE	Percent	SE	Percent	SE	Percent	SE	Percent	SE	Percent	SE	Percent	SE	Percent	SE
2003–2004	16.5	0.9	16.0	1.4	12.5	1.8	12.8	2.5	20.4	2.5	17.6	1.3	15.3	1.9	16.4	2.3
2005–2006	14.5	0.9	15.0	1.5	9.8	1.6	11.5	1.2	13.3	2.1	14.1	2.4	17.6	1.4	17.3	2.1

*Significant increasing trend for all trends (total, boys, girls at each BMI level) (P<0.05)

[a]85th percentile ≤ BMI-for-age <95th percentile; BMI-for-age ≥95th percentile. BMI (body mass index) is weight in kilogram divided by height and meters squared. The 85th and 95th percentiles are based on the 2000 CDC growth charts and represent the revised version of the 1977 NCHS growth charts

[b]US National Health Examination Survey (1963–1965; 1966–1970); National Health and Nutrition Examination Survey (I, 1971–1974; II, 1976–1980; III, 1988–1994; 1999–2000; 2001–2002; 2003–2004; 2005–2006)

[c]1966–1970: 12–17 years

Note: *SE* standard error

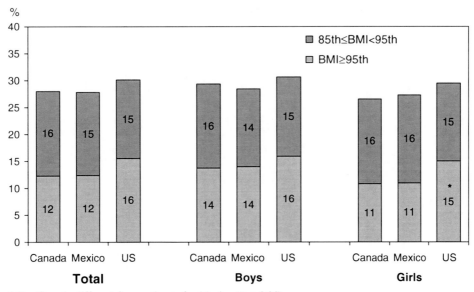

* Significantly different from estimate for Mexico ($P < 0.05$)

Fig. 5.1 Prevalence of high body mass index (BMI)-for-age among children aged 2–19 years, Canada (2004), Mexico (2006) and United States (2005–2006). *Sources*: 2004 Canadian Community Health Survey: Nutrition; Mexican National Health and Nutrition Survey 2006; US National Health and Nutrition Examination Survey 2005–2006

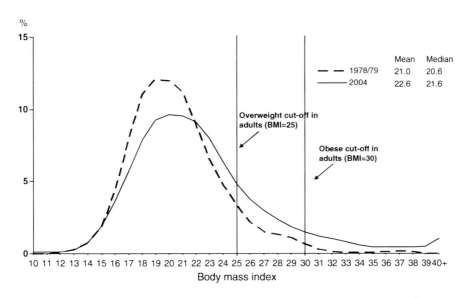

Fig. 5.2 Percentage distribution of children aged 12–19 years, by body mass index (BMI), Canada excluding territories, 1978/1979 and 2004. *Sources*: 2004 Canadian Community Health Survey: Nutrition; 1978/1979 Canada Health Survey

Socio-Demographic Differences

Although high BMI is a problem for the general population, some sub-groups of the population experience a greater prevalence than other groups. Prevalence estimates may vary by race/ethnic group, sex, age group, income, and/or education level. Moreover, the classifications used to define race/ethnic groups, income or education levels may vary between countries. The results shown below reflect the usual sub-group classifications made in Canada, Mexico and the US.

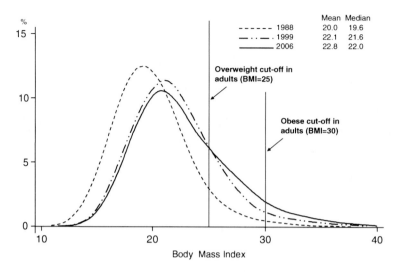

Fig. 5.3 Percentage distribution of girls aged 12–19 years, by body mass index (BMI), Mexico, 1988, 1999 and 2006. *Sources*: 1988 Mexican National Nutrition Survey; 1999 Mexican National Nutrition Survey; 2006 Mexican National Health and Nutrition Survey

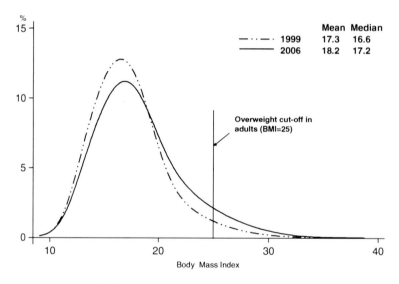

Fig. 5.4 Percentage distribution of children aged 6–11 years, by body mass index (BMI), Mexico, 1999 and 2006. *Sources*: 1999 Mexican National Nutrition Survey; 2006 Mexican National Health and Nutrition Survey

Race/Ethnicity

In the Canadian data, race and ethnicity were classified into four groups including: Whites, Blacks, Off-reserve Aboriginal children (North American Indian, Métis or Inuit), and Southeast/East Asians, with an "Other" category to capture the remainder of the population. Off-reserve Aboriginal children and youth were the most likely to have high BMI, with 25% being at or above the 95th percentile of BMI-for-age (Table 5.4). These numbers were significantly higher than the overall prevalence estimates for the total population (12% at or above the 95th percentile). The CCHS does not sample Aboriginal children living on reserves so no estimates are available for this group.

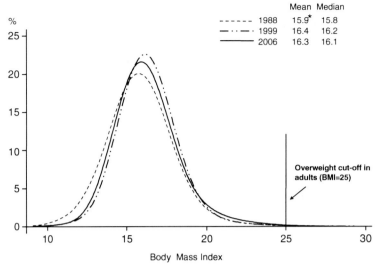

* Two to four age group only

Fig. 5.5 Percentage distribution of children aged 2–5 years, by body mass index (BMI), Mexico, 1988, 1999 and 2006. *Sources*: 1988 Mexican National Nutrition Survey; 1999 Mexican National Nutrition Survey; 2006 Mexican National Health and Nutrition Survey

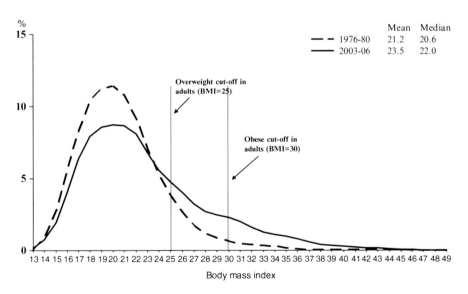

Fig. 5.6 Percentage distribution of adolescents ages 12–19 years, by body mass index (BMI), US, 1976–1980 and 2003–2006. *Sources*: US National Health and Nutrition Examination Survey II 1976–1980; US National Health and Nutrition Examination Survey 2003–2006

For Mexico, ethnic differences based on non-indigenous and indigenous classifications are shown in Table 5.5. Indigenous is defined as anyone living in a household where at least one person speaks an indigenous language. The prevalence is significantly higher among the non-indigenous children compared to the indigenous children. More than 13% of non-indigenous children and teens 2–19 years of age were at or above the 95th percentile of BMI-for-age in 2006 compared to 7.2% of indigenous children and teens.

Table 5.4 Prevalence of high body mass index (BMI)-for-age[a] among children aged 2–19 years by race/ethnicity, Canada excluding territories, 2004[b]

Race/ethnicity	n	BMI≥85th		85th≤BMI <95th		BMI≥95th	
		Percent	SE	Percent	SE	Percent	SE
Total	9,539	28	0.8	15.7	0.7	12.3	0.5
White	8,108	28.6	0.9	16.1	0.7	12.5	0.6
Black	135	33.8[c]	0.6	16.4[c]	4.4	17.4[c]	4.9
Southeast/East Asian	359	16.7*,[c]	2.7	7.8*,[c]	1.8	8.9[c]	0.2
Off-reserve Aboriginal	290	42.8*	5.5	17.5[c]	3.9	25.3*,[c]	4.6
Other	646	26.5	2.6	17.1	2.2	9.4	1.5

*Significantly different from estimate for total ($P<0.05$)
[a] BMI-for-age ≥85th percentile; 85th percentile ≤ BMI-for-age <95th percentile; BMI-for-age ≥95th percentile. BMI (body mass index) is weight in kilogram divided by height and meters squared. The 85th and 95th percentiles are based on the 2000 CDC growth charts and represent the revised version of the 1977 NCHS growth charts
[b] 2004 Canadian Community Health Survey: Nutrition
[c] Use with caution (coefficient of variation between 16.6 and 33.3%)

In 2003–2006, there were large disparities by race-ethnicity in the US (Table 5.6). Among girls, non-Hispanic Blacks were significantly more likely to have high BMI compared to non-Hispanic Whites and the prevalence of high BMI was significantly higher in Mexican American girls 6–11 years than in non-Hispanic White girls of the same age group. Among boys, Mexican Americans were more likely to have high BMI compared to non-Hispanic White boys.

A comparison between the majority populations (White) in Canada and the US shows an insignificant difference in prevalence of high BMI among children and teens 2–19 years of age. In Canada, 12.5% (SE=0.6) had high BMI compared to 14.7% (SE=1.3) in the US. A comparison between the prevalence of high BMI in Mexico among the non-indigenous majority group with that among Mexican Americans (a minority group) in the US, however, shows a significant difference ($P<0.05$). In Mexico 13.1% (SE=0.4) of 2–19 years old had a high BMI while 20.9% (SE=1.3) of Mexican American children in the US were above the same cut-point.

Sex and Age

Demographic differences in prevalence of high BMI can be seen in the most recent data from Mexico and the US. In Mexico in 2006, the prevalence of high BMI was significantly higher among boys than girls 2–19 years of age ($P<0.0001$) (Table 5.5). This was true for 2–5 year old children, 6–11 year old children and 12–19 year old teens. In the US in 2003–2006, the prevalence of high BMI increased with age (Table 5.6). The highest prevalence was among school-age children and adolescents; 12.5% of pre-school age children 2–5 years, 17.0% of school-age children 6–11 years and 17.6% of adolescents 12–19 years were at or above the 95th percentile of BMI-for-age in 2003–2006. Unlike in the US, in Canada in 2004 (Table 5.1) and in Mexico (Table 5.5) the differences across age groups for either sex were not significant.

Socio-Economic Status

Body size is often associated with socio-economic status. However, the magnitude and the direction of the association tend to differ by level of economic development, sex and race/ethnicity

Table 5.5 Prevalence of high body mass index (BMI)-for-age[a] among children age 2–19 years by age and ethnicity, Mexico, 2006[b]

| Sex | Age (years) | Total | | | Ethnicity | | | | | |
| | | | | | Non-Indigenous | | | Indigenous | | |
		n	Percent	SE	n	Percent	SE	n	Percent	SE
All	2–19	34,832	12.4	0.4	30,809	13.1*	0.4	4,023	7.2	0.7
	2–5	7,126	11.0	0.6	6,321	11.0	0.6	805	10.6[c]	2.4
	6–11	13,132	14.6	0.5	11,503	15.6*	0.6	1,629	7.5	1.1
	12–19	14,574	11.5	0.5	12,985	12.3*	0.6	1,589	5.3	0.7
Boys	2–19	17,290	14.0	0.5	15,331	14.7*	0.6	1,959	8.3	1.0
	2–5	3,621	12.3	0.9	3,224	12.4	0.9	397	11.8[c]	2.7
	6–11	6,575	16.6	0.7	5,768	17.6*	0.8	807	9.3[c]	1.8
	12–19	7,094	12.9	0.9	6,339	13.8*	1.0	755	5.8[c]	1.1
Girls	2–19	17,542	10.9	0.4	15,478	11.5*	0.5	2,064	6.1[c]	1.0
	2–5	3,505	9.6	0.8	3,097	9.7	0.7	408	[d]	
	6–11	6,557	12.7	0.8	5,735	13.7*	0.9	822	5.9[c]	1.0
	12–19	7,480	10.1	0.6	6,646	10.8*	0.7	834	4.7[c]	0.9

*Significantly different from estimate for Non-Indigenous versus Indigenous groups

[a] BMI-for-age ≥95th percentile. BMI (body mass index) is weight in kilogram divided by height and meters squared. The 95th percentile is based on the 2000 CDC growth charts and represent the revised version of the 1977 NCHS growth charts

[b] Mexican National Health and Nutrition Survey 2006

[c] Use with caution (coefficient of variation between 16.6 and 33.3%)

[d] Too unreliable to be published (coefficient of variation greater than 33.3%)

Table 5.6 Prevalence of high body mass index (BMI)-for-age[a] among children age 2–19 years by age and race/ethnicity, US, 2003–2006[b]

Sex	Age (years)	Total			Race-ethnicity								
					Non-Hispanic White			Non-Hispanic Black			Mexican American		
		n	Percent	SE	n	Percent	SE	n	Percent	SE	n	Percent	SE
All	2–19	8,168	16.3	0.9	2,195	14.7	1.3	2,696	20.7	1.0	2,583	20.9	1.3
	2–5	1,771	12.5	1.0	498	10.8	1.6	517	14.9	1.3	558	16.7	2.3
	6–11	2,096	17.0	1.3	558	15.0	1.9	673	21.3	1.8	671	23.7	2.0
	12–19	4,301	17.6	1.2	1,139	16.0	1.7	1,506	22.9	1.1	1,354	21.1	1.4
Boys	2–19	4,118	17.0	1.1	1,113	15.6	1.5	1,397	17.4	1.0	1,279	23.2	1.6
	2–5	875	12.8	1.2	260	11.1	2.2	254	13.3	2.5	269	18.8	2.8
	6–11	1,013	18.0	1.7	265	15.5	2.8	335	18.6	2.6	321	27.5*	2.1
	12–19	2,230	18.2	1.5	588	17.3	2.0	808	18.4	1.3	689	22.1	2.2
Girls	2–19	4,050	15.5	1.1	1,082	13.7	1.4	1,299	24.1	1.3	1,304	18.4	1.5
	2–5	896	12.2	1.4	238	10.4	2.0	263	16.6	2.3	289	14.5	2.7
	6–11	1,083	15.8	1.4	293	14.4	2.1	338	24.0*	2.0	350	19.7	2.6
	12–19	2,071	16.8	1.5	551	14.5	2.0	698	27.7*	1.9	665	19.9*	1.4

* Significantly different from estimate for non-Hispanic Whites ($P < 0.05$) with Bonferroni correction

[a] BMI-for-age ≥95th percentile. BMI (body mass index) is weight in kilogram divided by height and meters squared. The 95th percentile is based on the 2000 CDC growth charts and represent the revised version of the 1977 NCHS growth charts

[b] National Health and Nutrition Examination Survey 2003–2006

(Cassidy 1991; Chang and Lauderdale 2005; Sobal and Stunkard 1989). In less developed countries, higher weight may be associated with wealth and prosperity, and there may be a positive association between socio-economic status and body size for both men and women. Historically in many contexts, greater body size, including tallness, increased muscularity and increased fatness, has symbolized power, dominance, wealth or high social standing. For men in developed countries, height is positively associated with socio-economic status but weight and BMI tend to be weakly, if at all, associated with socio-economic status. For women in developed countries, however, weight and BMI have a strong inverse association with socio-economic status. The slender body that in the past might have reflected economic deprivation, limited access to food, or the necessity for hard physical labor now may require expenditures of time, money and effort to achieve. The finding in several studies that obesity is negatively predictive of subsequent education and earnings for women but not for men may reflect the stronger association between obesity and low socio-economic status at baseline for women than for men (Gortmaker et al. 1993; Sargent and Blanchflower 1994). The relationship between socio-economic status and weight in children is less well studied and less consistent.

The prevalence of high BMI according to household income quintiles for Canadian children and youth 2–19 years of age is provided in Fig. 5.7. Household income quintiles were derived by dividing total household income from all sources in the previous 12 months by Statistics Canada's Low Income Cut-Off (LICO) specific to the number of people in the household and the size of the community. This provides, for each respondent, a relative measure of their household income to the household incomes of all other respondents. There is no significant relationship between household income and high BMI for Canadian boys, but for girls the prevalence of high BMI was significantly lower in the highest income quintile compared to all other quintiles.

In Mexico, the prevalence of high BMI is significantly higher among boys 2–19 years of age in the highest household living conditions quintile compared to the first, second and third quintiles (Fig. 5.8). Among girls, those in the lowest quintile had a significantly lower prevalence of high BMI compared to those in the highest quintile. The living conditions score was computed using household characteristics and possession of goods through principal components analysis (PCA). We used the first component of the PCA which explained 46% of the variance. The variables in the model were floor material, ceiling material, total number of rooms in the household, possession of refrigerator, washing machine and stove as well as the number of electric appliances in the household (radio, TV, video player, telephone, and computer). The living conditions score was divided into quintiles to categorize the wellbeing condition; thus, subjects in quintile 1 had the lowest living condition and quintile 5 the highest condition.

Figures 5.9 and 5.10 contain estimates of the prevalence of high BMI among US children 2–19 years of age by poverty income ratio (PIR) quintile. Results are shown for total boys and total girls to be comparable to results from Canada and Mexico. Results are also shown by race/ethnic group because differences in the relationship between PIR and high BMI prevalence have been reported (Ogden et al. 2007). PIR is the ratio of household income to the poverty threshold, as defined by the US Census Bureau appropriate for family size. Poverty thresholds are updated for changes in prices but do not take into account differences in cost of living around the country. In the US, the prevalence of high BMI was significantly higher among all boys and non-Hispanic Black boys in the lowest PIR quintile (first) compared to the highest (fifth) quintile. Among all boys and non-Hispanic White boys in the second quintile the prevalence of high BMI was higher compared to the highest (fifth) PIR quintile. Among girls only one significant difference was found, all girls in the lowest PIR quintile had a higher prevalence than all girls in the highest PIR quintile. Nonetheless, there are no significant trends (quadratic or linear) in the prevalence of high BMI by PIR quintile.

Socio-economic status can also be assessed by education level. Table 5.7 depicts the prevalence estimates of high BMI according to the highest level of education in the household in Canada. Although there was a trend of decreasing BMI with increasing education, the only significant association was found for those with BMIs ≥ the 85th percentile. At this lower cut-point, the prevalence

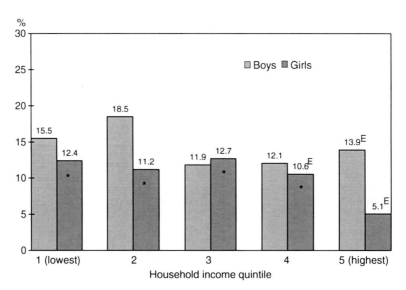

* Significantly different from estimate for quintile 5 (*P* < 0.05)

Fig. 5.7 Prevalence of high body mass index (BMI)-for-age (BMI ≥ 95th percentile) among children aged 2–19 years, by household income (total household income from all sources in previous 12 months divided by Statistics Canada's Low Income Cut-Off specific to number of people in household and size of community), Canada excluding territories, 2004. *E* use with caution (coefficient of variation between 16.6 and 33.3%). *Source:* 2004 Canadian Community Health Survey: Nutrition

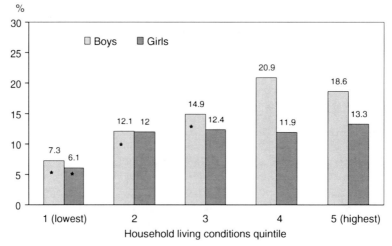

* Significantly different from estimate for quintile 5 (*P* < 0.05)

Fig. 5.8 Prevalence of high body mass index (BMI)-for-age (BMI ≥ 95th percentile) among children aged 2–19 years, by household living conditions (household living conditions derived using Principal Components Analysis which included housing characteristics and possession of goods) in Mexico, 2006. *Source:* Mexican National Health and Nutrition Survey 2006

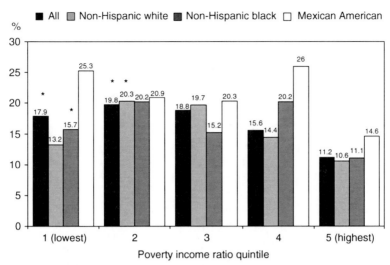

* Significantly different from estimate for quintile 5 ($P < 0.05$) with
Bonferroni correction

Fig. 5.9 Prevalence of high body mass index (BMI)-for-age (≥ 95th percentile) among boys aged 2–19 years, by poverty income ratio (ratio of household income to the poverty threshold accounts for family size and inflation) and race/ethnicity, United States, 2001–2006. *Source*: US National Health and Nutrition Examination Survey, 2001–2006

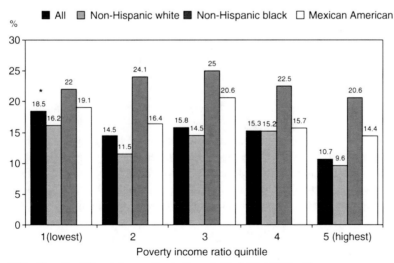

* Significantly different from estimate for quintile 5 ($P < 0.05$) with
Bonferroni correction

Fig. 5.10 Prevalence of high body mass index (BMI)-for-age (BMI ≥ 95th percentile) among girls aged 2–19 years, by poverty income ratio (ratio of household income to the poverty threshold accounts for family size and inflation) and race/ethnicity, United States, 2001–2006. *Source*: US National Health and Nutrition Examination Survey, 2001–2006

Table 5.7 Prevalence of high body mass index (BMI)-for-age[a] among children aged 2–19 years by sex and highest level of education in household, Canada excluding territories, 2004[b]

	n	BMI≥85th		85th≤BMI<95th		BMI≥95th	
		Percent	SE	Percent	SE	Percent	SE
All	9,539	28	0.8	15.7	0.7	12.3	0.5
Secondary graduation or less	1,813	32.5*	1.8	18.2	1.6	14.3	1.3
Some postsecondary	738	29	3.2	16.6	2.7	12.4	1.9
Postsecondary graduation	6,835	26.9	0.9	15	0.7	11.9	0.6
Boys	4,736	29.4	1.2	15.7	0.9	13.8	0.9
Secondary graduation or less	898	34.9*	2.7	20.4*	2.5	14.5	2.0
Some postsecondary	363	29.7[c]	5.0	15.3[c]	4.3	14.4[c]	3.1
Postsecondary graduation	3,398	28.3	1.4	14.8	1.0	13.5	1.0
Girls	4,803	26.6	1.1	15.8	0.9	10.8	0.7
Secondary graduation or less	915	29.9	2.4	15.9	2.1	14.0	1.9
Some postsecondary	375	28.2	3.8	17.9[c]	3.3	10.3[c]	2.1
Postsecondary graduation	3,437	25.5	1.3	15.3	1.0	10.2	0.9

*Significantly different from estimate for postsecondary graduation ($P < 0.05$)
[a] BMI-for-age ≥85th percentile; 85th percentile ≤BMI-for-age <95th percentile; BMI-for-age ≥95th percentile. BMI (body mass index) is weight in kilogram divided by height and meters squared. The 85th and 95th percentiles are based on the 2000 CDC growth charts and represent the revised version of the 1977 NCHS growth charts
[b] 2004 Canadian Community Health Survey: Nutrition
[c] Use with caution (coefficient of variation between 16.6 and 33.3%)

of BMI ≥85th percentile for those living in a household where the highest level of education was a postsecondary degree (college or university) was significantly lower than for those where the highest educational attainment was secondary school or less.

In Mexico, there were significant differences in prevalence of high BMI (BMI ≥95th percentile) among boys (but not girls) by the education level of the household head. Boys in households where the head had more than a high school education were significantly more likely to have high BMI compared to those in households where the head of household had less than a high school education (Table 5.8).

Table 5.9 contains prevalence estimates of high BMI by categories of education of the household head by sex and race/ethnicity in the US. The prevalence of high BMI among non-Hispanic Black girls in households with greater than a high school education was significantly lower than the prevalence in households with only a high school education. This was the only significant difference found when comparing prevalence estimates between households with greater than a high school education to households with less education.

Although socio-economic status is measured differently in each country, the relationship between socio-economic status and high BMI among children and teens 2–19 years of age appears to be different in Mexico compared to Canada and the US. In Mexico, the relationship between household living conditions and high BMI is positive among both boys and girls while in Canada there is an inverse relationship between household income and high BMI only among girls. In the US, the relationship is not so clear. Among girls there was a significant difference between quintile groups only when analyzing the entire population but not when looking at race/ethnic groups separately. Among boys, non-Hispanic Whites and non-Hispanic Blacks in the lower PIR quintiles were significantly more likely to have high BMI compared to the highest PIR quintile. There were no significant trends within group. Analyses of high BMI based on education of household head show slight relationships that are not consistent across countries. In Canadian boys, a significant inverse relationship was found only at the BMI level between the 85th and 95th percentiles. In Mexican boys, there was a significant positive relationship between high BMI and education of household head while in the US, non-Hispanic Black girls in households with greater than a high school education were less likely to have high BMI compared to those in households with only a high school education.

Table 5.8 Prevalence of high body mass index (BMI)-for-age[a] among children age 2–19 years by sex, education level of household head and Ethnicity, Mexico, 2006[b]

Sex	Education	Total			Ethnicity Non-Indigenous			Indigenous		
		n	Percent	SE	n	Percent	SE	n	Percent	SE
All	Total	34,633	12.4	0.4	30,637	13.1	0.4	3,996	7.1	0.8
	<High school	28,199	11.6	0.4	24,505	12.3	0.4	3,694	6.8	0.8
	High school	4,037	16.8	1.5	3,854	17.0	1.5	183	12.0[c]	2.9
	>High school	2,397	14.6	1.0	2,278	14.7	1.0	119	12.2[c]	3.6
Boys	Total	17,203	14.0	0.5	15,250	14.8	0.6	1,953	8.3	1.0
	<High school	13,935	12.6*	0.5	12,132	13.4*	0.5	1,803	7.6	1.0
	High school	2,080	20.0	2.5	1,991	20.1	2.6	89	17.5[c]	4.8
	>High school	1,188	19.0	1.7	1,127	19.1	1.8	61	[d]	
Girls	Total	17,430	10.9	0.4	15,387	11.5	0.5	2,043	6.1[c]	1.0
	<High school	14,264	10.6	0.5	12,373	11.3	0.5	1,891	6.0[c]	1.0
	High school	1,957	13.5	1.3	1,863	13.7	1.3	94	[d]	
	>High school	1,209	10.4	1.2	1,151	10.5	1.3	58	[d]	

*Significantly different from estimate for more than high school education ($P < 0.05$)

[a] BMI-for-age $\geq$95th percentile (BMI: body mass index, weight in kilograms divided by height in meters squared)

[b] National Health and Nutrition Survey 2005–2006

[c] Use with caution (coefficient of variation between 16.6 and 33.3%)

[d] Too unreliable to be published (coefficient of variation greater than 33.3%)

Note: SE standard error

Table 5.9 Prevalence of high body mass index (BMI)-for-age[a] among children age 2–19 years by sex, education level of household head and race/ethnicity, US, 2003–2006[b]

Sex	Education	Total			Non-Hispanic White			Non-Hispanic Black			Mexican American		
		n[c]	Percent	SE	n[c]	Percent	SE	n[c]	Percent	SE	n[c]	Percent	SE
All	Total	8,168	16.3	0.9	2,195	14.7	1.3	2,696	20.7	1.0	2,583	20.9	1.3
	<High school	2,553	18.9	1.3	247	16.2	3.2	802	21.4	1.2	1,343	22.5	1.3
	High school	1,956	19.3	1.6	607	18.5	1.9	651	25.0	2.2	532	18.8	2.8
	>High school	3,321	13.9	1.0	1,280	12.8	1.3	1,148	17.9	1.2	564	18.5	2.5
Boys	Total	4,118	17.0	1.1	1,113	15.6	1.5	1,397	17.4	1.0	1,279	23.2	1.6
	<High school	1,250	18.6	1.5	120	15.3	4.0	405	17.2	1.5	652	24.7	2.0
	High school	990	19.3	1.9	315	19.0	2.4	324	20.2	2.0	261	21.4	3.8
	>High school	1,699	15.3	1.5	653	14.3	1.8	617	16.6	1.5	278	19.8	2.3
Girls	Total	4,050	15.5	1.1	1,082	13.7	1.4	1,299	24.1	1.3	1,304	18.4	1.5
	<High school	1,303	19.2	1.9	127	17.1	4.7	397	25.6	2.0	691	20.2	2.0
	High school	966	19.4	2.0	292	18.0	2.0	327	29.6*	3.2	271	15.9	2.2
	>High school	1,622	12.5	1.2	627	11.3	1.3	531	19.4	1.8	286	17.2	3.6

*Significantly different from estimate for >high school (P<0.05) with Bonferroni correction

[a] BMI-for-age ≥95th percentile (BMI: body mass index, weight in kilograms divided by height in meters squared)

[b] National Health and Nutrition Examination Survey 2003–2006

[c] Number of respondent with non-missing data for BMI. Pregnant girls were excluded

Note: SE standard error

Behavioral Aspects of Obesity

Obesity is a complex condition determined ultimately by a balance of energy intake and energy expenditure. Clearly, individual behaviors, genetics, along with social, cultural and environmental factors must play important roles in the incidence and prevalence of obesity. Genetic factors, however, are unlikely to explain the current increases in the prevalence of overweight and obesity occurring around the world. It is likely that a gene-environment interaction, in which genetically susceptible individuals respond differentially to an environment with increased availability of palatable energy-dense foods and reduced opportunities for energy expenditure, contributes to our current high prevalence of obesity (Ogden et al. 2007).

Diet

Poor eating habits are often established during childhood (Birch and Fisher 1998) and children often do not consume healthy diets (Eaton et al. 2008). Figure 5.11 depicts the prevalence of high BMI-for-age among Canadian children aged 12–19 years by daily fruit and vegetable consumption levels. Children and youth who consumed fruit and vegetables less than three times daily were significantly more likely to be overweight than those who consumed them five or more times daily (prevalence of 15 and 9% respectively). In the United States, in 2007 only 21.4% of high school students ate fruits and vegetables five or more times per day (Healthy People 2010 objective, http://www.healthypeople.gov/). Boys were more likely to consume the five or more fruits and vegetables per day compared to girls (Eaton et al. 2008). In the US, the prevalence of high BMI among teens 12–19 years of age was higher among those who consumed less than three servings of fruits and vegetables per day compared to those who consumed five or more servings per day (Fig. 5.12).

Changes in the composition of the diet have also been recorded. In Mexico, adolescents consume 20.1% of their energy from energy containing beverages. Total beverage consumption increased significantly between 1999 and 2006 among Mexican adolescents (Barquera et al. 2008). Moreover,

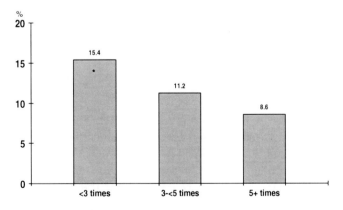

Number of times of daily fruit and vegetable consumption

* Significantly different from estimate for five or more times ($P < 0.05$)

Fig. 5.11 Prevalence of high body mass index (BMI)-for-age (BMI ≥ 95th percentile) among children aged 12–19 years, by daily fruit and vegetable consumption, Canada excluding territories, 2004. *Source*: 2004 Canadian Community Health Survey: Nutrition

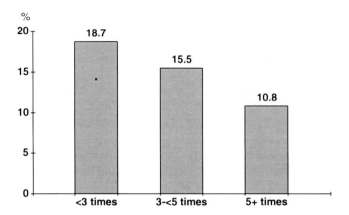

Servings of daily fruit and vegetable consumption

* Significantly different from estimate for five or more servings ($P < 0.01$)

Fig. 5.12 Prevalence of high body mass index (BMI)-for-age (BMI ≥ 95th percentile) among children aged 12–19 years, by daily fruit and vegetable consumption, US, 2003–2006. *Source*: 2003–2006 US National Health and Nutrition Examination Survey

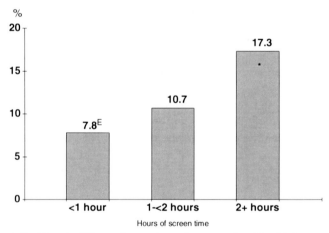

Hours of screen time

* Significantly different from estimate for one or less ($P < 0.05$);
  E use with caution (coefficient of variation between 16.6 and 33.3%)

Fig. 5.13 Prevalence of high body mass index (BMI)-for-age (BMI ≥ 95th percentile) among children aged 6–11 years, by daily hours of screen time, Canada excluding territories, 2004. *Source*: 2004 Canadian Community Health Survey: Nutrition

in the US, there has been an increase in soda consumption among 6–11 and 12–19 year olds and a decrease in milk consumption among 6–11 year olds between 1977–1978 and 2001–2002 (Sebastian et al. 2006). In the US, 33.8% of high school students drank soda in the previous 7 days (based on questionnaire data from the 2007 Youth Risk Behavior System) (Eaton et al. 2008).

Sedentary Behaviors

Many adolescents also participate in sedentary activities such as watching television or videos, playing video games or using a computer. Canadian data on screen time and high BMI for children aged

6–11 years are displayed in Fig. 5.13. There was a gradient between daily hours of screen time and prevalence of high BMI for this age group, with those who watched more than 2 h per day being significantly more likely to have high BMI than those who watched 1 or fewer hours daily.

In Mexico, teenage boys who spent 1–2 h or 2 or more hours involved in screen activities were more likely to have high BMI compared to those who spent less than 1 h per day involved in screen activities (Fig. 5.14). Similarly, in the US 12–19 year old teens were more likely to have high BMI if they spent 2 or more hours involved in screen activities compared to if they spent less than 1 h per day (Fig. 5.15). There was no difference in prevalence of high BMI by amount of screen time between boys and girls in the US.

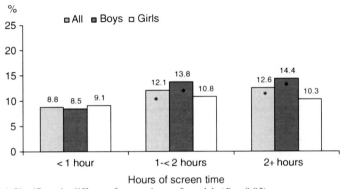

* Significantly different from estimate for <1 h (*P* < 0.05)

Fig. 5.14 Prevalence of high body mass index (BMI)-for-age (BMI ≥ 95th percentile) among children aged 12–19 years, by daily hours of screen times, Mexico, 2006. *Source*: Mexican national Health and Nutrition Survey 2006

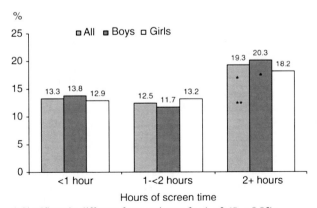

* Significantly different from estimate for 1-<2 (*P* < 0.05);
** Significantly different from estimate for <1 (*P* < 0.05)

Fig. 5.15 Prevalence of high body mass index (BMI)-for-age (≥ 95th percentile) among children aged 12–19 years, by daily hours of screen time, US, 2003–2006. *Source*: 2003–2006 US National Health and Nutrition Examination Survey

Conclusions

The prevalence of high BMI-for-age among children and teens in North America is a public health concern. The prevalence has increased in Canada, Mexico and the US over the past several decades, although it is not clear whether these increases will continue. Differences can be seen between sub-groups and between countries, however a shift in the entire distribution of BMI has occurred in each country. These increases are currently not well understood and further research is needed to identify the reasons for these changes, as well as their potential impact.

Acknowledgements The authors would like to thank Claudia Ivonne Ramirez Silva and Eric Monterubio Flores for their programming assistance with the Mexican data.

References

Barlow, S.E., & Dietz W.H. (1998). Obesity evaluation and treatment: Expert Committee recommendations. The Maternal and Child Health Bureau, Health Resources and Services Administration and the Department of Health and Human Services. *Pediatrics, 102(3)*, E29.

Barquera, S., Hernandez-Barrera, L., Tolentino, M.L., Espinosa, J., Ng, S.W., Rivera, J.A., & Popkin, B.M. (2008). Energy intake from beverages is increasing among Mexican adolescents and adults. *Journal of Nutrition, 138(12)*, 2454-2461.

Birch, L.L., & Fisher, J.O. (1998). Development of eating behaviors among children and adolescents. *Pediatrics, 101(3 Pt 2)*, 539-549.

Cassidy, C.M. (1991). The good body: when big is better. *Medical Anthropology, 13*, 181-213.

Centers for Disease Control and Prevention (2009). Data sets and related documentation. (March 15, 2009); http://www.cdc.gov/nchs/about/major/nhanes/datalink.htm.

Chang, V.W., & Lauderdale, D.S. (2005). Income disparities in body mass index and obesity in the United States, 1971-2002. *Archives of Internal Medicine, 165(18)*, 2122-2128.

Cole, T.J., Freeman, J.V., & Preece, M.A. (1998). British 1990 growth reference centiles for weight, height, body mass index and head circumference fitted by maximum penalized likelihood. *Statistics in Medicine, 17*, 407-429.

Cole, T.J., Bellizzi, M.C., Flegal, K.M., & Dietz, W.H. (2000). Establishing a standard definition for child overweight and obesity worldwide: international survey. *British Medical Journal, 320*, 1240-1243.

Connor Gorber, S., Tremblay, M., Moher, D., & Gorber, B. (2007). A comparison of direct vs. self-report measures for assessing height, weight and body mass index: a systematic review. *Obesity Reviews, 8*, 307-326.

Davis, H., & Gergen, P.J. (1994). Mexican-American mothers' reports of the weights and heights of children 6 months through 11 years old. *Journal of the American Dietetic Association, 94(5)*, 512-516.

Dibley, M.J., Goldsby, J.B., Staehling, N.W., & Trowbridge, F.L. (1987). Development of normalized curves for the international growth reference: historical and technical considerations. *American Journal of Clinical Nutrition, 46(5)*, 736-748.

Dietz, W.H., & Robinson, T.N. (1998). Use of the body mass index (BMI) as a measure of overweight in children and adolescents. *Journal of Pediatrics, 132*, 191-193.

Eaton, D.K., Kann, L., Kinchen, S., Shanklin, S., Ross, J., Hawkins, J., Harris, W.A., Lowry, R., McManus, T., Chyen, D., Lim, C., Brener, N.D., & Wechsler, H. (2008). Centers for Disease Control and Prevention (CDC). Youth risk behavior surveillance – United States, 2007. *MMWR Surveillance Summaries, 57(4)*, 1-131.

Flegal, K.M., Tabak, C.J., & Ogden, C.L. (2006). Overweight in children: definitions and interpretation. *Health Education Research, 21(6)*, 755-760.

Gortmaker, S.L., Must, A., Perrin, J.M., Sobol, A.M., & Dietz, W.H. (1993). Social and economic consequences of overweight in adolescence and young adulthood. *New England Journal of Medicine, 329*, 1008-1012.

Hamill, P.V., Drizd, T.A., Johnson, C.L., Reed, R.B., & Roche, A.F. (1977). NCHS growth curves for children birth-18 years. United States. *Vital and Health Statistics Series, 11(165):i–iv*, 1-74.

Himes, J.H., & Dietz, W.H. (1994). Guidelines for overweight in adolescent preventive services: recommendations from an expert committee. The Expert Committee on Clinical Guidelines for Overweight in Adolescent Preventive Services. *American Journal of Clinical Nutrition, 59(2)*, 307-316.

Krebs, N.F., Himes, J.H., Jacobson, D., Nicklas, T.A., Guilday, P., & Styne, D. (2007). Assessment of child and adolescent overweight and obesity. *Pediatrics, 120(Suppl 4)*, S193-S228. Review.

Kuczmarski, M.F., Kuczmarski, R.J., & Najjar, M. (2001). Effects of age on validity of self-reported height, weight, and body mass index: findings from the Third National Health and Nutrition Examination Survey, 1988-1994. *Journal of the American Dietetic Association, 101(1)*, 28–34.

Kuczmarski, R.J., Ogden, C.L., Guo, S.S., Grummer-Strawn, L.M., Flegal, K.M., Mei, Z., Wei, R., Curtin, L.R., Roche, A.F., & Johnson, C.L. (2002). 2000 CDC Growth Charts for the United States: methods and development. *Vital and Health Statistics Series, 11, 246*, 1–190.

McDowell, A., Engel, A., Masse, J.T, & Maurer, K. (1981). Plan and operation of the Second National Health and Nutrition Examination Survey, 1976-1980. *Vital and Health Statistics Series, 1(15)*, 1–144.

Miller, H.W. (1973). Plan and operation of the health and nutrition examination survey. United States – 1971-1973. *Vital and Health Statistics Series, 1(10a)*, 1–46.

National Center for Health Statistics (1994). Plan and operation of the Third National Health and Nutrition Examination Survey, 1988-94. Series 1: programs and collection procedures. *Vital and Health Statistics Series, 1(32)*, 1–407.

Ogden, C.L., Flegal, K.M., Carroll, M.D., & Johnson, C.L. (2002). Prevalence and trends in overweight among US children and adolescents, 1999-2000. *Journal of the American Medical Association, 288*, 1728–1732.

Ogden, C.L., Carroll, M.D., & Flegal, K.M. (2003). Epidemiologic trends in overweight and obesity. *Endocrinology and Metabolism Clinics of North America, 32(4)*, 741–760, vii. Review.

Ogden, C.L., Yanovski, S.Z., Carroll, M.D., & Flegal, K.M. (2007). The epidemiology of obesity. *Gastroenterology, 132(6)*, 2087–2102. Review.

Ogden, C.L., Carroll, M.D., & Flegal, K.M. (2008). High body mass index for age among US children and adolescents, 2003-2006. *Journal of the American Medical Association, 299(20)*, 2401–2405.

Olaiz, G., Rivera-Dommarco, J., Shamah, T., Rojas, R., Villalpando, S., Hernández, M., & Sepúlveda, J. (2006). *Encuesta Nacional de Salud y Nutrición 2006.* Cuernavaca (Mexico): Instituto Nacional de Sauld Pública.

Perry, G.S., Byers, T.E., Mokdad, A.H., Serdula, M.K., & Williamson, D.F. (1995). The validity of self-reports of past body weights by U.S. adults. *Epidemiology, 6(1)*, 61–66.

Resano-Pérez, E., Méndez-Ramírez, I., Shamah-Levy, T., Rivera, J.A., & Sepúlveda-Amor, J. (2003). Methods of the National Nutrition Survey 1999. *Salud pública de México [online], 45(suppl 4)*, 558–564.

Rivera, J.A, Barquera, S., Campirano, F., Campos, I., Safdie, M., & Tovar, V. (2002). Epidemiological and nutritional transition in Mexico: rapid increase of non-communicable chronic diseases and obesity. *Public Health Nutrition, 5(1A)*, 113–122.

Rowland, M. (1990). Self-reported weight and height. *American Journal of Clinical Nutrition, 52*, 1125–1133.

Sargent, J.D., & Blanchflower, D.G. (1994). Obesity and stature in adolescence and earnings in young adulthood. Analysis of a British birth cohort. *Archives of Pediatric and Adolescent Medicine, 148*, 681–687.

Sebastian, R.D., Cleveland, L.E., Goldman, J.D., & Moshfegh, A.J. (2006). Trends in the food intakes of children 1977-2002. *Consumer Interest Annual, 52*, 433–434.

Sepúlveda, A., Lezana, M.A., Tapia, R., Valdespino, J., Madrigal, H., & Kumate, J.(1990). Estado nutricional de preescolares y mujeres en México: Resultados de una encuesta probabilística nacional. *Gaceta Médica de México, 126*, 207–225.

Shields, M. (2006). Overweight and obesity among children and youth. *Health Reports, 17(3)*, 27–42.

Sobal, J., & Stunkard, A. J. (1989). Socioeconomic status and obesity: a review of the literature. *Psychological Bulletin, 105*, 260–275.

Statistics Canada. (2005). Population health surveys. Ottawa: Statistics Canada (January 13, 2009); http://www.statcan.ca/english/concepts/hs/index.htm#content.

Tremblay, M.S., Katzmarzyk, P.T., & Willms, J.D. (2002). Temporal trends in overweight and obesity in Canada, 1981-1996. *International Journal of Obesity, 26*, 538–543.

United Nations Statistics Division (2009). (June 17, 2009); http://unstats.un.org/unsd/default.htm.

Health and Welfare Canada, Statistics Canada (1981). *The Health of Canadians: Report of the Canada Health Survey.* Ottawa: Minister of Supply and Services Canada.

World Health Organization (2006). *WHO child growth standards. Length/height-for-age, weight-for-age, weight-for-length, weight-for-height and body mass index-for-age. Methods and development.* Geneva: World Health Organization.

World Bank, Data and Statistics (2009). Key development data & statistics. (June 17, 2009); http://web.worldbank.org/WBSITE/EXTERNAL/DATASTATISTICS/0,,contentMDK:20535285~menuPK:1192694~pagePK:64133150~piPK:64133175~theSitePK:239419,00.html.

Chapter 6
Epidemiology of Obesity in Children in South America

Cecilia Albala and Camila Corvalan

Introduction

South America is experiencing rapid epidemiologic and nutrition transitions. In the last two to three decades, profound demographic, socio-economic and environmental changes have occurred in the region (Popkin 1994). As a result, dietary and physical activity patterns of the population have changed, influencing the epidemiologic and nutritional profiles of the countries. The epidemiologic situation in the Americas is now characterized by a reduction of communicable diseases, maternal, and perinatal diseases, and a progressive increase of non-communicable chronic diseases (i.e., cardiovascular diseases, diabetes and cancer) and injuries as causes of mortality, morbidity and disability (Albala and Vio 1995). At the same time, the nutritional profile of the region has dramatically changed. Low birth weight, wasting, stunting, and nutrient deficiencies have decreased and obesity and overweight increasingly arise as the main nutritional problems in all age groups and even among low-income and indigenous people (Albala et al. 2001).

However, these changes have occurred at different speeds within the region portraying a picture of high variability among the different countries. Some countries, such as Uruguay and Chile, are in the advanced stages of the demographic, epidemiologic and nutrition transitions while others, such as Peru or Bolivia, still present high infant mortality rates, significant prevalence of infectious diseases and persistence of stunting, anemia, and micronutrient deficiencies. Early life undernutrition (i.e., low birth weight) as well as chronic undernutrition (i.e., stunting) may contribute to exacerbate obesity and nutrition-related chronic disease risk later in life (Duran et al. 2006; Sawaya et al. 2003). Thus, the coexistence of yesterday`s unsolved problems with the emerging challenges of obesity, chronic diseases and injuries poses additional difficulties for ensuring healthy life in the region (Frenk et al. 1991).

According to the 2004 report of the International Obesity Task Force (IOTF), more than 20% of school-age children in the Americas have excess weight (Lobstein et al. 2004). Moreover, in most countries childhood obesity is worsening at a dramatic rate. The World Health Organization (WHO) global estimates predict that if the current trends persist, by 2050 one out of four children will be obese and almost 40% will be overweight. Current evidence suggests that overweight in children persists into adulthood. More than half of the children who are overweight at 2–5 years of age and 80% of children who are overweight at 7–11 years will remain overweight at age 12 years (Nader

C. Albala (✉) and C. Corvalan
Instituto de Nutrición y Tecnología de los Alimentos, Universidad de Chile,
Av. El Líbano 5524, Casilla 138-11, Santiago, Chile
e-mail: calbala@uchile.cl

L.A. Moreno et al. (eds.), *Epidemiology of Obesity in Children and Adolescents*,
Springer Series on Epidemiology and Public Health 2, DOI 10.1007/978-1-4419-6039-9_6,
© Springer Science+Business Media, LLC 2011

et al. 2006); similar tracking from childhood to adulthood has been described for obese children with obese parents (Whitaker et al. 1997). Moreover, obese children are more likely to develop similar metabolic complications and cardiovascular disease as adults (Baker et al. 2007; Bibbins-Domingo et al. 2007; Freedman et al. 2001; Srinivasan et al. 2002). If current obesity trends persist among adolescents, it is estimated that by 2035 cardiovascular disease will increase to 5–16% with more than 100,000 excess cases attributable to the increased obesity (Bibbins-Domingo et al. 2007). Childhood obesity is also associated with several concurrent medical and psychological problems. Insulin resistance, hypertension, dyslipidemia, type 2 diabetes and the metabolic syndrome are increasingly diagnosed in obese young people (Eisenmann 2003; Freedman et al. 1999) among many other diseases. Obese children are also at risk of developing psychosocial problems such as depression, shame, low self esteem, self-blame, etc. that may impair their social and academic performance (Schwartz and Puhl 2003). Overall, the social and economic cost of obesity and its related problems are staggering (Powers et al. 2007).

The aim of this paper is to display a picture of childhood obesity in Latin South America and to provide a general overview of some of its risk factors in the context of the nutrition transition that the region is experiencing.

Geographic Region

According to the Pan-American Health Organization (PAHO) America is divided into three main regions: North America, the Caribbean, and Latin America. The South portion of Latin America in turns encompasses three sub regions: Brazil, the Southern Cone (Argentina, Uruguay, Chile and Paraguay) and the Andean Area (Bolivia, Colombia, Peru, Venezuela and Ecuador).

Socio-economic and demographic characteristics of countries of the South part of Latin America are presented in Table 6.1 and Table 6.2, respectively. In terms of socio-economic conditions, on average, countries of this sub region are located in an intermediate position worldwide and in a high position within developing countries. Demographic indicators also reflect a higher degree of development compared to other regions worldwide. However, within the region there are important differences in the level of socio-demographic development. Countries of the southern cone are the most advanced into the demographic, epidemiologic and nutrition transition, with the exception of Paraguay. Correspondingly, people in these countries have better socio-economic condition and higher life expectancy than the rest of the countries of the region. Countries of the southern cone present lower infant, maternal, and perinatal mortality rates and lower infectious diseases whereas morbidity and mortality from chronic diseases are more common than in other countries. Brazil, Colombia, and Venezuela are in an intermediate position while Bolivia, Peru, Ecuador and Paraguay are at an early stage of the demographic, epidemiologic and nutrition transitions.

Methods

This chapter is based on descriptive cross-sectional population-based data. Data were obtained from multiple sources: national surveys conducted from 2000 onwards that were publically available; governmental data and publications when they were available at the web; World Health Organization (WHO) and Pan American Health Organization (PAHO) databases and publications; databases from non-governmental organizations; and published articles compiled trough Medline, Scielo and Lilacs.

Table 6.1 Socio-economic characteristics of the south region of Latin America (WHO 2008)

	Year	Argentina	Bolivia	Brazil	Chile	Colombia	Ecuador	Paraguay	Peru	Uruguay	Venezuela
HDI (ranking)	1990 (UNDP 2007)	0.813	0.606	0.723	0.788	0.729	0.714	0.718	0.71	0.806	0.762
		(38)	(117)	(70)	(40)	(75)	(89)	(95)	(87)	(46)	(74)
	2008 (UNDP 2008)	0.860	0.723	0.807	0.874	0.787	0.807	0.752	0.788	0.859	0.826
		(46)	(111)	(70)	(40)	(80)	(72)	(98)	(79)	(47)	(61)
GDP US	1990	6,850	1,600	5,150	4,430	4,310	2,330	3,690	3,020	5,510	4,630
PPP	2006	15,390	2,890	8,800	11,270	7,620	4,400	5,070	6,080	11,150	7,440
H20/L20 (PAHO 2007)	2000–2005	17.9	42	21	15.8	21	17.6	25.8	15.3	10.1	15.8
% Urban population (UNDP 2007)	1990	87	56	75	83	69	55	49	69	89	84
	2006	90	65	85	88	73	63	59	73	92	94
Drinking water access %	2006	96	86	91	97	93	95	77	84	100	89
Access to sanitation %	2006	91	43	77	94	78	84	70	72	100	83
% Literacy (≥ 15 years)	2000–2005	97.2	86.7	88.6	95.7	92.8	91	93.5	87.9	100	93
Calories availability (FAO 2007)	2003	2,959	2,219	3,146	2,872	2,567	2,641	2,524	2,579	2,883	2,272

HDI human development index; *GDP PPP* gross domestic product at purchasing power parity; *H20/L20* ratio of share in total income/expenditure of the highest quintile group to the lowest quintile group

Table 6.2 Demographic characteristics of the south region of Latin American countries 1990–2006 (WHO 2008)

	Year	Argentina	Bolivia	Brazil	Chile	Colombia	Ecuador	Paraguay	Peru	Uruguay	Venezuela
IMR (per 1,000 live births)	1990	24	89	48	18	26	43	33	41	22	27
	2006	14	50	19	8	17	21	19	24	13	18
Mortality <5 years (per 1,000 live births)	1990	28	125	57	21	35	57	41	78	25	33
	2006	17	61	20	9	21	24	22	25	15	21
LBW (%)	2000–2002	7	9	10	5	9	16	9	11	8	7
TFR (per woman)	1990	3	4.9	2.8	2.6	3	3.3	4.5	3.9	2.5	3.4
	2006	2.3	3.6	2.3	1.9	2.3	2.8	3.2	2.5	2.1	2.6
Mortality 15–60 year rate (per 1,000 pop)	1990	150	277	212	147	211	214	119	178	147	148
	2006	124	208	176	91	131	166	132	136	125	142
Men	1990	198	307	272	196	268	254	173	204	195	178
	2006	162	242	230	98	176	206	123	153	164	187
Women	1990	103	248	150	98	152	173	99	152	98	117
	2006	86	176	121	60	87	123	101	118	88	95
Life expectancy at birth (year)	1990	72	58	62	72	68	67	73	67	72	72
	2006	75	66	72	78	74	73	75	73	75	74
Men	1990	69	57	63	69	65	64	71	65	69	70
	2006	72	64	68	75	71	70	72	71	72	71
Women	1990	76	59	70	76	71	69	75	69	76	74
	2006	78	67	75	81	78	76	78	75	79	78

IMR infant mortality rate; *TFR* total fertility rate; *LBW* low birth weight

Socio-Economic and Demographic Indicators

General socio-economic and demographic information were obtained from the World Health Statistics 2008 (WHO 2008), and PAHO Health in the Americas: basic indicators 2007 (PAHO 2007). Human development indexes were obtained from United Nations Development Programme (UNDP) (UNDP 2007, 2008).

Obesity Estimates

Pre-school children were defined as children 0–4.99 years of age. Prevalence of obesity at this age was obtained from WHO global data base on child growth and malnutrition (WHO 2009a). Data for obesity trends in pre-school children were abstracted from previous reports of WHO and published papers.

School age children were defined as children 5–9.99 years of age, except in the case of Venezuela where those data were available for 7–14 years old children only. Excess weight estimates for school children comes from published papers and national data sources.

Adolescence was defined as the period between 10 and 18 years of age, except in the case of Brazil where those data were available for the 10–19 years old age range. Data on excess weight prevalence in adolescents come from published papers and available national data sources.

Obesity Definition

In pre-school children, excess weight was defined based on z-scores (i.e., standard score that indicates the number of standard deviations (SD) over or below the mean). Obesity was defined as weight for-height z-score (WHZ)$>+2$SD and overweight as WHZ$>+1$SD of the WHO Child Growth Standards (World Health Organization (WHO) 2006). Survey data prior to 2006 were analyzed using the National Centre for Health Statistics (NCHS WHO) international reference population (Hamill et al. 1979).

In school age children and adolescents available information was based on various definitions of excess weight (i.e., WHO 2006 (WHO 2006), NCHS/WHO 1978 (Hamill et al. 1979), Centers for Disease Control (CDC) (Kuczmarski et al. 2002), IOTF (Cole et al. 2000) and Must criteria (Must et al. 1991)).

Obesity Risk Factors

Breastfeeding data were obtained from the global data bank on breastfeeding and complementary feeding (WHO 2009b) and national health surveys.

Physical activity information was not available from official web sites or representative reports. Thus, we used non-comparable information available from published papers.

Dietary intake information was mainly abstracted from FAO statistical yearbook (FAO 2007) and published papers.

In women, obesity was defined as body mass index (BMI) ≥ 30 and overweight as a BMI ≥ 25. This information was available from IOTF and national surveys.

Results

Prevalence of Obesity in Pre-School Children

Table 6.3 shows figures from the 1990s and the latest available data for the ten countries of the Latin American region. As shown, in the 1990s, Peru, Argentina and Brazil had the highest prevalence (9.0, 7.3, and 6.6%, respectively), while the lowest prevalence is observed in Colombia and Venezuela (4.5 and 3.0% respectively). In the last two decades the trends in the prevalence of obesity in pre-school children has increased in all countries of the region with the exception of Venezuela. As it is depicted in Table 6.3, presently the Southern Cone as a whole has the highest prevalence. In Paraguay obesity among pre-schoolers reaches a prevalence of 14.2% and it is the highest in South America. In the Andean region, Peru and Bolivia have the highest prevalence while Ecuador, Colombia and Venezuela have the lowest. Brazil with a prevalence of 7% is in an intermediate position.

Prevalence of Obesity in School Children

In the region, anthropometric measurements in school age children are less systematically collected than in pre-school children. The figures presented in Table 6.4 come from different sources but almost all are from official governmental organizations or ministries. In some countries with a national surveillance system there are annual data available as in Chile, while in others, national data come from cross-sectional surveys such as in Colombia, Ecuador, Paraguay, Uruguay, and Venezuela. In Argentina, Bolivia, Brazil, and Peru we were unable to find national data, therefore we present latest estimates from specific samples. This lack of consistency in the sample population and in the obesity definition used in each of the countries did not allow us to validly compare obesity prevalence among countries. Nonetheless, and considering this limitation, it can be observed that at this age the general picture is similar to that described for pre-school children, with countries of the Southern Cone of Latin America presenting the highest obesity prevalence of the region. Information about obesity trends was available only in a few countries and indicated that there is a consistent upward trend. In Peru for example the prevalence of overweight in the

Table 6.3 Trends in the prevalence of obesity[a] in pre-school children from the south region of Latin America in the last decade, by country

Andean sub region	1990–1998 (WHO 2008)	2000–2007 (WHO 2009a)
Bolivia	6.5 (1998) (Lobstein et al. 2004)	9.2 (2003–2004)
Colombia	4.5 (1995)	5.1 (2004–2005)
Ecuador		5.1 (2004)
Peru	9.9 (1996)	11.8 (2000)
Venezuela	3.0 (1997) (Lobstein et al. 2004)	3.2 (2000)
Southern Cone		
Argentina	7.3 (1994) (de Onis and Blossner 2000)	9.9 (2004–2005)
Chile	6.2 (1996)	9.8 (2007)
Paraguay	6.3 (1990)	14.2 (2002) (PAHO 2007)
Uruguay	6.2 (92–93) (PAHO 2007)	9.4 (2004)
Brazil	6.6 (1996)	7.3 (2006–2007)

Reference population = 1978 NCHS/WHO for 1990–2005 estimates
Reference population = WHO 2006 for 2006–2007 estimate
[a] Obesity = weight for height >2SD

Table 6.4 Prevalence of excess weight in school children from the south region of Latin America, by country

Andean sub region	Age (years)	Year	Sample	Definition	% Overweight	Definition	% Obesity
Bolivia (Perez-Cueto et al. 2009)	5–7	2007	NR	85th ≤ BMI ≤ 95th (WHO 2007)	24.0	BMI ≥ 95th (WHO 2007)	6.0
Colombia (Instituto colombiano de bienestar familiar (ICBF) 2006)	5–9	2005	National			WHZ ≥ 2 SD (NCHS/WHO 1978)	4.3
Ecuador (Yépez 2005)	7.5–8.5	2001	National	85th ≤ BMI ≤ 95th	8.0	BMI ≥ 95th	6.0
Peru (Pajuelo et al. 2004)	6–10	2004	NR	85th ≤ BMI ≤ 95th (Must 1991)	16.5	BMI ≥ 95th (Must 1991)	13.9
Venezuela (Instituto Nacional de Nutrición Gobierno Bolivariano de Venezuela 2005)	7–14	2005	National	WHZ ≥ 90th (NCHS/WHO 1978)	19.3		
Southern Cone							
Argentina (Bejarano et al. 2005)	4–10	2000	NR	85th ≤ BMI ≤ 95th (CDC 2000/IOTF)	17.5/17.0	BMI ≥ 95th (CDC 2000/IOTF)	6.7/11.9
Chile (Junta Nacional de auxilio escolar y becas (JUNAEB) Gobierno de Chile 2008)	6–8	2008	NR-National			WHZ ≥ 2 SD (NCHS/WHO 1978)	20.8
Uruguay (Pisabarro et al. 2000)	9	2000	National	85th ≤ BMI ≤ 95th (Must 1991)	21.8	BMI ≥ 95th (Must 1991)	10.0
Paraguay (Sistema de Vigilancia Nutricional (SISVAN) 2008, 2009)	6–8	2008	National	85th ≤ BMI ≤ 95th (CDC 2000)	11.4	BMI ≥ 95th (CDC 2000)	5.1
Brazil (Triches and Giugliani 2005)	8–10	2003	NR	85th ≤ BMI ≤ 95th (Must 1991)	16.9	BMI ≥ 95th (Must 1991)	7.5

NR non representative

population under 15 years of age rose from 8.5% in 1990 to 11.3% in 2000 (PAHO, 2007) while in Chile prevalence of obesity in first graders increased from ~5% in 1990 to ~19% in 2005 (Kain et al. 2003; Vio et al. 2008).

Prevalence of Obesity in Adolescents

In the case of adolescents, representative national data were available for most of the countries, except for Argentina, Chile, Peru, and Paraguay (Table 6.5). Most of this information comes from national nutritional surveillance systems and it was available through governmental web sites. For Argentina, Chile, and Peru we present the latest estimates from specific samples; for Paraguay we were unable to find valid data. Estimates were derived from study samples with different age ranges and used different definitions of obesity what, as in school age children, makes them difficult to compare. Nonetheless, overall, the obesity distribution in adolescents of the region indicated that the highest prevalence were observed in countries of the Southern Cone followed by Brazil and the Andean sub region, thus confirming the picture observed at earlier ages.

What Do We Know About Key Risk Factors?

At the individual level, obesity has an undeniable genetic component. However, genetic predisposition cannot explain differences in obesity prevalence within and between populations. Modifiable factors involved in the large increase in childhood obesity observed in the last decades can be grouped into three main groups of causes. First, there are contextual factors such as cultural, environmental and socio-economic factors (i.e., low education level of mothers, poverty, accelerated urbanization, etc.) that have dramatically changed the living conditions of the population promoting positive energy balance. Second, there are behavioral factors associated with increased energy intake (i.e., raise in soda and snack consumption, enlarged portion sizes, parental feeding styles that promote overeating, etc.) and decreased physical activity (i.e., TV viewing, decreased exercise, etc.). Finally, there are developmental factors mainly related to early nutrition such as poor nutrition of the mother, obesity in pregnant women, low birth weight, duration of breastfeeding and child malnutrition (Albala et al. 2002; WHO/PAHO 2007; World Health Organization (WHO) 2003). For more details on determinants of childhood obesity please refer to the corresponding chapters of Part II of this book.

Urbanization and Socio-Economic Conditions

The economic growth, the achievements in education and the rapid urbanization have produced dietary changes and a progressive decrease of physical activity during work and leisure time, primary causes of the explosion of obesity in the region (Uauy et al. 2008). The urbanization process began earlier in Argentina, Chile, Uruguay Venezuela and Brazil, with more than 75% of the population living in urban settlements previous to the 1970s. Nowadays urban living is a common phenomenon in the whole region reaching 76.4% in the Andean Sub Region, 85.6% in Brazil and 88.1% in the Southern Cone (Table 6.1). On the one hand, this process had positive effects in increasing access to drinking water and sanitation, better literacy rates and education and more access to housing and health services. On the other hand, urbanization produces dramatic changes in lifestyles increasing sedentarism and turning to diets rich in fat, animal products, sugar and salt coupled with low

Table 6.5 Prevalence of excess weight in adolescents of the south region of Latin America, by country

Andean sub region	Age (years)	Year	Sample	Definition	% Overweight	Definition	% Obesity
Bolivia (Perez-Cueto et al. 2009)	12–18	2005–2007	National	BMI (IOTF)	13.2	BMI (IOTF)	2.5
Colombia (Instituto colombiano de bienestar familiar (ICBF) 2006)	10–17	2005	National	85th ≤ BMI ≤ 95th (CDC 2000)	10.3		
Ecuador (Yépez 2005)	12–18	2006	National	85th ≤ BMI ≤ 95th	13.7	BMI ≥ 95th	8.5
Peru (based on Pajuelo (2003))	10–15	2003	NR	85th ≤ BMI ≤ 95th (Must 1991)	18.2	BMI ≥ 95th (Must 1991)	5.0
Venezuela (Instituto Nacional de Nutrición Gobierno Bolivariano de Venezuela)	7–14	2005	National	WHZ ≥ 90th (NCHS/WHO 1978)	19.3		
Southern Cone							
Argentina (Poletti and Barrios 2007)	10–15	2007	NR	BMI (IOTF)	17.1	BMI (IOTF)	4.5
Chile (Bustos et al. 2010)	10–18	2006	NR	85th ≤ BMI ≤ 95th (CDC 2000)	18.2	BMI ≥ 95th (CDC 2000)	9.8
Uruguay (Pisabarro et al. 2000)	12	2000	National	85th ≤ BMI ≤ 95th (Must 1991)	18.7	BMI ≥ 95th (Must 1991)	4.8
Brazil (Instituto Brasileiro de Geografia e Estatística 2006)	10–19	2002–2003	National	BMI (IOTF)	16.7	BMI (IOTF)	2.3

NR non representative data

consumption of cereals, legumes, and other fiber-rich foods, such as vegetables and fruits. All these changes promote a positive energy balance that is reflected in an increase in obesity prevalence.

Data from different countries in the region confirm that obesity increases with urbanization. For example, in Colombia in 2005 for the 10–17 years old age group, overweight was 7.2% in rural regions while reached 11.6% in urban regions (Instituto colombiano de bienestar familiar (ICBF) 2006). In Peru, several studies published by Pajuelo (Pajuelo 2003; Pajuelo et al. 2000; Pajuelo et al. 2001) show that in 2000 overweight and obesity were at least twice times higher in urban than rural children (9.8% vs. 21.4% overweight, and 2.2% vs. 12.4% obesity). Recent reports of Bolivia national estimates also confirm that childhood obesity is higher in the urban areas (Perez-Cueto et al. 2009).

The socio-economic distribution of obesity depends on the level of development of the countries. At initial stages of the nutrition transition, excess weight tends to concentrate in groups of high socio-economic status (SES). As the transition moves into further stages, obesity starts to affect medium and low SES groups. Finally, in a post-transitional situation, obesity is concentrated in low SES groups (Monteiro et al. 2004). This trend is consistent with what is observed in Latin America. Data from countries facing early stages of the transition such as Bolivia, Ecuador, and Peru indicate that overweight and obesity is more frequent in high than low SES groups (OPS Ecuador 2007; Perez-Cueto et al. 2009; Yépez 2005; Yépez et al. 2008) while in countries in more advanced stages such as Brazil, Uruguay or Chile there is no clear association between SES and obesity or obesity tends to be higher among low SES children. In Brazil, the 2004–2005 follow-up of the 1993 Pelotas Cohort Study showed that obesity was more prevalent among high SES adolescents than in those with low SES (Matijasevich et al. 2009). However, the opposite situation was observed in the case of women from the 1982 Pelotas Cohort Study. In this study, 18 years old women with high SES had lower prevalence of obesity than women from low SES. The same situation has been described by Monteiro et al. (2007), who in the last years observed a decrease in the prevalence of obesity among females of higher income and an increase in females of low income. Unfortunately, the observed trend in Brazil, where the obesity epidemic is shifting toward poor people, is being observed in other Latin American countries.

Sedentary Behavior

WHO reports that sedentary lifestyle is one of the main contributory factors to increasing obesity rates (World Health Organization (WHO) 2002). According to the WHO report, 30–60% of the population of the Latin American region does not achieve the minimum recommended levels of physical activity (World Health Organization (WHO) 2003). The rapid urbanization of the countries of the region has contributed to achieving these alarming rates of physical inactivity. The expansion of the cities has led to an increase in the amount of time spent commuting to work or school. On the one hand, insecurity and the reduction of public spaces and parks contribute to decreasing active recreational exercise time as well as increasing the time spent watching TV or in front of a computer. On the other hand, technical appliances that are increasingly more accessible to all population, save time but also decrease physical activity (Vio et al. 2008).

Although it is very difficult to have comparable measurements of physical activity among countries, all the available data evidence a high prevalence of sedentary behavior in the Region. The last two national surveys done in Chile (Ministerio de Salud-Instituto Nacional de Estadísticas 2004, 2007) demonstrated that 90% or more of the population can be defined as sedentary. Only 8.6% of the interviewed performed at least 30 min of exercise three times per week in 2000 and 10.8% in 2006. Women were more inactive than men in their leisure time, particularly if they belonged to low SES groups. In both surveys the main reasons to be inactive were: lack of time (33%), no interest

(23.3 to 25.2%), health reasons (19.5 to 20.1%) and lack of places to exercise (14 to 9%). In Argentina, the National Survey 2007 (Ministerio de Salud. Presidencia de la Nacion Argentina, 2007) showed that only 18.6% of the women between 10 and 49 years performed three or more sessions of moderate or vigorous physical activity per week. The 2004 National Health Survey conducted in Colombia reported that 12.5% of adolescents (12–17 years) and 23.5% of adults (18–69 years) regularly practice vigorous PA. In the group of adolescents, 42.9% do not exercise at all, being the same situation observed in 79% of the adults. In Brazil, during 2002–2003 a survey to identify risk factors in the population 15 years and older was conducted in 15 state capitals of the country. The highest proportion of individuals classified as insufficiently active was found in Paraiba (54.5%) and the lowest in Para (28.2%). The National Health Survey conducted in Bolivia in 2003 (Gutiérrez Sardán et al. 2004) showed up that 41% women and 74% of men reported exercising at least 10 min during leisure time in the last week. In Peru, the 2006 Food and Nutrition Survey of the National Institute of Health indicated that 40% of the assessed population practiced little physical activity (Ministerio de Salud. Instituto Nacional de Salud (INS), Centro Nacional de Alimentación y Nutrición (CENAN) (2006)).

Dietary Factors

Presently, dietary factors are important risk factors for the main causes of death and disease in South American countries. As income increases, so does overall energy intake and total fat, especially saturated fat. With the exception of Venezuela and Bolivia, the availability of total calories and calories from fat, has increased in the last two decades in the entire region. The largest increase took place in Peru (20%) followed by Ecuador, Brazil and Colombia (Table 6.6). The consumption of cereals, legumes and other fiber-rich foods such as vegetables and fruits remain stable or decline in the same period (Albala et al. 2003; Popkin 1993). According to the FAO food balance sheets a decrease in the consumption of cereals and pulses was observed in Chile and Brazil between 1979 and 1999. A decrease in the consumption of fruits and vegetables has been also observed in Chile (Albala et al. 2003; Uauy et al. 2001). Trends in household food expenditure by income quintile in Chile in the last decade show a decrease in the consumption of bread while sweetened soft drinks have doubled or tripled in all socio-economic groups (Albala et al. 2002). In Table 6.7, we present the last available data on dietary components for the South American countries. Bolivia, Peru, Paraguay and Ecuador (i.e., the least urbanized countries) show the highest consumption of tubers, roots, fruits and vegetables while more urbanized countries such as Brazil, Chile, Colombia, and Uruguay present higher consumption of meats, cereals, and sugar than the rest of the countries of the region.

Breastfeeding

The duration of breastfeeding is a crucial factor in child nutrition. Several studies have shown that maintaining exclusive breastfeeding for 6 months is associated with lower infant morbidity and mortality as well as with a faster postpartum recovering (Kramer and Kakuma 2002). Furthermore, exclusive breastfeeding appears to be a protective factor against obesity and overweight in children (Bergmann et al. 2003; Scanferla de Siqueira and Monteiro 2007; Simon et al. 2009). WHO appraisals for South America, made by Léuer and De Onis, estimate that 40% of women exclusively breastfed for at least 6 months (de Onis and Blossner 2000; Lauer et al. 2004). These values are consistent with the prevalence described in Table 6.8. In all countries breastfeeding rates at 4 months are under 50%, with the exception of Peru and Chile.

Table 6.6 Dietary energy, protein, and fat consumption in the south region of Latin America, by country 1980–2002 (FAO 2007)

	Kcal/day			Fats g/person/day			Proteins g/day		
	1979–1981	2001–2003	Difference (%)	1979–1981	2001–2003	Difference (%)	1979–1981	2001–2003	Difference (%)
Argentina	3,210	2,980	−7.2	116	100	−13.8	107	94	−12.2
Bolivia	2,130	2,220	+4.2	52	58	+11.5	55	57	+3.6
Brazil	2,680	3,060	+14.2	65	93	+43.1	63	83	+31.7
Chile	2,670	2,860	+7.1	60	85	+41.7	71	80	+12.7
Colombia	2,290	2,580	+12.7	47	65	+38.3	49	60	+22.5
Ecuador	2,360	2,710	+14.8	60	99	+65	50	57	+14
Paraguay	2,580	2,530	−1.9	70	87	+24.3	75	69	−8
Peru	2,130	2,570	+20.7	38	48	+26.3	54	67	+24.1
Uruguay	2,850	2,850	0	103	86	−16.5	86	86	0
Venezuela	2,760	2,350	−14.9	78	68	−12.8	70	62	−11.4

Table 6.7 Share of dietary components in total energy consumption of countries of the south region of Latin America, 2001–2003 (% kcal/person/day) (FAO 2007)

	Vegetal oils	Animal fats	Cereals	Sugar	Meat and offal	Milk, eggs and fish	Roots and tubers	Pulses	Fruits and vegetables
Argentina	10.1	2.4	33.1	14.9	17	9.5	3.7	0.3	5.0
Bolivia	8.7	1.8	38	12.9	11.7	3.0	8.3	1.0	10.1
Brazil	10.5	1.8	30.5	18	12.2	7.5	4.4	5.1	4.6
Chile	8.8	1.2	40.2	15.8	13	7.0	3.7	1.3	4.8
Colombia	10.7	2.2	33.3	18.6	6.5	8.3	7.4	2.6	8.3
Ecuador	18.6	3.1	30.8	16.4	7.8	7.3	2.6	1.5	10.0
Paraguay	13.3	3.0	29.5	9.2	8.6	7.1	13.8	4.0	4.1
Peru	5.3	3.2	40.5	14.5	4.3	5.4	13.3	2.6	6.7
Uruguay	6.4	2.0	40.5	11.4	14.8	11.5	4.4	0.9	4.4
Venezuela	14.4	1.6	36.2	15.5	8.2	6.5	6.7	1.9	6.7

Table 6.8 Prevalence of early life obesity risk factors in countries from the south region of Latin

	LBW %2000–2002 (WHO 2008)	Stunting <5 %	Breastfeeding at 4 months % (WHO 2008)	Obesity in women % (WHO 2008)
Argentina	7	8.2	25.9	17.5
Bolivia	9	32.5	34	11.2
Brazil	10	7.1	40	13.8
Chile	5	2.1	59.4	29.3
Colombia	9	16.2	34	10.5
Ecuador	16	29	42	14.6
Paraguay	9	10.9	22.1	35.7
Peru	11	31.3	73	23
Uruguay	8	13.9		18
Venezuela	7	12.8	11	

LBW low birth weight

Maternal Obesity

It has been proposed that mothers who are obese at the time of their pregnancy and during the breastfeeding period maintain higher concentrations of glucose and free fatty acids what in turn affects fetal metabolism, tissue growth, and hormonal regulation and possibly inducing lasting epigenetic changes (Lawlor et al. 2008; Plagemann 2008). These changes would define permanent changes in appetite control, neuroendocrine function, fuel metabolism and energy partitioning during early development potentially leading to greater adiposity and risk of obesity in later life. If this hypothesis is substantiated it would imply that the obesity epidemic will progress through generations irrespective of other changes (Ebbeling et al. 2002). This should be a matter of concern for the region considering that presently in all the countries maternal obesity is higher to 10% and in some countries such as in Chile, Paraguay, and Peru is even close to 30% (Table 6.8).

Low Birth Weight and Stunting

Low birth weight (LBW, birth weight below 2,500 g) and stunting (height-for-age below 2 SD of the mean) are still prevalent in some countries of the region, particularly in those that are just initiating the nutrition transition (Table 6.8). Several studies have demonstrated that birth weight is positively associated with body mass index at age 25–30 years (Stein et al. 2005; Victora et al. 2008). However, the association is stronger for lean mass than for fat mass; thus the link with BMI may represent an association between birth weight and lean mass rather than with adiposity. In Brazil, it has been demonstrated that early malnutrition leading to stunted linear growth is accompanied by an increased risk of obesity later on, as consumption of energy dense foods and inactivity during work and leisure have become common (Sawaya and Roberts 2003). In Table 6.8 it is possible to observe that the prevalence of stunting is inversely associated with the degree of development of the country. The highest estimates are observed in countries such as Ecuador, Bolivia and Peru in which almost one third of the children under five years are stunted. Also, besides Brazil, these countries have the highest prevalence of LBW (Table 8).

Conclusions

Obesity is increasing in the whole region at an alarming speed. Obesity constitutes the first nutrition problem in Chile, Argentina and Uruguay (Pisabarro et al. 2000) and one of the most important public health issues in almost all countries of the region. Countries at early stages of the nutrition transition have the challenge of simultaneously dealing with high rates of childhood obesity as well as stunting and LBW. This is compounded to the actual epidemic of obesity in women what further exacerbates the problem (Kain et al. 2003; Uauy et al. 2008). In most of these countries the prevalence of overweight and obesity in children is higher at higher SES but this is likely to change as countries improve their economic conditions (Peña and Bacallao 2000). The increasing urbanization with cities becoming larger and less secure discourages outdoor activities and recreational games for children that have been replaced by more hours watching television. Besides, urban life brings the people closer to fast food, cheaper, palatable and more accessible than traditional food. Thus, as countries move further into the nutrition transition it is likely that childhood obesity will increase if no action is taken. Urgent and effective actions are needed to tackle the obesity epidemic. Comprehensive actions implemented at all levels and with the participation of all sectors of the community are needed to ensure healthy eating and physical activity in children and their families.

References

Albala, C., & Vio, F. (1995). Epidemiological transition in Latin America: the case of Chile. *Public Health, 109(6)*, 431–442.
Albala, C., Vio, F., Kain, J., & Uauy, R. (2001). Nutrition transition in Latin America: the case of Chile. *Nutrition Reviews, 59(6)*, 170–176.
Albala, C., Vio, F., Kain, J., & Uauy, R. (2002). Nutrition transition in Chile: determinants and consequences. *Public Health Nutriton, 5(1A)*, 123–128.
Albala, C., Vio, F., & Uauy, R. (2003). The global burden of nutritional disease: The case of Latin America. In M.J.G. Farthing & D. Mahalanabis (Eds.), *The control of food and fluid intake in health and disease* (Vol. 51). Philadelphia: Lippincott Williams & Wilkins.
Baker, J.L., Olsen, L.W., & Sorensen, T.I. (2007). Childhood body-mass index and the risk of coronary heart disease in adulthood. *New England Journal of Medicine, 357(23)*, 2329–2337.
Bejarano, I., Dipierri, J., & Alfaro, E. (2005). Evolución de la prevalencia de sobrepeso, obesidad y desnutrición en escolares de San Salvador de Jujuy. *Archivos Argentinos de Pediatría, 103(2)*, 101–109.
Bergmann, K.E., Bergmann, R.L., von Kries, R., Böhm, O., Richter, R., Dudenhausen, J.W., & Wahn, U. (2003). Early determinants of childhood overweight and adiposity in a birth cohort study: role of breast-feeding. *International Journal of Obesity and Related Metabolic Disorders, 27(2)*, 162–172.
Bibbins-Domingo, K., Coxson, P., Pletcher, M.J., Lightwood, J., & Goldman, L. (2007). Adolescent overweight and future adult coronary heart disease. *New England Journal of Medicine, 357(23)*, 2371–2379.
Bustos, P., Saez, K., Gleisner, A., Ulloa, N., Calvo, C., & Asenjo, S. (2010). Metabolic syndrome in obese adolescents. *Pediatric Diabetes, 11(1)*, 55–60.
Cole, T.J., Bellizzi, M.C., Flegal, K.M., & Dietz, W.H. (2000). Establishing a standard definition for child overweight and obesity worldwide: international survey. *British Medical Journal, 320(7244)*, 1240–1243.
de Onis, M., & Blossner, M. (2000). Prevalence and trends of overweight among preschool children in developing countries. *American Journal of Clinical Nutrition, 72(4)*, 1032–1039.
Duran, P., Caballero, B., & de Onis, M. (2006). The association between stunting and overweight in Latin American and Caribbean preschool children. *Food and Nutrition Bulletin, 27(4)*, 300–305.
Ebbeling, C.B., Pawlak, D.B., & Ludwig, D.S. (2002). Childhood obesity: public-health crisis, common sense cure. *Lancet, 360(9331)*, 473–482.
OPS Ecuador (2007). *La equidad en la mira: la salud pública del Ecuador durante las últimas décadas* Quito, Ecuador.
Eisenmann, J.C. (2003). Secular trends in variables associated with the metabolic syndrome of North American children and adolescents: a review and synthesis. *American Journal of Human Biology, 15(6)*, 786–794.
Instituto Brasileiro de Geografia e Estatística (2006). *Pesquisa de Orçamentos Familiares 2002-2003. Análise da disponibilidade domiciliar de alimentos e do estado nutricional no Brasil.* Retrieved August, 2009, from http://www.ibge.gov.br/home/estatistica/populacao/condicaodevida/pof/2003medidas/default.shtm.
FAO (2007). Statistical yearbook 2004. Retrieved March, 2009, from http://www.fao.org/statistics/yearbook.
Freedman, D.S., Dietz, W.H., Srinivasan, S.R., & Berenson, G.S. (1999). The relation of overweight to cardiovascular risk factors among children and adolescents: the Bogalusa Heart Study. *Pediatrics, 103(6 Pt 1)*, 1175–1182.
Freedman, D.S., Khan, L.K., Dietz, W.H., Srinivasan, S.R., & Berenson, G.S. (2001). Relationship of childhood obesity to coronary heart disease risk factors in adulthood: the Bogalusa Heart Study. *Pediatrics, 108(3)*, 712–718.
Frenk, J., Frejka, T., Bobadilla, J.L., Stern, C., Lozano, R., Sepúlveda, J., & José, M. (1991). The epidemiologic transition in Latin America. *Boletín de la Oficina Sanitaria Panamericana, 111(6)*, 485–496.
Gutiérrez Sardán, M., Ochoa, L.H., & Castillo Guerra, W. (2004). *Encuesta Nacional de Demografía y Salud 2003 (ENDSA 2003)*. La Paz, Bolivia.
Hamill, P.V., Drizd, T.A., Johnson, C.L., Reed, R.B., Roche, A.F., & Moore, W.M. (1979). Physical growth: National Center for Health Statistics percentiles. *American Journal of Clinical Nutrition, 32(3)*, 607–629.
Instituto colombiano de bienestar familiar (ICBF). (2006). *Encuesta nacional de la situacion nutricional en Colombia 2005*. Bogotá, Colombia.
Instituto Nacional de Nutrición Gobierno Bolivariano de Venezuela. (2005). *Anuario SISVAN 2005*. Retrieved August 2009, from http://www.inn.gob.ve/webinn/.

Junta Nacional de auxilio escolar y becas (JUNAEB) Gobierno de Chile. (2008). *Mapa Nutricional Año 2008.* Retrieved August 2009, from http://www.junaeb.cl/home/mapa_nutricional.htm.

Kain, J., Vio, F., & Albala, C. (2003). Obesity trends and determinant factors in Latin America. *Cadernos de Saúde Pública, 19 Suppl 1,* S77–S86.

Kramer, M.S., & Kakuma, R. (2002). Optimal duration of exclusive breastfeeding. *Cochrane Database of Systematic Reviews* (1), CD003517.

Kuczmarski, R.J., Ogden, C.L., Guo, S.S., Grummer-Strawn, L.M., Flegal, K.M., Mei, Z., Wei, R., Curtin, L.R., Roche, A.F., & Johnson, C.L. (2002). 2000 CDC Growth Charts for the United States: methods and development. *Vital and Health Statistics Series, 11, 246,* 1–190.

Lauer, J.A., Betran, A.P., Victora, C.G., de Onis, M., & Barros, A.J. (2004). Breastfeeding patterns and exposure to suboptimal breastfeeding among children in developing countries: review and analysis of nationally representative surveys. *BMC Medicine, 2,* 26.

Lawlor, D.A., Timpson, N.J., Harbord, R.M., Leary, S., Ness, A., McCarthy, M.I., Frayling, T.M., Hattersley, A.T., & Smith, G.D. (2008). Exploring the developmental overnutrition hypothesis using parental-offspring associations and FTO as an instrumental variable. *PLoS Medicine, 5(3),* e33.

Lobstein, T., Baur, L., & Uauy, R. (2004). Obesity in children and young people: a crisis in public health. *Obesity Reviews, 5 Suppl 1,* 4–104.

Matijasevich, A., Victora, C.G., Golding, J., Barros, F.C., Menezes, A.M., Araujo, C.L., & Smith, G.D. (2009). Socioeconomic position and overweight among adolescents: data from birth cohort studies in Brazil and the UK. *BMC Public Health, 9,* 105.

Ministerio de Salud. Instituto Nacional de Salud (INS), & Centro Nacional de Alimentación y Nutrición (CENAN). (2006). *Encuesta Nacional de Indicadores Nutricionales, Bioquímicas, Socioeconómicos y Culturales Relacionados con las Enfermedades Crónico Degenerativas.* Lima, Peru.

Ministerio de Salud. Presidencia de la Nacion Argentina. (2007). *Encuesta Nacional de Nutricion y Salud.* Buenos Aires, Argentina.

Ministerio de Salud-Instituto Nacional de Estadísticas (2004). *Encuesta Nacional de Salud (ENS) 2003.* Santiago, Chile.

Ministerio de Salud-Instituto Nacional de Estadísticas (2007). *II Encuesta Nacional de Salud y de Calidad de Vida.* Santiago, Chile.

Monteiro, C.A., Moura, E.C., Conde, W.L., & Popkin, B.M. (2004). Socioeconomic status and obesity in adult populations of developing countries: a review. *Bulletin of the World Health Organization, 82(12),* 940–946.

Monteiro, C.A., Conde, W.L., & Popkin, B.M. (2007). Income-specific trends in obesity in Brazil: 1975-2003. *American Journal of Public Health, 97(10),* 1808–1812.

Must, A., Dallal, G.E., & Dietz, W.H. (1991). Reference data for obesity: 85th and 95th percentiles of body mass index (wt/ht2) and triceps skinfold thickness. *American Journal of Clinical Nutrition, 53(4),* 839–846.

Nader, P.R., O'Brien, M., Houts, R., Bradley, R., Belsky, J., Crosnoe, R., Friedman, S., Mei, Z., & Susman, E.J. (2006). Identifying risk for obesity in early childhood. *Pediatrics, 118(3),* e594–601.

PAHO (2007). Health in the Americas 2007. Retrieved March 2009, from http://new.paho.org/hq/index.php?option=com_content&task=view&id=44&Itemid=191.

Pajuelo, J. (2003). El sobrepeso y la obesidad en adolescentes. *Diagnostico, 42(1),* 17–22.

Pajuelo, J., Villanueva, M., & Chávez, J. (2000). La Desnutrición Crónica, el Sobrepeso y la Obesidad en Niños de Areas Rurales del Perú. *Anales de la Facultad de Medicina, 61(3),* 201–206.

Pajuelo, J., Morales, H., & Novak, A. (2001). La desnutrición crónica, el sobrepeso y obesidad en niños de 6 a 9 años en áreas urbanas del Perú. *Diagnóstico (Perú), 40(4),* 202–209.

Pajuelo, J., Canchari, E., Carrera, J., & Leguia, D. (2004). La circunferencia de la cintura en niños con sobrepeso y obesidad. *Anales de la Facultad de Medicina, 65(3),* 167–171.

Peña, M., & Bacallao, J. (2000). Obesidad y pobreza: un desafío pendiente en Chile (Obesity and poverty: a pending challenge in Chile). In Panamerican Health Organization (PAHO) (Ed.), *Obesity and poverty. A new Public Health challenge* (Vol. Scientific Publication No. 576). Washington, DC: Panamerican Health Organization (PAHO).

Perez-Cueto, F.J., Botti, A.B., & Verbeke, W. (2009). Prevalence of overweight in Bolivia: data on women and adolescents. *Obesity Reviews, 10(4),* 373–377.

Pisabarro, R., Irrazábal, E., & Recalde, A. (2000). Primera encuesta nacional de sobrepeso y obesidad (ENSO I). *Revista Médica del Uruguay, 16,* 31–38.

Plagemann, A. (2008). A matter of insulin: developmental programming of body weight regulation. *Journal of Maternal-Fetal and Neonatal Medicine, 21(3),* 143–148.

Poletti, O., & Barrios, L. (2007). Obesidad e hipertensión arterial en escolares de la ciudad de Corrientes, Argentina. *Archivos Argentinos de Pediatria, 105(4),* 293–298.

Popkin, B.M. (1993). Nutritional patterns and transitions. *Population Development Review, 19,* 138–157.

Popkin, B.M. (1994). The nutrition transition in low-income countries: an emerging crisis. *Nutrition Reviews, 52(9),* 285–298.

Powers, K.A., Rehrig, S.T., & Jones, D.B. (2007). Financial impact of obesity and bariatric surgery. *Medical Clinics of North America, 91(3)*, 321–338, ix.

Sawaya, A.L., & Roberts, S. (2003). Stunting and future risk of obesity: principal physiological mechanisms. *Cadernos de Saúde Pública, 19 Suppl 1*, S21–S28.

Sawaya, A.L., Martins, P., Hoffman, D., & Roberts, S.B. (2003). The link between childhood undernutrition and risk of chronic diseases in adulthood: a case study of Brazil. *Nutrition Reviews, 61(5 Pt 1)*, 168–175.

Scanferla de Siqueira, R., & Monteiro, C.A. (2007). Breastfeeding and obesity in school-age children from families of high socioeconomic status. *Revista de Saúde Pública, 41(1)*, 5–12.

Schwartz, M.B., & Puhl, R. (2003). Childhood obesity: a societal problem to solve. *Obesity Reviews, 4(1)*, 57–71.

Simon, V.G., Souza, J.M., & Souza, S.B. (2009). Breastfeeding, complementary feeding, overweight and obesity in pre-school children. *Revista de Saúde Pública, 43(1)*, 60–69.

Sistema de Vigilancia Nutricional (SISVAN) 2008. (2009). Asuncion, Paraguay.

Srinivasan, S.R., Myers, L., & Berenson, G.S. (2002). Predictability of childhood adiposity and insulin for developing insulin resistance syndrome (syndrome X) in young adulthood: the Bogalusa Heart Study. *Diabetes, 51(1)*, 204–209.

Stein, A.D., Thompson, A.M., & Waters, A. (2005). Childhood growth and chronic disease: evidence from countries undergoing the nutrition transition. *Maternal and Child Nutrition, 1(3)*, 177–184.

Triches, R.M., & Giugliani, E.R. (2005). Obesity, eating habits and nutritional knowledge among school children. *Revista de Saúde Pública, 39(4)*, 541–547.

Uauy, R., Atalah, E., & Kain, J. (2001). The nutrition transition: New nutritional influences on child growth. In R. Martorell & F. Haschke (Eds.), *Nutrition and growth* (Vol. 47). Philadelphia: Lippincott Williams & Wilkins.

Uauy, R., Kain, J., Mericq, V., Rojas, J., & Corvalan, C. (2008). Nutrition, child growth, and chronic disease prevention. *Annals of Medicine, 40(1)*, 11–20.

UNDP (UN development programme) (2007). Human development index trends 2007. Retrieved March 2009, from http://origin-hdr.undp.org/en/media/hdr_20072008_tables.pdf.

UNDP (UN development programme) (2008). Human development indices: A statistical update. Retrieved March 2009, from http://hdr.undp.org/en/statistics.

Victora, C.G., Adair, L., Fall, C., Hallal, P.C., Martorell, R., Richter, L., Sachdev, H.S., & Maternal and Child Undernutrion Study Goup. (2008). Maternal and child undernutrition: consequences for adult health and human capital. *Lancet, 371(9609)*, 340–357.

Vio, F., Albala, C., & Kain, J. (2008). Nutrition transition in Chile revisited: mid-term evaluation of obesity goals for the period 2000-2010. *Public Health Nutrition, 11(4)*, 405–412.

Whitaker, R.C., Wright, J.A., Pepe, M.S., Seidel, K.D., & Dietz, W.H. (1997). Predicting obesity in young adulthood from childhood and parental obesity. *New England Journal of Medicine, 337(13)*, 869–873.

WHO/PAHO (2007). *The regional strategy on an integrated approach to the prevention and control of chronic diseases including diet, physical activity, and health.* Retrieved March 2009, from http://www.paho.org/English/AD/dpc/nc/reg-strat-cncds.pdf.

World Health Organization (WHO) (2002). *Sedentary lifestyle: A Global Public Health Problem.* Geneva:WHO.

World Health Organization (WHO) (2003). *Diet, nutrition and the prevention of chronic diseases. Report of a joint WHO/FAO Expert Consultation.* WHO Technical Report Series no. 916. Geneva: WHO.

World Health Organization (WHO) (2006). *WHO child growth standards: Methods and development: Length/height-for-age, weight-for-age, weight-for-length, weight-for-height and body mass index-for-age.* Geneva: WHO.

World Health Organization (WHO) (2008). *World health statistics 2008. Part 2: Global indicators.* Retrieved March 2009, from www.who.int/whosis/whostat.

World Health Organization (WHO) (2009a). *Global database on child growth and malnutrition.* Retrieved March 2009, from http://www.who.int/nutgrowthdb/database/en/.

World Health Organization (WHO) (2009b). *WHO global data bank on breastfeeding and complementary feeding.* Retrieved March 2009, from http://www.who.int/research/iycf/bfcf/.

Yépez, R. (2005). La obesidad en el Ecuador en tempranas edades de la vida. *Revista de la Facultad de Ciencias Médicas, 30*, 20–24.

Yépez, R., Carrasco, F., & Baldeon M.E. (2008). Prevalence of overweight and obesity in Ecuadorian adolescent students in the urban area. *Archivos Latinoamericanos de Nutrición, 58(2)*, 139–143.

Chapter 7
Epidemiology of Obesity in Children and Adolescents in Australia, New Zealand and the Pacific Region

Kylie Hesketh, Karen Campbell, and Rachael Taylor

Introduction

Australia, New Zealand and the Pacific Region define a large area in the southern hemisphere comprising multiple countries with disparate characteristics. Defining the Pacific Region is challenging as there is no consensus on which countries are included. Thus, the World Bank includes The Federated States of Micronesia, Fiji, Kiribati, Palau, the Republic of the Marshall Islands, Samoa, the Solomon Islands, Tonga and Vanuatu (The World Bank 2009). According to the World Health Organization (World Health Organisation 2009), the Western Pacific Region in addition to the aforementioned countries also includes Cook Islands, Nauru, Niue, Palau Papua and Papua New Guinea, and additional countries which fit into the Asia Pacific Region, not included in this chapter. While Australia and New Zealand are relatively wealthy, developed countries, the countries encompassing the Pacific Region are more socio-economically diverse. In contrast cultural and ethnic diversity is high in Australia and New Zealand while countries in the Pacific Region, with the exception of Fiji, tend to be relatively ethnically homogeneous. A further distinguishing feature of the areas covered in this chapter is political stability, which is high in Australia and New Zealand but less so in many of the countries encompassing the Pacific Region.

The epidemiology of overweight and obesity is well described in Australia and New Zealand. This is not the case in the Pacific Region, with no nationally representative data available for many of the smaller Pacific Region countries. Similar patterns of obesity prevalence have been documented in Australia and New Zealand over recent decades, indicating that more than half the adult population and approximately one quarter of the child and adolescent populations are currently overweight or obese. Secular trend data suggest these rates of overweight and obesity have increased over recent decades. Obesity prevalence amongst Pacific Region populations tends to be higher than in Australia and New Zealand, but coexists with issues of undernutrition, particularly amongst children.

While many studies conducted in Australia and New Zealand describe the prevalence of overweight and obesity and associations with potential risk factors, studies involving nationally representative samples in these countries are sparse with no systematic regular national data collection in Australia or New Zealand. The available nationally representative studies investigating the prevalence of overweight and obesity provide limited information on associations with potential risk factors.

K. Hesketh (✉) and K. Campbell
Centre for Physical Activity and Nutrition Research, Deakin University, Melbourne, Australia
e-mail: kylie.hesketh@deakin.edu.au

R. Taylor
Edgar National Centre for Diabetes Research, University of Otago, Dunedin, New Zealand

L.A. Moreno et al. (eds.), *Epidemiology of Obesity in Children and Adolescents*,
Springer Series on Epidemiology and Public Health 2, DOI 10.1007/978-1-4419-6039-9_7,
© Springer Science+Business Media, LLC 2011

This chapter describes evidence from nationally representative studies on the prevalence of overweight and obesity in children and youth in Australia and New Zealand and, where available, provides information on associations with potential risk factors. With no nationally representative data available for countries within the Pacific Region, estimates from large scale prevalence studies are reported.

Geographic Area

The geographic area encompassing Australia, New Zealand and the Pacific Region consists of more than 85 million square kilometers of land mass. Each country within this region is an island, or series of islands. Australia makes up the vast majority of the total land mass, although much of the land area is sparsely populated, with most of the population inhabiting the coastal areas. The combined population of Australia, New Zealand and the Pacific Region exceeds 33 million people. Approximately two thirds of this total population inhabits Australia (>20 million), with the next most populous country being Papua New Guinea (>6 million) followed by New Zealand (>4 million) (see Table 7.1).

This is a culturally diverse region. Within Australia 2.5% of the population are indigenous (Aboriginal or Torres Strait Islander) and 25% of the population have recently immigrated, mainly from Europe or Asia. The remaining majority of inhabitants are Australian born but represent the cultural diversity of a predominantly immigrant nation, with a high proportion of second-, third- and subsequent-generation Australians of predominantly European background (Australian Bureau of Statistics 2006). This cultural diversity has implications for the prevalence of overweight and obesity, with the rates of these conditions known to be higher amongst certain cultural and ethnic groups, for example, higher amongst Mediterranean peoples who are populous in Australia. New Zealand has a much larger indigenous population than Australia. More than one quarter of the New Zealand population identify as either Maori or Pacific, with the remainder predominantly of European or Asian descent. While information is available for only a few Pacific Region countries, the majority of these are primarily inhabited by indigenous peoples: Tonga 98% indigenous (Tonga Department of Statistics 2006); Cook Islands 90% indigenous (Secretariat of the Pacific Community Noumea New Caledonia 1999); Vanuatu 99% indigenous (Vanuatu National Statistics Office 1999). The exception is Fiji where 57% of the population are indigenous, 38% Indian and the remainder born in other countries (Fiji Islands Bureau of Statistics 2007).

Disparities in wealth and health across the countries comprising these regions are highlighted by rankings on the Human Development Index (HDI), which provides a composite measure of the achievements of a country on three broad dimensions of human development. These dimensions are: (1) living a long and healthy life, as measured by life expectancy at birth; (2) knowledge or education, as measured by adult literacy rates and gross primary, secondary and tertiary level education enrolment; and (3) standard of living, as measured by gross domestic product per capita in purchasing power parity. Australia ranks highest in the region and second internationally, with New Zealand also ranked amongst the high human development countries (20th internationally). Only six Pacific Region Countries have a ranking on the HDI (ranging from 94th to 148th internationally), all classified as having medium human development. Thus while Australia and New Zealand are clearly classified as developed nations, many of the countries comprised within the Pacific Region fall within the classification of developing nations.

The per capita gross domestic product of Australia ($38,100) and New Zealand ($27,900) far exceeds that of any of the Pacific Region countries ($1,900 to $9,100). This is reflected in general health statistics, with infant mortality of less than 5 per 1,000 live births in Australia and New Zealand, compared with much higher rates in most of the Pacific Region countries. The highest infant mortality rates are recorded in Papua New Guinea, with in excess of 45 per 1,000 live births.

Table 7.1 Demographics table

	Area (Km²)[a]	Population (N)*	Population <15 years (%)	GDP per capita ($)***[a]	Human development index ranking[b]	Life expectancy at birth (years)[a]	Crude birth rate (per 1,000 population)***[a]	Infant mortality (per 1,000 live births)[a]
Australia	7,686,850	20,700,000[c]	19.6[d]	$38,100	2	82.0	12.6	4.8
New Zealand	268,680	4,143,279[e]	20.7[a]	$27,900	20	80.4	14.1	4.9
Pacific region								
Cook Islands	236.7	11,870[a]	27.1[a]	$9,100	–	74.2	16.7	16.9
Fiji	18,270	944,720[a]	30.3[a]	$3,900	108	70.7	22.2	11.6
Kiribati	811	112,850[a]	37.6[a]	$3,200	–	63.2	30.3	43.5
Marshall Islands	181.3	64,522[a]	38.6[a]	$2,500	–	71.2	31.5	25.5
Micronesia	702	107,434[a]	34.8[a]	$2,200	–	70.9	23.7	26.1
Nauru	21	14,019[a]	34.7[a]	$5,000	–	64.2	24.3	9.3
Palau	458	20,796[a]	22.9[a]	$8,100	–	71.2	17.4	13.1
Papua New Guinea	462,840	6,057,263[a]	36.9[a]	$2,200	148	66.3	28.1	45.2
Samoa	2,944	219,998[a]	37.6[a]	$4,900	94	71.9	28.2	24.2
Solomon Islands	28,450	595,613[a]	39.5[a]	$1,900	135	73.7	28.5	19.0
Tonga	748	120,898[a]	32.8[a]	$4,600	99	70.7	21.8	11.6
Vanuatu	12,200	218,519[a]	30.7[a]	$4,600	126	64.0	22.0	7.6

*Australia: June 2006 estimate; New Zealand: March 2006 estimate; Pacific Region: July 2009 estimate; **2008 estimate
[a](Central Intelligence Agency 2009)
[b](United Nations Development Programme 2009)
[c](Australian Bureau of Statistics 2006)
[d](Australian Bureau of Statistics 2005)
[e](Statistics New Zealand 2006)

These trends in infant mortality are also reflected in life expectancies across countries. In both Australia and New Zealand the average life expectancy of the population exceeds 80 years. This is notably higher than in the Pacific Region countries where average life expectancy ranges between 63 and 74 years. Crude birth rates for Australia and New Zealand (12.6 and 14.1 per 1,000 population, respectively) are lower than for the Pacific Region countries (range: 16.7 to 31.5 per 1,000 population). As would be expected with higher life expectancy and lower birth rates, the number of youth (aged under 15 years) as a proportion of the total population is lower in Australia (19.6%) and New Zealand (20.7%) than in Pacific Region countries (22.9 to 39.5%).

Prevalence of Overweight and Obesity

For all studies reported here, overweight and obesity are defined based on the age- and sex-specific body mass index cut-off points recommended by the International Obesity Task Force (Cole et al. 2000). Table 7.2 provides an overview and comparison of the prevalence of overweight and obesity by different countries in the region.

Australia

The most recent nationally representative data on the prevalence of overweight and obesity in Australian children and adolescents come from three recent population-based studies: the 2007–2008 National Health Survey (Australian Bureau of Statistics 2009) which included children aged 5–17 years of age; the 2007 Australian National Children's Nutrition and Physical Activity Survey (Commonwealth of Australia 2008) which involved children 2–16 years of age; and the Longitudinal Study of Australian Children (LSAC) (Soloff et al. 2005) which involved children 4–5 years of age.

The 2007–2008 National Health Survey was conducted between August 2007 and June 2008. It is the seventh in a series of national surveys assessing the health of Australians which have been conducted by the Australian Bureau of Statistics since 1977, but the first to collect anthropometric data on children. This survey collected information on a broad range of health-related issues from residents in more than 15,800 randomly selected private homes across Australia. Within each of these homes, one adult (aged 18 years and over) and one child were randomly selected for inclusion in the survey. This sample closely approximated the socio-demographic characteristics of the wider population, however, population weights were applied to the data.

Table 7.2 Prevalence of overweight and obesity by country

Classification	Australia[a]		New Zealand[b]		Fiji[c]		Tonga[c]	
	Boys	Girls	Boys	Girls	Boys	Girls	Boys	Girls
Thin	5	5	2	3	21	17	1	1
Healthy weight	73	72	69	67	62	58	67	46
Overweight	17	18	21	21	13	20	24	38
Obese	5	6	8	9	4	6	7	15[d]

[a]2007 Australian National Children's Nutrition and Physical Activity Survey data for 2–16 year old children (Commonwealth of Australia 2008). *Note: while 2007/2008 National Health Survey provides slightly more recent data, it does not present data stratified by sex and therefore is not included in this table*
[b]2006/2007 New Zealand National Health Survey data for 2–14 year old children (Ministry of Health 2008)
[c]2005/2006 Obesity Prevention in Communities Study data for 12–18 year old children (Utter et al. 2008)
[d]Significant difference between boys (7%) and girls (15%)

The 2007 Australian National Children's Nutrition and Physical Activity Survey was conducted between February and August 2007 and involved a total of 4,487 children aged 2–16 years from across Australia. Households containing children 2–16 years of age were randomly sampled using random digit dialing. One child from each eligible household participated. Approximately 500 girls and 500 boys were sampled from each of the age groups: 2–3, 4–8, 9–13, 14–16 years. In addition, one state (South Australia) funded the collection of data from an additional 400 children in that state. This survey was limited by the fact that the sample was not representative of the Australian population in terms of cultural diversity or socio-economic diversity. The resultant sample contained a lower proportion of non-Australian born caregivers (parents or guardians), families speaking a language other than English at home, and children of indigenous background, than were reported in 2006 national Census data (Australian Bureau of Statistics 2006). In addition, the sample appeared to underrepresent socio-economically disadvantaged families by having a substantially higher proportion of tertiary educated caregivers and households in the higher income brackets than would be expected based on national Census data. Population weights were applied to data from the 2007 Australian National Children's Nutrition and Physical Activity Survey to minimize the impact of these sampling biases.

The first wave of the Longitudinal Study of Australian Children (LSAC) was conducted between March and November 2004. It collected data from two cohorts of children: 5,107 infants aged 3–19 months (not discussed here as overweight and obesity prevalence was not investigated in this cohort) and 4,983 children aged 4–5 years (59% of those selected for the sample participated). Children were sampled from 311 postal areas across Australia that were randomly selected with probability proportional to size, stratified by state or territory and by a capital city vs. rest of state dichotomy. An average of 40 children were selected from each postal area in larger states and an average of 20 children selected from postal areas in smaller states and territories. The resultant sample was broadly representative of the Australian population although children whose parents had completed secondary school were slightly overrepresented and children living in single parent families were underrepresented. Population weights were applied to the data.

Findings from the 2007 to 2008 National Health Survey

Height, weight and waist circumference data were collected from children in the 2007–2008 National Health Survey by trained assessors during face-to-face interviews in the home. National prevalence estimates of overweight and obesity, stratified by age groupings, are presented in Table 7.3. Proportions of children overweight and obese in this cohort were not presented stratified by sex and age concurrently, although child and adolescent datas were presented by sex. Overall, 17% of 5–17 year old children were classified as overweight and 8% as obese. Proportions of children classified above the healthy weight range (i.e. overweight or obese) were similar for boys (26%) and girls (24%), however, the proportion of boys who were obese (10%) was higher than the proportion of girls (6%) (Australian Bureau of Statistics, 2009). The prevalence of overweight and obesity increased across the age groupings included in the study. While waist circumference was measured in this survey, crude average waist circumference measurements were reported which do not allow classification of overweight and obesity.

Findings from the 2007 Australian National Children's Nutrition and Physical Activity Survey

Height, weight and waist circumference data were collected from children in the 2007 Australian National Children's Nutrition and Physical Activity Survey by trained assessors during face-to-face

Table 7.3 Prevalence (%)[a] of Australian children classified as overweight and obese[b] by age[c] from the 2007 to 2008 National Health Survey

	Age group (years)				
	5–7	8–11	12–15	16–17	Total
Overweight (%)	14	16	20	19	17
Obese (%)	8[d]	7	7	13	8
Total number of children ('000)	566	737	742	365	2,410

Adapted from the 2007/2008 National Health Survey (Australian Bureau of Statistics 2009)
[a]Population weights applied
[b]Classified using International Obesity Task Force cut-off points (Cole et al. 2000)
[c]Data not available stratified by sex
[d]Estimate has a relative standard error of 25 to 50% and should be used with caution

Table 7.4 Prevalence (%)[a] of Australian children classified as overweight and obese[b] by age and sex from the 2007 Australian National Children's Nutrition and Physical Activity Survey

	Age group (years)				
	2–3	4–8	9–13	14–16	Total
Boys					
Overweight	17	13	18	19	17
Obese	4	5	7	6	5
Waist-to-height ratio >50%	n/a	16[c]	18	13	n/a
Girls					
Overweight	14	15	23	16	18
Obese	4	6	7	7	6
Waist-to-height ratio >50%	n/a	14[c]	18	13	n/a

Adapted from the 2007 Australian National Children's Nutrition and Physical Activity Survey (Commonwealth of Australia 2008)
n/a not applicable
[a]Population weights applied
[b]Classified using International Obesity Task Force cut-off points (Cole et al. 2000)
[c]Data for 5–8 year olds; there are no guidelines for defining overweight by waist girth for those younger than 5 years of age

interviews in the home. Additional information on food intake and activity levels was collected during a subsequent telephone interview. National prevalence estimates of overweight and obesity, for boys and girls in each of the age groups sampled are presented in Table 7.4. Overall, approximately 5% of Australian children were found to be underweight, 17% overweight and 6% obese. With an additional 5% classified as thin (underweight), almost three quarters (72%) of these children were of a healthy weight (Commonwealth of Australia 2008).

While there is less agreement on appropriate cut-off points to define overweight and obesity using waist circumference measurements, a commonly applied definition of excess weight assessed by waist circumference for those aged 5 years and above is a waist-to-height ratio greater than 50% (Ashwell and Hsieh 2005). This is the definition applied in the 2007 Australian National Children's Nutrition and Physical Activity Survey. Proportion of children exceeding 50% waist-to-height ratio are presented for boys and girls in each of the sampled age groups in Table 7.4. Note that the proportion exceeding the ratio is not presented for the 2–4 years age groups as there is no agreed cut-off point for young children. For Australian children aged 5–16 years, approximately one sixth had waist circumferences which exceeded the 50% waist-to-height ratio.

Significant inverse associations between physical activity level (measured by a 4-day computer assisted activity recall) and weight category were found for children aged 9–16 years. Physical activity level was not assessed for younger children. Children aged 9–16 years who were thin (underweight) or obese tended to report lower physical activity levels than children who were classified as being of healthy weight. Physical activity levels for children who were overweight were similar to levels for children who were classified as being of healthy weight. Reporting biases may have influenced this subjective physical activity data.

Associations between total energy intake (measured by food recall using a three pass 24 h recall interview methodology) and weight category were found for 2–16 year old children. Obese children tended to report lower energy intakes than healthy weight children. This may reflect reporting biases or methodological issues inherent in the use of a single day's food recall. No differences were noted in energy intake between healthy weight children and either thin (underweight) or overweight children.

Findings from the Longitudinal Study of Australian Children (2004)

Height, weight and waist circumference were collected from children in the Longitudinal Study of Australian Children by trained assessors during face-to-face interviews in the home. Prevalence estimates for overweight and obesity in these 4–5 year old children were 15% and 6% respectively (Wake et al. 2007). Prevalence was higher for girls (17% overweight and 6% obese) than boys (14% overweight and 5% obese). The prevalence of overweight and obesity was higher amongst the 181 children of Aboriginal or Torres Strait Islander (indigenous) descent included in the sample (17% overweight and 11% obese) and also amongst the 613 children who spoke a language other than English at home (17% overweight and 8% obese). There was evidence of a socio-economic gradient in overweight and obesity prevalence. Prevalence of overweight and obesity by maternal education level (one measure of socio-economic position) is presented in Table 7.5. Similar results were seen for other measures of socio-economic position. Children of lower socio-economic position, as indicated independently by each of maternal education, family income, postal area level socio-economic disadvantage (Socio-Economic Indices For Areas (SEIFA)), and highest family occupation class, had higher odds of being classified as overweight or obese. With no agreed definition of excess weight by waist circumference, average crude waist circumference measurement for 4–5 year old children was reported in the Longitudinal Study of Australian Children. The average waist circumference measurement was 54.6 cm, with average measurements being almost identical for boys and girls.

Table 7.5 Prevalence (%)[a] of Australian 4–5 year old children classified as overweight and obese[b] by maternal education category (measure of socio-economic position) from the Longitudinal Study of Australian Children (2004)

| | Maternal education level | | | |
	Did not complete secondary school	Completed secondary school	Tertiary education	Total
Overweight	16	15	14	15
Obese	6	5	5	6

Adapted from the Longitudinal Study of Australian Children (2004) (Wake et al. 2007)
[a]Population weights applied
[b]Classified using International Obesity Task Force cut-off points (Cole et al. 2000)

Secular Trends

Australia does not have a regular national monitoring or surveillance system for childhood overweight and obesity and does not regularly collect national data on body mass index, diet or activity levels in children and adolescents. Prior to the 2007 Australian National Children's Nutrition and Physical Activity Survey and the 2007–2008 National Health Survey, a national survey including assessment of children's adiposity had not been conducted for over a decade, since the 1995 National Nutrition Survey, and prior to that in the 1985 Australian Health and Fitness Survey. While the sampling frames of these surveys were quite different, all had trained assessors measure height and weight from which body mass index was derived and provide some evidence of secular trends in weight status in the Australian child and adolescent population (see Table 7.6).

Sampling methodologies of the 2007 Australian National Children's Nutrition and Physical Activity Survey and the 2009–2008 National Health Survey are reported above. Sampling for the 1995 National Nutrition Survey involved a systematically selected subsample of private homes involved in the 1995 National Health Survey. Data collection from 2,962 2–18 year old children occurred between February 1995 and March 1996. Sampling for the 1985 Australian Health and Fitness Survey involved a random sample of 109 schools selected proportional to total number of children enrolled, followed by a systematic selection of 15 students within each age and sex category. Data collection from 8,492 7–15 year old children occurred between May and October 1985.

Table 7.6 Secular trends in prevalence of overweight and obesity in Australian children across different studies from 1985 to 2007

		Age group (years)				
		2–3	4–6	7–11	12–15	16–18
Boys						
1985 Australian Health and Fitness Survey	Overweight			9.7	8.8	
	Obese			1.5	1.9	
1995 National Nutrition Survey	Overweight	14.6	10.4	11.6	20.0	18.9
	Obese	2.4	3.0	3.7	6.1	6.8
2005 Longitudinal Study of Australian Children	Overweight		14			
	Obese		5			
2007 Australian National Children's Nutrition and Physical Activity Survey[a]	Overweight	17	13	18	19	
	Obese	4	5	7	6	
2007–2008 National Health Survey[b]	Overweight			15	19	
	Obese			8	13	
Girls						
1985 Australian Health and Fitness Survey	Overweight			11.0	10.1	
	Obese			1.9	1.3	
1995 National Nutrition Survey	Overweight	16.5	15.3	17.2	14.5	14.7
	Obese	6.1	4.2	6.3	4.4	6.0
2005 Longitudinal Study of Australian Children	Overweight		17			
	Obese		6			
2007 Australian National Children's Nutrition and Physical Activity Survey	Overweight	14.0	15.0	23.0	16.0	
	Obese	4.0	6.0	7.0	7.0	
2007–2008 National Health Survey	Overweight			17	20	
	Obese			6	6	

[a]Actual age ranges for data in this study are 2–3 years, 4–8 years, 9–13 years, 14–16 years
[b]Actual age ranges for data in this study are 5–12 years, 13–17 years

For boys, secular increases in the prevalence of overweight and obesity were observed across the 1995 and 2007 national surveys for 2–3 and 4–6 year old children (4–8 years in 2007 survey). For girls, there was no clear secular trend amongst these age groups. Data were not available for younger children in the 1985 dataset.

Substantial increases in the prevalence of overweight and obesity were observed in 7–11 year old children (9–13 years in 2007 survey) across 1985, 1995, and 2007 in boys and girls. Increases were also seen across this 12 year period in 12–15 year old girls (14–16 year olds in 2007), although for boys substantial increases in overweight and obesity prevalence observed between 1985 and 1995 did not appear to continue, with suggestion of a plateau between 1995 and 2007.

While differences in study methodologies and sample representativeness between the four national surveys makes conclusions on secular trends in national overweight and obesity prevalence difficult, it is clear that the prevalence of overweight and obesity in Australian children and adolescents has increased over recent decades.

New Zealand

Data on the prevalence of overweight and obesity in New Zealand children are available from two recent nationally representative samples; the 2002 national Children's Nutrition Survey (Ministry of Health 2003) and the 2006/2007 New Zealand Health Survey (Ministry of Health 2008). Although only 22% of New Zealand children identify as Maori and 10% as Pacific Islanders (Statistics New Zealand 2002), these groups were over-sampled in both surveys to ensure that robust national estimates could be obtained for key outcomes (Ministry of Health 2008). The Children's Nutrition Survey used a two-stage sampling frame to recruit approximately equal numbers of children aged 5–14 years into each of three main ethnic groups: Maori, Pacific, and New Zealand European & Others, and trained interviewers completed all anthropometric measurements at school. The New Zealand Health Survey used a multi-stage, stratified, probability proportionate to size design to recruit children aged 2–14 years, through home visits. In this latter survey, Asian peoples were included as a separate fourth ethnic group, due to recent rapid increases in this sector of the New Zealand population. Ethnicity was self-reported in both samples, using national Census questions.

Table 7.7 reports the prevalence of overweight and obesity according to age and sex from the more recent New Zealand Health Survey (Ministry of Health 2008). Overall, one in five children were overweight (21%) and a further one in twelve (8%) were obese. Sexual dimorphism in the prevalence of overweight or obesity was not apparent, with no sex differences in prevalence, adjusted for age.

Marked differences in the prevalence of overweight and obesity were apparent by ethnic group (Table 7.8). Approximately one in twenty Asian or European/other children were obese, whereas obesity was considerably more common in Maori (12%) and especially Pacific (23%) children. Comparable patterns were observed in the prevalence of overweight. One in six Asian and one in five European/other children had BMI (body mass index) values indicating that they were overweight, compared with one in four Maori and as many as one in three Pacific children. Standardized rate ratios indicate that Pacific children were greater than 2.5 times more likely to be obese than the total population, and Maori children approximately 1.5 times more likely (Ministry of Health 2008). By contrast, Asian (0.71) and European/other (0.67) children were less likely to be obese than the total population of children aged 2–14 years.

These ethnic disparities are even more marked when investigating the prevalence of extreme obesity, defined as a BMI greater than the 99th age and sex-specific percentile of US reference data (Kuczmarski et al. 2000). Based on the Children's Nutrition Survey data of children aged 5–14 years (Ministry of Health 2003), 10% of Pacific females and 11% of Pacific males had extreme obesity

Table 7.7 Unadjusted prevalence (%) of New Zealand children classified as overweight and obese[a] by age and sex from the 2006/2007 New Zealand Health Survey

| | Age group (years) | | | |
	2–4	5–9	10–14	Total
Boys				
Overweight	22	20	21	21
Obese	8	8	8	8
Girls				
Overweight	26	19	21	21
Obese	9	8	9	9

Adapted from the New Zealand Health Survey (Ministry of Health 2008)
[a]Classified using International Obesity Task Force cut-off points (Cole et al. 2000)

Table 7.8 Age-standardized prevalence (%) of New Zealand children classified as overweight and obese[a] by ethnic group and sex from the 2006/2007 New Zealand Health Survey

| | Ethnic group | | | |
	Maori	Pacific	Asian	European/other
Boys				
Overweight	25	31	17	19
Obese	11	21	5	6
Girls				
Overweight	26	32	12	20
Obese	12	26	7	5

Adapted from the New Zealand Health Survey (Ministry of Health 2008)
[a]Classified using International Obesity Task Force cut-off points (Cole et al. 2000)

(Goulding et al. 2007). While the level of extreme obesity was still of concern in Maori children (4% in girls, 6% in boys), equating to another 6,000 children nationwide, the prevalence was considerably reduced compared with Pacific youth. Finally, extreme obesity was rare in New Zealand European & Other children, being less than 1% in both sexes (Goulding et al. 2007).

Social class is related to obesity in New Zealand children (Ministry of Health 2008), as measured using the New Zealand Deprivation Index (NZDep2006) (Salmond et al. 2007). NZDep2006 shows a graduated scale of deprivation based on variables that reflect eight types of deprivation (including income, home ownership, family support, employment, qualifications and transport). A score of one represents the least deprived 10% of areas (rather than individuals) while ten is given to the most deprived 10% of areas (Salmond et al. 2007). Data from the 2006/2007 New Zealand Health Survey show that children living in areas of high neighborhood deprivation (NZDep2006 quintile 5) were significantly more likely ($P < 0.05$) to be obese than children living in all other areas (quintiles 1–4), in both sexes. Fourteen percent of boys and 16% of girls in the most deprived quintile were obese compared with 5–6% of children in the least deprived areas (adjusted for age). It is difficult to tease out the relative influence of ethnicity and deprivation in these statistics, given that children from the ethnic minorities are over represented in the more deprived areas (Table 7.9).

Little data are available examining the links between behavioral indicators of energy balance and overweight in nationally representative samples of New Zealand children. Analyses utilizing the Children's Nutrition Survey data (Ministry of Health 2003) have investigated several potential dietary and lifestyle determinants of body weight in children aged 5–14 years (Utter et al. 2007).

Table 7.9 Age-standardized prevalence (%) of New Zealand children classified as overweight and obese[a] by area-level deprivation from the 2006/2007 New Zealand Health Survey

	Quintile of New Zealand deprivation index				
	1	2	3	4	5
	Least deprived				Most deprived
Boys	5	5	8	8	14
Girls	6	5	7	9	16
Total	6	5	7	9	15

Adapted from the New Zealand Health Survey (Ministry of Health 2008)

[a]Classified using International Obesity Task Force cut-off points (Cole et al. 2000)

After controlling for demographics, mean BMI was significantly higher in children who had higher sweet beverage intakes ($P=0.03$), those who bought school food from the dairy/takeaway shops more often ($P=0.02$), and in children who skipped breakfast ($P<0.01$). Similarly, increased television viewing ($P=0.02$) or decreased participation in physical activity ($P=0.04$) were associated with higher BMI values. After controlling for all other behaviors in the model, only buying school food from the dairy/takeaway shops and skipping breakfast remained significantly associated with BMI.

Secular Trends

It is widely acknowledged that the prevalence of obesity has increased dramatically in children throughout the world over the past 10 to 20 years (Lobstein et al. 2004). Suitable data are not available within New Zealand to inform discussions regarding secular trends prior to the first national survey in children in 2002 (Ministry of Health 2003). By this time much of the increase in prevalence in overweight and obesity had already been observed internationally (see remaining chapters in Part I of this book). Examination of our two national prevalence surveys (Ministry of Health 2003, 2008) demonstrates that the prevalence of obesity in children did not change between 2002 and 2006/2007 in either sex; 8% of boys aged 5–14 years were classified as obese at both time points, whereas in girls, 10% were obese in 2002 compared with 9% in the latest survey (Table 7.10).

Pacific Region

The capacity to report the prevalence of overweight and obesity in children and adolescents in the Pacific countries is very limited, with data only available for Fiji and Tonga. These data were collected as part of the Obesity Prevention In Communities project (OPIC) commenced in 2005 (Utter et al. 2008). The primary aim of the OPIC study is to evaluate the effectiveness of community-based obesity prevention strategies at sites in Fiji, Tonga, New Zealand and Australia. It uses a quasi-experimental study design to compare secondary school students attending schools in intervention areas with students at comparison schools in control areas and thus these data are not necessarily representative of the entire adolescent population.

Height, weight and waist circumference data were collected from children and adolescents in 2005/2006 for the OPIC study. Measurements were taken by trained assessors during face-to-face interviews at the children's schools.

Table 7.10 Secular trends in prevalence of overweight and obesity in New Zealand children across two studies from 2002 to 2006/2007

		Age group (years)			
		2–4	5–9	10–14	Total
Boys					
2002 Children's	Overweight		18	24	20
Nutrition	Obese		9	10	9
Survey[a]					
2006/2007 New	Overweight	22	20	21	21
Zealand	Obese	8	8	8	8
Health					
Survey					
Girls					
2002 Children's	Overweight		23	22	23
Nutrition	Obese		10	12	11
Survey[a]					
2006/2007 New	Overweight	26	19	21	21
Zealand	Obese	9	8	9	9
Health					
Survey					

[a]Actual age ranges for data in this study are 5–6 and 7–10 years (combined here under 5–9 category), and 11–14 years

Findings from the 2005/2006 Obesity Prevention in Communities Study for Fiji

Fiji, in contrast to Tonga, is an ethnically heterogeneous community with two distinct ethnic groups, indigenous Fijians and Indo-Fijians, comprising the bulk of the population. Reflecting this, 43% of students identified their ethnicity as indigenous and 52% as Indo-Fijian. Five percent of students identified their ethnicity as "other".

As shown in Table 7.11, ethnic differences in the prevalence of overweight and obesity were observed in Fiji with the indigenous students being most likely to be overweight and obese (22% of boys and 39% of girls), while the Indo-Fijian students were least likely to classified as overweight or obese (13% of boys and 13% of girls). Few differences in obesity by sex were observed.

While more than three-quarters of students in Fiji (89% boys; 76% girls) had a waist-to-height ratio within the healthy range (<0.5), this did differ by ethnicity with 67% of indigenous Fijian females and 93% of indigenous Fijian males having waist-to-height ratios less than 0.5 compared to 83% of Indo-Fijian females and 87% of Indo-Fijian males.

Findings from the 2005/2006 Obesity Prevention in Communities Study for Tonga

Approximately 10% of students in Tonga were classified as obese (Table 7.11). However, the prevalence of obesity was significantly higher among girls (15%) than boys (7%). This increased prevalence in girls was also pronounced in the figures for overweight with 38% of girls and 24% of boys classified as overweight.

Assessments of waist-to-height ratios for Tongan students showed that around half of all girls had ratios greater than 0.5 (unhealthy). In contrast, the prevalence in boys was substantially lower with 15% of boys falling into the unhealthy category.

Table 7.11 Age-standardized prevalence (%) of Fijian and Tongan adolescents classified as overweight and obese[a] by ethnic group and sex from the 2005/2006 Obesity Prevention in Communities Study

| | Ethnic group | | | | |
| | Fiji | | | | Tonga |
	Indigenous	Indo-Fijian	Others	Total	
Participants (n)	3,104	3,767	366	7,237	2,535
Boys					
Overweight	18	9	23	13	24
Obese	4	4	9	4	7
Waist-to-height ratio > 50%	7	13	18	11	15
Girls					
Overweight	31	10	22	20	38
Obese	8	3	8	6	15
Waist-to-height ratio > 50%	33	17	27	24	49

Adapted from the Obesity Prevention in Communities Study (Utter et al. 2008)
[a]Classified using International Obesity Task Force cut-off points (Cole et al. 2000)

Secular Trends

No secular data on overweight and obesity prevalence are available for any of the Pacific countries.

Conclusions

Overweight and obesity is commonly observed in children and adolescents in Australia, New Zealand and the Pacific region, with the prevalence being higher amongst children and adolescents in the Pacific region and of Pacific descent living in New Zealand. There is evidence of secular increases in overweight and obesity in children and adolescents in Australia, however, the available data are sparse. National surveys for New Zealand do not suggest secular increases in the prevalence of overweight and obesity in children in that country. While New Zealand regularly collects data on overweight and obesity prevalence through their national health survey, Australia does not have regular, frequent, national data collections to monitor rates of overweight and obesity. Further while both Australia and New Zealand collect national data on potential risk factors for the development of overweight and obesity including diet and physical activity, such data are generally not collected in conjunction with weight status data in Australia. In New Zealand, while potential risk factor data are collected they have not been analyzed in conjunction with weight status data, precluding conclusions about associations. What can be elicited from the available data is that overweight and obesity are likely to be socio-economically patterned, with children and adolescents from lower socio-economic families more likely to be overweight or obese. Further, there are distinct ethnic disparities in the prevalence of overweight and obesity in New Zealand children and adolescents. Those of Maori and Pacific descent are not only substantially more likely to be overweight or obese, but also tend to represent the more severe cases of excess weight, with extreme obesity experienced almost exclusively by Maori and Pacific youth.

Data for the Pacific region is almost non-existent. No nationally representative data are available and no data were identified for the majority of countries making up the Pacific region. Given the countries grouped within the Pacific region are heterogeneous in terms of geographic, social and economic circumstances, data from one country within this region may not accurately reflect the picture of childhood overweight and obesity in the entire region. Children and adolescents of Pacific descent living in New Zealand have been identified as being of particularly high risk for overweight and obesity. Thus data on indigenous Pacific children and adolescents is important as it may assist in explaining the reasons for this increased risk.

In conclusion, the data summarized in this chapter highlight the need for regular and frequent collections of nationally representative data on the prevalence and associated risk factors of overweight and obesity in children and adolescents in this region. This information is vital for understanding the epidemiology of overweight and obesity in this region. It is also imperative to inform national planning for prevention and treatment strategies.

Acknowledgments Kylie Hesketh is supported by a National Heart Foundation of Australia Career Development Award. Karen Campbell is supported by a Victorian Health Promotion Foundation Fellowship. Rachael Taylor is supported by the Karitane Products Society Fellowship.

References

Ashwell, M., & Hsieh, S.D. (2005). Six reasons why the waist-to-height ratio is a rapid and effective global indicator for health risks of obesity and how its use could simplify the international public health message on obesity. *International Journal of Food Science & Nutrition, 56(5)*, 303–307.

Australian Bureau of Statistics (2005). *Population by age and sex, Australia* (September 5, 2008); http://www.abs.gov.au/ausstats/abs@.nsf/productsbytitle/1F51406DCEEBAC14CA256EC7007B5B4E?OpenDocument.

Australian Bureau of Statistics (2006). *A picture of the nation: the statistician's report on the 2006 census.* Catalogue No. 2070.0.

Australian Bureau of Statistics (2009). *National Health Survey 2007-2008.* Catalogue No. 4364.0.

Central Intelligence Agency (2009). *The world factbook.* (August, 2009); https://www.cia.gov/library/publications/the-world-factbook/index.html.

Cole, T.J., Bellizzi, M.C., Flegal, K.M., & Dietz, W.H. (2000). Establishing a standard definition for child overweight and obesity worldwide: international survey. *British Medical Journal, 320(7244)*, 1240–1243.

Commonwealth of Australia (2008). *2007 Australian National Children's Nutrition and Physical Activity Survey: Main findings,* Commonwealth of Australia.

Fiji Islands Bureau of Statistics (2007). *2007 census of population and housing.* (August 2009); http://www.statsfiji.gov.fj/Census2007.

Goulding, A., Grant, A.M., Taylor, R.W., Williams, S.M., Parnell, W.R., Wilson, N., & Mann, J.I. (2007). Ethnic differences in extreme obesity. *Journal of Pediatrics, 151*, 542–544.

Kuczmarski, R.J., Ogden, C.L., Grummer-Strawn, L.M., Flegal, K.M., Guo, S.S., Wei, R., Mei, Z., Curtin, L.R., Roche, A.F., & Johnson, C.L. (2000). *CDC growth charts: United States. Advance data from Vital and Health Statistics: n. 314.* Hyattsville, Maryland: National Center for Health Statistics.

Lobstein, T., Baur, L., & Uauy, R. for the IASO International Obesity Taskforce (2004). Obesity in children and young people: a crisis in public health. *Obesity Reviews, 5(Suppl 1)*, 4–85.

Ministry of Health (2003). *NZ Food NZ Children: Key results of the 2002 National Children's Nutrition Survey.* Wellington, New Zealand.

Ministry of Health (2008). *A Portrait of Health: Key results of the 2006/07 New Zealand Health Survey.* Wellington, New Zealand.

Salmond, C., Crampton, P., & Atkinson, H. (2007). *NZDep2006 Index of Deprivation.* Wellington, New Zealand: Department of Public Health, University of Otago.

Secretariat of the Pacific Community Noumea New Caledonia (1999). *Cook Islands Population Profile Based on 1996 Census: a guide for planners and policy-makers.*

Soloff, C., Lawrence, D., & Johnstone, R. (2005). *The Longitudinal Study of Australian Children (LSAC). Sample design. LSAC Technical Paper No. 1,* Australian Institute of Family Studies.

Statistics New Zealand (2002). *2001 census of population and dwellings; population and dwelling statistics.* Wellington, New Zealand.

Statistics New Zealand (2006). *QuickStats about New Zealand's population and dewllings-population counts.* (May 18, 2007); http://www.stats.govt.nz/Census/2006CensusHomePage/QuickStats/quickstats-about-a-subject/nzs-population-and-dwellings/population-counts.aspx.

The World Bank (2009). *Pacific Islands brief.* (August, 2009); http://web.worldbank.org/WBSITE/EXTERNAL/COUNTRIES/EASTASIAPACIFICEXT/PACIFICISLANDSEXTN/0,,contentMDK:20212765~menuPK:44189 5~pagePK:1497618~piPK:217854~theSitePK:441883~isCURL:Y,00.html.

Tonga Department of Statistics (2006). *Tonga statistics population census 2006.* Analytical Report Volume 2.

United Nations Development Programme (2009). *Human development report 2009-HDI rankings.* (December, 2009); http://hdr.undp.org/en/statistics/.

Utter, J., Scragg, R., Schaaf, D., Fitzgerald, E., & Wilson, N. (2007). Correlates of body mass index among a nationally representative sample of New Zealand children. *International Journal of Pediatric Obesity, 2,* 104–113.

Utter, J., Faeamani, G., Malakellis, M., Vanualailai, N., Kremer, P., Scragg, R., & Swinburn, B. (2008). *Lifestyle and obesity in South Pacific youth: Baseline results from the Pacific Obesity Prevention in Communities (OPIC) project in New Zealand, Fiji, Tonga and Australia.* Auckland, University of Auckland.

Vanuatu National Statistics Office (1999). *Population statistics: population by ethnicity 1999.* (June 26, 2009). http://www.spc.int/prism/country/vu/stats/social/population/ethnicity.htm.

Wake, M., Hardy, P., Canterford, L., Sawyer, M., & Carlin, J.B. (2007). Overweight, obesity and girth of Australian preschoolers: prevalence and socio-economic correlates. *International Journal of Obesity, 31(7),* 1044–1051.

World Health Organisation (2009). *Regional office for the Western Pacific: Countries and areas.* (August, 2009); http://www.wpro.who.int/countries/countries.htm.

Chapter 8
Prevalence and Etiology: Middle East and North Africa (MENA) Countries

Hafez Elzein and Sima Hamadeh

Introduction

The increasing prevalence of obesity at an alarming rate in many parts of the world probably has multiple underlying etiologies. Obesity is generally attributed to a combination of genetic and/or environmental factors. In children, genetic, prenatal and perinatal factors have a great effect on individual predisposition, practices and behaviors, contributing to a long-term positive energy balance.

Risk Profile in Developing Countries

It is clear that obesity does not discriminate between geographical location, economic level, sex and age. Emerging data from developing countries indicate that the prevalence of obesity among children and adolescents is escalating more rapidly today than in industrialized countries. This pattern appears to mimic what occurred in the USA between 1980 and 2007 where the percentage of overweight children age 6–11 years more than doubled from 7 to over 15%, while the percentage of overweight adolescents age 12–19 years tripled in the same period from 5 to 15% (Kelishadi 2007; Kuczmarski et al. 2000). In the 1990s, this emerging pattern in developing countries has been largely ignored in health strategies developed at national and international levels (WHO, Geneva 1997) but nowadays research interest and studies in this area are rapidly expanding (http://www.ucsfhealth.org).

The prevalence of chronic or non-communicable disease (NCD) is also increasing more rapidly in developing countries than industrialized countries (Kelishadi 2006), where according to the World Health Organization (WHO) estimates, by 2020, approximately three-quarters of all death in the developing countries will be related to NCD (Onis 2004). Obesity and/or overweight are major risk factors for chronic diseases and play a central role in the "insulin resistance" or "metabolic syndrome", which includes hyperinsulinemia, hypertension, and hyperlipidemia and type-2 diabetes mellitus. It also correlates strongly with increased risk of atherosclerotic cardiovascular disease (Kelishadi 2007;

H. Elzein (✉)
Faculty of Medicine, American University of Beirut, Beirut 1107 2020, Lebanon
e-mail: hafezezein@aol.com

L.A. Moreno et al. (eds.), *Epidemiology of Obesity in Children and Adolescents*, Springer Series on Epidemiology and Public Health 2, DOI 10.1007/978-1-4419-6039-9_8, © Springer Science+Business Media, LLC 2011

Papandreou et al. 2008), stroke, sleep apnoea syndrome (Papandreou et al. 2008), and some forms of cancer (Kelishadi 2006; Papandreou et al. 2008; WHO Geneva 1997; WHO Europe 2005, 2007).

However, little is known about the prevalence of childhood obesity and the pediatric metabolic syndrome in the developing countries because of the limited number of studies (Kelishadi 2007; Papandreou et al. 2008), the variety of definitions and cut-offs used, and the different age groups studied which makes comparisons difficult (Kelishadi 2007). In summary, the rapid progress of urbanization and demographic trends in developing countries is associated with a cluster of NCD and unhealthy lifestyle described as "Lifestyle Syndrome" (Monteiro et al. 2002, 2004). Among developing countries, the prevalence of childhood obesity is highest in the Middle East and Central and Eastern Europe (James 2004).

Overweight Standards

There is no universal consensus on a cut-off point for defining overweight or obesity in children and adolescents; for example, the 85th percentile for children in the US corresponds to the 95th percentile for Brazilian children and the 90th percentile for British children (Abdulbari 2006). Usually, clinical and epidemiological studies are assessed by indicators based on weight and height, such as body mass index (BMI) defined as weight (kg)/height (m^2) (http://www.ucsf-health.org).

For children and teens, BMI ranges are defined so that they can take into account normal differences in body composition related to sex and age. Additionally, these ranges above a normal weight have different labels, for example: "at risk of overweight" and "overweight" (Kelishadi 2007).

In general, overweight and obesity status were defined in the literature by using the following three sets of criteria, all of which were used in studies of childhood obesity in the Middle East North Africa (MENA) region:

- First, the US Centers for Disease Control and Prevention (CDC) defines "overweight" as being at or above the 95th percentile of BMI for age, and "at risk of overweight" as being between the 85th and 95th percentiles of BMI for age (Kuczmarski et al. 2000). US population statistics were used to derive the CDC cut-off values (http://www.cdc.gov/nccdphp/dnpa/obesity/childhood).
- Second, the European Childhood Obesity Group classifies "overweight" as being at or above the 85th percentile of BMI and "obesity" as being at or above the 95th percentile of BMI (Flodmark et al. 2004). European population was used to derive these cut-offs values.
- Finally, the International Obesity Task Force (IOTF), in their definition, used cut-off points of 25 kg/m^2 for adult overweight and 30 kg/m^2 for adult obesity. These cut-off points are based on pooled international data in contrast to the other two definitions given above (Cole et al. 2000).

However, BMI cannot distinguish fat mass from muscle mass, nor can it represent the fat distribution; hence, it may not be the only measure to predict NCD (American Academy of Pediatrics Policy Statement 2003). Though there is no universal cut-off for waist circumference some studies used waist circumference above 75th percentile for age and sex to define abdominal obesity (Katzmarzyk et al. 2004; Moreno et al. 2002).

Risk Profile in the MENA Region

The risk profile in the MENA region appears to be similar to the general risk profile for obesity in developing countries. In the last decades, the Eastern Mediterranean Region (EMR) experienced a transition from a traditional to a westernized lifestyle accompanied by a similarly rapid epidemiologic transition (Kelishadi 2006). The Middle East, located in this region, has the highest dietary energy surplus of the developing countries (Kelishadi 2006, 2007) as they transition in that direction with large shifts in dietary and physical activity patterns (Abdulbari 2006; Gittelsohn and Kumar 2007; James 2004; Kelishadi 2006, 2007; Lafta et al. 2007; Lasserre et al. 2007; Marsh et al. 2007; Mokhtar et al. 2001; WHO Europe 2005, 2007). As a result, a rise in NCD risk factors is occurring in different age groups (Kelishadi 2006) especially among adolescents (Kelishadi 2007).

Based on the secular trends observed in different countries, it is estimated that by 2010 approximately 41% of children in the EMR (compared to 38% in the European region, 27% in the Western Pacific region and 22% in the Southeast Asian region) will be overweight or obese. In other words, it is estimated that during the next 3–4 years, approximately 1/10 children in the Eastern Mediterranean will be obese; compared to 1/7 for American children (Wang and Lobstein 2006). In Iran, the prevalence of childhood obesity and overweight is reported to be lower than in Arabic countries of the EMR (Kelishadi 2006). Concurrently, many developing countries especially in the MENA region are still grappling with the public health effects of malnutrition and micronutrient deficiencies (Kelishadi 2006; Mokhtar et al. 2001).

Through a qualitative and quantitative systematic review, the present chapter compares and analyzes the results of published research studies on the prevalence of overweight and obesity among children and adolescents living in MENA region. We will use a meta-analysis approach to integrate findings across these publications. We will attempt to outline the factors (geographical, environmental, economic, sex and age) that act separately or jointly as best predictors of the variation of obesity prevalence and etiology in the MENA region.

Geographic Area

The term MENA, for "Middle East and North Africa" covers an extensive region extending from Iran in southwest Asia to Morocco in northwest Africa. It generally includes all the Arab Middle East and North Africa countries, as well as Iran and Israel but not Turkey. The countries of the MENA region can be grouped into three sub-regions (Whitaker and Dietz 1998).

Near East

The Near East is also known as Levant. This sub-region includes: Lebanon, Syria, Palestine, Israel and Jordan but excludes Turkey (http://icf.at/?id=6174).

Gulf Region and Arabian Peninsula

This sub-region includes all the six countries of the Gulf Cooperation Council (GCC): Saudi Arabia, United Arab Emirates (UAE), Kuwait, Bahrain, Qatar and Oman, plus three of their neighbors: Yemen, Iraq and Iran (http://icf.at/?id=6174).

North Africa

This sub-region covers four of the five Maghreb countries (Tunisia, Morocco, Libya, and Algeria) plus Egypt and Sudan (http://icf.at/?id=6174).

Socio-demographic and Economic Characteristics

The MENA region spans an area of 14.8 million km², roughly one-tenth of the earth's land surface. It is comprised of 20 countries (Whitaker and Dietz 1998) inhabited by slightly more than 300 million people (WDI, World Bank, 2008). It is the least populated developing region in the world (5% proportion of world population in 2001) with 36.4% below the age of 15 (Levin and Govek 1998). The population of the MENA region comprises 6% of the total world population and is equivalent in number to one third of the population of China Republic, almost equivalent to the population of the European Union, and is one and a quarter times larger than the population of the United States (Whitaker and Dietz 1998). However, the region has the second-highest population growth rate with a 2.2% annual average growth rate between 1990 and 2001, second only to Sub-Saharan Africa (WDI, World Bank 2008). The crude birth rate and the crude death rate in 2006 were 25 and 6‰, respectively (http://www.dcp2.org/pubs/GBD). Infant mortality and under-five mortality rates have declined in recent years and are below the averages for the developing world. Life expectancy at birth in the MENA region in 2006 was 70 years, which is above the developing world average (WDI, World Bank 2008).

The socio-demographic and economic characteristics of the MENA region are summarized in Table 8.1 below.

While rates of extreme poverty in MENA are low, these rates have slightly increased since 1990. Purchasing power parity (Gross National Income (GNI) per capita) was $6,710 in 2006 (WDI, World Bank 2008). Economic growth in the MENA region was the lowest among developing regions in 2006 at 5.1% (WDI, World Bank 2008). The top performers in the region in 2006 were Morocco (8% growth) and Egypt (6.8% growth). But Iran, which accounted for 20% of the region output, grew at 4.6% and Algeria, which accounted for 16% of the region's output, grew by only

Table 8.1 Summary of socio-demographic and economic characteristics

Area	14.8 million km²
Number of countries	20 countries
Population (in 2008)	>300 million (6% of world population)
Population below the age of 15	36.4%
Growth rate	2.2%
Life expectancy at birth (in 2006)	70 years
Crude birth rate (in 2006)	25 ‰
Crude death rate (in 2006)	6 ‰
Infant mortality and under 5 mortality	Below the averages of the developing world
Mildly underweight	35%
Moderately to severe underweight	21%
Purchasing power parity (in 2006) (Growth National Income (GNI) per capita)	6,710$
Economic growth (in 2006)	5.1%
Sources of economic stability	70% of the world's oil reserves and 46% of the world's natural gas reserves

3% (WDI, World Bank 2008). The MENA region has vast reserves of petroleum (70% of the world's oil reserves) and natural gas (46% of the world's natural gas reserves) that makes it a vital source of global economic stability (Whitaker and Dietz 1998). As of 2007, eight of the twelve OPEC nations are within the MENA region (Whitaker and Dietz 1998).

Methods

A quantitative and qualitative systematic review on the prevalence of overweight and obesity, among children and adolescents living in the MENA region was carried out through an electronic search of the literature from 1996 to 2008 (Medline, PubMed, Google scholar and WHO). Only two reference articles published prior to 1996 were used.

The criteria for inclusion of the studies were

1. Publication in English language
2. Publication date between late 1990s and 2008
3. Study location inside the MENA region
4. Focus on children and adolescents of MENA countries (few studies included adults as well)

The keywords used in this review were "children," "adolescents." "youth," "non communicable diseases," "obesity," "overweight," "BMI," "body composition," "anthropometric measures," "body circumference," "dietary intake," "prevention," "WHO-MENA," "developing countries," "low and middle income countries" "Middle East countries", "North African countries" as well as the names of individual countries.

We identified 51 articles published since 1996. Five studies were in males only (2 children, 2 adolescents and 1 university students), 10 were in females only (6 adolescents and 4 adults) and 36 used mixed sex (10 children, 11 adolescents, 2 children and adolescents, 6 adults, 2 university students and 5 all the population of the country). The articles used in this meta-analysis covered 13 of the 20 countries in the MENA region distributed as follows: 4 in Lebanon, 1 in Syria, 2 in Bahrain, 1 in Iraq, 3 in Kuwait, 11 in Iran, 3 in Qatar, 4 in Saudi Arabia, 2 in UAE, 1 in Northern Africa, 6 in Tunis, 3 in Morocco, 5 in Egypt, 1 in Egypt/Lebanon/Kuwait and 5 in Israel.

A descriptive summary of these studies is provided by the three sub-regions: Near East, Gulf and North Africa in Tables 8.2–8.4, respectively. One study was done in three countries one from each of the three sub-regions is summarized separately in Table 8.5.

The summarized data was supplemented by WHO surveys and reports documenting prevalence and association with demographic, environmental, socio-economic and psychological problems among children and adolescents living in this region. For many parameters, data for the entire MENA region does not exist, and therefore, published data from a number of member countries was integrated in this systematic search.

Prevalence of Overweight and Obesity

The data in Tables 8.2–8.4 are sorted by country within the three main sub-regions of MENA (Near East, Gulf and Arabian peninsula, and North Africa). The first author, year of publication, sample size, key obesity-related parameters and summary of results are presented. The data in Table 8.5 are the summary of two studies comparing the prevalence of overweight and obesity between Egypt and other countries. The first study compared the prevalence between Egypt and Mexico. The second study compared the prevalence between three countries of the MENA region, each from a different sub-region: Egypt (North Africa), Lebanon (Near East) and Kuwait (Gulf and Arabian Peninsula).

Table 8.2 Profile of (childhood) obesity (Ob), overweight (Ow) and underweight (Uw) in countries of the Near East sub-region

Country	Study (no. of subjects)	Age (years)	Prevalence % (obesity, overweight and underweight)	Variables	Outcomes
Lebanon	Sibai et al. (2003) (2,104)	≥3	• 3–19 years: Boys: Ob 7.5, Ow 22.5; Girls: Ob 3.2, Ow 16.1 • ≥20 years: Males: Ob 14.3, Ow 57.7; Females: Ob 18.8, Ow 49.4 (WHO criteria)	– BMI – Body fat – Waist circumference	– All variables increased to mid age (40–60 years) and declined thereafter – Significant association between no exercise and children obesity – Adult obesity higher among least educated, family history of obesity and non-smokers – Ob and Ow higher in males, except in females ≥20 years
Lebanon	Jabre et al. (2005) (234)	6–8	Boys: Ob 7.0, Ow 26.0; Girls: Ob 6.0, Ow 25.0 (IOTF criteria)	– Age/sex – Household and family size – Single/2 parent family – Parental education and work – Physical activity – Dietary intake	– High proportion of Ow in 6–8-year-old children in Beirut – Reduced physical activity is the most significant factor associated with childhood overweight
Lebanon	Chakar and Salameh (2006) (12,299)	10–18	Boys Girls Total Non-Ob: 61.1 76.8 68.1 At risk: 28.8 19.0 24.4 Ob: 10.1 4.2 7.5 (CDC criteria)	– BMI	– Ob is 2.5 times higher in boys – Risk and prevalence of Ob lower with age in girls but not in boys – Risk of Ob and prevalence of Ob in Lebanese adolescents of private schools are high
Lebanon	Yahia et al. (2008) (220)	20±1.9	Males: Ob 12.5, Ow 37.5, Uw 1.0; Females: Ob 3.2, Ow 13.6, Uw 6.4 (NIH guidelines)	– Age – Weight – Height – BMI – % Body fat – Meal frequency – Dietary intake	– 64.7% of students are normal weight – Females have healthier eating habits: Daily breakfast intake and meal frequency – Intake of colored vegetables and fruits is common among students

Location	Reference (n)	Age	Variables	Results	Findings
Syria "Aleppo"	Maziak et al. (2007) (2,038)	18–65	– Weight – Height – BMI – Blood pressure (BP) – CVD (physician-diagnosed) – Mortality due to CVD in the past 5 years – Smoking (cigarettes or water pipes)	Males: Ob 28.8 Females: Ob 46.4 Total: Ob 38.2 (WHO criteria)	– Prevalence of CVD: 4.8% – CVD mortality 45% of overall in the past 5 years – 49% of CVD deaths before age 65 years, more males than females – Hypertension: 40.6% (47.7% males, 34.9% females) – Smoking: 38.7% (63.6% males, 19.2% females) – Main CVD risk factors: Older age, male sex and low education
Israel, "Jews and Arabs"	Keinan-Boker et al. (2005) (3,246)	25–64	– Weight and height – BMI – Age – Origin – Education level	• 55–64 years: Males: Ob 22.4 Females: Ob 40.4 • Females education level: Jewish (academic): Ob 13.6 Arab (basic): Ob 57.3 (WHO criteria)	– High Ob rates (comparable to those in USA), especially among older Arab women (55–64 years) – Ob is more prevalent in females – Ob increased with age – Significant risk factors for Ob: in males: Age in females: age, education, origin – Education level is negatively associated with Ob
Israel	Bar Dayan et al. (2005) (76,732)	17	– Weight and height – Education level – NCD (hypertension, diabetes type 2)	Males: Ob 4.1 Ow 12.4 Females: Ob 3.3 Ow 11.4 (Criteria used: Low weight <18 kg/m^2 Normal weight 18–25 kg/m^2 Overweight 25–30 kg/m^2 Obesity 30–40 kg/m^2 Morbidly obese >40 kg/m^2)	– Low prevalence of Ob but an alarming high prevalence of Ow – Ob is correlated with high prevalence of hypertension, diabetes type 2 and lower education level – A significant difference between sexes in the hypertension and diabetes type 2 prevalence
Israel	Kaluski and Berry (2005) (2,782)	25–64		Total: Ob 22.9 Ow 39.3 (WHO criteria)	– Ow is more common in males – Ob is more prevalent in females – Israeli Arab population is more obese than Jewish one
Israel	Israeli et al. (2006) (560,588)	16.5–19	– BMI – Systolic blood pressure (SBP) – Diastolic blood pressure (DBP)	Males: Ob 3.3 Ow 10.9 Females: Ob 3.2 Ow 11.1 (Ow defined as BMI 25 to ≤30, Ob defined as BMI >30)	– BMI doesn't increase with age – Prevalence of prehypertension is higher in obese subjects – A significant increase in the mean SBP and DBP with age and BMI – Prehypertension is very common among Israeli adolescents

Table 8.3 Profile of (childhood) obesity (Ob), overweight (Ow) and underweight (Uw) in countries of the Gulf and Arabian Peninsula sub-region

Country	Study (no of subjects)	Age (years)	Prevalence % (obesity, overweight and underweight)	Variables	Outcomes

Bahrain	Hamadeh (2000) (61.2% of 620,378)	Bahraini population	(WHO criteria)	– BMI
				– Physical activity
				– Daily fruits and vegetables intake
					– Prevalence of Ob higher among females in all age groups
					– Ow is higher among males
					– Age group 30–79:
					  males are more engaged in PA
					  males and females similar in daily intake of fruits and vegetables

Bahrain	Al-Sendi et al. (2003) (506)	12–17	Males: Ob 21.0 Females: Ob 35.0 (WHO criteria) Males: Ob 15.0 Females: Ob 18.0 (IOTF criteria Must et al. 1991)	– Age – Weight, height – Triceps and subscapular skinfolds	– Higher prevalence in adolescent obesity than was previously reported, especially in girls – Must et al. (1991) and IOTF criteria (Cole et al. 2000) BMI reference values are more practical for use in adolescents surveys than the WHO criteria
Iraq, "Baghdad"	Lafta et al. (2007) (5,361)	7–13	Ob: 4.1 Ow: 12.4 (ITOF criteria)	– Age/sex – BMI – Parental obesity – Physical activity – Watching TV – Eating while watching TV	– Obesity increases with age: a significant linear correlation – Ob and Ow higher in girls – Risk factors: sex, physical activity, parental obesity and family size – Most children watch TV daily and 60% eat while watching
Kuwait	Al-Isa and Moussa (1999) (3,473)	3–5	(NCHS/CDC references)	– Age and birth order – Weight and height – Parental education and work – Family income – Number of servants – Eating habits – Grandparents and number of persons living at home – Number of siblings – SES – Dental status	– Ow and Ob associated with: age, birth order, sex, parents education, region, dental status, eating regular meals and SES – In males, factors are: age, region, eating regular meals, no. of person living at home and SES – In females, factors are: dental status, governorate, number of servants and SES

Location	Reference (n)	Age	Variables	Values/Criteria	Findings
Kuwait	Moussa et al. (1999) (460 obese)	6–13	– Biochemical variables: serum lipids, lipoproteins, apolipoproteins, insulin – Blood pressure	(NCHS reference)	– Obese children have abnormal biochemical variables and BP – Obesity associated with family history of obesity, diabetes, respiratory and bone diseases – Physical activity and parental social class are not significant
Kuwait	Al-Isa (2004) (14,659)	10–14	– Weight – Height	Males: Ob 14.7, Ow 30.0 Females: Ob 13.1, Ow 31.8 (NCHS criteria)	– No change pattern with age in Ow and Ob in both sexes – Ow was lower in males but Ob was higher compared to females
Iran, "Kerman"	Janghorbani and Parvin (1998) (1,000)	14–21	– Weight, height, BMI – Chest, waist, abdomen, hip and thigh circumference – Criteria used: very Uw <15 Uw 15–19.9 Desirable weight 20–24.9 (Grade 1) Ow 25–29.9 (Grade 2) Ow 30–39.9 (Grade3) Ow ≥40	Girls: very Uw 1.6, Uw 54.6, (Grade 1) Ow 4.6, (Grade 2) Ow 0.7, (Grade 3) Ow 0.0 (NCHS criteria)	– Low prevalence of Ow among Iranian young women – Mean BMI: 19.8 – Mean WHR: 0.8 – Mean abdomen-to-hip ratio: 0.8 – Mean chest-to-hip ratio: 0.9
Iran, "Tehran"	Azizi et al. (2001) (421)	10–19	– Total energy intake (TEI) – % of energy derived from protein, carbohydrate and fat – % of energy supplied by each meal and snack	Boys: Ob 5.1, Ow 10.7 Girls: Ob 2.8, Ow 18.4 (BMI cut-offs values for adolescents)	– Diet not different between Ow/Ob and normal weight – In boys: BMI linked to TEI and daily energy distribution – In girls: BMI linked to daily energy distribution only
Iran, "Isfahan"	Kelishadi et al. (2001) (4,500)	2–18	– Serum lipid levels – High density lipoprotein cholesterol (HDL) – Blood pressure – BMI	In 1993: Ob 0.2, Ow 4.0 In 1999: Ob 0.35, Ow 8.0	– Prevalence of obesity is low – Twofold rise in Ow in 5 years, especially in school-aged and adolescent girls – Serum lipid levels higher than standard in both sexes and in all age groups (1993, 1999) – HDL lower than standard – No cases of diabetes mellitus – No difference in hypertension

(continued)

Table 8.3 (continued)

Country	Study (no of subjects)	Age (years)	Prevalence % (obesity, overweight and underweight)	Variables	Outcomes
Iran, "Isfahan"	Kelishadi et al. (2003) (2,000)	11–18	Boys: Ob 1.9, Ow 7.4; Girls: Ob 2.9, Ow 10.7; Mean BMI: Urban areas 25.4, Rural areas 23.2 (CDC critera)	– BMI – Physical activity (PA) – Family income – Area of residency – Mother education – Mean total energy intake – Watching TV – Serum lipid levels – Blood pressure	– Ob and Ow higher in girls – Mean BMI is different between rural and urban areas – BMI >85th percentile higher in families with average income and less-educated mothers – Similar mean total energy intake for normal, Ow and Ob – Regular PA is low – Time watching TV is high – BMI: Significant linear association with freq of rice, bread, fast foods, pasta and fat/salty snacks – BMI: Significant correlation with triglyceride, HDL and SBP
Iran, "Tabriz"	Gargari et al. (2004) (1,518)	14–20 Girls only	NHANES I, IOTF: Uw 8.0, ---; Ob 3.6, 3.9; Ow 11.1, 10.1; Total (Ob and Ow): 14.6, 14	– BMI	– Ob, Ow and Uw are present – Prevalence of Ob and Ow in Tabriz high-school girls higher than in many parts of Iran, but lower than in some neighboring countries such as Saudi Arabia
Iran, "Tehran"	Mohammadpour-Ahranjani et al. (2004) (2,321)	11–16	Total: Ob 7.8, Ow 21.1; Boys: Ow 18.8; Girls: Ow 23.1 (NCHS/CDC)	– Weight, height – BMI	– Ow higher among girls – Risk of Ob is not associated with age for both sexes – Mean BMI higher than in early 1990s in Tehrani adolescents especially among girls
Iran	Kolahdooz et al. (2004) (16,418)	<3	Not reported	– Dietary intake (type and daily/weekly frequency) – Area of residency	– Snacks is the major component of children's diet – Snacks from natural products replaced with industrial and processed products due to industrialization, increased media coverage and lifestyle changes
Iran	Sheikholeslam et al. (2004) (review of 3 national surveys in 1995, 1999 and 2002)	40–69 years	Males: Ob and Ow 50.0; Females: Ob and Ow 66.0	– NCD (CVD, hypertension, diabetes, hyperlipedimia) – Dietary intake – PA	– Fat and CHO are 30 and 40% more than recommended respectively – 80 to 90% of edible oils are hydrogenated – Mean trans fatty acid intake (15.6 to 30 g/day) much higher than recommended amount (<5 g/day) – 70 to 80% are inactive – NCD is a public health problem

Country	Study (sample)	Age/population	Prevalence (criteria)	Variables	Findings
Iran, "Islamshahr"	Soutoudeh et al. (2005) (1,003)	10–65 Women only	• Adolescent females: Ow (or at risk) 19.0 • Adult females: Ob or Ow 66.8 (IOTF criteria)	– BMI – WHR – Marital status – Occupation – Literacy – Parity – Daily meal and snack consumption	– Highest OW % was in 50–59 years – Ob and Ow are similar in urban and rural areas – Central obesity (WHR ≥85th) is 35.7% in all females – BMI higher in married women and those with <8 years education – WHR higher in women with <8 years of education or >6 parity – Mean BMI and WHR higher in with no daily snack consumption
Iran	Kelishadi et al. (2007) (211,111)	6–18	(CDC criteria)	– BMI – Physical activity – Dietary pattern – Parental education – Parental occupation – History of breastfeeding – History of family obesity and chronic diseases – Birth weight	– PA is higher among boys, in rural than urban, and in intermediate than high school students – PA significantly related to frequency of consumption of all food groups – BMI inversely associated with: frequency of consumption of vegetables and plant proteins (boys) and dairy products, fruits and high PA (girls) – OW significantly related with: boys: low fruit consumption, time spent on PA and energy spent girls: time spent on PA and energy spent

Iran	Kelishadi et al. (2008) (89,532)	>15	Total:
			  Morbid Ob Ob Ow
			  3.4 10.8 28.6
			BMI ≥25 kg/m²:
			Males: 37.0 Females: 48.0
			Urban: 46.7 Rural: 35.5 (WHO criteria)
				– BMI
				– Abdominal obesity
				– Area of residency
					– Abdominal Ob prevalence:
					Males: 9.7 Females: 43.4
					Urban: 28.5 Rural: 23.0
					– Ow, Ob and abdominal Ob are more prevalent in 45–64 years group

Qatar	Abdulbari et al. (2006) (593)	14–19	Boys: Ow 33.1 (IOTF criteria)	– BMI – Educational level – Living condition – Family size – Frequent dieting	– Extreme dieters: 10.1% – Intermediate dieters: 37.4% – Among the dieters: 34% are Ow – Extreme dieters: more psychological and sleeping problems, always tired and felt like crying – TV (61.7%) is the main source of information on diet

(continued)

Table 8.3 (continued)

Country	Study (no of subjects)	Age (years)	Prevalence % (obesity, overweight and underweight)	Variables	Outcomes
Qatar	Abdulbari (2006) (3,923)	12–17	Boys: Ob 7.9, Ow 28.6, Uw 8.6 Girls: Ob 4.7, Ow 18.9, Uw 5.8 (IOTF criteria for obesity and overweight) (CDC criteria for underweight)	– BMI – Parental education – Type of house – No of rooms/house	– Qatari adolescents are at high risk for Ow and Ob – Uw prevalence is highest at 16 years boys: 10.5% and 17 years girls: 8.9% – Ob prevalence is highest at 12 years boys: 11.7% and 13 years girls: 6.4% – The 95th percentile curve is above the IOTF standard curve for boys and below it for girls
Qatar	Abdulbari and Ihab (2006) (566)	14–19	• Adolescent females: Ob 1.8, Ow 13.4 • Adult Qatari population: Males: Ob 34.6, Ow 34.4 Females: Ob 45.3, Ow 33.0	– BMI – Hypertension – Smoking status – PA – Medical conditions – Family medical history – Dietary patterns – Living condition – Education level – Frequent dieting – Source of diet information – Psychological factors	– Adolescent female dieters: 39.9% are intermediate and 8.3% are extreme – Dieting is not associated with age but with BMI – Extreme dieting is strongly associated with peer perception and self perception of figure – Diet education sources: TV, magazine and radio – Main source of information for the extreme dieters: TV (43.6%)
Saudi Arabia	Al-Nuaim et al. (1996) (9,061)	6–18	Boys: Ob 15.8, Ow 11.7 (NCHS/CDC standard values)	– Age – Weight and height – BMI – Socio-demographic characteristics – Location of school	– A significant regional variation of Ow and Ob distribution: the highest in Riyadh (18%) and the lowest in Sabea (11.1%) – A high prevalence of childhood Ob is found when compared to NCHS/CDC

Country	Study (sample)	Age	Variables/Methods	Values	Findings
Saudi Arabia	El-Hazmi and Warsy (2002) (12,701)	1–18	– BMI	Boys: Ob 6.0, Ow 10.7; Girls: Ob 6.74, Ow 12.7 (IOTF criteria)	– Ow increase with age – Ob: the maximum prevalence for both boys and girls is in the 2–3 years age group, a decrease is found up to 8–13 years age group, and then increase again up to the 18 years age – The highest frequency is in the Eastern Province, the lowest in the Southern Province – The highest Ow: boys (15–16 years)/girls (17–18 years) – The highest Ob: boys and girls (2–3 years) – The lowest Ob: boys (10–11 years)/girls (9–10 years)
Saudi Arabia	Al-Rukban (2003) (894)	12–20	– Weight and height – BMI – Socio-demographic characteristics – Dietary and PA history – Obesity-related knowledge and behavior – Family medical history – Past medical history	Boys: Ob 20.5, Ow 13.8 (CDC criteria)	– Family history and lack of PA are associated with adolescent obesity – 20% of Ow participants did not think they are Ow – Ob is an important public health problem among male adolescents in Riyadh
Saudi Arabia	Al Turki (2007) (701)	≥18 years	– Weight and height – BMI	Males: Normal 45.8, Ob 23.3, Ow 31.0 (WHO classification)	– Changing in eating habits and PA explain the rising prevalence of Ob in Saudi Arabia – Prevention of Ow and Ob among university male students should be planned in early childhood
United Arab Emirates (UAE)	Al-Hourani et al. (2003) (898)	11–18	– BMI – Triceps skinfold thickness (TSF) – Mid-upper arm circumference	Adolescent females: Ow 9.0, at risk of Ow 14.0 (NHANES reference data)	– Mean BMI and TSF at all ages were higher than the 50th percentile (median) of the NHANES reference data – 27% (11 years) and 28% (12 years) are above the TSF 90th percentile and a high prevalence of Ow
United Arab Emirates (UAE)	Al-Haddad et al. (2005) (16,391)	4–18	– BMI	Males: Ob 7.7, Ow 17.1; Females: Ob 7.1, Ow 20.1 (IOTF criteria)	– Ob among UAE youth is 2–3 times greater than the recently published international standards • <9 years: Ob and Ow (among both sexes) are below Cole et al. international standards • 9–18 years: a consistent increase in Ow and Ob (among both sexes)

Table 8.4 Prevalence of (childhood) obesity (Ob), overweight (Ow) and underweight (Uw) in the North African sub-region

Country	Study (no of subjects)	Age (years)	Prevalence % (obesity, overweight and underweight)	Variables	Outcomes
Northern Africa	Mokhtar et al. (2001) Morocco (M: 17,320) Tunisia (T: 2,760)	M: ≥18 T: 20–60	• Morocco: Males: Ob 5.7, Females: Ob 18.0 • Tunisia: Males: Ob 6.7, Females: Ob 22.7 (WHO/NCHS references)	– BMI – Area of residency – Educational level – Daily energy and macronutrient intakes	– Prevalence of Ob: M: 12.2% T: 4.4% – Ob is higher among females than among males in both countries – Ob among females has tripled over the past 20 years – Half of females are Ow or Ob (BMI >25): M: 50.9%, T: 51.3% – Ow increases with age, particularly among girls – Ow and Ob are greater for women in urban areas and with lower educational levels – Obese females consume more calories and CHO than normal weight females – Fat intake is high in T: 31% – CHO intake is high in M: 65–67%
Tunis	Ben Mami Ben Miled et al. (2000) (951)	6–12	Total: Ob 5.25	– Weight (wt) and height (ht) – BMI – Birth order – Parental Ob history – Dietary intake	– Wt and ht are more than 3 standard deviations (SD) compared to the normal – 66% have 1 or 2 obese parents – 74% are the oldest or the youngest child in the family – Food intake is rich in sugar and protein – Dietetic troubles are common
Tunis, "Sousse"	Ghannem et al. (2001) (793)	Rural school-children	Total: Ob 4.0 (Criteria used: Ow >25 kg/m² Ob >27 kg/m²)	– Sex – CVD – Lipid serum levels – Blood pressure – Smoking	– Prevalence of hypertension: 11.2%, hypercholesterolemia: 2.9%, hypertriglyceridaemia: 1.0%, HDL: 0.6% and Ob: 4.0%; no significant sex difference – Smoking (4%) has sex difference: boys: 7.3%, girls: 1.2%
Tunis, "Ariana"	Ben Slama et al. (2002) (3,148)	6–10	Total: Ob 3.7	– Weight – Present size of parents – Children life habits	Risk factors of the child Ob are: – Parents' Ob – Short length of sleep (<8 h) – Erosion between meals – Daily consumption of sugary food and sparkling drinks
Tunis, "Sousse"	Laouani Kechrid et al. (2004) (600)	>60	Total: Ob 24.2	– Blood pressure (BP) – BMI – NCD (diabetes, hypertension, CVD)	– Prevalence of HBP: 69.3% and diabetes: 23% – 51.7% of hypertension patients are non compliant and uncontrolled

Location	Reference	Age	Prevalence	Measures	Findings
Tunis, "Monastir"	Ben Salem et al. (2006) (3,033)	Infants	• 3 months: Ob 6.2 • 9 months: Ob 11.6 Total: wasting and Uw <10% (NCHS reference)	– Weight-for-age – Height-for-age – Weight-for-height – BMI	– Prevalence of growth retardation increased with age – Anthropometrical parameters distribution in Monastir infants is different from NCHS reference curve
Tunis	Blouza-Chabchoub et al. (2006) (1,050)	13–17	Total: Ob 5.1 (NHANES criteria)	– Weight and height – BMI – Food intake – SES – Family history of Ob	– Highest Ob for both sexes is at age 13–14 years – Ob is more important in males of high SES – 51% of obese adolescents have family history of obesity – 96% have abnormal alimentary behavior – 52% have excess caloric intake – 82% have an excess of lipid
Morocco	Benjelloun (2002)	Early childhood	<5 (1997): Uw 10.0, Stunting 23.0 Ow <3 (1987): Ow 3.0 <3 (1997): Ow 9.0 Adults (1984): Ow 26.0 Adults (1998): Ow 36.0 1984 1998 Ow Males: 19.0 25.0 Females: 32.0 45.0 Urban: 30.0 40.0 Rural: 20.0 29.0 Ob: 4.0 10.0 (IOTF criteria)	– BMI – Area of residency – Dietary intake – SES – Education level	– Ow is directly associated with SES and inversely with education – Ow is higher among females and among urban than rural – Ow and Ob are major health problems in Morocco – Undernourishment persists among children <5 years – Dietary habits: increased animal products intake, high intake of cereals and sugars (mainly sugar in tea), rise of meat and vegetables consumption accompanied with a steady bread consumption
Morocco, "Urban Sahraoui of South Morocco"	Rguibi and Belahsen (2004) (249)	≥15	Total: Ob 49.0, Ow 30.0 (WHO criteria)	– Weight and height – BMI – Waist circumference (WC) – Hip circumference (HC) – Calorie intake – PA – Marital status – Education level – Desire to lose weight	– Ow and Ob high in younger ages – Abdominal Ob is high and increase with age – 68% with WHR >85th – 76% with WC ≥88 – Ob associated with calorie intake, time spent in walking and in traditional sedentary occupation – Ob higher among married females and not influenced by education – Small % of female population expressed desire to lose weight

(continued)

Table 8.4 (continued)

Country	Study (no of subjects)	Age (years)	Prevalence % (obesity, overweight and underweight)	Variables	Outcomes
Morocco	Rguibi and Belahsen (2007) (Moroccan population)	Adults	Total: • 1984/1985: Ob 4.1 • 1998/1999: Ob 10.3 • 2000: Ob 13.3 Males: Ob 8.0 Females: Ob 22.0 (WHO criteria)	– Weight and height – BMI – Area of residency – Education level	– Ob increased among Moroccan population over the past 15 years, more prevalent in urban areas – Excessive weight is positively associated with age and negatively with education level
Egypt	Bakr et al. (2002) (317)	Medical students at Ain Shams university	Total: Uw 9.5 Normal 41.3 Ob 2.5 Ow 36.9 (CDC criteria)	– Weight and height – BMI – Mid upper arm circumference (MUAC) – Mid arm muscle circumference (MAMC) – Triceps skinfold thickness (TSF) – Lifestyle factors – Food frequency consumption – Family history of obesity	– About half of medical students are Ow and Ob – MUAC and MAMC higher in males – TSF of females is higher – All food group items are consumed fairly – 64% have regular meals – Males practice sports and play computer more than females – Watching TV higher in females – Lifestyle factors responsible for Ob: longer time on computer, eating more during stress and snaking between meals
Egypt, "Cairo and surrounding rural areas"	Jackson et al. (2003) (340)	Adolescent school girls	Ob 13.0 Ow 35.0 (CDC criteria)	– Weight, height and BMI – Waist and hip circumference (WC and HC) – Body image – Areas of residency – SES	– Ow is more prevalent in urban and high SES girls – Girls' perceptions of how their mother viewed their bodies differed from how the girls viewed their own bodies

Egypt, "Alexandria" 2005 (82)	Kharboush et al. (2005) (172 families)	Females: (WHO criteria)	Ob	60.0	– Weight and height – Stool, urine and blood analysis – Education level – Occupation – Female to male comparison – Sex ratio of some parameters – Ill health and diseases	– Ill health rate increased with age (36% in girls to 90% in females >45 years) compared to 71% among older males – Females are head of the family in 19.8% of families – Wives participated in family income in 18% families – Female to male sex ratio is low for <6 and >60 years
Egypt (E)	Asfaw (2007)	Mothers			(WHO criteria) – BMI – Micronutrient deficiency	The odds of Ow/Ob are 80.8% higher for micronutrient deficient mothers than for non-deficient (all other variables constant)

Table 8.5 Comparison of the prevalence of childhood obesity (Ob) and overweight (Ow) between Egypt and Mexico; and between Egypt, Lebanon and Kuwait

Country	Study (no of subjects)	Age (years)	Prevalence % (obesity, overweight and underweight)	Variables	Outcomes
Egypt (E) and Mexico (Me)	Salazar-Martinez et al. (2006) (E = 15,02; Me = 10,537)	11–19	• Total: Me E Ob 7.9 6.2 Ow 19.8 12.1 Ob male 11.0 6.0 Ob female 9.0 8.0 Ow male 18.0 7.0 Ow female 21.0 18.0 (CDC criteria)	– BMI – Age – Education level – Area of residency – PA – Vitamin intake – Smoking	– In Me: the most consistent correlates of BMI are age, educational level, smoking, vitamin intake and PA – In E: the most consistent correlates of BMI are age and rural residence
Egypt (E), Lebanon (L) and Kuwait (K)	Jackson et al. (2007) (Total = 922: E = 340 L = 336 K = 245)	10–19 (adolescent girls)	IOTF Must CDC Egypt: Ob 11.2 11.2 13.5 Ow 35.9 35.9 34.4 Lebanon: Ob 2.1 2.7 2.7 Ow 18.8 15.5 16.4 Kuwait: Ob 12.2 13.5 14.3 Ow 33.1 31.0 31.0	– Age – Weight and height – BMI for age with 3 ref.: Must et al. (1991), IOTF criteria and CDC 2000 – Waist circumference (in E and L) – WHR (in E and L) – Daily dietary intake	– Ow and Ob are highest in Kuwait and lowest in Lebanon (height, weight and BMI) – Ow proportion varied by country, reference and age – In E, the mean waist and WHR are higher than in L – Mean energy intake is highest in E and lowest in K – Mean intake of protein and fat is highest in E – Significant correlation between BMI and calorie intake in L and E – The three reference standards differed in estimating Ow more than Ob – IOTF criteria gave the lowest percentage estimate of Ob, while the CDC 2000 gave the highest

Near East Sub-region

Nine studies from three countries of the Near East sub-region are summarized in Table 8.2. Four studies from Lebanon focused on the risk factors (social, biological, demographic, etc.) for obesity, while one study from Syria and four studies from Israel focused on the relationship between obesity and chronic diseases (CVD, hypertension, diabetes). In Lebanon, obesity and overweight were higher in males, except in adult females ($\geq$20 years). Reduced physical activity was the most significant factor associated with childhood overweight. Risk and prevalence of obesity decreased with age in girls but not in boys. Risk and prevalence of obesity in Lebanese adolescents of private schools were high. Females have healthier eating habits: daily breakfast intake and meal frequency. The study done in Aleppo – Syria focused on profiling cigarette smoking, found a high prevalence of obesity (38.2 %) which was a significant risk factor for CVD. In Israel, overweight was more common in males and obesity was more common in females. In addition obesity increased with age and correlates with low education level and origin: Arab females were more obese (57.3%) than Jewish females (13.6%). Pre hypertension was very common among Israeli adolescents.

Gulf and Arabian Peninsula Sub-region

A summary of 26 studies from six countries of this sub-region is presented in Table 8.3.

In Bahrain, the prevalence of adolescent obesity was higher than was previously reported, especially in girls. In general, prevalence of obesity was higher among females in all age groups but overweight was higher among males. Males were more engaged in physical activity and daily intake of fruits and vegetables is similar in both sexes.

In Iraq, the prevalence of obesity and overweight was higher in females. It increased with age and was associated with different risk factors (sex, physical activity, parental obesity and family size). It is important to notice that most children watch TV daily and 60% ate while watching.

Studies done in Kuwait showed that prevalence of overweight was lower but prevalence of obesity was higher in males compared to females. Also, obesity risk factors were different among males and females. Overall, obesity and overweight were positively associated with age, birth order, sex, parental education, region, dental status, eating regular meals, family history and socio-economic status (SES). Conversely, the three studies showed that physical activity and parental social class were not significant.

Iranian studies showed that obesity, overweight and underweight were present but the results may change between the different regions of the same country. The prevalence of overweight, obesity and underweight was higher in urban than rural areas. These studies showed the increasing prevalence of obesity and overweight in the Iranian population with time, which was higher in females than in males, especially in adult females. The analysis of the Iranian lifestyle and food habits demonstrated that there was a significant linear association between BMI and frequency of rice, bread, fast foods, pasta and fat/salty snacks. Time watching TV was high and exercising was low, especially among girls.

Studies in Qatar showed that obesity prevalence was highest among 12-year-old boys (11.7%) and 13-year-old girls (6.4%). Boys were more at risk than girls. Almost, all Qatari adolescents were intermediate to extreme dieters. Extreme dieting was strongly associated with peer perception and self-perception of figure. Diet education sources were TV (followed by 43.6% of extreme dieters), magazine and radio.

In the Kingdom of Saudi Arabia, significant regional variation of overweight and obesity distribution was detected. The highest frequency was in the Eastern Province (Riyadh 18%), the lowest in the Southern Province (Sabea 11.1%). Overweight increased with age (the highest in boys 15–16 years old and in girls 17–18 years old). Conversely, the highest prevalence of obesity for both boys and girls was in the 2–3 years age group, with a decrease up to the 8–13 years age group, followed by an increase up to an age of 18 years. Family history, lack of physical activity and changing in eating habits were associated with adolescent obesity which becomes an important public health problem among male adolescents in Riyadh.

In the UAE, results were compared to NHANES reference data and international standards by the IOTF (Cole et al. 2000). Mean BMI and TSF at all ages were higher than the 50th percentile of the NHANES reference data. On the other hand, obesity among UAE youth was 2–3 times greater than the recently published international standards.

North Africa Sub-region

A summary of 14 studies from three countries of this sub-region is presented in Table 8.4.

The prevalence of obesity in Morocco (12.2%) was higher than in Tunis (4.4%) and higher among females than males in both countries. Half of the females had a BMI >25 (50.9% in Morocco and 51.3% in Tunis) especially those living in urban areas and those having lower educational levels. Fat intake was high in Tunis (31%) and carbohydrates intake was high in Morocco (65–67%). Overweight increased with age, particularly among girls.

In Tunis, prevalence of obesity varied between the areas and increased with time. The highest prevalence for both sexes was observed at age 13–14 years but it was more frequent in males of high SES. 51% of obese adolescents had a family history of obesity. 96% had abnormal alimentary behavior (52% had excess caloric intake and 82% had an excess of fat consumption).

Obesity increased among Moroccan population over the past 15 years and was more prevalent among females and in urban areas. Excessive weight was a major health problem in Morocco and it was positively associated with age and SES but negatively with education level. Dietary habits such as high intake of animal products, cereals and sugars (mainly sugar in tea), increase of meat and vegetables consumption accompanied by steady bread consumption were responsible of increased obesity. However, it was important to underline that undernourishment persists among children below the age of 5 years.

In Egypt, overweight was more prevalent in urban and high SES girls. Body image perception differs between girls and their mothers. An interesting study described the excessive weight among medical students and showed that about half of them were overweight and obese. Although they consumed fairly all food group items and the majority had regular meals (64%) their lifestyle was responsible of obesity (longer time working with the computer, eating more during stress and snacking between meals).

Cross-regional Studies

Two studies compared profiles of obesity in multiple countries not from the same sub-region, and they are summarized in Table 8.5.

The first study compared obesity profiles in Egypt and Mexico. In Egypt, BMI correlated with age and rural area, while in Mexico it correlated with age, educational level, smoking, vitamin intake and physical activity.

The second study compared obesity profiles in Egypt, Lebanon and Kuwait, one country from each sub-region of the MENA region. The prevalence of overweight and obesity was highest in Kuwait and lowest in Lebanon. Mean waist circumference and waist-to-hip ratio (WHR) were higher in Egypt than in Lebanon. Mean energy intake was highest in Egypt (especially from protein and fat) and lowest in Kuwait. A significant correlation between BMI and calorie intake was found in Lebanon and Egypt. Furthermore, this study showed that using different standard references resulted in wider discrepancies in estimating the prevalence of overweight than the prevalence of obesity. Besides, reference values by the IOTF (Cole et al. 2000) gave the lowest percentage estimate of obesity, while the CDC charts (Kuczmarski et al. 2000) gave the highest.

Overall, the prevalence of overweight among pre-school children varied from near 3% in UAE and Iran to 8.6% in Egypt. Among older children and adolescents (6–18 years), the prevalence of overweight ranged between 6.3% in Bahrain to 31.8% in Kuwait among girls; and between 4.9% in Saudi Arabia to 30% in Kuwait among boys. The prevalence of obesity in the same age groups ranged from near 3% in UAE and Iran to 35.1% in Bahrain among girls; and from 2.1% in Iran to 21% in Bahrain among boys. In almost all MENA countries, obesity and overweight increased with age and became more prevalent among females than males.

Risk Factors Studied

The analysis of 51 representative articles from 13 MENA countries showed an increasing prevalence of overweight and obesity from childhood to adulthood, although rates of early childhood malnutrition remained relatively high.

In this descriptive summary we tracked the socio-demographic and physiological variables of common interest in the published literature from studies in the MENA countries. The results are summarized in Table 8.6.

In this systematic search we found that BMI, dietary and calories intake, educational level and physical activity are the major factors of interest in the MENA countries. However, only six studies measured waist circumference and waist-to-hip ratio; and three studies measured triceps and

Table 8.6 Most common overweight and obesity parameters: a summary

Variables	Countries (n)	Number of studies
BMI	All the MENA countries (13)	51
Waist circumference, waist to hip ratio	Lebanon, Iran, Morocco, Egypt (4)	6
Triceps and subscapular skinfolds, mid upper arm circumference	Bahrain, UAE, Egypt (3)	3
Physical activity	Lebanon, Bahrain, Iraq, Iran, Qatar, Morocco, Saudi Arabia, Egypt, Kuwait (8)	11
Dietary and caloric intake	Lebanon, Bahrain, Iraq, Kuwait, Iran, Qatar, Saudi Arabia, Tunis, Morocco (9)	23
Educational level	Lebanon, Iran, Morocco, Israel, Egypt, Kuwait, Tunis (7)	16
Area of residence	Iran, Morocco, Tunis, Egypt (4)	7
SES	Lebanon, Iran, Qatar, Morocco, Saudi Arabia, Egypt, Kuwait, Tunis (8)	7
Family history of obesity	Iraq, Kuwait, Qatar, Saudi Arabia, Tunis, Egypt, Iran (7)	9
Family size	Lebanon, Iraq, Kuwait, Qatar (4)	4
Birth weight, breastfeeding	Iran	2
Frequency and level of dieting	Qatar	2
Order of birth	Kuwait and Tunis	2
Desire to lose weight	Morocco	1

subscapular skinfolds and mid upper arm circumference. These measures should be more integrated into future studies since they explain the fat distribution in the body. Family history of obesity, area of residence, SES and family size are also documented in several studies. Conversely, birth weight, breastfeeding, frequency and level of dieting, order of birth and desire to lose weight were not enough reported. Genetic factors were absent.

Several of the studies summarized above revealed that obese children have less moderate to vigorous physical activity than non-obese children, which in turn is associated with increased TV watching. Increased TV watching was described to coincide with lower consumption of fruits and vegetables and with extra calorie intake from sweets and soft drinks during viewing, especially among 13-year-old boys of lower socioeconomic status. Familial environment and parental habits such as family food culture (eating together), parenting practices and the availability of alternatives (pre-prepared or takeaway food) are likely to mediate the role of TV and food consumption.

An association of obesity with parental education, BMI, SES and obesity in children also emerged in this literature review. A significant inverse relationship was found between the educational level of both parents as well as maternal employment and the prevalence of obesity in children. Also, a direct relationship was observed between the BMI of mothers and food habits of their daughters and boys, while the BMI of fathers was associated with frequency of activities of their sons only.

Obesity is apparently more acceptable in the Arabic values than in western culture, especially among children where obesity is considered a sign of healthiness and high social class. This pattern may have been assisted by increased abundance of fast foods that are generally cheaper, but have high caloric value. Such practices may be attributed to the general inadequacies of health education and awareness about the health risks associated with obesity.

Overall, factors that have been linked to childhood and adolescent obesity in the MENA region are similar to those reported elsewhere in the world and include family lifestyle (smoking, poor eating habits, sedentary lifestyle), environmental factors (increased availability of fast foods, media and advertisement, increased use of the internet and video games and peer influences) and a family history of obesity (http://www.ucsfhealth.org).

These findings emphasize that in addition to community-based lifestyle modification, culturally relevant family-based interventions especially focusing on mother's beliefs and behavior are needed to prevent obesity in children and adolescents and its long-term consequences. Special emphasize should be directed at families with a medical and/or history of obesity.

Conclusions

The prevalence of overweight and obesity among children and adolescents living in the MENA region appears to be increasing in parallel with a changing socio-demographic landscape and the adoption of western-style environmental influences (dietary, lifestyle and economic). Our review showed that the mean GDP was $6,710 in 2006, which is consistent with the finding that the prevalence of obesity increases rapidly when a country's GDP reaches about $5,000 (Lasserre et al. 2007).

Actions are needed at different levels. Short-term intervention and long term prevention efforts are being attempted to varying degrees in some countries of the MENA region through increased awareness, school-based and community-based interventions, as well as family involvement. Efforts to use advertising targeted at children and adolescents to promote healthy food and lifestyle and to replace young people's TV viewing time with alternative activities would offer a sound short term strategy. Prevention of overweight and obesity in early childhood can in the long run, attenuate the high prevalence of excessive weight among older adults in MENA region.

It was difficult to make comparisons of obesity across age groups because published studies used different population age structures and BMI references. Hence, further studies on overweight and obesity in the MENA region are needed to clarify the most appropriate reference to use to classify overweight and obesity. Additional variables should be studied such as the media impact, body image, peer influence, sources of diet information, socio-psychological factors, different types of cuisine and cultural beliefs and attitudes.

We hope that the results of this descriptive summary would contribute to guiding health planners and administrators to develop proper tools for obesity management in the countries of the MENA region. National Health Accounts (NHA) is one such tool designed for health sector policy makers and managers to aid them in their efforts to improve health system performance (NHA 2003). Many countries in the MENA region (Egypt, Iran, Jordan, Lebanon, Morocco, Tunisia, Yemen, Djibouti, Gulf countries and Syria) are in the process of reforming their health systems to reveal the areas in need of more health care funding and awareness (NHA 2003). Overweight and obesity appears to be gaining steam as a key health issue to be targeted by such plans.

Genetic studies are another area where a significant amount of research in needed in the MENA region. Worldwide studies suggested that pre-disposition to obesity seems to be caused by a complex interaction between over 250 obesity-associated genes and perhaps perinatal factors. Studies that focus on the specific genetic profile pertinent to the peoples of this region would be of great relevance to any plan to combat this emerging health problem.

References

Abdulbari, B. (2006). Prevalence of obesity, overweight, and underweight in Qatari adolescents. *Food and Nutrition Bulletin, 27*, 39–45.

Abdulbari, B., & Ihab, T. (2006). Prevalence of overweight, obesity, and associated psychological problems in Qatari's female population. *Obesity Reviews, 7*, 139–145.

Abdulbari, B., Abdulaziz, K., Ihab, T., & Osman, S. (2006). Prevalence of dieting, overweight, body image satisfaction and associated psychological problems in adolescent boys. *Nutrition and Food Science, 36*, 295–304.

Al-Haddad, F., Little, B., & Abdul Ghafoor, A.G. (2005). Child obesity in United Arab Emirates schoolchildren: A national study. *Annals of Human Biology, 32*, 72–79.

Al-Hourani, H.M., Henry, C.J.K., & Lightowler, H.J. (2003). Prevalence of overweight among adolescent females in the United Arab Emirates. *American Journal of Human Biology, 15*, 758–764.

Al-Isa, A.N. (2004). Body mass index, overweight and obesity among Kuwaiti intermediate school adolescents aged 10–14 years. *European Journal of Clinical Nutrition, 58*, 1273–1277.

Al-Isa, A.N., & Moussa, M.A. (1999). Factors associated with overweight and obesity among Kuwaiti kindergarten children aged 3–5 years. *Nutrition and Health, 13*, 125–139.

Al-Nuaim, A.R., Bamgboye, E.A., & Al-Herbish, A. (1996). The pattern of growth and obesity in Saudi Arabian male school children. *International Journal of Obesity and Related Metabolic Disorders, 20*, 1000–1005.

Al-Rukban, M.O. (2003), Obesity among Saudi male adolescents in Riyadh, Saudi Arabia. *Saudi Medical Journal, 24*, 27–33.

Al-Sendi, A.M., Shetty, P., & Musaiger, A.O. (2003). Prevalence of overweight and obesity among Bahraini adolescents: a comparison between three different sets of criteria. *European Journal of Clinical Nutrition, 57*, 471–474.

Al Turki, Y.A. (2007). Overweight and obesity among university students, Riyadh, Saudi Arabia. *Middle East Journal of Family Medicine, 5*, 1–3.

American Academy of Pediatrics Policy Statement (2003). Prevention of pediatric overweight and obesity. *Pediatrics, 112*, 424–430.

Asfaw, A. (2007). Micronutrient deficiency and the prevalence of mothers' overweight / obesity in Egypt. *Economics and Human Biology, 5*, 471–483.

Azizi, F., Allahverdian, S., Mirmirian, P., Rahmani, M., & Mohammadi, F. (2001). Dietary factors and body mass index in a group of Iranian adolescents: Tehran lipid and glucose study-2. *International Journal for Vitamin and Nutrition Research, 71*, 123–127.

Bar Dayan, Y., Elishkevits, K., Grotto, I., Goldstein, L., Goldberg, A., Shvarts, S., Levin, A., Ohana, N., Onn, E., & Levi, Y. (2005). The prevalence of obesity and associated morbidity among 17-year-old Israeli conscripts. *Public Health, 119*, 385–389.

Ben Mami Ben Miled, F., Dakhli, S., Blouza, S., & Achour, A. (2000). Obesity in children. *Tunis Medicine, 78*, 162–166.

Ben Salem, K., Mandhouj, O., Letaief, M., Mtar, A., & Soltani, M. (2006). Distribution of anthropometrical parameters in infants in the Monastir region, Tunisia. *Eastern Mediterranean Health Journal, 12 (Suppl 2)*, S168–S177.

Ben Slama, F., Achour, A., Belhadj, O., Hsairi, M., Oueslati, M., & Achour, N. (2002). Obesity and lifestyle in a population of male school children aged 6 to 10 years in Ariana (Tunisia). *Tunis Medicine, 80*, 542–547.

Benjelloun, S.. (2002). Nutrition transition in Morocco. *Public Health Nutrition, 5*, 135–140.

Bakr, E.M., Ismail, N.A., & Mahaba, H.M. (2002). Impact of lifestyle on the nutritional status of medical students at Ain Shams University. *Journal of the Egyptian Public Health Association, 77*, 29–49.

Blouza-Chabchoub, S., Rached-Amrouche, C., Jamoussi-Kammoun, H., & Bouchaa, N. (2006). Frequency and risk factors of obesity in Tunisian adolescents. *Tunis Medicine, 84*, 714–716.

Centers for Disease Control and Prevention. Division of Nutrition, Physical Activity and Obesity. Atlanta (December 2008); http://www.cdc.gov/nccdphp/dnpa/obesity/childhood

Chakar, H., & Salameh, P. (2006). Adolescent obesity in Lebanese private schools. *European Journal of Public Health, 16*, 648–651.

Cole, T.J., Bellizi, M.C., & Flegal, K.M. (2000). Establishing a standard definition for child overweight and obesity worldwide: international survey. *British Medical Journal, 320*, 1240–1243.

Disease Control Priorities Project. Global burden of disease and risk factors. (November 2008); http://www.dcp2.org/pubs/GBD

El-Hazmi, M., & Warsy, A. (2002). The prevalence of obesity and overweight in 1–18-year-old Saudi children. *Annals of Saudi Medicine, 22*, 303–307.

Flodmark, C.E., Lissau, I., & Moreno, L.A.. (2004). New insights into the field of children and adolescents' obesity: the European perspective. *International Journal of Obesity and Related Metabolic Disorders, 28*, 1189–1196.

Gargari, B.P., Behzad, M.H., Ghassabpour, S., & Ayat, A. (2004). Prevalence of overweight and obesity among highschool girls in Tabriz, Iran in 2001. *Food and Nutrition Bulletin, 25*, 288–291.

Ghannem, H., Trabelsi, L., Gaha, R., Harrabi, I., & Essoussi, A.S. (2001). Study of cardiovascular disease risk factors among rural schoolchildren in Sousse, Tunisia. *Eastern Mediterranean Health Journal, 7*, 617–624.

Gittelsohn, J., & Kumar, M.B. (2007). Preventing childhood obesity and diabetes: is it time to move out of the school? *Pediatric Diabetes, 8 (Suppl. 9)*, 1–15.

Hamadeh, R.R. (2000). Non-communicable diseases among the Bahraini population: a review. *Eastern Mediterranean Health Journal, 6*, 1091–1097.

International Cablemakers Federation. MENA Definition. Vienna (November 2008); http://icf.at/?id=6174

Israeli, E., Schochat, T., Korzets, Z., Tekes-Manova, D., Bernheim, J., & Golan, E. (2006). Prehypertension and obesity in adolescents: a population study. *American Journal of Hypertension, 19*, 708–712.

Jabre, P., Sikias, P., Khater-Menassa, B., Baddoura, R., & Awada, H. (2005). Overweight children in Beirut: prevalence estimates and characteristics. *Child: Care, Health and Development, 31*, 159–165.

Jackson, R.T., Rashed, M., & Saad-Eldin, R. (2003). Rural urban differences in weight, body image, and dieting behavior among adolescent Egyptian schoolgirls. *International Journal of Food Sciences and Nutrition, 54*, 1–11.

Jackson, R.T., Rashed, M., Hwalla, N., & Al-Somaie, M. (2007). Comparison of BMI for age in adolescent girls in 3 countries of the Eastern Mediterranean Region. *Eastern Mediterranean Health Journal, 13*, 1–10.

James, P. (2004). Obesity: The worldwide epidemic. *Clinics in Dermatology, 23*, 276–280.

Janghorbani, M., & Parvin, F. (1998). Prevalence of overweight and thinness in high-school girls in Kerman, Iran. *International Journal of Obesity and Related Metabolic Disorders, 22*, 629–633.

Kaluski, D.N., & Berry, E.M. (2005). Prevalence of obesity in Israel. *Obesity Reviews, 6*, 115–116.

Katzmarzyk, P.T., Srinivasan, S.R., & Chen, W. (2004). Body mass index, waist circumference, and clustering of cardiovascular disease risk factors in a biracial sample of children and adolescents. *Pediatrics, 114*, e198–e205.

Keinan-Boker, L., Noyman, N., Chinich, A., Green, M.S., & Nitzan-Kaluski, D. (2005). Overweight and obesity in Israel: findings of the first national health and nutrition survey (MABAT). *Israel Medical Association Journal, 7*, 219–223.

Kelishadi, R. (2006). Global Dimension of Childhood Obesity in the Eastern Mediterranean region. In R.K. Flamenbaum (Ed). *Global dimensions of childhood obesity* (pp. 71–89). New York: Nova Science Publishers.

Kelishadi, R. (2007). Childhood overweight, obesity, and the metabolic syndrome in developing countries. *Epidemiologic Reviews, 29*, 62–76.

Kelishadi, R., Hashemipour, M., Sarraf-Zadegan, N., & Amiri, M. (2001). Trend of atherosclerosis risk factors in children of Isfahan. *Asian Cardiovascular and Thoracic Annals, 9*, 36–40.

Kelishadi, R., Pour, M.H., Sarraf-Zadegan, N., Sadry, G.H., Ansari, R., Alikhassy, H., & Bashardoust, N. (2003) Obesity and associated modifiable environmental factors in Iranian adolescents: Isfahan Healthy Heart Program-Heart Health Promotion from Childhood. *Pediatrics International, 45*, 435–442.

Kelishadi, R., Hashemipour, M., Sadeghi, M., Roohafza, H.R., Tavasoli, A.A., & Khosravi, A. (2005). The impact of familial factors on obesity in Iranian children and adolescents. *Journal of Pediatric Neonatal, 2,* 16–23.

Kelishadi, R., Ardalan, G., Gheiratmand, R., Gouya, M.M., Razhagi, E.M., Delavari, A., Majdzadeh, R., Heshmat, R., Motoghian, M., Barekati, H., Mahmoud-Arabi, M.S., & Riazi, M.M. (2007). Association of physical activity and dietary behaviours in relation to the body mass index in a national sample of Iranian children and adolescents: CASPIAN study. *Bulletin of the World Health Organization, 85,* 19–26.

Kelishadi, R., Alikhani, S., Delavari, A., Alaedini, F., Safaie, A., & Hojatzadeh, E. (2008). Obesity and associated lifestyle behaviors in Iran: findings from the First National Non-Communicable Disease Risk Factor Surveillance Survey. *Public Health Nutrition, 11,* 246–251.

Kharboush, I.F., Youssef, A.A., Makhlouf, M.M., Zaghloul, A.A., El-Hamid, A.A., & El Masry, A.G. (2005). Women health in poor urban settings in Alexandria. *Journal of the Egyptian Public Health Association, 80,* 321–348.

Kolahdooz, F., Sheikholeslam, R., Naghavi, M., & Abdollah, Z. (2004). Junk food consumption: an indicator of changing dietary habit in Iranian children. *Asia Pacific Journal of Clinical Nutrition, 13,* S121.

Kuczmarski, R.J., Ogden, C.L., & Grummer-Strawn, L.M. (2000). CDC growth charts: United States. *Advanced Data, 314,* 1–27.

Lafta, R.K., Al Saffar, A.J., Eisa, S.A., Hayyawi, A.H., & Abdulhameed, F.N. (2007). Obesity in children: A sample from Baghdad. *Qatar Medical Journal, 16,* 10–15.

Laouani Kechrid, C., Hmouda, H., Ben Naceur, M.H., Ghannem, H., Toumi, S., & Ajmi, F. (2004). High blood pressure for people aged more than 60 years in the district of Sousse. *Tunis Medicine, 82,* 1001–1005.

Lasserre, A., Chiolero, A., Paccaud, F., & Bovet, P. (2007). Worldwide trends in childhood obesity. *Swiss Medical Weekly, 137,* 157–158.

Levin, B.E., & Govek, E. (1998). Gestational obesity accentuates obesity in obesity-prone progeny. *American Journal of Physiology, 275,* R1374–1379.

Marsh, H., Hau, K.T., Sung, R.Y.T., & Yu, C.W. (2007). Childhood obesity, gender, actual-ideal body image discrepancies, and physical self-concept in Hong-Kong children: cultural differences in the value of moderation. *Developmental Psychology, 43,* 647–662.

Maziak, W., Rastam, S., Mzayek, F., Ward, K.D., Eissenberg, T., & Keil, U. (2007). Cardiovascular health among adults in Syria: a model from developing countries. *Annals of Epidemiology, 17,* 713–720.

Mohammadpour-Ahranjani, B., Rashidi, A., Karandish, M., Eshraghian, M.R., & Kalantari, N. (2004). Prevalence of overweight and obesity in adolescent Tehrani students, 2000–2001: an epidemic health problem. *Public Health Nutrition, 7,* 645–648.

Mokhtar, N., Elati, J., Chabir, R., Bour, A., Elkari, K., Schlossman, N., Caballero, B., & Aguenaou, H. (2001). Diet culture and obesity in Northern Africa. *The Journal of Nutrition, 131,* 887S–892S.

Monteiro, C.A., Conde, W.L., & Popkin, B.M. (2002). Is obesity replacing to undernutrition? Evidence from different social classes in Brazil. *Public Health Nutrition, 5,* 105–112.

Monteiro, C.A., Conde, W.L., Lu, B., & Popkin, B.M. (2004). Obesity and inequities in health in the developing world. *International Journal of Obesity, 28,* 1181–1186.

Moreno, L.A., Pineda, I., & Rodriguez, G. (2002). Waist circumference for the screening of the metabolic syndrome in children. *Acta Paediatrica, 91,* 1307–1312.

Moussa, M.A., Shaltout, A.A., Mourad, M., Alsheikh, N., Agha, N., & Galal, D.O. (1999). Factors associated with obesity in Kuwaiti children. *European Journal of Epidemiolology, 15,* 41–49.

Must, A., Dallal, G.E., & Dietz, W.H. (1991). Reference data for obesity: 85th and 95th percentile of body mass index and triceps skinfold thickness. *American Journal of Clinical Nutrition, 53,* 839–846.

National Health Accounts (NHA) (2003). National Health Accounts and its relevance to policymaking in the Middle East and North Africa. *NHA Regional Policy Brief,* 1–4.

Onis, M. (2004). The use of anthropometry in the prevention of childhood overweight. *International Journal of Obesity and Related Metabolic Disorders, 28,* S81–S85.

Papandreou, C., Abu Murad, T., Jideh, C., Abdeen, Z., Philalithis, A., & Tzanakis, N. (2008). Obesity in Mediterranean region (1997–2007): a systematic review. *Obesity Reviews, 9,* 389–399.

Rguibi, M., & Belahsen, R. (2004). Overweight and obesity among urban Sahraoui women of South Morocco. *Ethnicity and Disease, 14,* 542–547.

Rguibi, M., & Belahsen, R. (2007). Prevalence of obesity in Morocco. *Obesity Reviews, 8,* 11–13.

Salazar-Martinez, E., Allen, B., Fernandez-Ortega, C., Torres-Mejia, G., Galal, O., & Lazcano-Ponce, E. (2006). Overweight and obesity status among adolescents from Mexico and Egypt. *Archives of Medical Research, 37,* 535–542.

Sheikholeslam, R., Mohamad, A., Mohamad, K., & Vaseghi, S. (2004). Non communicable disease risk factors in Iran. *Asia Pacific Journal of Clinical Nutrition, 13,* S100.

Sibai, A., Hwalla, N., Adra, N., & Rahal, B. (2003). Prevalence and covariates of obesity in Lebanon: Findings from the first epidemiological study. *Obesity Research, 11,* 1353–1361.

Soutoudeh, G., Khosravi, Sh., Khajehnasiri, F., & Khalkhali, H.R. (2005). High prevalence of overweight and obesity in women of Islamshahr, Iran. *Asia Pacific of Journal of Clinical Nutrition, 14,* 169–172.

University of California, San Francisco Medical Center. (October 2008); http://www.ucsfhealth.org
Wang, Y., & Lobstein, T. (2006). Worldwide trends in childhood over-weight and obesity. *International Journal of Pediatric Obesity, 1*, 11–25.
Whitaker, R.C., & Dietz, W.H. (1998). Role of the prenatal environment in the development of obesity. *Journal of Pediatrics, 132*, 768–776.
World Development Indicators (WDI), World Bank (2008). Middle East and North Africa: regional data from the WDI database. *Regional Fact Sheet from the World Development Indicators 11 April 2008,* 1–2.
World Health Organization (WHO) (1997). Obesity: Preventing and managing the global epidemic. *Report of a WHO Consultation on Obesity,* Geneva: World Health Organization.
World Health Organization (WHO) Europe (2005). The challenge of obesity in the WHO European Region. *Fact sheet EURO/13/05* 2005, 1–6.
World Health Organization (WHO) Europe (2007). European environment and health information system. Prevalence of excess body weight and obesity in children and adolescents. *Fact sheet No.2.3 2007,* 1–4.
Yahia, N., Achkar, A., Abdallah, A., & Rizk, S. (2008). Eating habits and obesity among Lebanese university students. *Nutrition Journal, 7,* 32.

Chapter 9
Prevalence of Overweight and Obesity in Japan

Masao Yoshinaga, Tomoko Ichiki, and Yoshiya Ito

Introduction

Three critical periods for the development of obesity have been reported: the fetal period; a period of adiposity rebound between ages 4 and 6; and during adolescence (Dietz 1994). The elementary school period is also reported to be a critical period for obesity in Japan; a rapid increase in the prevalence of obesity during the elementary school period was evident in 1989/1990 (Yoshinaga et al. 2004). However, little is known about the characteristics of this rapid increase in Japanese children and adolescents.

This chapter will discuss the prevalence of overweight and obesity in Japanese children and adolescents between 1977 and 2007 by cross-sectional analysis of population-based samples. Time trends of the prevalence of overweight and obesity of 5, 8, 11, 14, and 17 year old males and females between 1977 and 2007 are also presented in detail. Time trends of obesity and severe obesity in pre-school-aged children between 1998 and 2007 are presented for a local area. Definition of overweight and obesity in this chapter is mainly based on the international body mass index (BMI) cut-off point for overweight and obesity (Cole et al. 2000). Socio-demographic and economic characteristics of Japan are described from most recent data available.

To help readers to understand the epidemiologic background of the prevalence of overweight and obesity in Japanese children and adolescents, total energy intake and intake of each macronutrient, prevalence of breast feeding, and the time trend of the prevalence of overweight in Japanese adult population are also presented.

M. Yoshinaga (✉)
Department of Pediatrics, National Hospital Organization Kagoshima Medical Center,
Shiroyama-cho 8-1, Kagoshima City 892-0853, Kagoshima, Japan
e-mail: m-yoshi@biscuit.ocn.ne.jp

T. Ichiki
Clinical Experimental Medicine, National Hospital Organization Kagoshima Medical Center,
Shiroyama- cho 8-1, Kagoshima City, 892-0853, Kagoshima, Japan

Y. Ito
Department of Clinical Medicine, The Japanese Red Cross Hokkaido College of Nursing, Akebono-cho 664,
Kitami City, Hokkaido, 090-0011, Japan

L.A. Moreno et al. (eds.), *Epidemiology of Obesity in Children and Adolescents*,
Springer Series on Epidemiology and Public Health 2, DOI 10.1007/978-1-4419-6039-9_9,
© Springer Science+Business Media, LLC 2011

Geographic Area

Definition

Japan is an island country in East Asia, located in the Pacific Ocean. Japan comprises over 6,000 islands, the largest of which are Honshu, Hokkaido, Kyushu and Shikoku, together accounting for 97% of its land area. Most of the islands are mountainous, many volcanic; for example, Japan's highest peak, Mount Fuji, was a volcano. Japan has the world's tenth largest population, with about 128 million people. The Greater Tokyo Area, which includes the capital city of Tokyo and several surrounding prefectures, is the largest metropolitan area in the world, with over 30 million residents (Japan 2008).

Socio-demographic and Economic Characteristics

Japan has the world's second largest economy by nominal Gross Domestic Product (GDP) (GDP. Japan 2008) and the third largest in purchasing power parity (Table 9.1). It is a member of the United Nations, G8, Organization for Economic Co-operation and Development (OECD) and Asia-Pacific Economic Cooperation (APEC), with the world's fifth largest defense budget. It is also the world's fourth largest exporter and sixth largest importer. It is a developed country with high living standards (eighth highest Human Development Index (HDI)) (Human Development Index, Japan 2008) and a world leader in technology, machinery, and robotics. Japan has one of the highest life expectancy rates in the world, at 81.25 years of age as of 2006. The Japanese population is rapidly aging, the effect of a post-war baby boom followed by a decrease in births in the later part of the twentieth century (Journal of Health and Welfare Statistics 2007). In 2004, about 19.5% of the population was over the age of 65 (Japan 2008).

Methods

Data Source

School-Aged Children and Adolescents

The Ministry of Education, Culture, Sports, Science and Technology in Japan performs the School Health Survey for height and weight since 1948 which is published as the Annual Report of School Health Survey by the Ministry. In these surveys, all children and adolescents in kinder-

Table 9.1 Basic demographic and economic characteristics of Japan

Area in km^2	377,944
Population (N) (2006)	127,770,000
Population below the age of 20 in % (2006)	18.7
GDP per captia by International Monetary Fund $	34,312
Population below poverty line in %	Not available
Human development index (rank order)	0.953 (eighth of 177 countries)
Life expectancy at birth in years (2006)	79 year (males)
	86 year (females)
Crude birth rate in %	8.7
Crude death rate in %	8.6
Infant mortality in %	2.6
Modest and severe wasting in %	Not available
Modest and severe stunting in %	Not available

garten and school undergo a mandatory medical examination performed by school doctors and nurses. Height and weight are measured by the school nurses in early April each year. Height is measured to the nearest 0.1 cm without shoes and weight is measured to the nearest 0.1 kg in underwear. The data have been collected each year by probability proportionate sampling. The Ministry collects information each year from 72,380 children aged 5 (from 1,645 kindergartens), 270,720 children aged 6–11 years (from 2,820 elementary schools), 225,600 adolescents aged 12–14 year (from 1,880 junior high schools), and 126,900 adolescents aged 15–17 years (from 2,820 high schools). These samples accounted for 4.7% of all children and adolescents in Japan in 2007 (Annual Report of School Health Survey 2007).

Pre-school-aged Children

There were few comprehensive data for pre-school-aged children in Japan. We obtained the data of subjects aged 3, 4, and 5 years from the Niigata Dietetic Association. The Niigata area is located in the northwest part of Japan, and it has a population of approximately 2,405,000 individuals. The Niigata Dietetic Association collects the data of about 40,000 children aged 3–5 years each year. These samples accounted for 91% of all pre-school-aged children in the Niigata area in 2006.

National Nutrition Survey

The Ministry of Health, Labor and Welfare in Japan performs the National Nutrition Survey in November every year. Households are selected by stratified random sampling methods. In the surveys, daily intake of foods is weighed by a member of the household, and the data are collected by a national registered dietitian at each house. The sample sizes were 520, 770, and 435 subjects of 1–6, 7–14, and 15–19 age groups, respectively, in 2004 (National Health and Nutrition Survey in Japan 2008a, b).

Methods of Data Retrieval and Compilation

School-Aged Children and Adolescents

Data for school-aged children and adolescents were obtained from the Annual Report of the School Health Survey (2007). The reports show the frequency per thousand children for height (every 1 cm) and weight (every 1 kg) for each age and sex. Data are expressed to one decimal place. The height and weight in the reports were input into computers by personnel of a temporary-employment agency or by those of our hospital, and re-checked against the frequency tables. Financial support for the data input was provided by several grants, as stated in the acknowledgements.

Pre-school-aged Children

Prevalence of obesity and severe obesity of pre-school-aged children in Niigata area was obtained from the annual reports of the Niigata Dietetic Association.

Nutrient Intakes in Infants, Children, and Adolescents

Total energy intake and intake of each macronutrient were obtained from the Almanac of Data on Japanese Children from 2006 to 2008 (Imperial Gift Foundation Boshi-Aiiku-Kai 2008).

Prevalence of Overweight and Obesity

Definition of Overweight and Obesity

Overweight and obesity for school-aged children and adolescents are defined by the international body mass index (BMI) cut-off point (Cole et al. 2000). BMI is calculated as (weight in kg)/(height in m)^2.

In the reports of the Niigata Dietetic Association, obesity is defined when a pre-school-aged child has a percent relative body weight (%RBW)$\geq 15\%$. Severe obesity is defined when a child has a %RBW$\geq 30\%$. The %RBW is calculated as (individual body weight) / (age-, sex-, and height-specific body weight from a reference population)$\times 100$ (Ito et al. 1996). The age-, sex-, and height-specific body weight was based on the reports of the Ministry of Health, Labor and Welfare (Ito et al. 1996).

Prevalence of Overweight and Obesity of School-Aged Children and Adolescents in 2007

Prevalence of overweight and obesity from 5 to 17 years old in both males and females in 2007 is shown in Fig. 9.1. Generally, age classes in Japanese elementary school, junior high school, and high

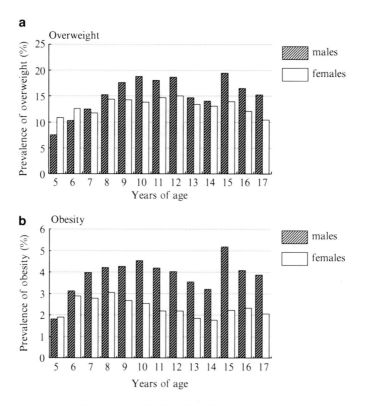

Fig. 9.1 Prevalence of overweight (**a**) and obesity (**b**) from 5 to 17 years old in males and females in 2007. Definition of overweight and obesity is based on the international BMI cut-off points for obesity. The data in Figs. 9.1–9.7 were obtained from the following database http://www.mhlw.go.jp/houdou/2006/05/h0508-1a.html (in Japanese)

school are 6–11, 12–14, and 15–17 years, respectively. Prevalence of overweight was higher in males than females from 7 years old through 17 years old. Prevalence of overweight in males increased throughout the elementary school period (Fig. 9.1a). Changes in the prevalence of overweight in females were not so prominent during school periods, compared with that in males.

Prevalence of obesity was more prominent in males than females from 6 years old through 17 years old. There was a prominent increase in the prevalence of overweight and obesity in 15 year-old boys. Entrance examinations for high school entry are mandatory for all students of 14 years old, with exception of a small number of private schools. Since a strong wish to enter some famous high schools has been present in Japan, especially in males, we suspect that more study and less physical activity may explain the increase in the prevalence of obesity of 15 year-old males (National Health and Nutrition Survey in Japan 2008a, b).

Time Trend of Prevalence of Overweight and Obesity of School-Aged Children and Adolescents Between 1977 and 2007

The time trend of the prevalence of overweight between 1977 and 2007 is shown in Fig. 9.2. The peak prevalence in 5 years old males occurred during the mid 1990s. Prevalence decreased thereafter. Among all age groups the prevalence in 11 year old males (the last year of the elementary school periods) was highest throughout the study period. Recently, the prevalence of overweight decreased

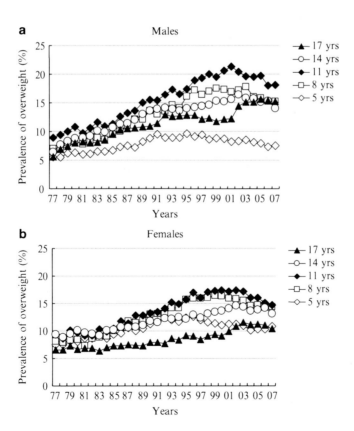

Fig. 9.2 Time trend of the prevalence of overweight in 5, 8, 11, 14, and 17 year old males (**a**) and females (**b**) from 1977 to 2007

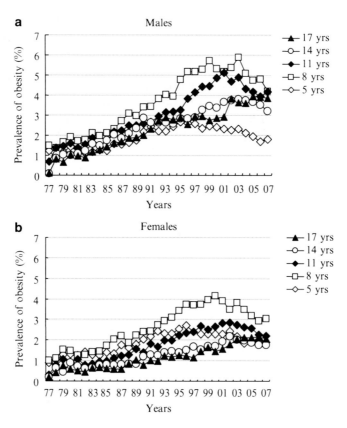

Fig. 9.3 Time trend of the prevalence of obesity in 5, 8, 11, 14, and 17 year old males (**a**) and females (**b**) from 1977 to 2007

in 8, 11, 14 year old males; however, prevalence of overweight still increased in 17 year old males. The change in the prevalence of overweight in females was smaller than that in males. The prevalence of overweight in 11 years old girls was higher than that of the other age groups after the early 1990s. Recently, the prevalence of overweight in 8 and 11 year old females was decreasing as was shown in males. Interestingly, the prevalence of overweight in 5 and 17 year old females was quite constant in recent years.

The prevalence of obesity was highest in 8 year olds in both males and females, and the prevalence of obesity was about 1.5 times higher in males than in females (Fig. 9.3). A prominent increase in the prevalence of obesity was present in early to mid 1990s, especially in males. Recently, the prevalence of obesity in 5, 8, 11, and 14 year olds was decreasing in both males and females.

Time Trend of Prevalence of Obesity and Severe Obesity of Pre-school-aged Children Between 1998 and 2007

The prevalence of obesity of 3-, 4-, and 5-year old boys and girls was almost similar between 1998 and 2007 (Fig. 9.4). However, prevalence of severe obesity in boys and 5-year old girls were gradually decreasing during the study periods (Fig. 9.5).

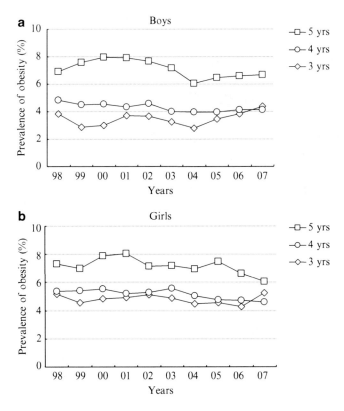

Fig. 9.4 Time trend of the prevalence of obesity of pre-school-aged children between 1998 and 2007

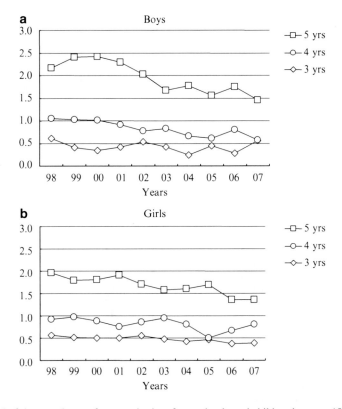

Fig. 9.5 Time trend of the prevalence of severe obesity of pre-school-aged children between 1998 and 2007

Risk Factors for Overweight and Obesity in Children and Adolescents

Total Energy Intake and Intake of Each Macronutrient

The National Nutrition Surveys (National Health and Nutrition Survey in Japan 2008a, b) showed that the total energy intake and intakes of protein and fat were similar in infants and children of 1–6 years of age, and that those in males were higher than those in females after the age of 7 years in 2004 (Fig. 9.6). The data suggest that one reason of sex difference of prevalence of overweight and obesity is the difference in energy intakes between sexes in children and adolescents.

Prevalence of Breastfeeding

Prevalence of breastfeeding and mixed feeding at 1 month was 42.4 and 52.5%, respectively, in 2005 in Japan. Prevalence of breastfeeding and mixed feeding at 3 months was 38.0 and 41.0%, respectively (Nutrition Survey in Infants 2006). The relationship between breastfeeding and prevention of obesity in children and adolescent is not clearly demonstrated in Japan.

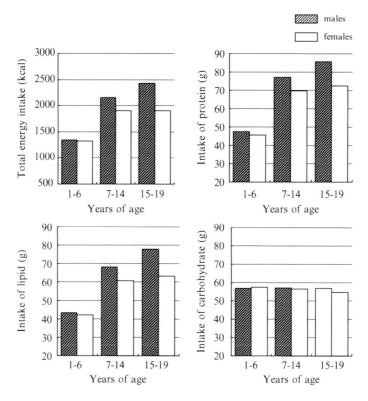

Fig. 9.6 Total calorie intake and intakes of protein, fat, and carbohydrate in infants, children, and adolescents. The total energy intake and intakes of protein, fat, and carbohydrate were similar between boys and girls aged 1–6 years old of age. However, the total energy intake and intakes of nutrients were higher in males than in females of children and adolescents aged 7–14 and 15–19 years of age

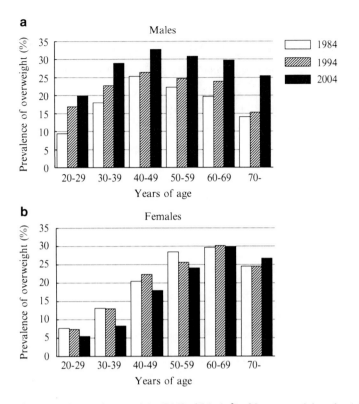

Fig. 9.7 Time trend of the prevalence of overweight (BMI ≥ 25 kg/m²) of Japanese adult males (**a**) and females (**b**) by age groups in 1984, 1994, and 2004

Prevalence of Overweight in Adults in Japan

The time trend of the prevalence of overweight (BMI ≥ 25 kg/m²) between 1984 and 2004 showed a rapid increase in the prevalence in males (Fig. 9.7). The data were based on the report published by the Ministry of Health, Labor and Welfare (National Health Nutrition Survey in Japan, 2006). The prevalence of overweight in males of the age group of 20–29 (19.9%) was much higher than that of 17 year old males in 2004 (15.1%, Fig. 9.2), indicating that the prevalence of obesity seriously increases from adolescence until the age group of 40–49 in males. The time trend of the prevalence of overweight in females showed a decrease from 1994 to 2004, except for the age group of greater than or equal to 70. The prevalence in the age group of 20–29 (5.4%) in 2004 was lower than that of 17 year old females in 2004 (11.2%, Fig. 9.2). We have no data to explain this decrease; however, wish to slim down may be greatest in the age group of 20–29 among all age groups. Thereafter the prevalence of overweight rapidly increased until the age group of 60–69 (29.9%).

Conclusions

This chapter shows that an explosive increase in the prevalence of overweight and obesity was present from 1977 (the first year of the study periods) until around 2000, especially in elementary school children; thereafter the prevalence was decreasing. The prevalence in 5 year old children decreased from late 1990s. On the other hand, the prevalence of overweight in adolescent males and male adults has been increasing. The data presented in this chapter suggest that Japan has started to reduce the problem of obesity in part, although the situation has not improved in the adolescent and adult population, especially not in males.

Acknowledgements This work was supported by the Foundation of Tanita Healthy Weight Promotion grants 2001 and 2004, the Chiyoda Mutual Life Foundation 2005, Mitsui Life Social Welfare Foundation 2007, and the Health and Labor Sciences Research Grants [Comprehensive Research on Cardiovascular and Life-style Related Diseases (H18-049)].

References

Annual Report of School Health Survey (2007). (http://www.mext.go.jp/b_menu/toukei/001/003/18/07031614/017.xls) (in Japanese) (December 1, 2008).

Cole, T.J., Bellizzi, M.C., Flegal, K.M., & Dietz, W.H. (2000). Establishing a standard definition for child at risk of overweight and overweight worldwide: international survey. *British Medical Journal, 320,* 1240–1243.

Dietz, W.H. (1994). Critical periods in childhood for development of obesity. *American Journal of Clinical Nutrition, 59,* 955–959.

GDP Japan (2008). http://ja.wikipedia.org/wiki/%E5%9B%BD%E3%81%AE%E5%9B%BD%E5%86%85%E7%B7%8F%E7%94%9F%E7%94%A3%E9%A0%86%E3%83%AA%E3%82%B9%E3%83%88#.E5.90.8D.E7.9B. AEGDP (December 1, 2008).

Human Development Index Japan (2008). http://hdrstats.undp.org/countries/country_fact_sheets/cty_fs_JPN.html (December 1, 2008).

Imperial Gift Foundation Boshi-Aiiku-Kai (2008). The National Health and Nutrition Survey in Japan. In: *Almanac of Data on Japanese Children.* Tokyo: Chuoh Publishing (in Japanese).

Ito, Y., Okuno, A., Murakami, Y., Uchiyama, M., Okada, T., Sakamoto, M. et al. (1996). Infantile standard height and weight curve for assessment of obesity. *Journal of Child Health, 55,* 752–756 (in Japanese).

Japan (2008). http://en.wikipedia.org/wiki/Japan (December 1, 2008).

Journal of Health and Welfare Statistics (2007). *Journal of Health and Welfare Statistics, 54,* 42 (in Japanese).

National Health and Nutrition Survey in Japan (2008a). http://www.mhlw.go.jp/houdou/2008/04/h0430-2.html (in Japanese) (December 1, 2008).

National Health and Nutrition Survey in Japan (2008b). http://www.mhlw.go.jp/houdou/2006/05/h0508-1a.html (in Japanese) (December 1, 2008).

Nutrition Survey in Infants (2006). http://www.mhlw.go.jp/houdou/2006/06/h0629-1.html (in Japanese) (December 1, 2008).

Yoshinaga, M., Shimago, A., Koriyama, C., Nomura, Y., Miyata, K., Hashiguchi, J., & Arima, K. (2004). Rapid increase in the prevalence of obesity in elementary school children. *International Journal of Obesity, 28,* 494–499.

Chapter 10
Social Epidemiology of Nutritional Burden Among Children and Adolescents in India

Jessica M. Perkins and S.V. Subramanian

Introduction

The increasing burdens of overweight and obesity in India, and their associated health consequences, have been receiving substantial attention (Bharati et al. 2007; Deepa et al. 2009; Gopalan 2001; Gopinath et al. 1994; Griffiths and Bentley 2001; Gupta et al. 2006a; Laxmaiah et al. 2007; Misra 2002; Misra et al. 2006b; Pednekar et al. 2008; Reddy et al. 2002; Sauvaget et al. 2008; Singh and Sharma 2005; Singh et al. 1995, 1999, 2003, 2007). Among children and adolescents in India, the documented prevalence of overweight and obesity has ranged from 1 to 24%, depending on the subgroup (Table 10.1). Fifteen percent of ever-married women and 12% of ever-married men between the ages of 15 and 49 in India in 2005–2006 were documented as overweight or obese (IIPS 2007). A consequence of obesity, coronary heart disease is predicted to rank first among the causes of death among adults in the Indian population by 2015 (Bulatao and Stephens 1992). Yet, India has one of the highest levels of undernutrition in the world, higher than most countries of sub-Saharan Africa (Black et al. 2008) despite the lower levels of poverty and infant and child mortality, as well as a faster rate of economic growth (Deaton and Dreze 2008).

Although India is currently experiencing an economic (as well as a social and nutritional) transition, it is still defined as a low income country and is still in the early stages of the nutrition transition (Kennedy et al. 2006; Ramachandran 2006). In rapidly developing economies, there is usually a paradoxical coexistence of the burden of underweight and overweight, often referred to as the double burden of nutrition (Kapoor and Anand 2002; Kennedy et al. 2006). The commonly held perspective in nutrition has been that in the initial stages of the nutritional transition, which accompanies rapid economic growth, the burden of overweight tends to fall on the high socio-economic status (SES) groups. The burden of overweight is posited to shift, however, to low SES groups as countries develop (Popkin 2004) with the double nutritional burden largely concentrated among low SES groups (Monteiro et al. 2004). This typical social patterning, found in most developed countries and some developing countries – where overweight and obesity most often occur among the lower socio-economic classes (and where there are low levels of underweight) does not yet apply to India.

J.M. Perkins
Department of Health Policy, Harvard University, Cambridge, MA, USA

S.V. Subramanian (✉)
Department of Society, Human Development and Health, Harvard School of Public Health,
677 Huntington Avenue, 7th floor, Boston, MA 02115, USA
e-mail: svsubram@hsph.harvard.edu

L.A. Moreno et al. (eds.), *Epidemiology of Obesity in Children and Adolescents*,
Springer Series on Epidemiology and Public Health 2, DOI 10.1007/978-1-4419-6039-9_10,
© Springer Science+Business Media, LLC 2011

163

Table 10.1 Information from small, non-nationally representative studies of overweight and obesity among children and adolescents in various parts of India

References	Age group/sex	N	Location	Year of data collection	Reference cut-off points	Overweight prevalence	Obesity prevalence	Combined prevalence
Dasgupta et al. (2008)	7–16 years/M only	800+	Kolkata, West Bengal	1982–1993, 1999–2002	85th percentile BMI cut-off according to WHO standards	Overweight increased from 4.7% in 1982 to 17.2% in 2002		
Aggarwal et al. (2008)	High school/ M & F	1,000	Ludhiana, Punjab	NA	IOTF age and sex specific BMI 85th and 95th percentiles	12.7% overall; 15% of boys; 10.2% of girls	3.4% obese	
Bhardwaj et al. (2008)	14–17 years/ M & F	3,493	New Delhi	2002, 2006	Author's criteria			Overweight/obesity increased from 16% in 2002 to 24% in 2006
Unnithan and Syamakumari (2008)	10–15 years/ M & F	3,886	Thiruvananthapuram education district of Kerala	NA	NA	21.3% of boys; 16.4% of girls	6.7% of boys; 3.8% of girls	
Kumar et al. (2008)	2–5 years/ M & F	425	Mangalore City	NA	Child Growth Standards from WHO	4.5% overall	1.4% overall	
Bharati et al. (2008a)	10–17 years/ M & F	2,555	Wardha City, Central India	NA	CDC BMI age and sex specific 85th and 95th percentile	3.1% for boys and girls	1.2% for boys and girls	
Kuriyan et al. (2007)	6–16 years/ M & F	598	Bangalore City	NA	IOTF standards			6.4% overall
Raj et al. (2007)	5–16 years/ M & F	20,000+	Ernakulam District, Kerala	2003, 2005	Sex- and age-specific BMI percentile cut-offs	Increased from 4.94% in 2003 to 6.57% in 2005 overall		
Sood et al. (2007)	9–18 years/ G only	794	Bangalore City	NA	CDC BMI age and sex specific 85th and 95th percentile for <18 years; IOTF for >17 years	13.10%	4.30%	
Mehta et al. (2007)	16–17 years/ G only	414	Delhi	2002	IOTF age and sex specific BMI 85th and 95th percentiles	15.20%	5.30%	
Laxmaiah et al. (2007)	12–17 years/ M & F	1,208	Hyderabad, Andhra Pradesh	NA	IOTF standards	6.1% of boys; 8.2% of girls	1.6% of boys; 1.0% of girls	

Study	Population	n	Location	Year	Criteria	Overweight	Obesity
Sidhu et al. (2006)	M & F	1,000	Ludhiana, Punjab	NA	NA	12.2% of boys; 14.3% of girls	5.92% of boys; 6.27% of girls
Gupta et al. (2006b)	11–17 years/ G only	1,000	Jaipur	1997, 2003	Sex- and age-specific BMI percentile cut-offs	10.9% in 1997; 10.5% in 2003	5.5% in 1997; 6.7% in 2003
Chhatwal et al. (2004)	9–15 years/ M & F	2,008	Ludhiana, Punjab	NA	Age- and sex-specific BMI ≥85th percentile based on WHO growth charts created from NHANES I; obese children also had to have TSFT ≥90th percentile	12.4% of boys; 15.7% of girls	9.9% of boys; 12.9% of girls
Ramachandran et al. (2002)	13–18 years/ M & F	4,700	Tamilnadu, India	NA	Expected status at age 18 of overweight (BMI ≥25) and obesity (BMI ≥30)	17.8% of boys; 15.7% of girls	3.6% of boys; 2.7% of girls

The purpose of this chapter is threefold: (1) to document the prevalence of overweight and obesity among children and adolescents in India (as well as underweight, stunting, and wasting because a far greater proportion of Indian youth face undernutrition problems in addition to a potentially increasing risk for overweight and obesity); (2) to report on the social epidemiology (social patterning) of nutritional status because weight status has been found to differ between subgroups; and (3) to summarize the available information on lifestyle risk factors for overweight/obesity among Indian youth. Given that India represents an amalgam of persona by most possible indicators of SES and that there is diversity across measures, any description of the social patterning of weight status should include discussion on clearly identified dimensions of SES (Braveman et al. 2005). Policy makers can use information across multiple SES spectrums as a foundation for planning preventive health care programs aimed at improving nutritional status among all different groups. This is especially important when we are looking at the possible co-existence of nutrition problems (both underweight and overweight in the same subgroup). Furthermore, if nutrition interventions are based on one set of SES-related patterns, but targeted at a different type of SES subgroup, the intervention may fail to produce results.

Although a few studies point to a general positive association between different measures of SES and the risk of overweight in India, the pattern of this association may differ depending on the measure. There are various dimensions along which the social distribution of overweight/obesity among children and adolescents can be discussed. The specific SES measure used to describe the prevalence of overweight and obesity in India is hugely salient. Many health and nutrition policies are based on evidence highlighting specific subgroups of society as at risk, and thus, target certain groups. As such, how SES is measured may affect research outcomes with implications on health policy and subsequent interventions (Braveman et al. 2005). If the evidence only takes into account one of the SES measures, then a policy may overlook serious risk among subgroups identified as at risk by other measures. The changing economic and social environment in India, coupled with an extremely diverse population, proposes a complex and dynamic social pattern of overweight/obesity in India. Moreover, India's regional heterogeneity and history of gender discrimination points to even greater possibility for a variety of nutrition patterns.

Socio-Demographic and Economic Characteristics of India

Bordering the Arabian Sea and the Bay of Bengal, India (comprised of 29 states) sits between Burma and Pakistan in Southern Asia covering 3,287,590 km² (CIA 2008). With a population growth rate of 1.7% between 1990 and 2005 (WB 2008), there were approximately 1,147,995,904 people in India in 2008 (CIA 2008) at which point there were 189.2 million males and 172.2 million females between the ages of 0 and 14 years. The median age was 25.1 years. In 2007, the estimated Gross Domestic Product (GDP) (purchasing power parity) was $2.989 trillion (the fourth largest economy in the world) although an estimated 25% of the population lived below the poverty line (CIA 2008). From 2008 estimates, the crude birth rate was 2.22%, the crude death rate was 0.64%, the infant mortality rate was 3.23%, and life expectancy was 69.25 years (CIA 2008).

Methods

Data

We compiled information on nutritional status from several studies investigating underweight and overweight prevalence as well as risk factors among various populations in India. Some of these studies used data from the Indian National Family Health Surveys 1998–1999 (NFHS-2) and

2005–2006 (NFHS-3) (IIPS and ORC-Macro 2000, 2007). These surveys covered various demographic and health aspects of women aged 15–49 years and their children aged 0–3 (NFHS-2) or under 5 years (NFHS-3), and were conducted in one of the 18 Indian languages in respondents' homes and had high response rates. We also referenced data from several small studies focused on nutritional outcomes, risk factors, and demographics from children and adolescents in specific areas (Aggarwal et al. 2008; Bharati et al. 2008a; Bhardwaj et al. 2008; Chhatwal et al. 2004; Dasgupta et al. 2008; Gupta et al. 2006b; Kumar et al. 2008; Kuriyan et al. 2007; Laxmaiah et al. 2007; Mehta et al. 2007; Raj et al. 2007; Ramachandran et al. 2002; Sidhu et al. 2006; Sood et al. 2007; Unnithan and Syamakumari 2008). All of the studies were published between 2002 and 2008.

Measures

For a basic description of the various measures of overweight and obesity, please refer to Chapter 3. This section details how the accuracy of various nutrition measures may differ for the Indian population as compared to other racial/ethnic groups. Much of the current knowledge regarding the variance in nutrition and body measurements for South Asians has focused on adults. It may be that those results are applicable to Indian children and adolescents as well. A major data limitation of many studies is the use of body mass index (BMI) as the only measure of nutritional status. Because of differences in body frame sizes and body proportions, at any given BMI, Indians may have a higher proportion of body fat and thus an elevated risk of some of the long-term consequences of obesity, in particular, diabetes and cardiovascular disease (Misra and Vikram 2004; Yajnik 2004). Even at birth, Indian babies exhibit a thin-fat phenomenon where they are centrally adipose, but thin in muscle which suggests that they preserve more fat than white babies of similar or larger size (Yajnik et al. 2002). Thus, a given BMI may confer a greater risk of obesity-related diseases, such as diabetes and cardiovascular disease, among Indians than in the populations in which the BMI standards were initially developed (Snehalatha et al. 2003). Waist circumference (WC) (Misra et al. 2006a) and waist-to-hip ratios (WHR) (Yusuf et al. 2005), consequently, have been suggested as better markers of obesity. Recent studies have shown that South Asians have the poorest correlation between WC and BMI when comparing them against Europeans, Chinese, and Aboriginal persons, although the correlation is still substantial (Razak et al. 2005). Furthermore, at any given WC (as well as at almost any given BMI level), South Asians also have more metabolic abnormalities than do Europeans (Misra et al. 2006a; Razak et al. 2005). Thus, South Asians not only tend to gain more abdominal obesity, but their cut-off for elevated WC should also be lowered (Misra et al. 2006a).

Indeed, for adults the relevance of BMI as a measure of obesity has been called into question on the basis of an international case-control study (Yusuf et al. 2005). However, note that BMI is a strong predictor of WC (Molarius et al. 1999), and these critiques of BMI, although central to analyses dealing exclusively with obesity, are not particularly applicable to the present discussion in which the focus is on the entire nutritional spectrum, including underweight. It is possible, however, that the social patterning of BMI will not adequately reflect the social patterning of body fat, such that persons in less favored socio-economic groups may have a higher proportion of body fat at a given BMI, as has been shown in populations from developed countries (Ness et al. 2006). Regarding children and adolescents, children with ancestral origin in South Asia manifest adiposity, insulin resistance and metabolic perturbations earlier in life as compared to other ethnic groups, and these derangements are of higher magnitude than for white Caucasian children (Bhardwaj et al. 2008).

Within the research conducted among Indian children and adolescents, various measures have been employed to obtain the prevalence of overweight and obesity. Measures using BMI have focused on cut-offs for overweight and obesity as indicated by the (1) age- and sex-specific BMI cut-offs that correspond to BMIs of 25 for overweight and 30 for obesity at age 18 or 85th and 95th percentiles, respectively, for those under 18 years as provided by the International Obesity Task Force (IOTF) (Cole 2002; Cole et al. 2000), (2) age- and sex-specific Child Growth Standards provided by the World Health Organization with overweight and obesity defined as BMI > 85th and 95th percentiles and WHO z-scores of weight-for-age, height-for-age and weight-for-height (WHO 2006), and (3) age- and sex-specific BMI percentile references as provided by the Centers for Disease Control (CDC) in the United States where overweight is represented by the 85th percentile and obesity the 95th percentile for up to 19 year olds (Kuczmarski et al. 2000). Others have looked at the percent of body fat, WC > 80 cm, or WHR > 0.85 to denote central obesity, and triceps skinfold test (TSFT) where those with TSFT > 90th percentile for age and sex were defined as obese.

Regarding undernutrition, the World Health Organization has created standards which are often used to represent various levels of undernutrition. They calculate stunting with height-for-age, wasting with weight-for-height, and underweight with weight-for-age using z-scores (WHO 2008). Below 2 standard deviations from the median of the reference population represents children who fall into one of these categories. If their z-score falls below 3 standard deviations, the children are considered to be severely affected. One study argues that the standard indices of stunting, wasting and underweight may underestimate problems. Based on anthropometric data from 24,396 children in India, they created an alternative composite index of anthropometric failure (CIAF), which provides a single, aggregated figure of the number of undernourished children in a population. Although stunting, wasting, and underweight may represent separate problems, the CIAF allows examination of the relationship between these types of anthropometric failures by defining subgroups of children and relating them to poverty and morbidity. They showed that children with multiple anthropometric failures are at a greater risk of morbidity and are more likely to come from poorer households (Nandy et al. 2005). No present studies however, of which we are aware, have used this measure to determine the extent of nutrition problems among children and adolescents in India.

Prevalence

Overweight and Obesity

There are very few nationally representative studies on the prevalence of and risk factors for overweight and obesity among youth in India. According to the NFHS-3, there were very few children under age 5 who were overweight (<1%) (IIPS and Macro-International 2007). There are, however, several small, non-representative studies (and a few city-representative studies) that have recently examined the prevalence of nutrition problems among specific populations of children and adolescents in India (see Table 10.1). Among 1,000 affluent adolescents in Ludhiana, Punjab, 12.24% of the boys and 14.31% of the girls were overweight, and 5.92% of the boys and 6.27% of the girls were obese (according to the CDC standards) (Sidhu et al. 2006). Among another 1,000 affluent adolescents in Ludhiana, the overall prevalence of obesity was 3.4% and the overweight prevalence was 15% among the boys and 10.2% among the girls according to the IOTF standards (Aggarwal et al. 2008).

The prevalence of overweight and obesity (according to CDC standards) among 794 affluent adolescent school girls (9–18 years old) in Bangalore City was 13.1 and 4.3%, respectively (Sood et al. 2007). Similarly, among 414 affluent girls (16–17 years old) in Delhi, 15.2% were overweight and 5.3% were obese according to International Obesity Task Force standards (Mehta et al. 2007).

Among 3,493 urban children from New Delhi aged 14–17 years, 24% were overweight or obese (cut-off based on an age-sex-specific 85th percentile distribution developed by the authors of the study – Misra et al., unpublished data 2006–2007) in 2006, which indicated an increase in the prevalence of overweight/obesity from 16% in 2002 (Bhardwaj et al. 2008).

Among 2,008 students aged 9–15 years, where half of them attended a mostly upper class school and the other half attended two schools of lower and middle class background in Ludhiana, the prevalence of overweight and obesity was 14.2 and 11.1%, respectively (Chhatwal et al. 2004). Overweight status was calculated using age- and sex-specific BMI ≥ 85th percentile based on WHO growth charts created from NHANES I (WHO 1995). (Note: this is an older method for calculating weight status and was based on the first version of the NHANES growth charts.) Obese children also had to have an age-sex-specific TSFT ≥ 90th percentile in addition to being above the 85th percentile in BMI.

Another study on 4,700 urban adolescents (aged 13–18) from Tamilnadu, India showed that the expected prevalence at age 18 of overweight (BMI ≥ 25) and obesity (BMI ≥ 30) was 17.8 and 3.6% for boys, respectively, and 15.8 and 2.7% for girls, respectively (Ramachandran et al. 2002).

Among 1,208 students aged 12–17 years in Hyderabad, India, the prevalence of overweight among girls and boys was 8.2 and 6.1%, respectively, according to IOTF standards (Laxmaiah et al. 2007).

Among 598 male and female children aged 6–16 years in Bangalore from lower to middle socio-economic status households, the prevalence of overweight and above was 6.4% according to IOTF standards (Kuriyan et al. 2007).

Among 3,886 adolescents aged 10–15 years in the Thiruvananthapuram education district of Kerala, 21.3% of males and 16.4% of females were overweight, and 6.7% of males and 3.8% of females were obese (Unnithan and Syamakumari 2008). The urban/rural breakdown of overweight and above for girls was 24.2 and 14.2%, respectively, and for boys the breakdown was 20.0 and 11.2%, respectively.

Among a random sample of 425 children aged 2–5 years old attending nursery schools in semi-urban south India (Mangalore City), the prevalence of overweight was 4.5% and obesity was 1.4% according to the Child Growth Standards provided by the WHO (Kumar et al. 2008). (There was no breakdown by sex available.)

The prevalence of overweight and obesity was 3.1 and 1.2%, respectively, among a random sample of 2,555 children aged 10–17 years in Wardha City, Central India according to CDC standards (Bharati et al. 2008a). There was no significant difference in the prevalence of overweight/obesity between boys and girls.

A study on childhood obesity trends among a representative sample of over 20,000 schoolchildren from one district in Kerala showed an increasing trend in only 2 years (Raj et al. 2007). They found that the proportion of overweight children (sex- and age-specific BMI percentile cut-offs) significantly increased from 4.9% of the total students in 2003 to 6.6% in 2005 (OR: 1.4; 95% CI: 1.3–1.5; $P < 0.0001$) for both sexes. This rising trend, however, was limited to children in private schools.

Among middle-class boys from West Bengal aged 7–16 years ($n = 816$ in 1982–1983 and $n = 1,187$ in 1999–2002), the prevalence of overweight (BMI ≥ 85th percentile according to the Who standards) increased from 4.7% in 1982–1983 to 17.2% in 1999–2002 (Dasgupta et al. 2008).

A cross-sectional study of 1,224 girls in 1997 and 915 in 2003 aged 11–17 years of low socio-economic status showed that 10.9% were overweight and 5.5% were obese in 1997 compared to an overweight prevalence of 10.5% and an obesity prevalence of 6.7% in 2003 (Gupta et al. 2006b).

Underweight, Stunting, and Wasting

Despite the increasing risk of overweight among children and adolescents in India, undernutrition remains the largest burden among Indian children and adolescents. Nationally representative data from the Indian National Family and Health Surveys 1–3 (1992–1993, 1998–1999, 2005–2006) have shown that the percentage of children under age 3 years (according to WHO standards) who

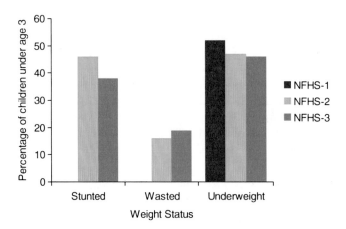

Fig. 10.1 The percentage of children under 3 years of age in three undernutrition-related weight status categories according to the NFHS 1–3 (IIPS 2007)

are wasted has increased to 19%, who are underweight has decreased to 46%, and who are stunted has decreased to 38% by 2005–2006 (see Fig. 10.1) (IIPS 2007). The 2005–2006 survey indicated similar results for children under age 5 years: 43% were underweight with 16% severely underweight; 48% were stunted with 24% severely stunted; 20% were identified as wasted (Arnold 2007; IIPS and ORC-Macro 2007). Similar to previous NFHS surveys, the 2005–2006 surveys revealed few differences between male and female children (Arnold 2007).

A nationally representative study of children 35 months or younger from rural India indicated that 48.3% suffered from stunting (chronic undernutrition) and 16.2% suffered from wasting (acute undernutrition) in 1998–1999 (Rajaram et al. 2007). This study revealed that prevalence of chronic undernutrition is greater than that of acute undernutrition and that a higher prevalence of chronic malnutrition (more than 50%) exists within many of the rural areas in the northern states compared with other regions of India.

Another nationally representative study of 26,360 children aged 0–35 months from all 26 Indian states in 1998–1999 showed similar findings (Bharati et al. 2008b).

Moreover, the NFHS-3 showed that undernutrition continues to be substantially higher in rural areas than in urban areas (IIPS and Macro-International 2007). However, even in urban areas, at least 40% of children under age 5 are stunted and 33% are underweight (IIPS and Macro-International 2007).

Unfortunately, there are no nationally representative studies on undernutrition prevalence among children older than age 5 and less than age 15. There are, however, several smaller studies. Among 3,886 adolescents aged 10–15 years in Thiruvananthapuram, Kerala 15.5% of males and 17.0% of females were underweight, and 1.9% of males and 3.1% of females were severely underweight, according to IOTF standards (Unnithan and Syamakumari 2008). The urban/rural breakdown of underweight and below for girls and boys was 14.1/26.0% and 5.9/25.2%, respectively.

India's tribal population, representing approximately 8% of the total population, is particularly vulnerable to undernutrition because of their isolation, inadequate facilities, and socio-economic disadvantage. Among almost 13,000 adolescents (aged 10–17 years) in 1998–1999 from various tribal areas of India, 63% of boys and 42% of girls were undernourished according to a cut-off of <5th BMI age-specific percentile (Rao et al. 2006).

Among middle-class boys from West Bengal aged 7–16 years ($n=816$ in 1982–1983 and $n=1,187$ in 1999–2002), the prevalence of stunting (height-for-age <3rd percentile) and thinness (BMI<5th percentile) had decreased, from 11.2 to 4.9%, respectively (Dasgupta et al. 2008).

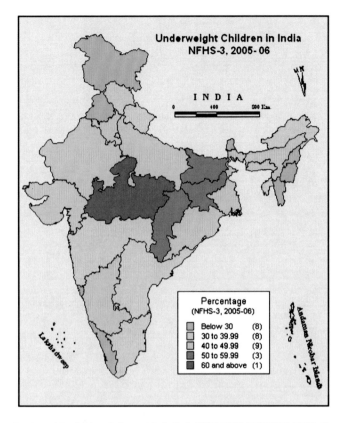

Fig. 10.2 Percentage of underweight children (<5 years) in India in 2005–2006 (MOHFW 2007). *Source*: MOHFW (2007)

Among cross sectional groups of low socio-economic status girls aged 11–17 years in Jaipur, the prevalence of wasting and stunting was 36.1 and 0.2%, respectively in 1997 and 27.7 and 0.3%, respectively, in 2003 (Gupta et al. 2006b).

In terms of geographic variation, in four Indian states the prevalence of underweight children under age 5 years is at least 50% (see Fig. 10.2) (MOHFW 2007). The underweight prevalence drops below 36% for only 12 (out of 29) Indian states (Table 10.2).

Dual Burden

The existence of the dual burden nutrition paradox – the occurrence of both undernutrition and overweight – is playing an important role in much of the nutrition transition literature as it becomes a salient dilemma for policymakers. This paradox can be explored at multiple levels such as within country, within SES groups, or within households. In many countries, both undernutrition and overweight problems exist across the general population. As a country's GDP increases, the population's diet shifts and physical activity reduces, and therefore, the prevalence of overweight increases (Popkin 2003; Popkin et al. 2002). As has been previously shown, there is a double burden of both overweight and underweight children in India at the country level.

Some research has explored the double burden paradox at the within group level, by examining the prevalence of both underweight and overweight within women in the highest wealth quintile (Subramanian et al. 2009). The ratio of underweight to overweight women was only

Table 10.2 Percentage of children under 5 years of age classified as malnourished according to three anthropometric indices of nutritional status: height-for-age, weight-for-height, and weight-for-age according to states, India, 2005–2006 (IIPS and Macro-International 2007)

State	Height-for-age			Weight-for-height				Weight-for-age			
	Percentage below −3 SD	Percentage below −2 SD[a]	Mean z-score (SD)	Percentage below −3 SD	Percentage below −2 SD[a]	Percentage above +2 SD	Mean z-score (SD)	Percentage below −3 SD	Percentage below −2 SD[a]	Percentage above +2 SD	Mean z-score (SD)
India	23.7	48.0	−1.9	6.4	19.8	1.5	−1.0	15.8	42.5	0.4	−1.8
North											
Delhi	20.4	42.2	−1.6	7.0	15.4	4.0	−0.5	8.7	26.1	1.0	−1.3
Haryana	19.4	45.7	−1.8	5.0	19.1	1.4	−1.0	14.2	39.6	0.2	−1.7
Himachal Pradesh	16.0	38.6	−1.5	5.5	19.3	1.1	−1.0	11.4	36.5	0.5	−1.6
Jammu and Kashmir	14.9	35.0	−1.3	4.4	14.8	2.3	−0.7	8.2	25.6	0.5	−1.3
Punjab	17.3	36.7	−1.5	2.1	9.2	1.5	−0.5	8.0	24.9	0.5	−1.2
Rajasthan	22.7	43.7	−1.7	7.3	20.4	1.6	−1.1	15.3	39.9	0.4	−1.7
Uttaranchal	23.1	44.4	−1.8	5.3	18.8	2.3	−0.9	15.7	38.0	0.3	−1.7
Central											
Chhattisgarh	24.8	52.9	−2.0	5.6	19.5	1.3	−1.1	16.4	47.1	0.0	−1.9
Madhya Pradesh	26.3	50.0	−2.0	12.6	35.0	1.0	−1.6	27.3	60.0	0.1	−2.3
Uttar Pradesh	32.4	56.8	−2.2	5.1	14.8	1.2	−0.8	16.4	42.4	0.1	−1.8
East											
Bihar	29.1	55.6	−2.1	8.3	27.1	0.3	−1.4	24.1	55.9	0.1	−2.2
Jharkhand	26.8	49.8	−1.9	11.8	32.3	0.6	−1.5	26.1	56.5	0.2	−2.2
Orissa	19.6	45.0	−1.7	5.2	19.5	1.7	−1.0	13.4	40.7	0.5	−1.7
West Bengal	17.8	44.6	−1.7	4.5	16.9	1.9	−0.9	11.1	38.7	0.5	−1.6
Northeast											
Arunachal Pradesh	21.7	43.3	−1.6	6.1	15.3	3.4	−0.7	11.1	32.5	0.6	−1.4
Assam	20.9	46.5	−1.8	4.0	13.7	1.2	−0.8	11.4	36.4	0.3	−1.6
Manipur	13.1	35.6	−1.4	2.1	9.0	2.2	−0.6	4.7	22.1	0.5	−1.2
Meghalaya	29.8	55.1	−2.0	19.9	30.7	2.6	−1.2	27.7	48.8	0.2	−2.0
Mizoram	17.7	39.8	−1.6	3.5	9.0	4.3	−0.3	5.4	19.9	1.2	−1.1

Nagaland	19.3	38.8	−1.4	5.2	13.3	4.7	−0.5	7.1	25.2	0.8	−1.2
Sikkim	17.9	38.3	−1.4	3.3	9.7	8.3	−0.1	4.9	19.7	1.3	−0.9
Tripura	14.7	35.7	−1.5	8.6	24.6	2.2	−1.2	15.7	39.6	0.1	−1.7
West											
Goa	10.2	25.6	−1.1	5.6	14.1	4.3	−0.7	6.7	25.0	1.9	−1.1
Gujarat	25.5	51.7	−2.0	5.8	18.7	1.2	−1.0	16.3	44.6	0.1	−1.8
Maharashtra	19.1	46.3	−1.8	5.2	16.5	2.8	−0.9	11.9	37.0	0.9	−1.6
South											
Andhra Pradesh	18.7	42.7	−1.7	3.5	12.2	2.2	−0.7	9.9	32.5	0.6	−1.5
Karnataka	20.5	43.7	−1.7	5.9	17.6	2.6	−1.0	12.8	37.6	0.5	−1.6
Kerala	6.5	24.5	−1.1	4.1	15.9	1.2	−0.9	4.7	22.9	0.4	−1.2
Tamil Nadu	10.9	30.9	−1.1	8.9	22.2	3.6	−1.0	6.4	29.8	1.9	−1.3

Note: Table is based on children who stayed in the household the night before the interview. Each of the indices is expressed in standard deviation units (SD) from the median of the 2006 WHO International Reference Population. Table is based on children with valid dates of birth (month and year) and valid measurements of both height and weight

Source: IIPS and Macro-International (2007)

[a]Includes children who are below −3 standard deviations (SD) from the Reference Population median

equal (or tilted towards more overweight women) among the highest wealth quintile and higher education groups. Among the lower classes, the prevalence of underweight women was much higher than overweight women. Although the situation appears to be changing in India as the prevalence of overweight or obese women in India has increased from 10.6 to 14.8% from 1998–1999 to 2005–2006 (IIPS 2007), the nutrition transition still appears to be split by SES (Subramanian et al. 2009). The beginning dual burden among the upper classes might be true for children in India as well, however.

Other researchers have found a significant presence of dual burden within households where at least one household member is underweight and one is overweight (Delisle 2008; Doak et al. 2000, 2005). The highest prevalence of dual burden households exists in middle Gross National Product (GNP) countries. However, this particular problem has yet to be explored in India. Given that India is not a country which falls in the middle range of GNP, the prevalence of dual burden households is probably much smaller.

Summary

The main message of the preceding discussion on the burden of overweight, underweight and the dual burden is that India continues to experience exceptionally high levels of undernutrition. That noted, the problem of overweight is beginning to emerge although its prevalence is relatively much smaller compared to underweight. And, as we show below, it is likely to be concentrated in the high SES groups. Thus, the dual burden of underweight and overweight remains socially segregated.

Social Epidemiology

This section documents the association between weight status and various socio-economic indicators (SES-related risk factors). Due to the dearth of studies on social epidemiological risk factors among Indian children and adolescents, the type of relationship between SES indicators and weight status is provided when available. However, many times the only information available is the prevalence of status stratified by level of the SES indicator.

Parental Indicators

Most studies looking at individual/household SES as a risk factor for nutrition problems among adults in India have focused on versions of the following six SES measures: household standard of living (sometimes referred to as income or wealth), individual education, caste, occupational status and living environment. Household wealth is usually defined in terms of ownership of material possessions. Significant milestones in the formal Indian education system are often used to create education categories such as 0 years (illiterate), 1–5 years (primary), 6–8 years (secondary), 9–12 years (higher), 13–15 years (college), and >15 years (postgraduate).

Caste identification is usually based on the household head and grouped as scheduled caste, scheduled tribe, other backward class or the general class. Scheduled castes are those whose members have suffered the greatest burden of deprivation within the caste system (Chitnis 1997). Scheduled tribes include approximately 700 officially recognized social groups that have historically been geographically and socially isolated and represent the "indigenous" groups in India

(Subramanian et al. 2006). Other backward class is a legislatively-defined group representing those who have historically suffered significant deprivation, but not as severe as scheduled castes and tribes. The general class is a residual category containing those not identifying themselves as members of legislatively recognized marginalized classes and constitute the "high" caste groups. Current occupation is often classified according to whether the person is not working, or working in a manual, non-manual, or agricultural profession. Living environment is characterized according to whether the household in which the person resides is located in a large city (population >1 million), small city (population 100,000–1 million), town (population <100,000), or village or rural area. Each of these measures provides important information on the complex picture of social determinants of both overweight and underweight in India.

Similar versions of the above measures, which are traditionally used for investigating nutrition patterns among adults, may also be used to measure weight and/or nutritional status among children and adolescents. Often, parental responses on any of the various SES indicators are used to represent the SES level for their children and to describe the SES pattern of an outcome for children. The following paragraph describes how child and adolescent overweight/obesity status is associated with various parental SES indicators.

Among adolescents in Tamilnadu, India (previously described), overweight was associated with higher income group (family owning transportation) and father's occupation (executive/professional position) (Ramachandran et al. 2002). Among West Bengalese boys, maternal education and family expenditure were positively associated with BMI (Dasgupta et al. 2008). Among the Hyderabad adolescents (described previously), 14.9% of high SES students were overweight and above as compared to 3.3% of low SES students (with SES indicated by a collection of parental variables) (Laxmaiah et al. 2007). Further, the prevalence of overweight and above was 9.1 and 7.4%, respectively, vs. 3.1% among students whose parental occupation was service or business compared to other parental professions (Laxmaiah et al. 2007). Among adolescents from Wardha City, Central India (described above), urban residence and father's or mother's service or business occupation were associated with increased risk of overweight/obesity (Bharati et al. 2008a).

Most of SES-related risk factors for adolescent underweight status are based on parental indicators as many of the studies on undernutrition in India have focused on children who are less than 5 years old. The prevalence of undernutrition (stunting, wasting and underweight) among children in rural India (study previously described) was greater among children with illiterate mothers, from households with a low standard of living, and who belonged to scheduled tribes and scheduled castes, and lowest among children of mothers with high school or more education and households with a medium or high standard of living (Rajaram et al. 2007). The results from this study showed that maternal characteristics, such as socio-economic and behavioral factors, were more highly associated with childhood nutritional status than program factors, such as receiving tetanus shorts or iron tablets (Rajaram et al. 2007). A nationally representative study of children aged between 0 and 35 months (previously described) showed that mother's education, state, and urban/rural living environment were associated with children's underweight (Bharati et al. 2008b). From the nationally representative NFHS-3 data, the risk of underweight for children under 5 years of age was negatively associated with household wealth and mother's education and child's inadequate nutrition was associated with scheduled caste/tribe identification and living in a rural area (Arnold 2007). (See Fig. 10.3 for underweight prevalence among children under 5 years by their household wealth status.) The study on India's tribal populations revealed a significant association between undernutrition and type of family, size of land holding and the household head's occupation, all indicators of socio-economic position (Rao et al. 2006).

As a side note, other maternal characteristics, such as maternal nutrition (Yajnik 2004) and maternal weight status (Bharati et al. 2008b), have been cited as determinants of children's weight status. Data from the NFHS-3 indicated that children's inadequate nutrition was associated with

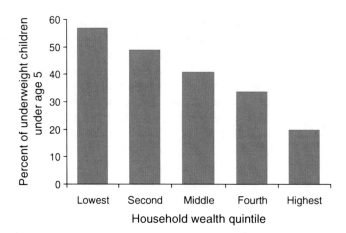

Fig. 10.3 The percentage of underweight children under 5 years old according to the 2005–2006 NFHS-3 household wealth quintile cut-off points (Arnold 2007)

short-birth intervals and higher-order births (Arnold 2007). Moreover, a nationally representative study found a suggested positive relationship between multiple incidents of domestic violence and mother and child's underweight (Ackerson and Subramanian 2008).

School Level Indicators

Many studies have examined how prevalence of weight status varies depending upon the SES level of schools that students attend. The following describes differences in overweight/obesity prevalence between students of differing school level SES in India. The study on adolescents in Hyderabad found that the prevalence of overweight and above was 9.6% among students in private schools vs. 3.2% among students in government schools (Laxmaiah et al. 2007). (Also, 9.9% of students who used vehicular transport were overweight and above as compared to 6.4% among students who walked or biked to school.) The prevalence of overweight and obesity among adolescent children in New Delhi (previously described study) was 29% in private schools and 11.3% in government funded schools (Bhardwaj et al. 2008). Similarly, 16% of children attending an affluent school in Ludhiana (as described above) were obese as compared to 6.4% in two less affluent schools (Chhatwal et al. 2004). Moreover, the proportion of overweight children in Kerala (previously described) was significantly higher in urban regions and in private schools compared to rural regions and government schools (Raj et al. 2007). Among a random sample of 5,087 students aged 5–18 years who attended a low income school in Delhi, the prevalence of overweight and obesity was 1.4 and 0.2%, respectively, according to IOTF standards as compared to prevalence of 6.7 and 0.6%, respectively, among a similar group of students who attended middle income schools ($n=5,134$) (Kaur and Kapil 2008). Among a random sample of students from Wardha City, attending an English medium school (vs. not) was associated with an increased risk for overweight/obesity (Bharati et al. 2008a).

State-Level Indicators

Recent research has also highlighted regional socio-economic determinants of overweight/obesity among adults that are related to the economic position of Indian states, such as a state's per capita consumption expenditure and a state level measure of inequality (Subramanian et al. 2007). These may be risk factors for nutritional status among children and adolescents as well.

Summary

The key message of the preceding discussion is that overweight is primarily concentrated among the high SES groups while underweight is primarily concentrated among low SES groups.

Lifestyle Risk Factors

There are several lifestyle risk factors for overweight and obesity related to the nutrition transition occurring in India (Shetty 2002), a transition which is directly connected to India's current economic transition as cited in the introduction. Many of the overweight and obesity risk factors for children and adolescents that have been studied represent decreased physical activity and increased consumption of energy-dense, nutrition poor food. Among 307 urban school children aged 7–15 years in Bangalore, an increase in socio-economic status was associated with an increase in the proportion of energy contributed by fat and saturated fat and a decrease in the energy contributed by carbohydrates (Swaminathan et al. 2007). They also found that energy intake increased with increased frequency of eating out. Among urban adolescents in Tamilnadu, India (previously described), low physical activity was associated with overweight (Ramachandran et al. 2002). Among lower to middle income adolescents in Bangalore (previously described), overweight (vs. not overweight) was significantly associated with watching television at least 1.5 h/day as compared to less than 45 min/day, consuming fried foods at least 6 times per week as compared to less than 2.5 times per week, and sleeping less than 8.4 h/day as compared to more than 9.5 h/day (Kuriyan et al. 2007). Among adolescents in Wardha City, participating in less than 30 min of outdoor games was associated with an increased risk of overweight/obesity (Bharati et al. 2008a). The incidence of overweight/obesity was significantly associated with eating meals outside the home among adolescents from Ludhiana (previously described) (Aggarwal et al. 2008). Further, overweight/obese adolescents had a higher mean score of replacing snacks for meals as compared to those of normal weight.

Unfortunately, there is no research that has reported nationally representative prevalence of lifestyle risk factors for nutritional and weight status among children in India. Further, there is a paucity of prevalence research on lifestyle risk factors among non-representative samples. However, we present some of the data that are available, which has primarily focused on dietary intake and physical activity. Among 510 students aged 12–18 years in New Delhi, 1/3 of boys and girls ate fast food more than 3 times per week, 31.5% of boys and 16.5% of girls added salt to their food, and only 39.4% of children consumed fruits on a daily basis (Singh et al. 2006). Fifty-four percent of boys and 69% of girls reported not engaging in sports at school or at home. Among this group of students, approximately 50% of boys and girls reported having a family history of hypertension and 23% of boys and 30% of girls reported a family history of obesity. Among the students in Hyderabad, the prevalence of overweight and obesity was higher among adolescents who participated in outdoor games (3.1%), household activities (4.7%), and watching less than 3 h of television per day (5.9%) compared to those who did not or watched more than 3 h/day (9.7, 18.6, and 10.4%, respectively) (Laxmaiah et al. 2007). Also, the prevalence of overweight and obesity was higher among those who liked to consume junk food (12.6%) as compared to those who did not (5.7%).

Conclusions

This chapter has strived to describe the current situation regarding the prevalence overweight and obesity (as well as stunting, wasting, and underweight) among youth in India and the associated risk factors. A major limitation of this chapter is that there are very few nationally representative studies that have examined these issues among children and adolescents in India. It is, thus, difficult to obtain figures at the national level. Moreover, although various studies have associated risk factors with weight status, they have not presented the prevalence of these risk factors. There is a need for more research on the national prevalence of various weight statuses among adolescents less than 20 years old in India and the associated risk factors.

The risk of overweight and obesity is increasing among children and adolescents in India. The increase follows a social gradient; more affluent youth, especially those in urban settings, are at increased risk for overweight problems than are less affluent youth, the latter who are at increased risk for underweight problems. Various risk factors associated with the nutrition and economic transitions are associated with adolescent weight status. Undernutrition, however, is still the largest burden for Indian youth. Despite the increase in overweight adolescents, almost half of the children under age 5 suffer from underweight, stunting, or wasting.

Acknowledgements SVS is supported by the National Institutes of Health Career Development Award (NHLBI K25 HL081275).

References

Ackerson, L.K., & Subramanian, S.V. (2008). Domestic violence and chronic malnutrition among women and children in India. *American Journal of Epidemiology, 167(10)*, 1188–1196.

Aggarwal, T., Bhatia, R.C., Singh, D., & Sobti, P.C. (2008). Prevalence of obesity and overweight in affluent adolescents from Ludhiana, Punjab. *Indian Pediatrics, 45(6)*, 500–502.

Arnold, F. (2007). *Nutrition in India: key findings from the 2005–06 National Family Health Survey (NFHS-3)*. India: Macro International.

Bharati, S., Pal, M., Bhattacharya, B., & Bharati, P. (2007). Prevalence and causes of chronic energy deficiency and obesity in Indian women. *Human Biology, 79(4)*, 395–412.

Bharati, D.R., Deshmukh, P.R., & Garg, B.S. (2008a). Correlates of overweight & obesity among school going children of Wardha city, Central India. *Indian Journal of Medical Research, 127(6)*, 539–543.

Bharati, S., Pal, M., & Bharati, P. (2008b). Determinants of nutritional status of pre-school children in India. *Journal of Biosocial Science, 40*, 801–814.

Bhardwaj, S., Misra, A., Khurana, L., Gulati, S., Shah, P., & Vikram, N.K. (2008). Childhood obesity in Asian Indians: a burgeoning cause of insulin resistance, diabetes and sub-clinical inflammation. *Asia-Pacific Journal of Clinical Nutrition, 17, Suppl 1*, 172–175.

Black, R.E., Allen, L.H., Bhutta, Z.A., Caulfield, L.E., de Onis, M., Ezzati, M., Mathers, C., & Rivera, J. (2008). Maternal and child undernutrition: global and regional exposures and health consequences. *Lancet, 371(9608)*, 243–260.

Braveman, P.A., Cubbin, C., Egerter, S., Chideya, S., Marchi, K.S., Metzler, M., & Posner, S. (2005). Socioeconomic status in health research: one size does not fit all. *JAMA, 294*, 2879–2888.

Bulatao, R.A., & Stephens, P.W. (1992). *Global estimates and projections of mortality by cause 1970–2015*. Washington: Population, Health and Nutrition Department, World Bank.

Chhatwal, J., Verma, M., & Riar, S. (2004). Obesity among pre-adolescent and adolescents of a developing country (India). *Asia-Pacific Journal of Clinical Nutrition, 13(3)*, 231–235.

Chitnis, S. (1997). Definition of the terms scheduled castes and scheduled tribes: a crisis of ambivalence. In V.A. Pai Panandiker (Ed.), *The politics of backwardness: reservation policy in India* (pp. 88–107). New Delhi: Konark.

CIA (2008). The world factbook: India. Retrieved September 25, 2008, 2008, from https://www.cia.gov/library/publications/the-world-factbook/geos/in.html#Intro

Cole, T.J. (2002). A chart to link child centiles of body mass index, weight and height. *European Journal of Clinical Nutrition, 56(12)*, 1194–1199.

Cole, T.J., Bellizzi, M.C., Flegal, K.M., & Dietz, W.H. (2000). Establishing a standard definition for child overweight and obesity worldwide: international survey. *British Medical Journal, 320(7244)*, 1240–1243.

Dasgupta, P., Saha, R., & Nube, M. (2008). Changes in body size, shape and nutritional status of middle-class Bengali boys of Kolkata, India, 1982–2002. *Economics and Human Biology, 6(1)*, 75–94.

Deaton, A., & Dreze, J. (2008). *Nutrition in India: facts and interpretations*. Princeton: Center for Health and Wellbeing, Princeton University.

Deepa, M., Farooq, S., Deepa, R., Manjula, D., & Mohan, V. (2009). Prevalence and significance of generalized and central body obesity in an urban Asian Indian population in Chennai, India (CURES: 47). *European Journal of Clinical Nutrition, 63*, 259–267.

Delisle, H.F. (2008). Poverty: the double burden of malnutrition in mothers and the intergenerational impact. *Annals of the New York Academy of Sciences, 1136*, 172–184.

Doak, C.M., Adair, L.S., Monteiro, C., & Popkin, B.M. (2000). Overweight and underweight coexist within households in Brazil, China and Russia. *The Journal of Nutrition, 130(12)*, 2965–2971.

Doak, C.M., Adair, L.S., Bentley, M., Monteiro, C., & Popkin, B.M. (2005). The dual burden household and the nutrition transition paradox. *International Journal of Obesity, 29*, 129–136.

Gopalan, C. (2001). Rising incidence of obesity, coronary heart disease and diabetes in the Indian urban middle class. Possible role of genetic and environmental factors. *World Review of Nutrition and Dietetics, 90*, 127–143.

Gopinath, N., Chadha, S.L., Jain, P., Shekhawat, S., & Tandon, R. (1994). An epidemiological study of obesity in adults in the urban population of Delhi. *The Journal of the Association of Physicians of India, 42(3)*, 212–215.

Griffiths, P., & Bentley, M. (2001). The nutrition transition is underway in India. *Journal of Nutrition, 131(10)*, 2692–2700.

Gupta, R., Misra, A., Pais, P., Rastogi, P., & Gupta, V.P. (2006a). Correlation of regional cardiovascular disease mortality in India with lifestyle and nutritional factors. *International Journal of Cardiology, 108(3)*, 291–300.

Gupta, R., Rastogi, P., & Arora, S. (2006b). Low obesity and high undernutrition prevalence in lower socioeconomic status school girls: a double jeopardy. *Human Ecology Special Issue, 14*, 65–70.

IIPS (2007). *National fact sheet India*. Mumbai: International Institute for Population Sciences.

IIPS & Macro-International (2007). *National Family Health Survey (NFHS-3), 2005–2006: India: Volume I*. Mumbai: International Institute for Population Sciences.

IIPS & ORC-Macro (2000). *National Family Health Survey, 1998–1999: India*. Mumbai: International Institute for Population Sciences.

IIPS & ORC-Macro (2007). *National Family Health Survey, 2005–2006: India*. Mumbai: International Institute for Population Sciences.

Kapoor, S.K., & Anand, K. (2002). Nutritional transition: a public health challenge in developing countries. *Journal of Epidemiology and Community Health, 56(11)*, 804–805.

Kaur, S., & Kapil, U. (2008). Prevalence of overweight and obesity in school children in Delhi. *Indian Pediatrics, 45(4)*, 330–331.

Kennedy, G., Nantel, G., & Shetty, P. (2006). *Assessment of the double burden of malnutrition in six case study countries*. Rome: Nutrition Planning, Assessment and Evaluation Service, Food and Agriculture Organization of the United Nations.

Kuczmarski, R.J., Ogden, C.L., Grummer-Strawn, L.M., Flegal, K.M., Guo, S.S., Wei, R., Mei, Z., Curtin, L.R., Roche, A.F., & Johnson, C.L. (2000). CDC growth charts: United States. *Advance Data, 314*, 1–27.

Kumar, H.N., Mohanan, P., Kotian, S., Sajjan, B.S., & Kumar, S.G. (2008). Prevalence of overweight and obesity among preschool children in semi urban South India. *Indian Pediatrics, 45(6)*, 497–499.

Kuriyan, R., Bhat, S., Thomas, T., Vaz, M., & Kurpad, A.V. (2007). Television viewing and sleep are associated with overweight among urban and semi-urban South Indian children. *Nutrition Journal, 6*, 25.

Laxmaiah, A., Nagalla, B., Vijayaraghavan, K., & Nair, M. (2007). Factors affecting prevalence of overweight among 12- to 17-year-old urban adolescents in Hyderabad, India. *Obesity (Silver Spring), 15(6)*, 1384–1390.

Mehta, M., Bhasin, S., Agrawal, K., & Dwivedi, S. (2007). Obesity amongst affluent adolescent girls. *Indian Journal of Pediatrics, 74(7)*, 619–622.

Misra, A. (2002). Overnutrition and nutritional deficiency contribute to metabolic syndrome and atherosclerosis in Asian Indians. *Nutrition, 18(7–8)*, 702–703.

Misra, A., & Vikram, N.K. (2004). Insulin resistance syndrome (metabolic syndrome) and obesity in Asian Indians: evidence and implications. *Nutrition, 20(5)*, 482–491.

Misra, A., Vikram, N.K., Gupta, R., Pandey, R.M., Wasir, J.S., & Gupta, V.P. (2006a). Waist circumference cutoff points and action levels for Asian Indians for identification of abdominal obesity. *International Journal of Obesity, 30*, 106–111.

Misra, A., Vikram, N.K., Sharma, R., & Basit, A. (2006b). High prevalence of obesity and associated risk factors in urban children in India and Pakistan highlights immediate need to initiate primary prevention program for diabetes and coronary heart disease in schools. *Diabetes Research and Clinical Practice, 71(1)*, 101–102.

MOHFW (2007). *2005–06 National Family Health Survey (NFHS-3) key findings*, from http://mohfw.nic.in/NFHS-3%20Key%20Findings.ppt. Accessed 6 June 2009.

Molarius, A., Seidell, J.C., Sans, S., Tuomilehto, J., & Kuulasmaa, K. (1999). Waist and hip circumferences, and waist-hip ratio in 19 populations of the WHO MONICA Project. *International Journal of Obesity and Related Metabolic Disorders, 23(2)*, 116–125.

Monteiro, C.A., Moura, E.C., Conde, W.L., & Popkin, B.M. (2004). Socioeconomic status and obesity in adult populations of developing countries: a review. *Bulletin of the World Health Organization, 82(12)*, 940–946.

Nandy, S., Irving, M., Gordon, D., Subramanian, S.V., & Smith, G.D. (2005). Poverty, child undernutrition and morbidity: new evidence from India. *Bulletin of the World Health Organization, 83(3)*, 210–216.

Ness, A., Leary, S., Reilly, J., Wells, J., Tobias, J., Clark, E., Davey Smith, G., & Team, A.S. (2006). The social patterning of fat and lean mass in a contemporary cohort of children. *International Journal of Paediatric Obesity, 1*, 56–61.

Pednekar, M.S., Hakama, M., Hebert, J.R., & Gupta, P.C. (2008). Association of body mass index with all-cause and cause-specific mortality: findings from a prospective cohort study in Mumbai (Bombay), India. *International Journal of Epidemiology, 37*, 524–535.

Popkin, B.M. (2003). The nutrition transition in the developing world. *Development Policy Review, 21(5–6)*, 581–597.

Popkin, B.M. (2004). The nutrition transition: an overview of world patterns of change. *Nutrition Reviews, 62(7 Pt 2)*, S140–S143.

Popkin, B.M., Lu, B., & Zhai, F. (2002). Understanding the nutrition transition: measuring rapid dietary changes in transitional countries. *Public Health Nutrition, 5(6A)*, 947–953.

Raj, M., Sundaram, K.R., Paul, M., Deepa, A.S., & Kumar, R.K. (2007). Obesity in Indian children: time trends and relationship with hypertension. *The National Medical Journal of India, 20(6)*, 288–293.

Rajaram, S., Zottarelli, L.K., & Sunil, T.S. (2007). Individual, household, programme and community effects on childhood malnutrition in rural India. *Maternal & Child Nutrition, 3(2)*, 129–140.

Ramachandran, P. (2006). *The double burden of malnutrition in India*. New Delhi: Nutrition Foundation of India.

Ramachandran, A., Snehalatha, C., Vinitha, R., Thayyil, M., Kumar, C.K., Sheeba, L., Joseph, S., & Vijay, V. (2002). Prevalence of overweight in urban Indian adolescent school children. *Diabetes Research and Clinical Practice, 57(3)*, 185–190.

Rao, K.M., Laxmaiah, A., Venkaiah, K., & Brahmam, G.N. (2006). Diet and nutritional status of adolescent tribal population in nine states of India. *Asia-Pacific Journal of Clinical Nutrition, 15(1)*, 64–71.

Razak, F., Anand, S., Vuksan, V., Davis, B., Jacobs, R., Teo, K.K., Yusuf, S. (2005). Ethnic differences in the relationships between obesity and glucose-metabolic abnormalities: a cross-sectional population-based study. *International Journal of Obesity, 29*, 656–667.

Reddy, K., Rao, A., & Reddy, T. (2002). Socioeconomic status and the prevalence of coronary heart disease risk factors. *Asia-Pacific Journal of Clinical Nutrition, 11(2)*, 98–103.

Sauvaget, C., Ramadas, K., Thomas, G., Vinoda, J., Thara, S., & Sankaranarayanan, R. (2008). Body mass index, weight change and mortality risk in a prospective study in India. *International Journal of Epidemiology, 37*, 990–1004.

Shetty, P.S. (2002). Nutrition transition in India. *Public Health Nutrition, 5(1A)*, 175–182.

Sidhu, S., Kaur, N., & Kaur, R. (2006). Overweight and obesity in affluent school children of Punjab. *Annals of Human Biology, 33(2)*, 255–259.

Singh, M., & Sharma, M. (2005). Risk factors for obesity in children. *Indian Pediatrics, 42(2)*, 183–185.

Singh, R.B., Ghosh, S., Niaz, A.M., Gupta, S., Bishnoi, I., Sharma, J.P., Agarwal, P., Rastogi, S.S., Beegum, R., Chibo, H., & Shoumin, Z. (1995). Epidemiologic study of diet and coronary risk factors in relation to central obesity and insulin levels in rural and urban populations of north India. *International Journal of Cardiology, 47(3)*, 245–255.

Singh, R.B., Beegom, R., Mehta, A.S., Niaz, M.A., De, A.K., Mitra, R.K., Haque, M., Verma, S.P., Dube, G.K., Siddiqui, H.M., Wander, G.S., Janus, E.D., Postiglione, A., & Haque, M.S. (1999). Social class, coronary risk factors and undernutrition, a double burden of diseases, in women during transition, in five Indian cities. *International Journal of Cardiology, 69(2)*, 139–147.

Singh, P., Pathak, P., & Kapil, U. (2003). Obesity amongst affluent adolescent in India. *Indian Journal of Pediatrics, 70(10)*, 844.

Singh, A.K., Maheshwari, A., Sharma, N., & Anand, K. (2006). Lifestyle associated risk factors in adolescents. *Indian Journal of Pediatrics, 73(10)*, 901–906.

Singh, R.B., Pella, D., Mechirova, V., Kartikey, K., Demeester, F., Tomar, R.S., Beegom, R., Mehta, A.S., Gupta, S.B., De Amit, K., Neki, N.S., Haque, M., Nayse, J., Singh, S., Thakur, A.S., Rastogi, S.S., Singh, K., & Krishna, A. (2007). Prevalence of obesity, physical inactivity and undernutrition, a triple burden of diseases during transition in a developing economy. The Five City Study Group. *Acta Cardiologica, 62(2)*, 119–127.

Snehalatha, C., Viswanathan, V., & Ramachandran, A. (2003). Cutoff values for normal anthropometric variables in Asian Indian adults. *Diabetes Care, 26*, 1380–1384.

Sood, A., Sundararaj, P., Sharma, S., Kurpad, A.V., & Muthayya, S. (2007). BMI and body fat percent: affluent adolescent girls in Bangalore City. *Indian Pediatrics, 44(8)*, 587–591.

Subramanian, S.V., Davey Smith, G., & Subramanyam, M. (2006). Indigenous health and socioeconomic status in India. *PLoS Medicine, 3(10)*, e421.

Subramanian, S.V., Kawachi, I., & Davey Smith, G. (2007). Income inequality and the double burden of under- and overnutrition in India. *Journal of Epidemiology and Community Health, 61(9)*, 802–809.

Subramanian, S.V., Perkins, J.M., & Khan, K.T. (2009). Do burdens of underweight and overweight coexist among lower socioeconomic groups in India?, *American Journal of Clinical Nutrition, 90*, 369–376.

Swaminathan, S., Thomas, T., Kurpad, A.V., & Vaz, M. (2007). Dietary patterns in urban school children in South India. *Indian Pediatrics, 44(7)*, 593–596.

Unnithan, A.G., & Syamakumari, S. (2008). Prevalence of overweight, obesity and underweight among school going children in rural and urban areas of Thiruvananthapuram educational district, Kerala (India). http://www.ispub. com/ostia/index.php?xmlFilePath=journals/ijnw/vol6n2/obesity.xml *The Internet Journal of Nutrition and Wellness, 6(2)*.

WB (2008). *India country overview 2007*. Retrieved September 25, 2008, 2008, from http://go.worldbank. org/0BXQ5J38J0

WHO (1995). *Physical status: the use and interpretation of anthropometry* (Technical Report Series No. 854). Geneva: World Health Organization.

WHO (2006). *The WHO child growth standards*. Retrieved May 12 2008, from http://www.who.int/childgrowth/en/

WHO (2008). *Cutoff points and summary statistics*. Retrieved January 12 2008, from http://www.who.int/nutgrowthdb/ about/introduction/en/index5.html

Yajnik, C.S. (2004). Obesity epidemic in India: intrauterine origins? *The Proceedings of the Nutrition Society, 63(3)*, 387–396.

Yajnik, C.S., Lubree, H.G., Rege, S.S., Naik, S.S., Deshpande, J.A., Deshpande, S.S., Joglekar, C.V., & Yudkin, J.S. (2002). Adiposity and hyperinsulinemia in Indians are present at birth. *Journal of Clinical Endocrinology and Metabolism, 87(12)*, 5575–5580.

Yusuf, S., Hawken, S., Ounpuu, S., Bautista, L., Franzosi, M.G., Commerford, P., Lang, C.C., Rumboldt, Z., Onen, C.L., Lisheng, L., Tanomsup, S., Wangai, P., Jr., Razak, F., Sharma, A.M., & Anand, S.S. (2005). Obesity and the risk of myocardial infarction in 27,000 participants from 52 countries: a case-control study. *Lancet, 366(9497)*, 1640–1649.

Chapter 11
Epidemiology of Obesity in Children and Adolescents in China

Youfa Wang, Jie Mi, Yexuan Tao, and Ping Chen

Introduction

Over the past three decades, China, the world's most populous country whose population accounts for one-fifth of the global population, has enjoyed impressive economic developments. People in China have experienced many dramatic changes in their lifestyles thanks to the increases in family income and availability of food as a result of China's economic reform and the growing global trade (CSSB 2008). Meanwhile, people's lifestyles are becoming more sedentary compared to decades ago. Compared to other groups, children and adolescents are likely to be affected to a greater extent by these changes, partially due to China's family planning policy, the so called "one child policy" initiated in the later 1970s, which enables parents and grandparents to provide their children with more resources and care.

Some recent studies, predominately published in Chinese, suggest that the prevalence of obesity has increased in China both in children and adults as well as the related chronic diseases (Ji and Working group on Obesity in China (WGOC) 2007; Ma et al. 2005; Mi et al. 2006; Wang et al. 2007). Nationally representative survey data show that between 1992 and 2002, the prevalence of overweight and obesity increased in all sex and age groups, and in all geographic areas. Using the World Health Organization (WHO) body mass index (BMI) cut points, among adults in China, the combined prevalence of overweight and obesity (BMI ≥ 25 kg/m^2) increased from 14.6 to 21.8% during this period, while based on the Chinese standard (BMI ≥ 24 kg/m^2), it increased from 20.0 to 29.9%. With the increase in obesity, obesity- and diet-related chronic diseases such as hypertension, Cardiovascular disease (CVD), and type 2 diabetes also increased over the past decade and became the most important preventable cause of death. For example, the prevalence of hypertension increased from 14.4% in 1991 to 18.8% in 2002 in adults (Wang et al. 2007). On the other hand, data collected from pre-school children show that undernutrition remains a major public health concern, particularly in poor and rural areas (Liu et al. 2008). Therefore, China is facing a double burden of both, an overnutrition and an undernutrition problem.

This chapter describes the current situation and the time trends of overweight and obesity among children and adolescents in China. We focused on representative data collected in large national surveys and results that are based on the recently released Chinese BMI reference (Ji and Working Group on Obesity in China (WGOC) 2005).

Y. Wang (✉), Y. Tao, and P. Chen
Center for Human Nutrition, Department of International Health, Bloomberg School of Public Health,
Johns Hopkins University, 615 North Wolfe Street, Baltimore, MD 21205, USA
e-mail: ywang@jhsph.edu

J. Mi
Department of Epidemiology, Capital Institute of Pediatrics, Beijing, China

L.A. Moreno et al. (eds.), *Epidemiology of Obesity in Children and Adolescents*,
Springer Series on Epidemiology and Public Health 2, DOI 10.1007/978-1-4419-6039-9_11,
© Springer Science+Business Media, LLC 2011

China's Socio-demographic and Economic Characteristics

China is the largest developing country with the fastest growing economy in the world (World Bank 2009; Wikipedia 2009) (see Table 11.1). China has about one-fifth of the global population. China's economy during the past 30 years has changed from a centrally planned system that was largely closed to international trade to a more market-oriented economy that has a rapidly growing private sector. China's Gross Domestic Product (GDP) has increased by more than tenfold since 1978, and China contributed one-third of global economic growth in 2004. In 2008, China's economy is the second largest in the world after that of the United States with a GDP of $7.8 trillion when measured on a purchasing power parity (PPP) basis. China has been the fastest-growing major nation for the past three decades with an average annual GDP growth rate above 10% since China initiated its economic reform in the late 1970s. Nevertheless, at present, China remains a low-to-medium income country.

Thanks to China's fast per capita income increase, an average annual rate of more than 8% over the last three decades, and the government's strong support for poverty reduction programs, poverty rate in China has drastically decreased. China alone accounted for over 75% of poverty reduction in the developing world over the last 20 years. On the other hand, this rapid economic growth has been accompanied by rising income inequalities.

China's economic reforms and development over the last three decades have also resulted in substantial improvements in people's daily life and in human development indicators. Adult illiteracy rate fell from 37% in 1978 to less than 10% in 2005; and, indicative of health indices, the infant mortality rate fell from 41 per 1,000 live births in 1978 to 23 in 2005. Life expectancy has

Table 11.1 Basic demographic and economic characteristics of the People's Republic of China

Characteristics	
Area	9,596,960 km^2
Population (2008)	1,330,044,544
Population proportion, 0–14 years	20.1%
Population proportion, 65 years and over	8.0%
Population growth rate (2008)	0.63%
Birth rate (/1000, 2008)	13.7
Death rate (/1000, 2008)	7.0
Infant mortality rate (/1000, 2002)	27.3
Life expectancy (2008)	73.2
Life expectancy, males (2008)	71.4
Life expectancy, females (2008)	75.2
Total fertility rate (children/women, 2008)	1.8
Literacy in total population (2000 census)	90.90%
Literacy in males (2000 census)	95.10%
Literacy in females (2000 census)	85.50%
GDP (nominal, 2008)	$4.42 trillion (ranked second in the world)
GDP (PPP, 2008)	$7.8 trillion (ranked second in the world)
GDP per capita (nominal, 2007)	$2,660 (ranked 104th in the world)
GDP per capita (PPP, 2007)	$5,300 (ranked 105th in the world)
GDP growth rate (2008)	9.0%
Population below poverty line (2004)	10%
Gini index (2004)	46.9
Labor force by major industrial sectors (2006)	Agriculture (43%), industry (25%), services (32%)

Data sources: CIA (2009), Wikipedia (2009), and World Bank (2009)

increased to 73.2 years by 2008. China enforced its "one child" policy since the late 1970s, as a result, Chinese children are enjoying more family resources and care than their early counterparts, and China is now one of the most rapidly aging countries in the world.

The two most important sectors of the Chinese economy have traditionally been agriculture and industry, which together employ more than 70% of the labor force and produce more than 60% of GDP. The two sectors have differed in many respects, and affect people's life differently. For example, technology, labor productivity, and incomes have advanced much more rapidly in industry than in agriculture. These disparities between the two sectors have resulted in an economic-cultural-social gap between the rural and urban areas, a major division in Chinese society, where in general, most urban residents have enjoyed better living standards and further improvements over the past two decades. It is estimated that more than 204 million Chinese, many in remote and resource-poor areas in the western and interior regions, still suffer from poverty, often without access to clean water, arable land, or adequate health and education services.

Classification of Obesity in Children and Adolescents in China

BMI is a simple and widely used method for estimating body fat mass and has been widely accepted as a useful measurement for overweight and obesity classification in both adult and child population (WHO 2000, 2004). However, different cut points for the classification of childhood obesity have been used across populations and studies and several international references have been developed and recommended for use (Cole et al. 2000; Kuczmarski et al. 2002). It is argued that the WHO BMI cut points are developed primarily based on data collected in Western populations, and may not be appropriate for some population groups such as some in the Asia Pacific areas (Misra 2003; WHO 2004; WHO, IASO, & IOTF 2000).

In China, for adults, BMI cut points of 24 (for overweight) and 28 (for obesity), lower than the WHO standard, have been recommended and used (Wang et al. 2007; Zhou and Cooperative Meta-Analysis Group of the Working Group on Obesity in China 2002). These Chinese BMI cut points were developed based on analysis of data collected from 239,972 Chinese adults in the 1990s. A BMI cut point of 24 was found having the best sensitivity (=62.07% for men and 63.15% for women) and specificity (=63.85% for men and 62.13% for women) for identifying health conditions including hypertension, diabetes and dyslipidaemia, while a BMI of 28 had a specificity around 90% (Zhou and Cooperative Meta-Analysis Group of the Working Group on Obesity in China 2002).

To define childhood obesity and for screening overweight and obesity in school-age children (7–18 years old), in 2004, the Working Group on Obesity in China (WGOC) published a national reference, which is a set of sex-age-specific BMI cut points (Table 11.2 and Fig. 11.1) (Ji and Working Group on Obesity in China (WGOC) 2005). Overall these BMI cut points are lower than those in the US CDC 2000 Growth Charts. The WGOC BMI reference was developed based on anthropometric data (height and weight) collected in the 2000 Chinese National Survey on Students Constitution and Health (CNSSCH) from 216,620 subjects aged 7–18 years old in 30 of China's 31 provinces (except for Taiwan). For children younger than 7 years old, the WGOC recommended to use the WHO's weight-for-height z-score (WHZ) standard $2 \leq WHZ < 3$ for overweight and ≥ 3 for obesity. Figure 11.1 shows that compared to their US counterparts, Chinese children and adolescents remain thinner; and the BMI cut points recommended in China are lower that the US 2000 CDC Growth Charts, but the differences become greater at older ages. The present chapter focused on results based on the Chinese WGOC BMI reference.

Table 11.2 Chinese body mass index (BMI) reference for overweight and obesity classification among school-age children

Age	Boys		Girls	
	Overweight	Obesity	Overweight	Obesity
7–7.9	17.4	19.2	17.2	18.9
8–8.9	18.1	20.3	18.1	19.9
9–9.9	18.9	21.4	19.0	21.0
10–10.9	19.6	22.5	20.0	22.1
11–11.9	20.3	23.6	21.1	23.3
12–12.9	21.0	24.7	21.9	24.5
13–13.9	21.9	25.7	22.6	25.6
14–14.9	22.6	26.4	23.0	26.3
15–15.9	23.1	26.9	23.4	26.9
16–16.9	23.5	27.4	23.7	27.4
17–17.9	23.8	27.8	23.8	27.7

Data source: Ji and Working Group on Obesity in China (WGOC) (2005)

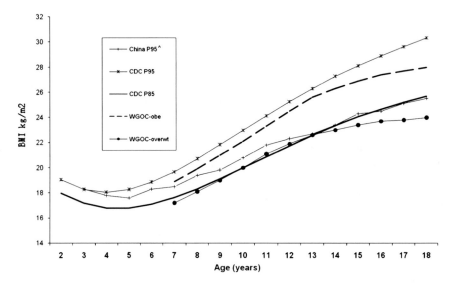

Fig. 11.1 Comparison of age-specific BMI percentiles in China (the 2002 national survey [The 2002 China National Health and Nutrition Survey, the 85th percentile was not provided.]), the US CDC 2000 Growth Chart, and the Chinese/WGOC BMI reference for classification of overweight and obesity in girls. ^The Chinese reference only covers school age children aged 7–17 years old. *WGOC* Working Group on Obesity in China (Ji and Working Group on Obesity in China (WGOC) 2005)

The Prevalence and Trends of Childhood Obesity in China

Good nationally representative data have been collected in China allowing for examining the time trend in childhood obesity. Many additional nationwide, regional and local surveys have been conducted recently and provide additional important information. The 2002 China National Health and Nutrition Survey provides the best, most recent national estimates, and shows that the combined prevalence of overweight and obesity in children aged 0–18 years was 4.1 and 2.1%, respectively. While in urban areas, among school-age children (≥7 years), the combined prevalence was 12.9%.

A most recent study shows that in northern coastal big cities, the combined prevalence had reached 32.5% in boys and 17.6% in girls (both ≥7 years) in 2005 (Ji and Cheng 2008), which is similar to that in some industrialized countries (Wang and Lobstein 2007).

Time Trends in the Prevalence of Childhood Obesity

Table 11.3 shows that the prevalence of obesity and overweight has increased between 1992 and 2002 in all sex and age groups. The nationwide combined prevalence increased by 31.7% from 3.9% in 1992 to 5.4% in 2002 in pre-school children (up to age 6), and increased by 17.9% from 5.7% in 1992 to 6.6% in 2002 in school-age children (7–17 years).

Table 11.4 shows the trends based on data collected in another series of representative cross-sectional surveys in metropolitan areas in China, the health examination data collected among elementary

Table 11.3 Changes in the prevalence (%) of overweight and obesity in Chinese children (0–17 years) between 1992 and 2002 based on nationally representative data[a]

Age group	Male 1992	2002	Inc %	Female 1992	2002	Inc %	Total 1992	2002	Inc %
Children, 0–6 year									
Overweight[b], %	2.4	3.4	36.0	2.2	3.4	47.8	2.3	3.4	41.7
Obesity, %	1.7	2.0	11.1	1.6	2.1	31.3	1.6	2.0	17.6
Combined prev, %	4.1	5.4	25.6	3.8	5.5	41.0	3.9	5.4	31.7
Children, 7–17 year									
Overweight[b], %	4.3	5.1	21.4	3.5	3.9	14.7	3.9	4.5	18.4
Obesity, %	1.8	2.5	47.1	1.9	1.7	-5.6	1.8	2.1	16.7
Combined prev, %	6.1	7.6	28.8	5.4	5.6	7.7	5.7	6.6	17.9

Data source: Ma et al. (2005)
[a]Based on the 1992 and 2002 Chinese National Nutrition and Health Survey. Overweight and obesity are defined based on the Chinese BMI reference
[b]Not include obesity

Table 11.4 Changes in prevalence (%) of overweight and obesity among Chinese children and adolescents (7–17 years old) in metropolitan areas (1985–2000)

Age (year)	Overweight[a] 1985	1991	1995	2000	Obesity 1985	1991	1995	2000	Overweight and obesity 1985	1991	1995	2000
Boys												
7–9.9	1.3	4.1	6.8	10.4	0.6	2.4	4.8	8.0	1.9	6.5	11.6	18.4
10–12.9	1.4	5.4	8.6	13.9	0.2	1.4	3.4	5.4	1.6	6.8	12.0	19.3
13–15.9	1.0	4.3	8.0	11.3	0.1	0.8	2.7	4.4	1.1	5.1	10.7	15.7
16–16.9	1.2	4.2	7.1	11.3	0.1	0.5	1.8	3.7	1.3	4.7	8.9	15.0
Total	1.2	4.5	7.6	11.7	0.2	1.3	2.9	5.4	1.4	5.8	10.5	17.1
Girls												
7–9.9	1.1	2.9	4.0	6.7	0.3	1.5	2.4	4.4	1.4	4.4	6.4	11.1
10–12.9	0.7	2.4	4.1	5.5	0.1	0.9	2.1	3.4	0.8	3.3	6.2	8.9
13–15.9	1.6	3.1	5.7	7.3	0.1	0.7	1.8	2.4	1.7	3.8	7.5	9.7
16–16.9	2.1	3.5	5.3	7.5	0.0	0.3	0.6	1.6	2.1	3.8	5.9	9.1
Total	1.4	2.9	4.8	6.8	0.1	0.9	1.8	2.9	1.5	3.8	6.6	9.7

Data sources: Ji and Working Group on Obesity in China (WGOC) (2008)
[a]Not include obesity

and secondary school students. The surveys have been conducted every 5 years since 1985 by the Chinese National Survey on Students Constitution and Health Association. In the metropolitan areas, the prevalence of overweight and obesity in boys and girls have increased remarkably, approximately by 10 times. The combined prevalence increased from 1.4% in 1985 to 17.1 in 2000 in boys, more rapidly than that in girls (from 1.5 to 9.7%).

The available data show large disparities between regions and groups, even among urban areas. In major cities, during recent years, the prevalence of childhood obesity has increased more dramatically than in inland cities. For example, in Shanghai and Beijing, the two largest cities in China, the prevalence has more than tripled between 1985 and 1995. The prevalence in 7–12-year-old boys in these two cities increased from 5.4 to 5.8 to 29.0% in 2000. In inland cities, the figure increased from 0.6 to 11.8% (see Table 11.5).

Sex and Age Differences

Overall, the national average prevalence was comparable in boys and girls among pre-school age children, but was higher in boys than in girls in school-age children (e.g., Table 11.3). Similarly, in metropolitan areas, it was much higher (almost doubled) in boys than that in girls in these age groups (e.g., Tables 11.4 and 11.5).

Urban and Rural Differences

Similar to the situation in some other developing countries, there are large urban-rural differences in the prevalence of overweight and obesity in China, and the prevalence in urban areas is higher, in particular in school-age children (Table 11.6). Our calculated urban to rural ratio indicates that almost all of the prevalence is higher in urban than rural areas, except for the prevalence of obesity in pre-school girls. In addition, urban boys and girls have higher mean BMI compared to their rural counterparts (Fig. 11.2). These are based on the 2002 China Nutrition and Health Survey data. Note that most major cities in China have both urban and rural residents. For example, Beijing includes urban (inside the city) and rural areas (city surrounding areas).

Table 11.5 Comparison of trends in combined prevalence (%) of overweight and obesity among children (7–17 years old) in Beijing, Shanghai, and inland cities: between 1985 and 2000

City/year	Boys		Girls	
	7–12 year	13–17 year	7–12 year	13–17 year
Beijing				
1985	5.8	4.8	4.3	5.1
1995	17.5	18.1	12.0	11.6
2000	29.0	25.0	17.3	14.6
Shanghai				
1985	5.4	2.7	2.2	2.8
1995	20.5	15.7	11.8	8.0
2000	28.9	17.2	15.3	9.6
Inland cities				
1985	0.6	0.7	2.2	1.8
1995	4.0	4.5	2.9	3.9
2000	11.8	8.8	6.2	6.5

Data source: Ji and Working Group on Obesity in China (WGOC) (2008)

Table 11.6 Urban-rural difference in the prevalence (%) of overweight^ and obesity in Chinese children (0–17 years): The 2002 Chinese National Nutrition and Health Survey

Sex	Age	Overweight^			Obesity			Overweight+obesity		
		Urban	Rural	Ratio[a]	Urban	Rural	Ratio[a]	Urban	Rural	Ratio[a]
Boys	0–17	7.9	3.4	2.3	4.1	1.7	2.4	11.9	5.1	2.3
	0–6	3.9	3.3	1.2	2.3	1.9	1.2	6.2	5.2	1.2
	7–17	10.4	3.4	3.1	5.2	1.6	3.3	15.6	5.0	3.1
Girls	0–17	5.4	3.7	1.7	2.7	1.5	1.8	8.1	4.6	1.8
	0–6	3.4	3.4	1.0	1.6	2.2	0.7	5.0	5.6	0.9
	7–17	6.6	3.0	2.2	3.4	1.1	3.1	10	4.1	2.4
All	0–17	6.6	3.3	2.0	3.4	1.6	2.1	10	4.9	2.0
	0–6	3.6	3.4	1.1	1.9	2.1	0.9	5.5	5.5	1.0
	7–17	8.5	3.2	2.7	4.4	1.4	3.1	12.9	4.6	2.8

Data source: Ma et al. (2005)

[a]Ratio=prevalence in urban area/that in rural area

^Not include obesity

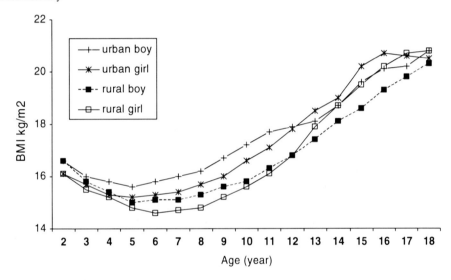

Fig. 11.2 Mean BMI in children aged 2–18 years old, by sex and urban-rural residence: the 2002 China Health and Nutrition Survey (data sources: Ma et al. 2005)

In China, usually people living in urban areas have better living standards, higher income, and more government-supported benefits such as retirement and healthcare than rural residents.

The Main Factors That Have Contributed to the Increase in Obesity in China

Obesity is believed to be the result of a number of biological, behavioral, cultural, social, and environmental factors and the complex interactions between them that promote a positive energy balance (Bray 1998; Davison and Birch 2001; WHO 2000). It is argued that the rapid increase in the prevalence of obesity worldwide over the past two decades probably suggests that environmental factors, but not genetic factors, are the major risk factors, because genetic factors cannot change so dramatically within such a short period (Hill and Peters 1998).

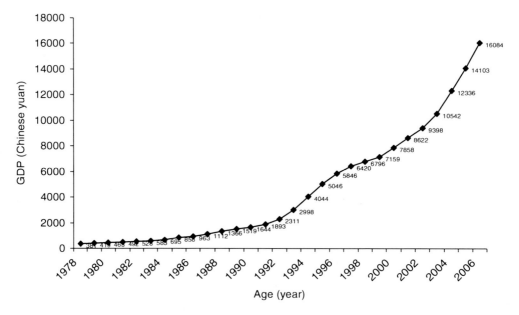

Fig. 11.3 Time trends in per capita gross domestic product (GDP, Chinese yuan) in China: 1978–2006 (data sources: CSSB 2008)

The rapid increase in the prevalence of overweight and obesity and the large disparities between population groups and regions in the prevalence and secular trends in China are particular a result of the rapid economic development and shifts in people's lifestyles and the differences in these shifts over the past two decades. Higher levels of parental education and family income have been found as significant risk factors for childhood obesity in China (Xie et al. 2007). The following highlights several such indicators and gives examples. China's per capita GDP has increased dramatically in the past two decades (Fig. 11.3). On one hand, this results in a steady increase in family income and improvements in people's living standards. On the other hand, this may have a number of unintended consequences such as shift in people's lifestyles.

Chinese citizens have experienced many dramatic changes in their lifestyles, including dietary intake and physical activity. The Chinese diet has shifted from a traditional dietary pattern, which typically contains quantities of plant foods including grains and vegetables, to the Western dietary pattern characterized by high intakes of meats, fat, and sugar (Du et al. 2004; Zhai et al. 2007). Nationally representative data show that the consumption of animal foods and dairy products have increased, while plant foods, including grains, fruit, and vegetable has steadily decreased, especially in urban areas. Consumption of cooking oil increased dramatically, especially of plant cooking oil (Fig. 11.4). The Western fast food industry has marketed aggressively in China, and Western fast food (which remains much more expensive than local food) and locally marketed and produced similar high-fat and energy-dense food are becoming an important part of urban children's diet. Often, parents and grandparents reward their children with meals at McDonald's (e.g., Jing 2000). Based on a recent report, by 2008, KFC has more than 2,200 outlets in some 450 cities and McDonald's has 950 outlets in China. Other Western fast food companies are entering the Chinese market more aggressively. For example, in April 2008 Burger King had just 12 outlets in mainland China, but soon the company announced plans to open between 250 and 300 outlets in China over the next 5 years (Economist 2008).

Changes in China have also contributed to the growing sedentary lifestyle among children in China. Among these changes, the major shifts include: first, children's greatly declined involvement in household work or farm work for children living in rural areas compared to the older cohorts, which

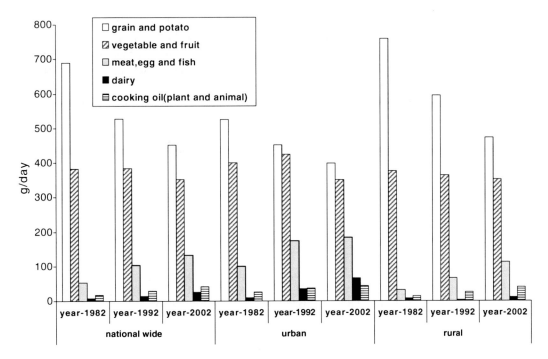

Fig. 11.4 Trends in food consumption (g/day per reference man) in China: 1982, 1992 and 2002. The 1982, 1992, and 2002 China National Health and Nutrition Survey. Reference man refers to adult men with light to medium physical activity (data source: Zhai et al. 2007)

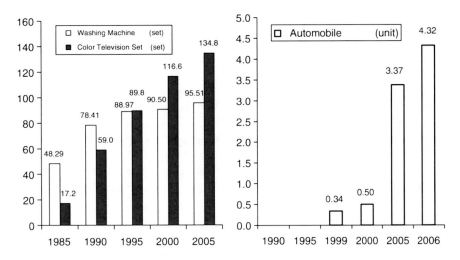

Fig. 11.5 Trends in household ownership of color television, washing machine, automobile (in urban areas) in China: sets/per 100 households (data sources: CSSB 2008)

are contributed by the one-child policy, shifts in parents' occupation, parents' higher expectation and the growing competition for students' academic performance, and the increasing availability and use of labor-saving devices at home such as washing machines (Fig. 11.5). For example, increased household ownership of a washing machine leads to less energy expenditure in housework. Second, children's screen time, such as time spent on watching television, playing computer and video games, has increased. For example, the television ownership increased from 17.2 per 100 urban households in 1985 to 134.8 to 2005 (Fig. 11.5). Third, changes in the means and options of transportation. For example, during recent years, much fewer young people ride bicycles or walk to schools, while more enjoy more convenient public transportation system, taxi, family-owned motorcycles and automobiles when travel. China's Bureau of Statistics started to include urban household automobile ownership in its yearly statistical books published since 1999. Urban household automobile ownership had increased by 1,160 times between 1999 and 2006 (Fig. 11.5). One study shows that 14% of the Chinese households acquired a motorized vehicle between 1989 and 1997. Another study shows that the odds of being obese were 80% higher for adults in households that own a motorized vehicle, compared to those that do not (Bell et al. 2002).

Discussion and Conclusions

China has experienced many rapid economic and social developments and changes over the past three decades. These have resulted in a number of major shifts in people's lifestyles, most of which have contributed to overconsumption of foods but reduced physical activity. Thus, no wonder, we are seeing a rapidly growing obesity epidemic in China. Recent data show that nationwide the average prevalence of overweight and obesity has reached 30% in adults, approximately 6–7% in children, while in major cities, the prevalence has reached over 50% in adults and approximately 20% in children (Ji and Working group on Obesity in China (WGOC) 2007; Mi et al. 2006; Wang et al. 2007).

Childhood obesity could track into adulthood and has a lot of health and financial consequences, for example, to increase the risks for hypertension, type 2 diabetes, coronary heart disease, and stroke, and increase healthcare costs. A recent study estimated that the total medical cost attributable to overweight and obesity was estimated at 21.11 billion Chinese Yuan (RMB, approximately US$2.74 billion), which accounted for 25.5% of the total medical costs for the four major obesity-related chronic diseases namely hypertension, type 2 diabetes, coronary heart disease and stroke, or 3.7% of China's national total medical costs in 2003 (Zhao et al. 2008). The researchers warned that the medical cost associated with overweight and obesity could increase to 37 billion Chinese Yuan (RMB, approximately US$4.8 billion), a 75% increase, if the epidemic developed speedily and the ratio of the prevalence of overweight to obesity approached 1.1:1. The study was based on the 2003 Third National Health Services Survey data from a large sample of 143,521 subjects, to derive direct medical costs including costs for outpatient visits, physician services, inpatient stays, rehabilitation services, nursing fees and medications. Recently another study warned that the economic costs related to the nutrition transition, in particular, the changing dietary and physical activity patterns and increase in obesity and overweight in China, may represent 4 to 8% of China's economy (Popkin 2008).

The United States can serve as an example to indicate the seriousness of the financial consequences of the obesity epidemic, and to show that the warnings made recently for China can become true if its growing obesity epidemic could not be controlled effectively. One of our recent studies projected that in the United States, medical costs attributable to overweight and obesity have already reached 72 to 82 billion US dollars and accounted for 12 to 13% of total US healthcare costs. The total healthcare costs attributable to obesity/overweight would double every decade to 860.7 to 956.9 billion US dollars by 2030, accounting for 16 to 18% of total US healthcare costs, if the obesity trend continues in the US (Wang et al. 2008a, b).

China already has had the largest number of overweight and obese people on earth. Timely attention and adequate effort should be made to prevent childhood obesity and to address the rapidly growing obesity epidemic in China. Comprehensive, national programs should be developed, in particular, while today China is making great effort and investing heavily to improve her citizen's health and access to healthcare service (e.g., the Healthy China 2020 Program). Multiple parties such as parents, children, health professionals, schools, media, food industry, and the central and local government agencies should all be involved for promoting healthy lifestyles and for the prevention of obesity. China should learn from the failure and successful experience of other countries in combating the obesity epidemic. Although there are many challenges for obesity prevention in China as the nation is facing many other public health challenges, there are emerging promising signs in this effort. For example, the work of the Working Group on Obesity in China has increased the attention of the general public and related health professionals on the obesity problem, the importance of using standardized references for classification as well as the screening of overweight and obesity among children and adults in China. Recently, in 2007 the Chinese State Council endorsed a report for child and adolescent health improvement, which recommended that every student should have at least 1h of physical activity each day in school.

References

Bell, A.C., Ge, K., & Popkin, B.M. (2002). The road to obesity or the path to prevention: motorized transportation and obesity in China. *Obesity Research, 10*, 277–283.

Bray, G.A. (1998). Obesity: a time bomb to be defused. *Lancet, 352*, 160–161.

Central Intelligence Agency (CIA) (2009). People's Republic of China. https://www.cia.gov/library/publications/the-world-factbook/geos/ch.html (assessed March 9, 2009).

China State Statistics Bureau (CSSB) (2008). *China statistical yearbook 2002 to 2008.* Beijing: China Statistics Press (in Chinese).

Cole, T.J., Bellizzi, M.C., Flegal, K.M., & Dietz, W.H. (2000). Establishing a standard definition for child overweight and obesity worldwide: international survey. *British Medical Journal, 320*, 1240–1243.

Davison, K.K., & Birch, L.L. (2001). Childhood overweight: a contextual model and recommendations for future research. *Obesity Reviews, 2*, 159–171.

Du, S., Mroz, T.A., Zhai, F., & Popkin, B.M. (2004). Rapid income growth adversely affects diet quality in China – particularly for the poor! *Social Science & Medicine, 59*, 1505–1515.

Economist (2008). Fast food in China: here comes a whopper – the world's second largest burger chain is gearing up in China (February 10, 2009); http://www.economist.com/business/displaystory.cfm?story_id=12488790.

Hill, J.O., & Peters, J.C. (1998). Environmental contributions to the obesity epidemic. *Science, 280*, 1371–1374.

Ji, C.Y., & Cheng, T.O. (2008). Prevalence and geographic distribution of childhood obesity in China in 2005. *International Journal of Cardiology, 131*, 1–8.

Ji, C.Y., & Working Group on Obesity in China (WGOC). (2005). Report on childhood obesity in China (1): body mass index reference for screening overweight and obesity in Chinese school-age children. *Biomedical and Environmental Sciences, 18*, 390–400.

Ji, C.Y., & Working group on Obesity in China (WGOC). (2007). Report on childhood obesity in China (4) prevalence and trends of overweight and obesity in Chinese urban school-age children and adolescents, 1985–2000. *Biomedical and Environmental Sciences, 20*, 1–10.

Ji, C.Y., & Working Group on Obesity in China (WGOC). (2008). The prevalence of childhood overweight/obesity and the epidemic changes in 1985–2000 for Chinese school-age children and adolescents. *Obesity Reviews, 9, Suppl 1*, 78–81.

Jing, J. (2000). *Feeding China's little emperors: food, children, and social change.* Stanford: Stanford University Press.

Kuczmarski, R.J., Ogden, C.L., & Guo, S.S. (2002). 2000 CDC growth charts for the United States: methods and development. National Center for Health Statistics. *Vital and Health Statistics, Series 11, 246*, 1–190.

Liu, A., Zhao, L., Yu, D., & Yu, W. (2008). Study on malnutrition status and changing trend of children under 5 years old in China. *Wei Sheng Yan Jiu, 37*, 324–326 (in Chinese).

Ma, G.S., Li, Y.P., Wu, Y.F., Zhai, F.Y., Cui, Z.H., Hu, X.Q., Luan, D.C., Hu, Y,H., & Yang, X.G. (2005). The prevalence of body overweight and obesity and its changes among Chinese people during 1992 to 2002. *Chinese Journal of Preventive Medicine, 39*, 311–315 (in Chinese).

Mi, J., Cheng, H., Hou, D.Q., Duan, J.L., Teng, H.H., & Wang, Y.F. (2006). Prevalence of overweight obesity among children and adolescents in Beijing in 2004. *Zhonghua Liu Xing Bing Xue Za Zhi, 27*, 469–474 (in Chinese).

Misra, A. (2003). Revisions of cutoffs of body mass index to define overweight and obesity are needed for the Asian-ethnic groups. *International Journal of Obesity and Related Metabolic Disorders, 27,* 1294–1296.

Ng, S.W., Zhai, F., & Popkin, B.M. (2008). Impacts of China's edible oil pricing policy on nutrition. *Social Science & Medicine, 66,* 414–426.

Popkin, B.M. (2008). Will China's nutrition transition overwhelm its health care system and slow economic growth? *Health Affairs, 27,* 1064–1076.

Wang, Y. (2004). Epidemiology of childhood obesity – methodological aspects and guidelines: what's new? *International Journal of Obesity, 28,* 21–28.

Wang, Y., & Lobstein, T. (2007). Worldwide trends in childhood obesity. *International Journal of Pediatric Obesity, 1,* 11–25.

Wang, Y., Beydoun, M.A., Liang, L., Caballero, B., & Kumanyika, S.K. (2008a). Will all Americans become overweight or obese? Estimating the progression and cost of the US obesity epidemic. *Obesity, 16,* 2323–2330.

Wang, Z., Zhai, F., Du, S., & Popkin, B. (2008b). Dynamic shifts in Chinese eating behaviors. *Asia-Pacific Journal of Clinical Nutrition, 17,* 123–130.

WHO (2000). Obesity: preventing and managing the global epidemic. Report of a WHO consultation. *WHO Technical Report Series, No. 894,* Geneva.

WHO (2004). WHO Expert Consultation. Appropriate body-mass index for Asian populations and its implications for policy and intervention strategies. *Lancet, 363,* 157–163.

WHO, IADO, & IOTF (2000). The Asia-Pacific perspective: redefining obesity and its treatment (December 20, 2001); http://www.asso.org.au/profiles/profs/reportsguides/obesity/371.

Wikipedia (2009). Economy of the People's Republic of China. http://en.wikipedia.org/wiki/Economy_of_the_People's_Republic_of_China (assessed March 9, 2009).

World Bank (2009). Country brief – China. http://web.worldbank.org/WBSITE/EXTERNAL/COUNTRIES/EASTASIAPACIFICEXT/CHINAEXTN/0,,menuPK:318960~pagePK:141132~piPK:141107~theSitePK:318950,00.html (assessed March 9, 2009).

Xie, B., Chou, C., Spruijt-Metz, D., Reynolds, K., Clark, F., Palmer, P.H., Gallaher, P., Sun, P., Guo, Q., & Johnson, C.A. (2007). Socio-demographic and economic correlates of overweight status in Chinese adolescents. *American Journal of Health Behavior, 31,* 339–352.

Yang, G., Kong, L., Zhao, W., Wan, X., Zhai, Y., Chen, L.C., & Koplan, J.P. (2008). Emergence of chronic noncommunicable diseases in China. *Lancet, 372,* 1697–1705.

Yang, X., & Zhai, F. (2006). *Report of the 2002 Chinese National Nutrition and Health Survey (3rd Report)* (pp. 87–88). Beijing: People's Health Press.

Zhai, F., Wang, H., Du, S., He, Y., Wang, Z., Ge, K., & Popkin, B.M. (2007). Lifespan nutrition and changing socioeconomic conditions in China. *Asia-Pacific Journal of Clinical Nutrition, 16, Suppl 1,* 374–382.

Zhao, W., Zhai, F., Hu, J., Wang, J., Yang, Z., Kong, L., & Chen, C. (2008). Economic burden of obesity-related chronic diseases in Mainland China. *Obesity Reviews, 9, Suppl 1,* 62–67.

Zhou, B.F., & Cooperative Meta-Analysis Group of the Working Group on Obesity in China (2002). Predictive values of body mass index and waist circumference for risk factors of certain related diseases in Chinese adults – study on optimal cut-off points of body mass index and waist circumference in Chinese adults. *Biomedical and Environmental Sciences, 15,* 83–96.

Chapter 12
Epidemiology and Clinical Profile of Obesity in Children and Adolescents: South-East Asia and Singapore

Ting Fei Ho

Introduction

Since 1980, the prevalence of obesity has more than trebled in many countries. In 2005, it is estimated that globally there are about 1.6 billion overweight adults and at least 400 million of them are obese (WHO Fact Sheet No. 311 2006). Such rapid increase in adult overweight and obesity is a worldwide problem, confined not only to developed countries but is also observed in developing countries. While the prevalence of overweight and obese adults in many Asian and South East Asian countries may be below that in Europe or the United States, the general trend of increasing prevalence is likewise observed.

Asia includes both developed and developing countries with a wide distribution of socio-economic, demographic, ethnic and cultural patterns. Some of the world's most populated countries are found in Asia. The People's Republic of China (PRC), for instance, covers almost 20% of the world's population. In the recent decades Asia has undergone tremendous socio-economic, demographic and epidemiologic changes. While malnutrition may still exist in some parts of Asia, overweight and obesity in childhood is emerging as a health problem in several of the Asian countries. Asia also has the largest number of people with diabetes and is likely to remain so for the next few decades (Roglic and King 2000). The causes of such a rising trend for obesity and diabetes are likely to be complex. However, the major contributing factors are urbanization and changes in lifestyle where traditional diets are replaced by diets rich in energy-dense foods and drinks and where physical activity levels are shifted towards a lower activity pattern and more sedentary behavior (Gill 2006).

This increase in prevalence of childhood and adult overweight and obesity comes with a heavy price. The cost of healthcare has significantly increased and is expected to increase even more because of the close association between obesity and various chronic diseases. It is estimated that the direct costs of obesity are around 7% of total health care costs for the US and about 1–5% for Europe (Colditz 1999; Seidell 1995). Loss of productivity and income arising from obesity can contribute a major economic burden. This is a matter of concern to many countries particularly in Europe and North America where some 2 to 8% of overall healthcare budgets are consumed by obesity and obesity-related problems (WHO Fact Sheet EURO/13/05 2005). Such a burden on healthcare costs as brought about by an increasing prevalence of obesity may be ill afforded by many developing Asian countries.

T.F. Ho (✉)
Weight Management Clinic, International Child & Adolescent Clinic, Gleneagles Hospital,
Annexe Block, #02-43, 6A Napier Road, Singapore 258500, Singapore
e-mail: tingfei28@gmail.com

L.A. Moreno et al. (eds.), *Epidemiology of Obesity in Children and Adolescents*,
Springer Series on Epidemiology and Public Health 2, DOI 10.1007/978-1-4419-6039-9_12,
© Springer Science+Business Media, LLC 2011

The prevalence of overweight and obesity in children and adolescents is also increasing rapidly both in high income as well as middle and low income countries. The rise in childhood obesity is particularly rapid in the recent years. There are about 155 million overweight children worldwide, of which about 30–45 million are obese (International Association for the Study of Obesity 2004). Globally, children are becoming overweight and obese at progressively younger ages (Rössner 2002). It is estimated that, worldwide, about 22 million children under the age of 5 are overweight and more than 75% of overweight and obese children live in middle and low income countries (WHO World Health Report 1998).

In this chapter, information on the geographical, social, demographic and economic profiles of some Asian and South East Asian countries is provided as a background to the presentation of the prevalence and risk factors of childhood obesity in these countries. Such information can be useful and important particularly for the planning and implementation of preventive measures and the management of childhood obesity.

Geographic, Socio-demographic and Economic Characteristics

Prevalence of overweight and obesity in children is partly influenced by socio-cultural factors in the respective country. In this section, the demographic and economic profile of various countries in Asia and South East Asia is highlighted. The entire surface area of Asia (Eastern, South Central, South Eastern, Western) makes up almost 46.8% of the total surface area of the world (United Nations Statistics Division 2005). The countries described in this section are selected based on the fact that there is available data that describe the changes or the status of childhood obesity in these various countries. These countries are Taiwan, Hong Kong, Korea, Thailand, Malaysia, Singapore, Vietnam and Philippines. Hopefully this information will complement our understanding of the development of childhood obesity in each country.

Some important geographic and demographic data for the various countries are presented in Table 12.1. These data are mainly derived from information available since the early 2000s and the text below will refer largely to data presented in Table 12.1.

Hong Kong

Hong Kong is now considered part of the PRC since 1997. But for a long time prior to 1997 it was under British rule. The economic and social trends of Hong Kong are therefore somewhat different from that of many parts of PRC.

The area of Hong Kong (1,100 km^2) is significantly smaller than that of the other Asian countries, surpassing only that of Singapore (704 km^2). It has a population of 6,857,000 with none living under the poverty line (living on < US$1 per day). Almost 14% of its population is below the age of 15 years.

Being a rather well-off country with a GDP per capita of US$27,640.32, Hong Kong has a relatively high life expectancy for males (79.5 years) and females (85.6 years). Its infant mortality rate (1.84 per 1,000 live births) is also the lowest amongst the other Asian countries.

Singapore

Singapore is a small country with an area of only 704 km^2 and a population of 4,326,000. Nevertheless, it enjoys a very high GDP per capita of US$29,474 and none of the population lives below the poverty line.

Table 12.1 Geographic, demographic and economic characteristics of selected Asian and South East Asian countries

	Hong Kong[a]	Singapore[a]	Taiwan[b]	Malaysia[a]	Korea (South)[a]	Philippines[a]	Thailand[a]	Vietnam[a]
Area in km²	1,100	704	35,980	330,250	98,480	300,000	514,000	329,560
Population (in thousands)	6,857 (2006)	4,326 (2005)	22,920 (2008 est.)	26,640 (2006)	48,050 (2006)	86,264 (2006)	63,444 (2006)	86,206 (2006)
Populations below the age of 15 in %	13.69 (2006)	19.3 (2006)	17.3 (2008 est.)	32.4 (2006)	18.0 (2006)	36.0 (2006)	21.0 (2006)	29.0 (2006)
GDP (gross domestic product) per capita (US $) at current market prices	27,640.32 (2006)	29,474 (2006)	15,978 (2005)	5,227.50 (2005)	16,309 (2005)	1,192 (2005)	2,750 (2005)	631 (2005)
Population below poverty line in % (% living on <US $1 per day)	Nil	Nil	0.95 (2007 est.)	<2.0 (1997)	<2.0 (1998)	14.8 (2003)	<2.0 (2000)	<2.0 (2000)
[c]Human development index (rank order)	22	28		63	25	102	81	114
Life expectancy at birth in years (males)	79.46 (2006)	78.0 (2006)	74.89 (2008 est.)	72.0 (2006)	75.0 (2006)	64.0 (2006)	69.0 (2005)	69.0 (2006)
Life expectancy at birth in years (females)	85.57 (2006)	81.8 (2006)	80.89 (2008 est.)	76.0 (2006)	82.0 (2005)	71.0 (2006)	75.0 (2006)	75.0 (2006)
Crude birth rate (per 1,000 population)	9.51 (2006)	10.1 (2006)	8.99 (2008 est.)	18.7 (2006)	10.3 (2005)	25.7 (2005)	16.3 (2005)	20.3 (2005)
Crude death rate (per 1,000 population)	5.46 (2006)	4.3 (2006)	6.65 (2008 est.)	4.5 (2006)	5.5 (2005)	5.1 (2005)	7.3 (2005)	6.1 (2005)
Infant mortality rate (per 1,000 live births)	1.84 (2006)	2.6 (2006)	5.45 (2008 est.)	6.6 (2006)	5.0 (2006)	24.0 (2006)	7.0 (2005)	15.0 (2006)

[a]Information taken from WHO Statistical Information System (2007)
[b]Information on Taiwan taken from The World Factbook (Central Intelligence Agency 2008)
[c]Information on Human development index extracted from Human Development Report 2007/2008 (United Nations Development Program 2008)

Its infant mortality rate is very low (2.6 per 1,000 live births), ranking just above that of Hong Kong. The life expectancy for males (78.0 years) and females (81.8 years) ranks just below that of Hong Kong.

Taiwan

Taiwan has an area of 35,980 km^2 with a population of 22,920,000. About 17% of its population is below the age of 15 years. The GDP per capita of US$15,978 is close to that of South Korea but lower than that of Singapore and Hong Kong. A small proportion (0.95%) of its population still lives below the poverty line.

The life expectancies of males and females in Taiwan are 74.9 and 80.9 years, respectively. Its infant mortality rate is about 5.45 per 1,000 live births.

Malaysia

The area of Malaysia is about 330,250 km^2. Being almost 10 times larger than Taiwan, Malaysia has a population (26,640,000) just slightly higher than that of Taiwan. About 32% of its population is below 15 years old.

The GDP per capita of Malaysia is US$5,227.50. Less than 2% of the population lives below the poverty line.

The life expectancies of males and females in Malaysia are 72.0 and 76.0 years, respectively. Its infant mortality rate (6.6 per 1,000 live births) is significantly higher than that of Hong Kong and Singapore and just slightly higher than that of Taiwan.

Korea (South)

The country of South Korea has an area of 98,480 km^2 and has a population of 48,050,000. Almost 18.0% of its population is below the age of 15 years.

The GDP of South Korea at US$16,309 per capita is slightly higher than that of Taiwan but below that of Hong Kong and Singapore. A small proportion (<2%) of the population lives below the poverty line.

Korea enjoys a relatively high life expectancy for both the males (75.0 years) and females (82.0 years). Its infant mortality rate of 5.0 per 1,000 live births is very close to that of Taiwan.

Philippines

The land area of Philippines (300,000 km^2) is rather similar to that of Malaysia. However, its population of 86,264,000 is more than 3 times that of Malaysia with about 36% of its population below 15 years of age.

In comparison with several South East Asian countries, Philippines has a rather low GDP of US$1,192 per capita and almost 14.8% of the population lives below the poverty line of less than US$1 per day.

The life expectancies for males (64.0 years) and females (71.0 years) are also lower than that in other South East Asian countries. Its infant mortality rate of 24.0 per 1,000 live births is significantly higher than that of its South East Asian neighbors.

Thailand

Thailand has an area of 514,000 km^2. It is larger than Philippines but has a smaller population of 63,444,000 with 21% of its population below 15 years of age.

It does not have as high a GDP compared to that of its close geographic neighbors like Singapore and Malaysia. Thailand's GDP per capita is US$2,750 and less than 2% of the population lives below the poverty line.

Comparatively, the life expectancy of males (69.0 years) and females (75.0 years) is relatively low while its infant mortality rate of 7.0 per 1,000 live births is close to that of Malaysia.

Vietnam

The area of Vietnam (329,560 km^2) and its population of 86,206,000 is comparable to that of Philippines. Approximately 29.0% of this population is below 15 years old.

Vietnam has one of the lowest GDP of only US$631 per capita in the South East Asian region and less than 2% of the population lives below the poverty line.

The life expectancies of males and females in Vietnam are similar to that of Thailand where males have a life expectancy of 69.0 years and females have a life expectancy of 75.0 years. The country has a relatively high infant mortality rate of 15.0 per 1,000 live births.

Summary

From the above it can be seen that countries in Asia and South East Asia have a wide diversity of geographic, socio-demographic and economic profiles. These characteristics can help us understand how various socio-demographic and economic factors are interrelated in the development of obesity in children of Asia and South East Asia.

Prevalence of Overweight and Obesity in Children

Urbanization, increasing affluence and changes in lifestyle have led to a dramatic transition towards a trend of increasing prevalence of overweight and obesity in many Asian countries. Some Asian countries like Singapore and Malaysia have intra-population ethnic diversities that can further contribute to such changes. The varied socio-cultural and dietary characteristics of various Asian countries have resulted in differences in the perception of body image and the associations between body mass index (BMI) and socio-economic status (Treloar et al. 1999). Furthermore, the distinct differences in economic, social and educational distributions between the urban and rural populations in some countries like Malaysia, Korea, Taiwan and Thailand can influence the patterns of infant feeding, diet and lifestyle of the various sub-groups in each population. Collectively, these can affect the development of overweight and obesity in adults and children.

Many Asian countries do not have comprehensive nationally representative data on the weight and health status of their populations as national surveys are not regularly or routinely conducted. This situation is gradually improving as the healthcare systems in many of the Asian countries become more organized and sophisticated. In spite of this inadequacy there are currently sufficient data to provide some insight into the status of overweight and obesity in children and adolescents in several Asian countries.

There is currently no single accepted consensus on the definition of overweight and obesity for children. The criteria used in various European and North American studies adhere to the cut-off values established by the International Obesity Task Force (IOTF). Currently, IOTF recommends the definition of child overweight and obesity based on percentile curves of BMI where the curves at age 18 years are drawn to pass through the cut-off values of 25 and 30 kg/m^2 for adult overweight and obesity (Cole et al. 2000). While BMI for age is commonly used for defining overweight and obesity, cut-off values may differ depending on the preference of the individual country (Cole et al. 2000; Guillaume 1999; Must et al. 1991).

Undoubtedly, childhood obesity does pose a public health problem for the twenty-first century even for Asia and South East Asia. Nevertheless, when we evaluate data and information from Asian countries, one must view these in the context where, unlike Western countries, obesity is often not considered an important health issue by government and healthcare authorities in many Asian countries. Malnutrition in infants and children remain a health concern in various Asian countries (Khor 2003). In recent years, there is a gradually increasing awareness of the clinical and public health impact of childhood obesity and its related health issues. This has led to increasing effort to study and assess the extent of the problem, its severity and the measures to prevent and manage this problem. Thus, it needs to be emphasized that study protocols and methodology for data collection and analysis across the various Asian countries may not be uniform and may not be entirely comparable. The diversities in social, demographic and economical characteristics of the regional populations in some countries can also introduce non-uniformity in the study cohorts. Nevertheless, the available information obtained from various sources serve as a useful and important baseline for study, evaluation and implementation of policies for management and control of childhood obesity in these countries.

Looking at data available from IOTF (International Association for the Study of Obesity 2008a) (Table 12.2), prevalence of obesity and overweight in children and adolescents in Asian countries

Table 12.2 Prevalence of obesity and overweight (combined) in Asian and South East Asian children

| Country | Year of survey | Childhood overweight (including obesity) | | | |
		Age range (years)	Boys (%)	Girls (%)	Cut-off
Hong Kong	1993	3–18	11.3 (obesity)	8.9 (obesity)	Weight-for-height standard
Korea (South)	2001	10–18	11.6 (obesity)	10.9 (obesity)	US CDC
Malaysia	2002	7–10	9.7 (obesity)	7.1 (obesity)	WHO
Singapore	1993	10 and 15	20.4	14.6	IOTF
Taiwan	2001	6–18	26.8	16.5	IOTF
Thailand	1997	5–15	21.1	12.6	85th percentile NHANES
Vietnam	2004	11–16	11.7 (overweight; boys + girls)		IOTF
England	2004	5–17	29	29.3	IOTF
Canada	2004	12–17	32.3	25.8	IOTF
USA	2003/2004	6–17	35.1	36	IOTF
Australia	2007	9–13	25.0	30.0	IOTF

Extracted from "global childhood overweight" (International Association for the Study of Obesity IASO; International Obesity Taskforce IOTF, London October 2008) (International Association for the Study of Obesity 2008a)
Data from England, North America and Australia are included for purpose of comparison

is generally lower than that reported in the West. The age groups studied varied between 5 and 18 years of age. The prevalence rates for overweight and obesity combined largely fall below 20% with the exception of Singapore, Taiwan and Thailand where prevalence rates for boys come close to or exceed 20% (Table 12.2).

Besides the collective data reported by IOTF, there are other individual studies that were reported in various journals. A review of various published papers, as presented below, shows prevalence rates that differ from those reported by IOTF. The lack of a universally agreed measurement and definition of obesity and overweight in children adds to the problem of uniformity of study protocols and comparability of data in children.

Taiwan

The population of Taiwan is largely Chinese in origin with a smaller proportion of indigenous people. In 1997, Chen (1997) reported a prevalence of obesity that ranged from 4.3 to 17.4% for children aged between 3 and 19 years. Here the author used a weight-for-height index for determination of obesity. During 1995–1996, the prevalence of obesity (defined as body weight >120% of mean age- and sex-specific body weight) for 12–15 year old boys and girls in Taipei city was 16.6 and 11.1% (Chu 2005). Using weight-for-height percentile curves derived from national growth reference values, Huang et al. (2003) noted that, in a nation-wide survey of boys and girls between the ages of 6.5–18.5 years, the prevalence of obesity was 18.5% in boys and 15.0% in girls. The higher prevalence of obesity in boys as compared to girls prevailed for all age groups. The authors also noted that the prevalence of obesity for both sexes has increased from 1997 to 2002 irrespective of sex (Huang et al. 2003). In the Nutrition And Health Survey In Taiwan (NAHSIT) of elementary school children it was noted that 15.5% of boys and 14.4% of girls were overweight. In addition, 14.7% of boys and 9.1% of girls were obese (Chu and Pan 2007). The authors also noted regional differences in prevalence rates of overweight and obesity for both boys and girls. There were more obese boys in the southern areas compared to the mountain area (23.3 vs. 4.3%). For girls, prevalence rates for overweight and obesity were highest in the central area (13.3%) and lowest in the southern area (2.6%).

The prevalence of obesity for children 12–15 years of age has increased from 1980 to 1996 (Chu 2005). Based on a definition of body weight >120% of mean age- and sex-specific body weight as obese, prevalence rates of obesity for the years 1980, 1986 and 1996 show an upward trend of increase from 12.4 to 14.8 and 15.6% for boys, respectively; 10.1 to 11.1 and 12.9% for girls, respectively (Chu 2005). Similar to the trend of increasing prevalence of obesity, a health survey reported by Chen et al. (2006) shows that overall prevalence of obesity for boys (aged 6–18 years old) was 19.8% in 1999 and 26.8% in 2001. For girls, the 1999 and 2001 prevalence rates for obesity were 15.2 and 16.5%, respectively. The NAHSIT of elementary school children conducted in the periods 1993–1996 and 2001–2002 showed that prevalence of obesity had doubled in girls and trebled in boys (Pan and Lee 2007).

Malaysia

The multi-ethnic composition of Malaysia comprises primarily of the Malay ethnic group and other bumiputras (65%). Thus the social and cultural characteristics are significantly different from that of other Asian and South East Asian countries like Taiwan, Korea, Thailand, Singapore and Philippines.

A survey of almost 6,000 children between 7 and 10 years of age using cut-off values for nutritional status recommended by WHO revealed that overall prevalence of obesity was 8.4%, with

9.7% for boys and 7.1% for girls (Tee et al. 2002). With regard to adolescents between 11 and 15 years of age, Zalilah et al. (2006) reported that overall prevalence rates for the three major ethnic groups in Malaysia (Malays, Chinese, Indians) were between 18 and 19%.

Korea (South)

In a cohort of 10–18 year old boys who participated in a survey between 1998 and 2001, Kim et al. (2006) defined obesity using BMI cut-off points proposed by the United States Centers for Disease Control and Prevention (Himes and Dietz 1994). Overweight was defined as ≥95th percentile. Prevalence of overweight was noted to have increased from 5.4% in 1998 to 11.3% in 2001 (Kim et al. 2006)

Thailand

Using a definition of childhood obesity as a weight-for-height Z score above two standard deviations of the National Center for Health Statistics/World Health Organization reference population median, Langendijk et al. (2003) found that prevalence of obesity in 7–9 year old Thai children was 10.8%. In 2001, Sakamoto et al. (2001) reported that prevalence of childhood obesity for second and third grade children was higher in the urban areas (22.7%) as compared to the rural areas (7.4%). In this study obesity was defined as weight-for-height greater than the 97th percentile (Sakamoto et al. 2001)

In Thailand, the prevalence of obesity in children has increased over the recent years. Likitmaskul et al. (2003) noted that prevalence of obesity for children and adolescents had increased from 5.8% in 1990 to 13.3% in 1996. In a 5-year follow-up from 1992 to 1997, prevalence of overweight for males (using the 85th percentile BMI cut-off point based on the United States first National Health and Nutritional Examination Survey reference for age and sex) increased from 12.4 to 21% (Mo-suwan et al. 2000). However, for girls, the prevalence decreased from 15.2% in 1992 to 12.6% in 1997 (Mo-suwan et al. 2000). In an earlier study, a trend of increasing prevalence of childhood obesity was already noted (Mo-suwan et al. 1993). Obesity was diagnosed as weight-for-height above 120% of the reference values for Bangkok children. Using this definition, the prevalence of obesity in 6–12 year old children increased from 12.2% in 1991 to 13.5% in 1992 and 15.6% in 1993 (Mo-suwan et al. 1993).

Vietnam

Dieu et al. (2007) defined obesity in children using age- and sex-specific BMI cut-off points proposed by the IOTF. The prevalence of overweight and obesity in preschool children in urban areas of Ho Chi Minh City were noted to be 20.5 and 16.3%, respectively. In another study, it was found that prevalence of overweight and obesity in adolescents in Ho Chi Minh City was significantly different between the wealthy urban districts and the semi-rural districts (Tang et al. 2007). The prevalence of overweight and obesity in adolescents living in wealthy urban districts were 8.2 and 0.6%, respectively, as compared to 1.6 and 0.2%, respectively, in the semi-rural districts (Tang et al. 2007).

Using IOTF age- and sex-specific BMI cut-off points to define overweight and obesity, Hong et al. (2007) noted that prevalence of overweight and obesity of adolescents in urban districts of Ho Chi Minh City had increased from 5.0 and 0.6% in 2002 to 11.7 and 2.0% in 2004, respectively. In a similar pattern, Tuan (Tuan et al. 2008) also reported an overall increase in overweight and obesity in the Vietnamese population aged 18–65 years old, from 1992 to 2002. Over the same period of time, the prevalence of underweight individuals had declined (Tuan et al. 2008).

Comparison of Prevalence of Overweight and Obesity in Children and Adults

In recent years, prevalence of adult overweight and obesity has increased in several Asian and South East Asian countries where overweight and obesity is traditionally low. BMI values of 25 to 29.9 and ≥30 are used in adults as criteria for adult overweight and obesity, respectively. However, the proposed BMI cut-off values for public health action in Asians are different due to the fact that Asian body composition tends towards more body fat for a given BMI (WHO Expert Consultation 2004).

Tables 12.2 and 12.3 show a comparison of prevalence of overweight and obesity in adults (International Association for the Study of Obesity 2008b) and children (International Association for the Study of Obesity 2008a) in various Asian and South East Asian countries (with prevalence of overweight and obesity in North America and some European countries included as comparison). For adults, the prevalence of overweight and obesity were separately reported, while for children these values were generally reported in combination, with some exceptions as listed in Table 12.2.

While it is not exactly accurate and valid to compare prevalence of adult overweight and obesity with that of children in each country due to the differences in definition and reporting, it can be seen that, generally, prevalence of overweight in adults were higher than prevalence of combined overweight and obesity in children in the respective Asian or South East Asian country. One exception is Thailand where prevalence of overweight adult male appeared to be lower than that of overweight (plus obesity) in Thai boys (Tables 12.2 and 12.3). Similarly, in Taiwan, the prevalence of overweight for both men and women combined was lower than that of overweight (plus obesity) in boys (Tables 12.2 and 12.3).

Summary

In the above section, it is seen that while prevalence of childhood overweight and obesity in Asia and South East Asia still lag behind that in the West, there is already an increasing trend of overweight and obesity even in some of the poorer countries where under-nutrition still exists. Boys seem to have a higher prevalence of overweight and obesity compared to girls. Within each country studied, the prevalence of overweight in adults is generally higher than that of overweight and obesity combined in children.

Risk Factors for Obesity

The rapid socio-economic and demographic changes in Asia and South East Asia can have an impact on the lifestyle, dietary practices and physical activity patterns of the populations. Changes in diet and physical activity may have a link with the rising prevalence in overweight and obesity observed in children and adults.

Table 12.3 Prevalence of overweight and obesity in Asian and South East Asian adults

Country	Year of data collection	Survey sample size	Age category (years)	Male		Female		Combined	
				Overweight % (BMI 25–29.9)	Obesity % (BMI 30+)	Overweight % (BMI 25–29.9)	Obesity % (BMI 30+)	Overweight % (BMI 25–29.9)	Obesity % (BMI 30+)
Hong Kong	1995/1996	2,875	25–74	33	5	27	7		
Korea (South)	1998	8,816	15–79	22.0	1.6	23.4	3.0		
Malaysia	1996	30,165	18+	20.1	4.0	21.4	7.6		
Philippines	1998	9,299	20+	14.9	2.1	18.9	4.4	16.9	3.3
Singapore	2004	4,168	18–69	28.6	6.4	22.6	7.3	25.6	6.9
Taiwan	1993–1996	3,046	20+					21.1	4.0
Thailand	1997	3,220	20–59	15.7	3.5	25.1	8.8	22.0	21.5
Vietnam	2001/2002		19+	4.4		6.6			
England	2007		16+	41.4	23.6	32.0	24.4		
Canada	2004	12,428	18+	42.0	22.9	30.2	23.2	36.1	23.1
USA	2003–2004	n/a	20+	39.7	31.1	28.6	33.2	34.1	32.2
Australia	2000	11,067	25+	48.2	19.3	29.9	22.2	39.0	20.8

Extracted from "Global Obesity Prevalence in Adults" (International Association for the Study of Obesity IASO; International Obesity Taskforce IOTF, London December 2008)
(International Association for the Study of Obesity 2008b)

Data from England, North America and Australia are included for purpose of comparison

Dietary Patterns

While there is a lack of information on the dietary patterns and the shifts in dietary habits in individual countries in Asia over the years, a shift from the traditional diets to diets high in sugars, animal and vegetable fats (Drewnowski and Popkin 1997) had been observed. This can be a significant contributor to the increase in prevalence of obesity. In high income countries like Singapore, Hong Kong and South Korea, the contribution of dietary fat to total energy increased from 8.8% in 1962 to 23.7% in 1996 (Gill 2005). In the China Health and Nutrition Surveys, Popkin et al. (1995) noted that higher fat and energy intake was associated with increased BMI. Urban residents had a lower energy intake, higher fat intake and lower physical activity when compared to rural residents.

Infant Feeding Practices

Exclusive breastfeeding of infants for 6 months is recommended by the World Health Organization (World Health Organization 2001). This is preferred over exclusive breastfeeding for 4 months followed by partial breastfeeding to 6 months. The primary reason relates to the control of infectious disease, particularly that of gastrointestinal infection, and the associated morbidity and mortality. While a large proportion of mothers in Asia may understand the requirements and benefits of such recommendations, many are not able to adhere to this due to various social and personal reasons.

In Taiwan, about 84% of the mothers who were employed and unemployed practiced initial breastfeeding. However, at 6 months, the breastfeeding rates had declined to 12.9 and 27.2% for the employed and unemployed mothers, respectively (Chuang et al. 2007). Maternal education, maternal age and sufficiency of breast milk were some factors influencing the practice of breastfeeding.

Similarly, breastfeeding was noted to be low over the past several decades in Hong Kong. In 1993, a survey of infants under 6 months old revealed that 36.1% had given up breastfeeding and were fed entirely on formula (Lee et al. 2007). Fifty-four percent had been exclusively formula-fed since birth. Thus, the remaining proportion of breastfed infants under 6 months old was very low at 9.6% (Lee et al. 2007). Various reasons are likely to discourage breastfeeding e.g., restricted food varieties, sore nipples, breast engorgement, perceived home confinement and inadequate milk supply (Lee et al. 2006a). In a longer follow-up study of over 3 years, Leung et al. (2006) noted that while 66.7% of mothers had initiated breastfeeding with a median duration of 1 month, only 13.4% met the WHO recommendations on breastfeeding.

A National Breastfeeding Survey conducted in Singapore in 2001 revealed that 94.5% mothers attempted breastfeeding after delivery. While 71.6% were still breastfeeding at 1 month the rate had fallen to 21% by 6 months (Foo et al. 2005).

In Bangkok, Thailand, almost 50 to 60% of mother practiced exclusive breastfeeding in the first 3 months of postpartum (Laisiriruangrai et al. 2008; Li et al. 1999). However, by 6 months postpartum, the rate of exclusive breastfeeding was low (11 to 14%) (Hangchaovanich and Voramongkol 2006; Laisiriruangrai et al. 2008). Mothers in the rural areas were more likely to practice exclusive breastfeeding with about 53% of infants still exclusively breastfed at 6 months (Panpanich et al. 2003).

While about 84% of mothers practiced exclusive breastfeeding at birth, only about 44% still breastfed exclusively at 16 weeks postpartum (Duong et al. 2005). Some studies revealed that mixed feeding with plain water, sugar water, premature introduction of semi-solid/solid food and other forms of complementary food could be issues of concern in infant feeding (Duong et al. 2004; Li et al. 2002b; Truong et al. 1995).

It can be seen that in various countries in Asia and South East Asia the rate of exclusive breastfeeding may be high in the initial first postpartum month but often declines rapidly in the subsequent months. The practice of breastfeeding generally falls short of the recommendations by the WHO. Various possible factors may be responsible for such a phenomenon. Factors like maternal educational level (Forman 1984; Scott et al. 2001a), maternal age (Ryan 1997; Vogel et al. 1999), employment status (Kearney and Cronenwett 1991; Noble 2001; Visness and Kennedy 1997), and support in terms of knowledge, information, physical and psychological conditions (Labarere et al. 2005; Raj and Plichta 1998; Scott et al. 2001b) are some important considerations.

Physical Activity

The level of physical activity has an important impact on the development of obesity in children and adults. However, data to support the pattern and the changes in physical activity level are rather lacking, particularly for countries in Asia.

Bell et al. (2002) noted that the odds of being obese were 80% higher for individuals in China who owned motorized vehicles than those who did not own such vehicles. In addition, men who recently acquired motor vehicles had a greater weight gain and twice the risk of becoming obese than those who did not recently acquire motor vehicles.

A recent meta-analysis was conducted for over 23.5 million 6–19 year old children and adolescents from seven Asian countries (PRC, Hong Kong, Japan, Korea, India, Singapore, Thailand) to review secular changes in their fitness test performances (Macfarlane and Tomkinson 2007). This study revealed that there was little change in the performance of power and speed of Asian children and adolescents in the recent decades. However, in the last 10–15 years, there was an alarming decline in cardiovascular endurance fitness in the youths across the Asian countries studied. Though information was scarce, two studies reported on the geographical variation in fitness test performance (Hatano et al. 1997; Meshizuka and Nakanishi 1972). Japanese children ranked first in fitness performance. Children from Hong Kong, Taiwan, Korea and Thailand ranked middle and children from Philippines and Vietnam had the worst performance index. Such data give us an insight into the level of fitness of youths in various Asian countries. In conjunction with the rising prevalence of obesity in children and adolescents, such information has some public health relevance.

Summary

Changes in dietary habits and physical activity patterns in Asia and South East Asia indicate that there is a trend towards diets that are high in fats and sugars and a lifestyle of lower physical activity resulting in a decline in cardiovascular endurance fitness for youths in several countries. Infant feeding practices tend to deviate from WHO recommendations and move towards shorter periods of breastfeeding. Various socio-economic factors may contribute to this trend.

Clinical Consequences of Childhood Obesity

Several large scale and long term studies have documented increased risk and mortality for obese children and adolescents who become obese adults (Mosberg 1989; Must et al. 1992; Nieto et al. 1992). More recently, an Australian study also confirms that adolescents who were obese and overweight had a higher risk for diseases like type II diabetes, cardiovascular disease and fatty liver disease (Denney-Wilson et al. 2008). While there is often no immediate morbidity or mortality linked to obesity in childhood or adolescence, it is known that many of these chronic diseases can begin early in childhood. For instance, atherosclerotic changes that are correlated with presence of cardiovascular risk factors can occur in young children and adolescents (Berenson et al. 1998; Mahoney et al. 1996).

In Asia, this association between childhood obesity and increased risk for chronic disease is no exception. Studies have increasingly documented the presence of cardiovascular abnormalities, insulin resistance, fatty liver disease in children and adolescents who are overweight or obese.

The association of BMI with chronic diseases is somewhat different for Asians as compared to Caucasians. It has been demonstrated that, given the same BMI, Asian adults have higher levels of percentage body fat compared to age- and sex-matched Caucasian adults (Deurenberg-Yap et al. 2000; Gurrici et al. 1998; Ko et al. 2001; Wang et al. 1994). Furthermore, in many Asian countries, the populations have increased prevalence of cardiovascular risk factors at BMI values considered normal by WHO (Deurenberg-Yap et al. 2001; Ishikawa-Takata et al. 2002; Lee et al. 2002; Li et al. 2002a; Moon et al. 2002; Reddy et al. 2002). Recognizing this fact, WHO has proposed BMI cut-off values associated with various levels of risk for cardiovascular diseases in Asian adults that are lower than that for Caucasian adults (Table 12.4) (WHO Expert Consultation 2004).

In children, there are anthropometric markers of central fat distribution that are reasonably well correlated with markers of metabolic disturbance (Freedman et al. 1999a, b). However, there are no well-defined BMI or anthropometric cut-off values that relate to obesity-related morbidity or mortality. Often, long term clinical or metabolic consequences of childhood obesity are difficult to study. The period between the origin and expression of diseases may take many years.

Hypertension

Elevation of blood pressure can occur in children and adolescents who are overweight or obese. In Singapore, preliminary studies in the mid 1980s revealed that systolic blood pressure was positively correlated with BMI (Ho 1987). It was also shown in the study of Lee et al. (2006b) that 32.8% of severely obese Singapore children and adolescents had hypertension. Chu et al. (1998) reported that

Table 12.4 Proposed BMI cut-off points[a] for public health action in Asians

Cardiovascular disease risk	Asian BMI cut-off points for action (kg/m^2)	Current WHO BMI cut-off points (kg/m^2)
	<18.5	<18.5
Low	18.5–22.9	18.5–24.9
Moderate	23.0–27.4	25.0–29.9
High	27.5–32.4	30.0–34.9
Very high	32.5–37.4	35.0–39.9
	≥37.5	≥40.0

[a] Contents of table adapted from WHO Expert Consultation (2004)

in a group of 12–16 year old Taiwanese adolescents, both obese boys and girls had significantly higher prevalence of hypertension compared to non-obese adolescents of the same age. More recently, a large cohort of 13,935 Taiwanese children and adolescents, aged 6–18 years, were surveyed in 2001 for weight, height, physical fitness and blood pressure (Chen et al. 2006). It was found that the risk of hypertension increased almost 2 times for the overweight/obese group that was fit and almost 3 times for the overweight/obese group that was unfit, when compared to the normal weight and fit children and adolescents. A study of Chinese children in the PRC revealed concurring findings where overweight and obese children between 15 and 17.9 years had a high risk of developing hypertension. The risk was 2.3 and 2.9 times higher than the normal weight children of the same age (Li et al. 2005). Sixteen percent of overweight or obese 15–18 year old adolescents had hypertension. A study of healthy adolescent Indian school children between the ages of 11–17 years revealed that prevalence of hypertension was 6.69% in urban areas and 2.56% in rural areas (Mohan et al. 2004). It was further shown that prevalence of hypertension increased with increased BMI in both urban and rural students. Prevalence of hypertension in urban normal weight students was 4.52%.Whereas in the overweight and obese urban students the prevalence of hypertension was 15.3 and 43.1%, respectively (Mohan et al. 2004).

Hyperlipidemia

Overweight or obesity in either adults or children has been known to be associated with hyperlipidemia. In Asia, several studies documented such an association as well. Overweight or obese adolescents in the PRC were found to have significantly increased risks for hypertriglyceridemia, low high-density lipoprotein (HDL) and dyslipidemia when compared to normal weight controls, after adjustment for age, sex, socio-economic status, location of stay, physical activity and dietary intake (Li et al. 2005). The prevalence for hypertriglyceridemia ($\geq$1.1 mmol/L) (18.2%), low HDL cholesterol (males <1.2 mmol/L; females <1.3 mmol/L) (56.1%) and dyslipidemia (61.9%) where either hypercholesterolemia, hypertriglyceridemia or low HDL cholesterol was present, were noted to be high in 15–18 year old PRC adolescents (Li et al. 2008). In Taiwan, Chu et al. (1998) had earlier reported that mean concentrations of lipids for obese 12–16 year old boys and girls were significantly higher than that of normal weight controls. The obese 12–16 year old boys and girls had higher ratio of total cholesterol to HDL cholesterol, lower HDL cholesterol concentrations and higher low-density lipoprotein (LDL) cholesterol, apolipoprotein A-I and apolipoprotein B concentrations when compared with their normal weight controls. In Singapore, studies in the mid 1980s revealed that obese children, aged 7–16 years, had elevated total cholesterol (35.6%), triglycerides (5.5%) and LDL cholesterol (26.0%) levels in blood (Ho 1987). These values are comparable to those reported more recently by Lee et al. (2006b) in severely obese Singapore children (mean age 11.1 years). In this study of 201 children and adolescents, 36.8% had elevated LDL cholesterol.

Insulin Resistance and Type 2 Diabetes

The increase in the prevalence of overweight or obesity in children, adolescents and adults worldwide contributes to a dismal outlook for the prevalence of type 2 diabetes mellitus (DM) and insulin resistance. The alarming increase in type 2 DM among youths is attributed to the increase in obesity in young people (Vivian 2006). In the United States the incidence of type 2 DM among adolescents is about 4 in 1,000 adolescents (Daniels et al. 2005).

In Asia, the rising trend of type 2 DM appears to have reached epidemic levels. There is also the perception that Asia may emerge as the epicenter of the epidemic of type 2 DM in the world (Sicree et al. 2003). Cases of type 2 DM have now greatly outnumbered cases of type 1 DM children and adolescents in the Asia-Pacific region (Cockram 2000). Clinically, the development of type 2 DM in Asia has some worrying differences compared to other parts of the world. Firstly, it has developed rapidly within a shorter time and in younger individuals (Alberti et al. 2004). In addition, Asians are developing type 2 DM at a much lower BMI (He et al. 1994; Ko et al. 1999). This has most likely led to differences in the prevalence of type 2 DM between different countries in Asia and the rest of the world. Table 12.5 and Fig. 12.1 show the discrepancy where prevalence of type 2 DM is higher than the prevalence of obesity in adults in various Asian countries. However, this pattern is the reverse for the United States where prevalence of adult obesity is 30% compared to a relatively lower prevalence of diabetes (8.2%).

Li et al. (2005) noted that obese adolescents in the PRC had significantly increased fasting blood glucose; 0.2% of 7–12 year olds and 0.4% of 12–18 year olds and adolescents were found to have diabetes (Li et al. 2008). Overweight adolescents were more likely to have hyperglycemia compared to normal weight adolescents, with an odds ratio of 2.3. Overweight and obese children had significantly higher levels of fasting blood glucose when compared to normal weight children (Li et al. 2008).

In Taiwan there was concurring observation where obese children and adolescents were found to have a higher level of fasting blood glucose compared to normal weight children (Chu et al. 1998). Mass screening of school students in Taiwan for glucosuria and examination of fasting blood samples showed significantly increased average rates of newly identified diabetes from 1993 to 1999 (Wei et al. 2003). The average rates per 100,000 boys (8.3%) and girls (12.0%) in 1993 had increased to peak rates of 14.7% for boys and 19.0% for girls in 1999 (Wei et al. 2003). Screening of fasting blood glucose and glucosuria in Taiwanese school children aged 6–18 years showed that

Table 12.5 Comparison of prevalence of overweight and obesity with prevalence of diabetes in adults from various countries

	Survey year	Prevalence of overweight adults (%)[a]	Prevalence of obese adults (%)[b]	Prevalence of diabetes (%)
USA	1999–2000	34.0	30.0	
	1999–2000			8.2
India	1998–1999	10.0	2.2	12.1
	2000			
Philippines	1998	16.9	3.3	5.1
	1996			
Taiwan	1993–1996	21.1	4.0	9.2
	1996			
Hong Kong	1996–1997	25.1	3.8	9.8
	1995–1996			
China	1999–2000	25.0	4.0	5.5
	2000–2001			
Singapore	1998	24.4	6.0	8.4
	1992			
Korea	2001	27.4	3.2	
	2001			7.6
Thailand	1998	28.3	6.8	11.9
	1995			

Contents of table adapted from Yoon et al. (2006)

[a] $25 \text{ kg/m}^2 \leq \text{BMI} < 30 \text{ kg/m}^2$

[b] $\text{BMI} \geq 30 \text{ kg/m}^2$

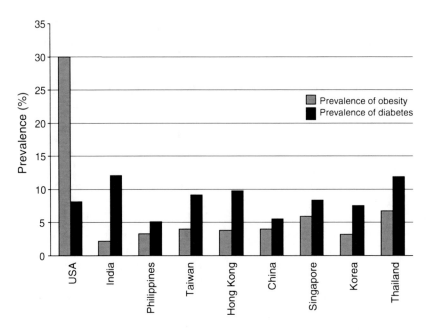

Fig. 12.1 Comparison of prevalence of obesity with prevalence of diabetes in adults in various countries adapted from Yoon et al. (2006)

the incidence of type 2 DM was sixfold higher than that of type 1 diabetes and obesity was the most important risk factor for type 2 DM (Chang et al. 2006).

In Thailand, the incidence of diabetes in children had been relatively low. However, from the period of 1986–1995 to the period of 1996–1999, the number of Thai children (mean age 11.6 years, mean BMI 27.8 kg/m^2) with type 2 DM has increased from 5 to 17.9% (Likitmaskul et al. 2003). This increase in type 2 DM was associated with an increase in the prevalence of obesity from 5.8% in 1990 to 13.3% in 1996.

Studies in Singapore revealed similar trends. The prevalence of type 2 DM in adults (age 18–69 years old) has risen from 2% in 1975 to 9.0% in 1998 (Lee 2000). Lee et al. (2006b) noted that 12.4% of severely obese children and adolescents with a mean age of 11.1 years and mean body fat of 40.7% had impaired glucose tolerance and 4.5% had type 2 DM.

A cross-sectional study of 271 Hong Kong school children between the ages of 9–12 years showed that overweight or obese children had an increased risk of hyperinsulinemia (Sung et al. 2003). Seventy-seven percent of overweight or obese children had insulin resistance.

Metabolic Syndrome

There is a fairly high prevalence of metabolic syndrome (MS) in South Asians (Mohan et al. 2001; Ramachandran et al. 2003). It is recognized that the definition of MS using standard criteria may not be optimal for South Asians and various criteria may need modification (Misra et al. 2005). Body composition and percentage body fat have strong correlation with MS in South Asians (Misra 2003; Deurenberg et al. 1998).

While some overweight or obese children have only isolated morbidity like hypertension, hyperlipidemia or type 2 DM, it is increasingly found that clustering of various cardiovascular risk factors can occur in overweight or obese children, just as in adults. In recent years, more and more studies have documented an increasing prevalence of MS in overweight/obese children and adolescents. Modifications of the National Cholesterol Education Program, Adult Treatment Panel III (NCEP, ATP III) have been used to define MS in children (Cook et al. 2003; de Ferranti et al. 2004). However, in Asian adolescents, the use of this definition has been less reliable in the identification of MS (Vikram et al. 2006). Identification of MS improved with the inclusion of BMI and fasting hyperinsulinemia (Vikram et al. 2006). In Indian children, increased thickness of subcutaneous fat might have significant correlation with insulin resistance (Misra et al. 2004).

In a cohort of obese adolescents in PRC, Li et al. (2005) noted that all obese adolescents had at least one cardiovascular risk factor. Of the obese adolescents, 83.3% of obese boys and all obese girls had MS, while only 15.5% normal weight boys and 18.8% normal weight girls had MS. In a health survey of PRC children aged 7–17 years (both obese and normal weight), overall prevalence of MS was 3.3%, with more than 50% of the children having at least one metabolic abnormality and 19.8% having at least two (Li et al. 2008).

In Taipei, although there was no clear definition of MS, 25% of obese boys between 12 and 16 years of age were found to have clustering of two or more cardiovascular risk factors other than obesity, and clustering of cardiovascular risk factors was also significantly higher in obese girls in contrast to non-obese girls (Chu et al. 1998). Ryu et al. (2007) studied Korean adolescents between 12 and 13 years old and noted that 22.3% of overweight adolescents versus 1.6% of normal weight adolescents had MS. Overweight status was an independent factor associated with MS with an odds ratio of 17.7.

In a cohort of 201 obese children in Singapore, 24.4% was found to have MS. Those children with MS were found to be more obese and with more severe insulin resistance (Lee et al. 2008).

Non-alcoholic Fatty Liver Disease (NAFLD)

NAFLD is a liver disease that is defined by both clinical and histopathological features (Brunt 2001). It is often associated with insulin resistance and obesity.

NAFLD is increasingly seen in adults in the recent years in concurrence with a rising prevalence of obesity. Prevalence of NAFLD in adults can vary from 5 to 29% (Ford et al. 2002). Similarly, NAFLD, which was previously considered rare in children, has also recently been detected in children. Among various studies of NAFLD in children, affected children of Hispanic and Asian ethnicity seem to be predisposed to more severe disease (Roberts 2002). However, studies of NAFLD in Asian children are still rather scarce. The study of de Silva et al. (2006) revealed that in obese Sri Lankan children almost 18% had non-alcoholic steatohepatitis (NASH). In Singapore, 26.4% of obese children were found to have elevated liver transaminases (Lee et al. 2008). Those children who had type 2 DM and impaired glucose tolerance were at increased risk of raised liver transaminases (Lee et al. 2008).

Summary

In summary, studies in Asian and South East Asian countries show concurring observations as in other parts of the world that various comorbidities associated with obesity can develop early in obese children. For instance, elevation of blood pressure, hyperlipidemia, insulin resistance, type 2 diabetes mellitus can occur singly or in clusters as in metabolic syndrome. Increased infiltration of fat in the liver causing non-alcoholic fatty liver disease has also been detected in obese children and this may have adverse consequences on liver function in the long term.

Conclusions

Overweight and obesity in children and adolescents in several Asian countries is noted to be increasing although the prevalence is generally not as high as that in the West. The diversity of socio-economic, demographic, geographic and ethnic patterns in Asia and South East Asia can contribute to the differences in prevalence rates of childhood overweight and obesity. Rapid changes in lifestyle, urbanization and socio-economic growth in various Asian and South East Asian countries can have a role to play in the rapid increase in prevalence of overweight and obesity in children. Diet and physical activity patterns have a tendency towards unhealthy trends of high fat and sugar intake and low physical activity with poor cardiovascular fitness levels in children and youths. In conjunction with the increase in prevalence of overweight and obesity in children in Asia and South East Asia, there is evidence of increasing comorbidities like elevation of blood pressure, hyperlipidemia, insulin resistance and type 2 diabetes mellitus and clustering of cardiovascular risk factors (metabolic syndrome).

The rising prevalence of childhood obesity in Asia and South East Asia, the associated development of chronic diseases and the impact on costs of healthcare deserve careful study and analysis so that prevention and management of overweight and obesity can be timely and effective. Organized research in these areas can address the current lack of data for proper analysis and interpretation. There is a need to derive a uniform definition of overweight and obesity in children so that comparison of data across different countries and groups can be possible. Insight into the ethnic or racial contribution towards the susceptibility to develop chronic diseases related to obesity can help in the development of specific and effective measures of prevention and management. Above all, there is a need to overcome cultural and ethnic misconceptions that obesity is harmless or even desirable.

References

Alberti, G., Zimmet, P., Shaw, J., Bloomgarden, Z., Kaufman, F., & Silink, M. (2004). Type 2 diabetes in the young: the evolving epidemic; the international diabetes federation consensus workshop. *Diabetes Care, 27*, 1798–1811.

Bell, A.C., Ge, K., & Popkin, B.M. (2002). The road to obesity or the path to prevention: motorized transportation and obesity in China. *Obesity Research, 10*, 277–283.

Berenson, G.S., Srinivasan, S.R., Bao, W., Newman, W.P. 3rd, Tracey, R.E., & Wattigney, W.A. (1998). Association between multiple cardiovascular risk factors and atherosclerosis in children and young adults. The Bogalusa Heart Study. *The New England Journal of Medicine, 338*, 1650–1656.

Brunt, E.M. (2001). Nonalcoholic steatohepatitis: definition and pathology. *Seminar in Liver Disease, 21*, 3–16.

Central Intelligence Agency. The World Factbook (2008). Washington DC (February 10, 2009); https://www.cia.gov/library/publications/the-world-factbook/geos/tw.html.

Chang, L.Y., Li, H.Y., Wei, J.N., & Chuang, L.M. (2006). Type 2 diabetes and obesity in children and adolescents: experience from studies in Taiwanese population. *Current Diabetes Reviews, 2*, 185–193.

Chen, W. (1997). Childhood obesity in Taiwan. *Zhonghua Min Guo Xiao Er Ke Yi Xue Za Zhi, 38*, 438–442.

Chen, L.J., Fox, K.R., Haase, A., & Wang, J.M. (2006). Obesity, fitness and health in Taiwanese children and adolescents. *European Journal of Clinical Nutrition, 60*, 1367–1375.

Chu, N.F. (2005). Prevalence of obesity in Taiwan. *Obesity Reviews, 6*, 271–274.

Chu, F.N., & Pan, W.H. (2007). Prevalence of obesity and its comorbidities among schoolchildren in Taiwan. *Asia Pacific Journal of Clinical Nutrition, 16(Suppl 2)*, 601–607.

Chu, N.F., Rimm, E.B., Wang, D.J., Liou, H.S., & Shieh, S.M. (1998). Clustering of cardiovascular disease risk factors among obese schoolchildren: the Taipei Children Heart Study. *American Journal Clinical Nutrition, 67*, 1141–1146.

Chuang, C.H., Chang, P.J., Hsieh, W.S., Guo, Y.L., Lin, S.H., Lin, S.J., & Chen, P.C. (2007). The combined effect of employment status and transcultural marriage on breast feeding: a population-based survey in Taiwan. *Paediatric and Perinatal Epidemiology, 21*, 319–329.

Cockram, C. (2000). The epidemiology of diabetes mellitus in the Asia-Pacific region. *Hong Kong Medical Journal, 6*, 43–52.

Colditz, G.A. (1999). Economic costs of obesity and inactivity. *Medicine and Science in Sports and Exercise, 31(11 Suppl)*, S663–S667.

Cole, T.J., Bellizzi, M.C., Flegal, K.M., & Dietz, W.H. (2000). Establishing a standard definition for child overweight and obesity worldwide: international survey. *British Medical Journal, 320*, 1240–1243.

Cook, S., Weitzman, M., Auinger, P., Nguyen, M., & Dietz, W.H. (2003). Prevalence of a metabolic syndrome phenotype in adolescents: findings from the third National Health and Nutrition Examination Survey, 1988–1994. *Archives of Pediatrics & Adolescent Medicine, 157*, 821–827.

Daniels, S.R., Arnett, D.K., Eckel, R.H., Gidding, S.S., Hayman, L.L., Kumanyika, S., Robinson, T.N., Scott, B.J., St Jeor, S., & Williams, C.L. (2005). Overweight in children and adolescents: pathophysiology, consequences, prevention, and treatment. *Circulation, 111*, 1999–2012.

de Ferranti, S.D., Gauvreau, K., Ludwig, D.S., Neufeld, E.J., Newburger, J.W., & Rifai, N. (2004). Prevalence of the metabolic syndrome in American adolescents: findings from the Third National Health and Nutrition Examination Survey. *Circulation, 110*, 2494–2497.

de Silva, K.S., Wickramasinghe, V.P., & Gooneratne, I.N. (2006). Metabolic consequences of childhood obesity – a preliminary report. *The Ceylon Medical Journal, 51*, 105–109.

Denney-Wilson, E., Hardy, L.L., Dobbins, T., Okely, A.D., & Baur, L.A. (2008). Body Mass Index, waist circumference, and chronic disease risk factors in Australian adolescents. *Archives of Pediatrics & Adolescent Medicine, 162*, 566–573.

Deurenberg, P., Yap, M., & van Staveren, W.A. (1998). Body mass index and percent body fat: a meta analysis among different ethnic groups. *International Journal of Obesity and Related Metabolic Disorders, 22*, 1164–1171.

Deurenberg-Yap, M., Schmidit, G., van Staveren, W.A., & Deurenberg, P. (2000). The paradox of low body mass index and high body fat percentage among Chinese, Malays and Indians in Singapore. *International Journal of Obesity and Related Metabolic Disorders, 24*, 1011–1017.

Deurenberg-Yap, M., Chew, S.K., Lin, V.F., Tan, B.Y., van Staveren, W.A., & Deurenberg, P. (2001). Relationships between indices of obesity and its co-morbidities in multi-ethnic Singapore. *International Journal of Obesity and Related Metabolic Disorders, 25*, 1554–1562.

Dieu, H.T., Dibley, M.J., Sibbritt, D., & Hanh, T.T. (2007). Prevalence of overweight and obesity in preschool children and associated socio-demographic factors in Ho Chi Minh City, Vietnam. *International Journal of Pediatric Obesity, 2*, 40–50.

Drewnowski, A., & Popkin, B.M. (1997). The nutrition transition: new trends in the global diet. *Nutrition Reviews, 55*, 31–43.

Duong, D.V., Binns, C.W., & Lee, A.H. (2004). Breast-feeding initiation and exclusive breast-feeding in rural Vietnam. *Public Health Nutrition, 7*, 795–799.

Duong, D.V., Lee, A.H., & Binns, C.W. (2005). Determinants of breast-feeding within the first 6 months post-partum in rural Vietnam. *Journal of Paediatrics and Child Health, 41*, 338–343.

Foo, L.L., Quek, S.J., Ng, S.A., Lim, M.T., & Deurenberg-Yap, M. (2005). Breastfeeding prevalence and practices among Singaporean Chinese, Malay and Indian mothers. *Health Promotion International, 20*, 229–237.

Ford, E.S., Giles, W.H., & Dietz, W.H. (2002). Prevalence of the metabolic syndrome among US adults: findings from the third National Health and Nutrition Examination Survey. *The Journal of the American Medical Association, 287*, 356–359.

Forman, M.R. (1984). Review of research on the factors associated with choice and duration of infant feeding in less-develop countries. *Pediatrics, 74*, 667–694.

Freedman, D.S., Dietz, W.H., Srinivasan, S.R., & Berenson, G.S. (1999a). The relation of overweight to cardiovascular risk factors among children and adolescents: the Bogalusa Heart Study. *Pediatrics, 103*, 1175–1182.

Freedman, D.S., Serdula, M.K., Srinivasan, S.R., & Berenson, G.S. (1999b). Relation of circumferences and skinfold thicknesses to lipid and insulin concentrations in children and adolescents: the Bogalusa Heart Study. *American Journal of Clinical Nutrition, 69*, 308–317.

Gill, T.P. (2005). Obesity in Asian populations. In P.G. Kopelman, I.D. Caterson & W.H. Dietz (Eds.), *Clinical obesity in adults and children* (pp. 431–442). Malden: Blackwell Publishing.

Gill, T. (2006). Epidemiology and health impact of obesity: an Asia Pacific perspective. *Asia Pacific Journal of Clinical Nutrition, 15(Suppl)*, 3–14.

Guillaume, M. (1999). Defining obesity in childhood: current practice. *American Journal of Clinical Nutrition, 70*, 126S–130S.

Gurrici, S., Hartriyanti, Y., Hautvast, J.G., & Deurenberg, P. (1998). Relationship between body fat and body mass index: differences between Indonesians and Dutch Caucasians. *European Journal of Clinical Nutrition, 52*, 779–783.

Hangchaovanich, Y., & Voramongkol, N. (2006). Breastfeeding promotion in Thailand. *Journal of the Medical Association of Thailand, 89(Suppl 4)*, S173–S177.

Hatano, Y., Hua, Z.D., Jiang, L.D., Fu, F.H., Zhi, C.J., & Wei, S.D. (1997). Comparative study of physical fitness of the youth in Asia and their attitude towards sports. *Journal of Physical Education and Recreation (Hong Kong), 3*, 4–11.

He, J., Klag, M.J., Whelton, P.K., Chen, J.Y., Qian, M.C., & He, G.Q. (1994). Body mass and blood pressure in a lean population in southwestern China. *American Journal of Epidemiology, 139*, 380–389.

Himes, J.H., & Dietz, W.H. (1994). Guidelines for overweight in adolescent preventive services: recommendations from an expert committee. The Expert Committee on Clinical Guidelines for Overweight in Adolescent Preventive Services. *American Journal of Clinical Nutrition, 59*, 307–316.

Ho, T.F. (1987). Childhood obesity in Singapore school children: Epidemiology, anthropometry and selected medical problems (MD Thesis, National University of Singapore, 1987).

Hong, T.K., Dibley, M.J., Sibbritt, D., Binh, P.N., Trang, N.H., & Hanh, T.T. (2007). Overweight and obesity are rapidly emerging among adolescents in Ho Chi Minh City, Vietnam, 2002–2004. *International Journal of Pediatric Obesity, 2*, 194–201.

Huang, Y.C., Wu, J.Y., & Yang, M.J. (2003). Weight-for-height reference and the prevalence of obesity for school children and adolescents in Taiwan and Fuchien Areas. *Journal of the Chinese Medical Association, 66*, 599–606.

International Association for the Study of Obesity IASO, International Obesity Task Force IOTF (2004). EU childhood obesity "out of control". IOTF Childhood Obesity Report May 2004. London: IASO International Obesity Task Force.

International Association for the Study of Obesity IASO, International Obesity Task Force IOTF (2008a). Global childhood overweight. London (October 2008); http://www.iotf.org/database/index.asp.

International Association for the Study of Obesity IASO, International Obesity Task Force IOTF (2008b). Global obesity prevalence in adults. London (December 2008); http://www.iotf.org/database/index.asp.

Ishikawa-Takata, K., Ohta, T., Moritaki, K., Gotou, T., & Inoue, S. (2002). Obesity, weight change and risks for hypertension, diabetes and hypercholesterolemia in Japanese men. *European Journal of Clinical Nutrition, 56*, 601–607.

Kearney, M.H., & Cronenwett, L. (1991). Breastfeeding and employment. *Journal of Obstetric, Gynecologic and Neonatal Nursing, 20*, 471–480.

Khor, G.L. (2003). Update on the prevalence of malnutrition among children in Asia. *Nepal Medical College Journal, 5*, 13–22.

Kim, H.M., Park, J., Kim, H.S., Kim, D.H., & Park, S.H. (2006). Obesity and cardiovascular risk factors in Korean children and adolescents aged 10–18 years from the Korean National Health and Nutrition Examination Survey, 1998 and 2001. *American Journal of Epidemiology, 164*, 787–793.

Ko, G.T., Chan, J.C., Cockram, C.S., & Woo, J. (1999). Prediction of hypertension, diabetes, dyslipidaemia or albuminuria using simple anthropometric indexes in Hong Kong Chinese. *International Journal of Obesity and Related Metabolic Disorders, 23*, 1136–1142.

Ko, G.T., Tang, J., Chan, J.C., Sung, R., Wu, M.M., Wai, H.P., & Chen, R. (2001). Lower BMI cut-off value to define obesity in Hong Kong Chinese: an analysis based on body fat assessment by bioelectrical impedance. *The British Journal of Nutrition, 85*, 239–242.

Labarere, J., Gelbert-Baudino, N., Ayral, A.S., Duc, C., Berchotteau, M., Bouchon, N., Schelstraete, C., Vittoz, J.P., Francois, P., & Pons, J.C. (2005). Efficacy of breastfeeding support provided by trained clinicians during an early, routine, preventive visit: a prospective, randomized, open trial of 226 mother-infant pairs. *Pediatrics, 115*, e139–e146.

Laisiriruangrai, P., Wiriyasirivaj, B., Phaloprakarn, C., & Manusirivithaya, S. (2008). Prevalence of exclusive breastfeeding at 3, 4 and 6 months in Bangkok Metropolitan Administration Medical College and Vajira Hospital. *Journal of the Medical Association of Thailand, 91*, 962–967.

Langendijk, G., Wellings, S., van Wyk, M., Thompson, S.J., McComb, J., & Chusilp, K. (2003). The prevalence of childhood obesity in primary school children in urban Khon Kaen, northeast Thailand. *Asia Pacific Journal of Clinical Nutrition, 12*, 66–72.

Lee, W.R. (2000). The changing demography of diabetes mellitus in Singapore. *Diabetes Research and Clinical Practice, 50(Suppl 2)*, S35–S39.

Lee, Z.S., Critchley, J.A., Ko, G.T., Anderson, P.J., Thomas, G.N., Young, R.P., Chan, T.Y., Cockram, C.S., Tomlinson, B., & Chan, J.C. (2002). Obesity and cardiovascular risk factors in Hong Kong Chinese. *Obesity Reviews, 3*, 173–182.

Lee, W.T., Lui, S.S., Chan, V., Wong, E., & Lau, J. (2006a). A population-based survey on infant feeding practice (0–2 years) in Hong Kong: breastfeeding rate and patterns among 3,161 infants below 6 months old. *Asia Pacific Journal of Clinical Nutrition, 15*, 377–387.

Lee, Y.S., Kek, B.L.K., Poh, L.K.S., Vaithinathan, R., Saw, S.M., & Loke, K.Y. (2006b). Characterisation of metabolic consequences in severely obese children. Paediatric endocrinology: looking into the future (pp. 92). Bangkok: Asia Pacific Paediatric Endocrine Society 2006 (4th Biennial scientific meeting Asia Pacific Paediatric Endocrine Society 2006, 1–4 Nov 2006, Cliff Resort Hotel, Pattaya, Thailand).

Lee, W.T., Wong, E., Lui, S.S., Chan, V., & Lau, J. (2007). Decision to breastfeed and early cessation of breastfeeding in infants below 6 months old – a population-based study of 3,204 infants in Hong Kong. *Asia Pacific Journal of Clinical Nutrition, 16*, 163–171.

Lee, Y.S., Kek, B.L.K., Poh, L.K.S., Saw, S.M., & Loke, K.Y. (2008). Association of raised liver transaminases with physical inactivity, increased waist-hip ratio and other metabolic morbidities in severely obese children. *Journal of Pediatric Gastroenterology and Nutrition, 47*, 172–178.

Leung, E.Y., Au, K.Y., Cheng, S.S., Kok, S.Y., Lui, H.K., & Wong, W.C. (2006). Practice of breastfeeding and factors that affect breastfeeding in Hong Kong. *Hong Kong Medical Journal, 12*, 432–436.

Li, Y., Kong, L., Hotta, M., Wongkhomthong, S.A., & Ushijima, H. (1999). Breast-feeding in Bangkok, Thailand: current status, maternal knowledge, attitude and social support. *Pediatrics International, 41*, 648–654.

Li, G., Chen, X., Jang, Y., Wang, J., Xing, X., Yang, W., & Hu, Y. (2002a). Obesity, coronary heart disease risk factors and diabetes in Chinese: an approach to the criteria of obesity in the Chinese population. *Obesity Reviews, 3*, 167–172.

Li, L., Thi Phuong Lan, D., Hoa, N.T., & Ushijima, H. (2002b). Prevalence of breast-feeding and its correlates in Ho Chi Minh City, Vietnam. *Pediatrics International, 44*, 47–54.

Li, Y.P., Yang, X.G., Zhai, F.Y., Piao, J.H., Zhao, W.H., Zhang, J., & Ma, G.S. (2005). Disease risks of childhood obesity in China. *Biomedical and Environmental Sciences, 18*, 401–410.

Li, Y., Yang, X., Zhai, F., Piao, J., Zhao, W., Zhang, J., & Ma, G. (2008). Childhood obesity and its health consequence in China. *Obesity Reviews, 9(Suppl 1)*, 82–86.

Likitmaskul, S., Kiattisathavee, P., Chaichanwatanakul, K., Punnakanta, L., Angsusingha, K., & Tuchinda, C. (2003). Increasing prevalence of type 2 diabetes mellitus in Thai children and adolescents associated with increasing prevalence of obesity. *Journal of Pediatric Endocrinology & Metabolism, 16*, 71–77.

Macfarlane, D.J., & Tomkinson, G.R. (2007). Evolution and variability in fitness test performance of Asian children and adolescents. *Medicine and Sport Science, 50*, 143–167.

Mahoney, L.T., Burns, T.L., & Stanford, W. (1996). Coronary risk factors in childhood and young adult life are associated with coronary artery calcification in young adults: the Muscatine Study. *Journal of the American College of Cardiology, 27*, 277–284.

Meshizuka, T., & Nakanishi, M. (1972). A report on the results of the ICSPFT performance test applied to the people in Asian countries. In U. Simri (Ed.), *Proceedings of the ACSPFT and the ICSPFT – 1972. Wingate Institute for Physical Education and Sport* (pp. 7–23). Israel.

Misra, A. (2003). Body composition and the metabolic syndrome in Asian Indians: a saga of multiple adversities. *The National Medical Journal of India, 16*, 3–7.

Misra, A., Vikram, N.K., Arya, S., Pandey, R.M., Dhingra, V., Chatterjee, A., Dwivedi, M., Sharma, R., Luthra, K., Guleria, R., & Talwar, K.K. (2004). High prevalence of insulin resistance in postpubertal Asian Indian children is associated with adverse truncal body fat patterning, abdominal adiposity and excess body fat. *International Journal of Obesity and Related Metabolic Disorders, 28*, 1217–1226.

Misra, A., Wasir, J.S., & Pandey, R.M. (2005). An evaluation of candidate definitions of the metabolic syndrome in adult Asian Indians. *Diabetes Care, 28*, 398–403.

Mohan, V., Shanthirani, S., Deepa, R., Premalatha, G., Sastry, N.G., & Saroja, R. (2001). Intra-urban differences in the prevalence of the metabolic syndrome in southern India – the Chennai Urban Population Study (CUPS No. 4). *Diabetic Medicine, 18*, 280–287.

Mohan, B., Kumar, N., Aslam, N., Rangbulla, A., Kumbkarni, S., Sood, N.K., & Wander, G.S. (2004). Prevalence of sustained hypertension and obesity in urban and rural school going children in Ludhiana. *Indian Heart Journal, 56*, 310–314.

Moon, O.R., Kim, N.S., Jang, S.M., Yoon, T.H., & Kim, S.O. (2002). The relationship between body mass index and the prevalence of obesity-related diseases based on the 1995 National Health Interview Survey in Korea. *Obesity Reviews, 3*, 191–196.

Mosberg, H.O. (1989). 40 year follow up of overweight children. *Lancet, ii*, 491–493.

Mo-suwan, L., Junjana, C., & Puetpaiboon, A. (1993). Increasing obesity in school children in a transitional society and the effect of the weight control program. *The Southeast Asian Journal of Tropical Medicine and Public Health, 24*, 590–594.

Mo-suwan, L., Tongkumchum, P., & Puetpaiboon, A. (2000). Determinants of overweight tracking from childhood to adolescence: a 5 y follow-up study of Hat Yai schoolchildren. *International Journal of Obesity and Related Metabolic Disorders, 24*, 1642–1647.

Must, A., Dallal, G.E., & Dietz, W.H. (1991). Reference data for obesity: 85th and 95th percentile of body mass index and triceps skinfold thickness. *American Journal of Clinical Nutrition, 53*, 839–846.

Must, A., Jacques, P.F., Dallal, G.E., Bajema, C.J., Dietz, W.H. (1992). Long term morbidity and mortality of overweight adolescents. A follow up of the Harvard Growth Study of 1922 to 1935. *The New England Journal of Medicine, 327*, 1350–1355.

Nieto, F.J., Szklo, M., & Comstock, G.W. (1992). Childhood weight and growth rate as predictors of adult mortality. *American Journal of Epidemiology, 136*, 201–213.

Noble, S. (2001). Maternal employment and the initiation of breastfeeding. *Acta Paediatrica, 90*, 923–928.

Pan, W.H, & Lee, M.S. (2007). The double malnutritional burden and regional disparities in Taiwan elementary school children: survey database and reference values. *Asia Pacific Journal of Clinical Nutrition, 16(Suppl 2)*, 478–506.

Panpanich, R., Vitsupakorn, K., & Brabin, B. (2003). Breastfeeding and its relation to child nutrition in rural Chiang Mai, Thailand. *Journal of the Medical Association of Thailand, 86,* 415–419.

Popkin, B.M., Paeratakul, S., Ge, K., & Zhai, F. (1995). Body weight patterns among the Chinese: results from the 1989 and 1991 China Health and Nutrition Surveys. *American Journal of Public Health, 85,* 690–694.

Raj, V.K., & Plichta, S.B. (1998). The role of social support in breastfeeding promotion: a literature review. *Journal of Human Lactation, 14,* 41–45.

Ramachandran, A., Snehalatha, C., Satyavani, K., Sivasankari, S., & Vijay, V. (2003). Metabolic syndrome in urban Asian Indian adults – a population study using modified ATP III criteria. *Diabetes Research and Clinical Practice, 60,* 199–204.

Reddy, K.S., Prabhakaran, D., Shah, P., & Shah, B. (2002). Differences in body mass index and waist: hip ratios in North Indian rural and urban populations. *Obesity Reviews, 3,* 197–202.

Roberts, E.A. (2002). Streatohepatitis in children. *Best Practice & Research Clinical Gastroenterology, 16,* 749–765.

Roglic, G., & King, H. (2000). Diabetes mellitus in Asia. *Hong Kong Medical Journal, 6,* 10–11.

Rössner, S. (2002). Obesity: the disease of the twenty-first century. *International Journal of Obesity and Related Metabolic Disorders, 26(Suppl 4),* S2-S4.

Ryan, A.S. (1997). The resurgence of breastfeeding in the United States. *Pediatrics, 99,* e12.

Ryu, S.Y., Kweon, S.S., Park, H.C., Shin, J.H., & Rhee, J.A. (2007). Obesity and the metabolic syndrome in Korean adolescents. *Journal of Korean Medical Science, 22,* 513–517.

Sakamoto, N., Wansorn, S., Tontisirin, K., & Marui, E. (2001). A social epidemiologic study of obesity among pre-school children in Thailand. *International Journal of Obesity and Related Metabolic Disorders, 25,* 389–394.

Scott, J.A., Landers, M.C.G., Hughes, R.M., & Binns, C.W. (2001a). Factors associated with breastfeeding at discharge and duration of breastfeeding. *Journal of Paediatrics and Child Health, 37,* 254–261.

Scott, J.A., Landers, M.C., Hughes, R.M., & Binns, C.W. (2001b). Psychosocial factors associated with the abandonment of breastfeeding prior to hospital discharge. *Journal of Human Lactation, 17,* 24–30.

Seidell, J.C. (1995). The impact of obesity on health status: some implications for health care costs. *International Journal of Obesity and Related Metabolic Disorders, 19(Suppl 6),* S13–S16.

Sicree, R., Shaw, J.E., & Zimmet, P.Z. (2003). The global burden of diabetes, In D. Gan (Ed.), *Diabetes atlas* (pp. 15–71). Brussels: International Diabetes Federation.

Sung, R.Y.T., Tong, P.C., Yu, C.W., Lau, P.W., Mok, G.T., Yam, M.C., Lam, P.K., & Chan, J.C. (2003). High prevalence of insulin resistance and metabolic syndrome in overweight/obese preadolescent Hong Kong Chinese children aged 9–12 Years. *Diabetes Care, 26,* 250–251.

Tang, H.K., Dibley, M.J., Sibbritt, D., & Tran, H.M. (2007). Gender and socio-economic differences in BMI of secondary high school students in Ho Chi Minh city. *Asia Pacific Journal of Clinical Nutrition 16,* 74–83.

Tee, E.S., Khor, S.C., Ooi, H.E., Young, S.I., Zakiyah, O., & Zulkafli, H. (2002). Regional study of nutritional status of urban primary schoolchildren. 3. Kuala Lumpur, Malaysia. *Food and Nutrition Bulletin, 23,* 41–47.

Treloar, C., Porteous, J., Hassan, F., Kasniyah, N., Lakshmanudu, M., Sama, M., Sja'bani, M., & Heller, R.C. (1999). The cross cultural context of obesity: an INCLEN multicentre collaborative study. *Health Place, 5,* 279–286.

Truong, S.A., Ngo, T.T., Knodel, J., Le, H., & Tran, T.T. (1995). Infant feeding practices in Viet Nam. *Asia-Pacific Population Journal, 10,* 3–22.

Tuan, N.T., Tuong, P.D., & Popkin, B.M. (2008). Body mass index (BMI) dynamics in Vietnam. *European Journal of Clinical Nutrition, 62,* 78–86.

United Nations Development Program (2008). Human Development Report 2007/2008. New York (18 December 2008); http://hdr.undp.org/en/statistics.

United Nations Statistics Division (2005). Demographic Yearbook 2005. New York: Department of Economic and Social Affairs, Statistical Office, United Nations.

Vikram, N.K., Misra, A., Pandey, R.M., Luthra, K., Wasir, J.S., & Dhingra, V. (2006). Heterogeneous phenotypes of insulin resistance and its implications for defining metabolic syndrome in Asian Indian adolescents. *Atherosclerosis, 186,* 193–199.

Visness, C.M., & Kennedy, K.I. (1997). Maternal employment and breastfeeding: findings from the 1988 National Maternal and Infant Health Survey. *American Journal of Public Health, 87,* 945–950.

Vivian, E.M. (2006). Type 2 diabetes in children and adolescents – the next epidemic? *Current Medical Research and Opinion, 22,* 297–306.

Vogel, A., Hutchison, B.L., & Mitchell, E.A. (1999). Factors associated with the duration of breastfeeding. *Acta Paediatrica, 88,* 1320–1326.

Wang, J., Thornton, J.C., Russell, M., Burastero, S., Heymsfield, S., & Pierson, R.N. Jr. (1994). Asians have lower body mass index (BMI) but higher percent body fat than do whites: comparisons of anthropometric measurements. *American Journal of Clinical Nutrition, 60,* 23–28.

Wei, J.N., Chuang, L.M., Lin, C.C., Chiang, C.C., Lin, R.S., & Sung, F.C. (2003). Childhood diabetes identified in mass urine screening program in Taiwan, 1993–1999. *Diabetes Research and Clinical Practice, 59,* 201–206.

WHO Expert Consultation (2004). Appropriate body mass index for Asian populations and its implications for policy and intervention strategies. *Lancet, 363*, 157–163.

WHO Fact Sheet EURO/13/05 (2005). The challenge of obesity in the WHO European Region. Geneva: World Health Organisation.

WHO Fact Sheet No. 311 (2006). Obesity and overweight (Sept 2006). Geneva: World Health Organisation.

WHO World Health Report (1998). Life in the 21st century: a vision for all (p. 132). Geneva: World Health Organisation.

World Health Organization (2001). The optimal duration of exclusive breastfeeding. Report of an Expert Consultation 28–30 March 2001. Geneva: WHO; http://www.who.int/nutrition/publications/infantfeeding/WHO_NHD_01.09/en/print.html.

World Health Organization (2007). WHO Statistical Information System. Geneva (February 6, 2009); http://www.who.int/whosis/en/index.html.

Yoon, K.H., Lee, J.H., Kim, J.W., Cho, J.H., Choi, Y.H., Ko, S.H., Zimmet, P., & Son, H.Y. (2006). Epidemic obesity and type 2 diabetes in Asia. *Lancet, 368*, 1681–1688.

Zalilah, M.S., Mirnalini, K., Khor, G.L., Merlin, A., Bahaman, A.S., & Norimah, K. (2006). Estimates and distribution of body mass index in a sample of Malaysian adolescents. *Medical Journal of Malaysia, 61*, 48–58.

Chapter 13
Childhood Obesity: Prevalence Worldwide - Synthesis Part I

Wolfgang Ahrens, Luis A. Moreno, and Iris Pigeot

Introduction

The first part of this book provides an overview of the worldwide prevalence of overweight and obesity and its key determinants in children and adolescents. However, such a comprehensive overview is hampered by several limitations. (1) While in some countries large scale systematic surveys were conducted that provide data that are nationally representative, in many countries of the world no or only small surveys were conducted. Most data refer to restricted study populations who were selected by varying sampling schemes which makes a judgment of their representativeness difficult. (2) Data were obtained during differing years such that time trends may in some cases mix up with geographic variations. (3) Comparability is further impaired by the restriction to certain age groups in some countries or by differing age categorizations. (4) The precise anthropometric methodologies may differ from country to country and from survey to survey since no commonly accepted standards exist for most measures (see Chapter 3). Although this may not be a major problem for weight and height that were obtained by measurements in the majority of the data presented in this book, there is still room for some degree of variation due to non-compliance with standard procedures or the use of non-calibrated instruments as described in Chapter 3. (5) Comparability across studies is severely impaired by the use of different reference systems used to define overweight and obesity during growth that take their age- and sex-dependency into account.

The comparison of determinants of overweight/obesity is even more difficult. Definitions of risk factors like socio-economic status (SES) are culturally dependant and the methods to assess these risk factors vary widely. This adds to the methodological variations in study design, sampling procedures and representativeness listed above. This heterogeneity makes it difficult to grasp similarities and differences of the main drivers of overweight/obesity in a cross-country comparison.

In this chapter we will compile the prevalence data on overweight/obesity reported by the authors in Part I of this book and we will complement them with data from the WHO Global Database on Child Growth and Malnutrition (WHO 2009) to provide a worldwide view of the obesity epidemic. We are aware of the double burden of over- and undernutrition that many developing countries are nowadays facing, but we have to leave this aspect aside in order not to detract from the focus of this book.

W. Ahrens (✉) and I. Pigeot
Bremen Institute for Prevention Research and Social Medicine (BIPS), University Bremen, Achterstrasse 30, 28359, Bremen, Germany
e-mail: ahrens@bips.uni-bremen.de

L.A. Moreno
GENUD (Growth, Exercise, Nutrition and Development) Research Group, E.U. Ciencias de la Salud, Universidad de Zaragoza, Zaragoza, Spain

L.A. Moreno et al. (eds.), *Epidemiology of Obesity in Children and Adolescents*, Springer Series on Epidemiology and Public Health 2, DOI 10.1007/978-1-4419-6039-9_13, © Springer Science+Business Media, LLC 2011

Methods

Database

The prevalence data compiled here are presented in more detail in Chapters 4 to 12. The resulting database was, as already mentioned in the introduction, quite heterogeneous. Apart from the problem that the considered age groups varied widely across countries data were not stratified by pre-school/ school children and adolescents in all countries. Moreover, prevalence data were not always stratified by overweight and obesity. Table 13.1 indicates in which country data were available for pre-school children, primary school children, adolescents and/or a combination of these groups and whether prevalence estimates for overweight and obesity were reported separately. The table also indicates which data were based on representative samples. In addition it gives an overview of the reference systems used in each country included in the above chapters. The various reference systems are defined in the next section and in Table 13.2. Despite the described limitations the obtained data provide a rough overview of the worldwide distribution of the overweight/obesity epidemic.

Comparability of Different Reference Systems

In Table 13.2 we give a descriptive overview of nine different reference systems that are commonly used to classify overweight/obesity in children and adolescents. The table provides details for most of the reference systems which are used throughout Chapters 4 to 12. Some data were based on internal standard reference systems (ISRS), some have applied the standard WHO criteria for adults (overweight body mass index (BMI) >25 kg/m^2; obesity BMI >30 kg/m^2; WHO 1995) and in some cases the classification criteria were unknown.

Several reference systems have been derived for the US, based on consecutive cross-sectional US representative health surveys NHES (National Health Examination Survey) and NHANES (National Health and Nutrition Examination Survey). The criteria published by Must et al. (1991) are based on the US NHANES I data collected between 1971 and 1974 and use the 85th and 95th percentiles to define overweight and obesity, respectively. The National Center for Health Statistics (NCHS) reference population, from 2 to 18 years of age, is based on data of NHES II and III and NHANES I conducted between 1960 and 1975. It provides smoothed age-specific percentiles for height, weight and other growth parameters (not including BMI) with upper cut-offs at the 90th and the 95th percentile of the distribution (Hamill et al. 1979). These data served as the basis for the NCHS/WHO international reference in the late 1970s (Waterlow et al. 1977). The adoption seemed to be justified by the growing evidence that the growth patterns of well-fed, healthy pre-school children from diverse ethnicities are quite similar (Habicht et al. 1974). The NCHS/WHO international reference that provided the cut-offs for the WHO Global Database on Child Growth and Malnutrition was replaced by the WHO Child Growth Standards in 2006 with substantial differences depending on age group, growth indicator, specific percentile or z-score curve, and the nutritional status of the index population (de Onis et al. 2006). However, WHO (2006) only provides references for children aged 0 to 5 years. Algorithms for converting prevalence estimates based on the NCHS reference into estimates based on the WHO Child Growth Standards have been published by Yang and de Onis (2008). Finally, the CDC growth charts for the United States (Kuczmarski et al. 2002) are based on the US surveys NHES II and III and NHANES I–III conducted between 1963 and 1994 and use the 85th and 95th percentiles of the sex-specific BMI growth curves as cut-offs for overweight and obesity, respectively.

Table 13.1 National representativeness, stratification by age and/or weight category and reference system used for prevalence data on overweight/obesity in countries covered in Chapters 4 to 12

Country/region	Age groups with reported prevalence estimates				Overweight/ obesity separately?	Reference system
	Preschoolers	School children	Adolescents	Age groups combined		
Europe						
Austria	6	10	15	–	No	K-H
Belgium 1	–	11	–	–	No	IOTF
Belgium 2	–	–	15	–	No	ISRS
Bulgaria	–	7–11	14–17	–	No	IOTF
Cyprus	2–5	10	15	–	No	IOTF
Czech Republic	–	7–11	14–17	–	No	IOTF
Denmark	–	11	–	–	No	IOTF
Estonia	–	9	15	–	No	IOTF
Finland	–	10	16	–	No	IOTF
France 1	3–5	6–12	–	–	No	IOTF
France 2	–	–	15	–	No	ISRS
Germany	3–6[b]	7–13[b]	14–17[b]	3–17[b]	No	K-H
Greece	1–5	10–12	12–14	–	No	IOTF
Hungary	5	10	15	–	No	IOTF
Iceland	–	9	–	–	No	IOTF
Ireland	4	8	15	–	No	IOTF
Italy	–	9	–	–	No	IOTF
Italy (north)	2–6	–	–	–	No	IOTF
Italy (south)	2–6	–	–	–	No	IOTF
Lithuania	4	7–13	14–18	–	No	IOTF
Malta	–	7–11	–	–	No	IOTF
Netherlands	4	10	15	–	No	IOTF
Norway	6	10	15	–	No	IOTF
Poland	–	7–9	16	–	No	IOTF
Portugal	–	8	13	–	No	IOTF
United Kingdom	4–5	10–11	15–17	–	No	IOTF
Slovakia 1	–	7–11	–	–	No	Not reported
Slovakia 2	–	–	15	–	No	ISRS
Spain	4–6	7–10	13–18	4–18	No	IOTF
Sweden	4	9	15	–	No	IOTF
Switzerland	–	6–12	–	–	No	IOTF
Turkey	6	9	12–13	–	No	IOTF
MENA						
Lebanon 1	–	6–8[b]	10–18[b]	–	Yes	IOTF
Lebanon 2	–	–	–	3–19[b]	Yes	ISRS
Israel 1	–	–	16–19[b]	–	Yes	WHO
Israel 2	–	7–8[b]	–	–	No	CDC
Israel 3	–	–	15[b]	–	Yes	ISRS
Bahrain	–	–	12–17[b]	–	–	IOTF
Iraq	–	7–13[b]	–	–	Yes	IOTF
Kuwait	–	–	10–14[b]	–	Yes	NCHS
Iran 1	–	–	14–20[b]	–	Yes	IOTF
Iran 2	–	–	14–21[b]	–	Yes	WHO
Iran 3	–	–	10–19[b]	–	Yes	Not reported
Iran 4	–	–	–	2–18[b]	Yes	Not reported
Iran 5	–	–	11–18[b]	–	Yes	CDC
Iran 6	–	–	11–16[b]	–	Yes	CDC

(continued)

Table 13.1 (continued)

Country/region	Age groups with reported prevalence estimates				Overweight/ obesity separately?	Reference system
	Preschoolers	School children	Adolescents	Age groups combined		
Qatar 1	–	–	12–17[b]	–	Yes	IOTF
Qatar 2	–	–	14–19[b]	–	Yes	Not reported
Saudi Arabia 1	–	–	–	6–18[b]	Yes	CDC
Saudi Arabia 2	–	–	–	1–18[b]	Yes	IOTF
Saudi Arabia 3	–	–	–	12–20[b]	Yes	CDC
Un. Arab Emirates	–	–	–	4–18[b]	Yes	CDC
Tunis	–	–	13–17[b]	–	–	CDC
Tunis 1	–	6–12[b]	–	–	–	Not reported
Tunis 2	–	6[b]	–	–	–	ISRS
Tunis 3	–	6–10[b]	–	–	–	Not reported
Morocco	3[b]	–	–	–	Yes	IOTF
Egypt	–	–	17[b]	–	Yes	CDC
North America						
Canada	2–5[b]	6–11[b]	12–19[b]	2–19[b]	Yes	CDC
Mexico	2–5[b]	6–11[b]	12–19[b]	2–19[b]	Yes	CDC
USA	2–5[b]	6–11[b]	12–19[b]	2–19[b]	Yes	CDC
South America						
Argentina 1	–	4–10	10–15	–	Yes	IOTF
Argentina 2	–	4–10	–	–	Yes	CDC
Bolivia 1	–	–	12–18[b]	–	Yes	IOTF
Bolivia 2	–	5–7[b]	–	–	Yes	WHO07
Brazil 1	–	–	10–19[b]	–	Yes	IOTF
Brazil 2	–	8–10[b]	–	–	Yes	Must
Chile 1	–	–	10–18	–	Yes	CDC
Chile 2	–	6–8	–	–	Yes	NCHS
Colombia	–	5–9[b]	–	–	Yes	NCHS
Ecuador	–	7–9[b]	12–18[b]	–	Yes	Must
Peru	–	6–10	10–15	–	Yes	Must
Uruguay	–	9[b]	12[b]	–	Yes	Must
Asia						
Russian Fed. 1	–	7–11	–	–	No	IOTF
Russian Fed. 2	–	–	10–18		No	Not reported
India						
Kolkata, West Bengal	–	–	–	7–16[b]	–	WHO
Ludhiana, Punjab 1	–	–	12	–	Yes	IOTF
Ludhiana, Punjab 2	–	–	–	NA	Yes	Not reported
Ludhiana, Punjab 3	–	–	–	9–15[b]	Yes	WHO
New Delhi 1	–	–	14–17[b]	–	No	ISRS
New Delhi 2	–	–	16–17[b]	–	Yes	IOTF
Kerala 1	–	–	10–15[b]	–	Yes	Not reported
Kerala 2	–	–	–	5–16[b]	–	Not reported
Mangalore City	2–5[b]	–	–	–	Yes	WHO07
Wardha City	–	–	10–17[b]	–	Yes	CDC
Bangalore City 1	–	–	–	6–16[b]	No	IOTF
Bangalore City 2	–	–	–	9–18[b]	Yes	CDC
Hyderabad	–	–	12–17[b]	–	Yes	IOTF
Jaipur	–	–	11–17[b]	–	Yes	Not reported
Tamilnadu	–	–	13–18[b]	–	Yes	IOTF

(continued)

Table 13.1 (continued)

Country/region	Age groups with reported prevalence estimates				Overweight/ obesity separately?	Reference system
	Preschoolers	School children	Adolescents	Age groups combined		
Japan	6[b]	10[b]	16[b]	–	Yes	IOTF
South Korea	–	–	10–18	–	–	CDC
Malaysia	–	7–10	–	–	–	WHO
Singapore	–	–	–	10 and 15	No	IOTF
Taiwan	–	–	–	6–18	No	IOTF
Thailand	–	–	–	5–15	No	ISRS
Vietnam	–	–	11–16	–	–	IOTF
China	0–6[b]	7–13[b]	13–17[b]	0–17	No	WGOZ
Pacific						
Australia 1	–	–	–	2–16[b]	Yes	IOTF
Australia 2	–	9–13	–	–	Yes	IOTF
New Zealand	2–4[b]	5–9[b]	10–14[b]	2–14[b]	Yes	IOTF
Fiji	–	–	13–16	–	Yes	IOTF
Tonga	–	–	13–16	–	Yes	IOTF

Ow Overweight; *Ob* Obesity; **K-H** Kromeyer-Hauschild for Germany, 90th and 97th percentiles; **IOTF** International Obesity Task Force for 6 countries (4 continents), 88th (female), 90th (male) and 99th percentiles; **ISRS** Internal Study Reference Standard; **NCHS** National Center for Health Statistics (NCHS) reference population; **WGOC** Working Group on Obesity in China (Ji and Working Group on Obesity in China) (WGOC) (2005) (<7 years: weight-for-height z-score (Ow: $2 \leq WHZ < 3$, Ob: WHZ ≥ 3); 7–18 years: 85th and 95th percentiles)
CDC: CDC growth charts for the United States 2000, 85th and 95th percentiles; **Must**: For the United States 1991, 85th and 95th percentiles; **WHO**: WHO criteria for adults (Ow: BMI >25 and Ob: BMI >30); **WHO07**: Child growths standards for 5–19 years
[a]Chapters 4 to 12 and the references therein
[b]Prevalence data considered as nationally representative

The Working Group on Obesity in China (WGOC) derived sex- and age-specific BMI cut-offs for 7–18 year old school children based on height and weight data collected in the 2000 Chinese National Survey on Students Constitution and Health (CNSSCH) with 216,620 subjects throughout China (Ji and Working Group on Obesity in China) (WGOC) (2005) using the 85th and 95th percentiles to define overweight and obesity, respectively. These BMI cut-offs were chosen to be lower than the US CDC 2000 Growth Charts in analogy to the Chinese cut-offs for adults (see Chapter 11). For Chinese children younger than 7 years old, the WGOC adopted the weight-for-height z-score (WHZ) of the WHO reference (WHO 2006) which defines overweight as $2 \leq WHZ < 3$ and obesity as WHZ ≥ 3.

The Kromeyer-Hauschild criteria are based on 17 pooled regional surveys in Germany between 1985 and 1999 and use the sex- and age-specific 90th and 97th percentiles as cut-offs (Kromeyer-Hauschild et al. 2001).

The criteria of the International Obesity Task Force (IOTF; Cole et al. 2000) use survey data from six countries in North and South America, Asia and Europe collected between 1963 and 1993. Percentile curves were drawn for each survey such that they passed through the BMI values of 25 and 30 kg/m^2 for adult overweight and obesity at age 18 years. The resulting curves were averaged to provide estimated age- and sex-specific cut-off points from 2 to 18 years.

Table 13.2 Overview of common reference systems used to classify overweight/obesity in various countries

Reference system	Geographic area	Study	Time period of data collection	Study size	Age	BMI category	Cut-off (percentile)
Must et al. (1991)	US	NHANES I	1971–1974	20,839 (all)	6–74 years	Overweight Obesity Obese men Obese women	≥85th ≥95th BMI=27.8 BMI=27.4
NCHS (Waterlow et al. 1977; Hamill et al. 1979)	US	NHES II (6–11 years) NHES III (12–17 years) NHANES I (1–17 years + subset 1–74 years)	1963–1965 1966–1970 1971–1974	Not reported	2–18	No age-specific BMI cut-offs[a]	
CDC 2000 (Kuczmarski et al. 2002)	US	NHES II NHES III NHANES I NHANES II NHANES III	1963–1965 1966–1970 1971–1974 1976–1980 1988–1994	3,632 boys; 3,487 girls 3,545 boys; 3,223 girls 3,533 boys; 3,532 girls 3,838 boys; 3,572 girls 2,207 boys; 2,302 girls Total: 16,755 boys; 16,116 girls	2–20 years	At risk of overweight Overweight	≥85th ≥95th
WHO Child Growth Standards (WHO 2006)	Brazil, Ghana, India, Norway, Oman, US	MGRS (Multicentre Growth Reference Study)	July 1997–December 2003	8,440 (all)	0–5 years	Overweight	≥85th ≥97th
WHO References 2007 (de Onis et al. 2007)		Reconstruction of the NCHS/WHO reference from 1977 (NHESII [6–11 years], NHESIII [12–17 years], NHANES I [0–74 years]), suppl. w/ data from the WHO Child Growth Standards	1997–2003 + since early 1960s (NHANES)	11,410 boys; 11,507 girls;	5–19 years	Obesity	

Reference	Country	Survey	Year	Sample	Age	Definition	
WGOC (Working Group on Obesity in China) (Ji 2005)	China	CNSSCH (Chinese National Survey on Students Constitution and Health)	2000	216,620 (all)	7–18 years	Overweight / Obesity	≥85th / ≥95th
Kromeyer-Hauschild (Kromeyer-Hauschild et al. 2001)	Germany	17 different regional studies	1985–1999	17,147 boys; 17,275 girls	0–18 years	Overweight / Obesity	≥90th / ≥97th
IOTF (Cole et al. 2000)	Brazil	2nd National anthropometric survey	1989	15,947 boys; 15,859 girls	Cut-offs from 2 to 18 years	Overweight	NA*
	Great Britain	Data pooled from five national growth surveys	1978–1993	16,491 boys; 5,731 girls		Obesity	NA*
	Hong Kong	National growth survey	1993	11,797 boys; 12,168 girls			
	Netherlands	Third Nationwide growth survey	1980	21,521 boys; 20,245 girls			
	Singapore	School health service survey	1993	17,356 boys; 16,616 girls			
	US	Data pooled from four national surveys 1963–1980		14,764 boys; 14,232 girls			
		Total: 97,876 boys, 94,851 girls					

a No BMI-for-age; only body weight by age, stature by age, weight by stature and head circumference for age growth charts. No definition for overweight and obesity (stature – body length [0–2 years], body height [>2 years])

* Estimated age- and sex-specific BMI values corresponding to 25 and 30 kg/m^2 at age 18

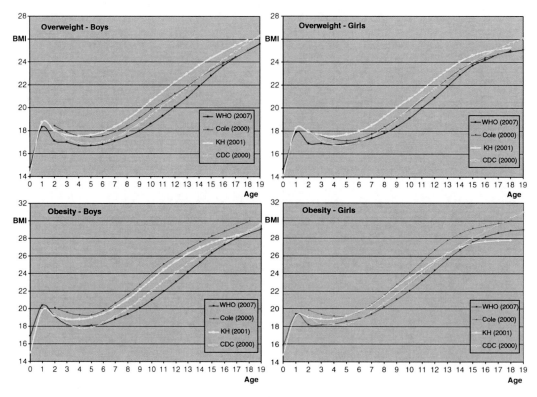

Fig. 13.1 BMI cut-offs by age and sex for common reference systems to classify overweight and obesity

The comparison of common reference systems used to classify overweight and obesity during growth is illustrated in Fig. 13.1. It shows that the WHO child growth charts use low cut-offs for the definition of both overweight and obesity in boys and girls. The IOTF criteria (Cole et al. 2000) which were most widely used in this book use relatively high cut-offs for obesity in boys and girls, leading to low prevalence estimates, while the same criteria lie in the middle for the definition of overweight for both sexes. The cut-offs based on the reference system by Kromeyer-Hauschild et al. (2001) are slightly below the IOTF cut-offs for obesity but they are the highest for overweight in both sexes. Thus the different reference systems used in various countries require a cautious interpretation of international comparisons.

Selection and Compilation of Data

Where available, preferably data generated by nationally representative surveys were selected by the authors, as e.g., for North America and Mexico, Australia and New Zealand, China, Japan and some European countries (for details see Table 13.1).

Data for South America included national surveys conducted since 2000. Data were extracted from governmental data available at the web, World Health Organization (WHO) and Pan American Health Organization (PAHO) databases and publications and databases from non-governmental organizations as well as published articles retrieved through MEDLINE, SciELO and LILACS.

For Europe and Russia, the data were compiled from published literature, personal communication with expert scientists, health agencies and existing databases. The literature search was done in MEDLINE and the ISI Web of Science and restricted to publications in English and French. Preferably, the most recent publications were selected, in particular cross-sectional and school-based studies with large and nationally representative samples with measured and not self-reported body weight and height using the IOFT cut-offs for BMI. For countries where the above criteria were not fulfilled, studies with self-reported data and with smaller sample sizes were accepted. These data were complemented by data from WHO and IOTF online databases for the prevalence of obesity.

A similar approach was used for the Mediterranean North African countries including the Middle East for which an electronic search of the literature from 1996 to 2008 was carried out in MEDLINE, PubMed, Google scholar and in the WHO databases.

The data for India were mainly obtained from surveys among various populations in India and were complemented by several small studies in specific areas published between 2002 and 2008.

Nationally representative data have been collected by the 2002 China National Health and Nutrition Survey. Additional data were obtained from recent nationwide, regional and local surveys.

In South-East Asia the situation was rather complex since many countries of this region do not conduct comprehensive national surveys regularly. Nevertheless, numerous sources provide data on the status of overweight and obesity in children and adolescents in several Asian countries.

For those countries for which data are not reported in the chapters of this book we obtained prevalence estimates from the WHO Global Database on Child Growth and Malnutrition wherever these were available. The WHO database is restricted to pre-school children. It compiles data on child growth and on the nutritional status of the world's children in a standardized way. It addresses the double burden of malnutrition and is designed to detect and monitor both undernutrition and overweight on a global basis. The data are obtained from population-based surveys that have to fulfill a given set of criteria to be included in this database. According to a standard procedure, all data are checked for validity and consistency and are re-analyzed to guarantee comparability of results. The WHO Child Growth Standards are used to obtain the z-score that describes the nutritional status of a given child. Upper and lower cut-offs of z-scores are defined for weight-for-age, height-for-age, weight-for-height and BMI-for-age. Prevalence values below and above these cut-offs are finally presented in the database. In 2003, the database included 412 national surveys from 138 countries and 434 sub-national surveys from 155 countries and covered 99 and 64% of the under 5 year olds in developing and developed countries, respectively. For more details on data sources, inclusion criteria and quality control (see de Onis and Blössner 2003).

Worldwide Prevalence of Overweight and Obesity

Geographic Distribution

The following maps summarize the data reported in Chapters 4 to 12 of this book, complemented by the WHO Global Database on Child Growth and Malnutrition for pre-school children. Colors from green to red illustrate increasing prevalence estimates and hatching indicates the reference system of the respective country. The categorization of prevalence estimates is chosen as to optimize the visual contrast between the countries. Therefore, the BMI categorization differs between maps showing prevalence estimates of obesity and those showing prevalence estimates of overweight and obesity combined. Some maps show prevalence estimates for preschoolers, school children and adolescents separately, where data were available. These categories do not always cover the same age groups as summarized in Table 13.1. The prevalence estimates for age groups combined (Figs. 13.2 and 13.3) were calculated as the arithmetic mean of the age-specific estimates if no pooled estimates were reported. If data were only reported for a single age group, as was the case for most African countries, these were taken in order to get an overall, though crude picture of the worldwide distribution.

Figure 13.2 demonstrates that the prevalence of both, obesity and overweight is highest in Western and industrialized countries, in the south of South America, in some MENA countries

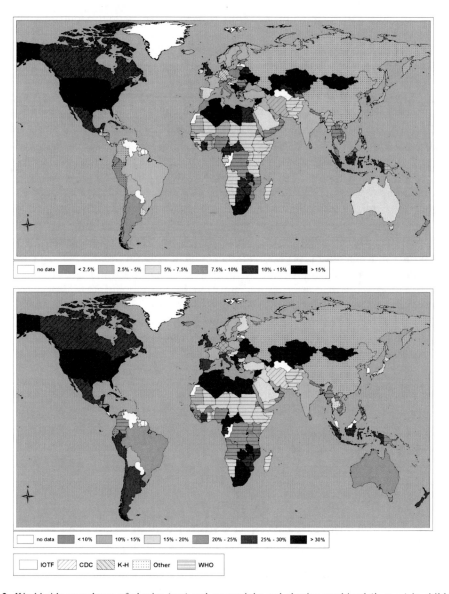

Fig. 13.2 Worldwide prevalence of obesity (*top*) and overweight and obesity combined (*bottom*) in children and adolescents

like Egypt, in south and central Africa, in central Asia, in Indonesia and in New Zealand. Within Europe (Fig. 13.3) the prevalence of overweight and obesity is highest in the south and east and in the UK.

The age-stratified maps (Fig. 13.4) reveal scarcity of data for school children and adolescents, especially for Africa. It is remarkable, though, that the prevalence of obesity and of overweight and obesity combined is already high among preschoolers. But this observation has to be put into

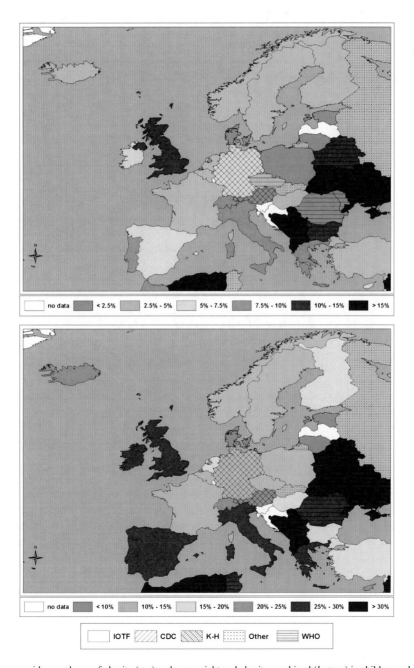

Fig. 13.3 Europe-wide prevalence of obesity (*top*) and overweight and obesity combined (*bottom*) in children and adolescents

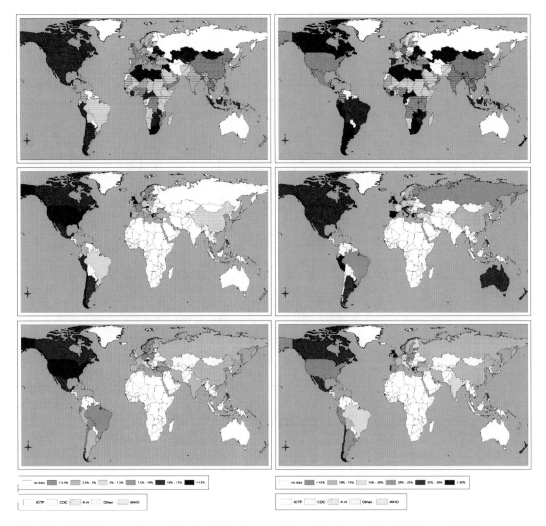

Fig. 13.4 Worldwide prevalence of obesity (*left*) and overweight and obesity combined (*right*) stratified by age-group, i.e., preschoolers (*top*), school children (*middle*) and adolescents (*bottom*)

perspective with regard to the reference system used. In preschoolers this was mostly the WHO child growth standards (WHO 2007) which uses lower cut-offs than most of the other systems, thus leading to higher prevalence estimates (cf. section on "Comparison of reference systems"). Figures 13.4–13.6 show that the prevalence of obesity and overweight increase by age in most countries where age-specific data are reported, particularly among boys. Generally, the prevalence of obesity and overweight tends to be higher in boys as compared to girls across all age categories (Fig. 13.6). Nevertheless, the overall ranking of high and low prevalence countries remains similar, regardless of which age-group is considered.

The interpretation of the maps is hampered by the fact that the time of data collection differed between the countries although all authors reported the most recent data available. Another limitation is the use of different reference systems to classify overweight and obese children which may distort ranking of countries.

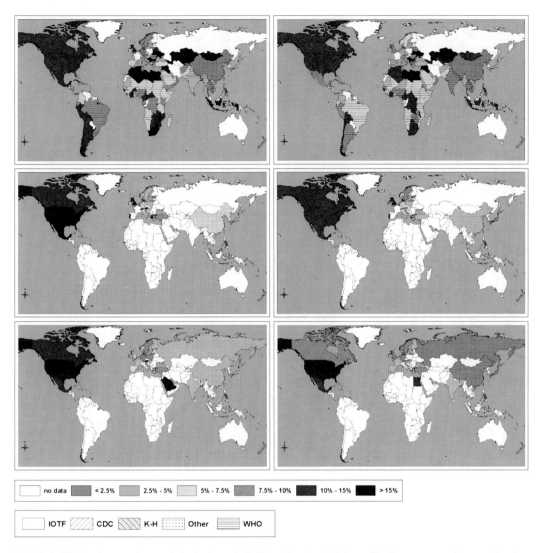

Fig. 13.5 Worldwide prevalence of obesity in male (*left*) and female (*right*) stratified by age-group, i.e., preschoolers (*top*), school children (*middle*) and adolescents (*bottom*)

Association with SES by Geographic Region

Part II of this book is devoted to the etiology of overweight and obesity and an overview of the most important risk factors will be given in the synthesis of Part II (see Chapter 26). Here we will only summarize the association of overweight and obesity with socio-economic status (SES) as one of its strongest determinants presented in the first part of this book. Figure 13.7 shows a negative association between SES and the prevalence of overweight and obesity in most industrialized countries like the US, Europe and Australia. In these countries a higher prevalence of overweight and obesity is observed in low SES groups. This is in contrast to South America, Asia and some North-African countries where a high SES is associated with a high prevalence of overweight and obesity.

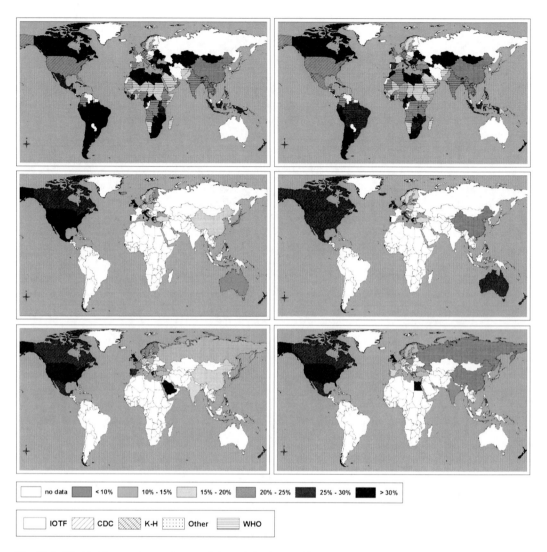

Fig. 13.6 Worldwide prevalence of overweight and obesity combined in male (*left*) and female (*right*) stratified by age-group, i.e., preschoolers (*top*), school children (*middle*) and adolescents (*bottom*)

It is important to note that SES is not measured the same way in the different countries. The assessment of SES is partly based on income, education, living in urban or rural areas or on a combination of various factors. Nevertheless, various indicators of SES are correlated and the direction of the association does not always change when the indicator is changed (e.g., Chapter 7). However, the choice of SES indicator has an influence on the strength and character of the association. Parental education most clearly shows an inverse relationship with children's obesity risk while the evidence for income or social class is less convincing (Shrewsbury and Wardle 2008; Chapter 21).

Consequently, in some countries, the association between prevalence of overweight and obesity and SES is not consistent because its direction differs by SES indicator or because it differs by region or ethnic group. Such countries and those where no association is apparent are summarized in the category "no association" in Fig. 13.7. It also becomes clear from Fig. 13.7 that information on the relationship between the prevalence of overweight and obesity and SES is missing in many countries.

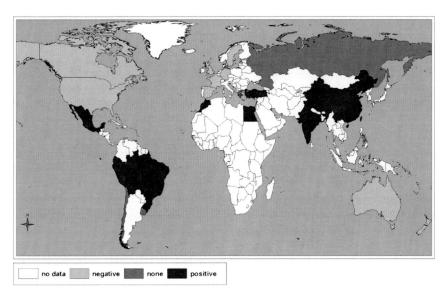

no data   negative   none   positive

Fig. 13.7 Worldwide association between socio-economic status and prevalence of overweight and obesity in children and adolescents

Conclusions and Outlook

Although it may be assumed that each of the studies investigating childhood obesity has been conducted according to the best quality standards available, the lack of a unified protocol to conduct such studies hampers the comparability of data between countries. Obvious limitations in that respect are the use of different reference systems, differing sampling schemes and different age groupings. More subtle limitations result from e.g., different measurement methods including self-reported weight and height.

Currently, the WHO Regional Office for Europe is establishing a standardized surveillance system, to fill the gap in comparable data on the nutritional status of primary school children across countries. Nationally representative samples of children aged 6–9 years are to be examined according to a common protocol. Children's body weight and height are to be measured by trained field-workers. Waist and hip circumference are included on a voluntary basis. The first data collection round was performed during the school year 2007/2008 in more than ten countries. It will be followed by further rounds at 2-year intervals (WHO 2010).

Nevertheless, some general trends emerge from the reported data: Although the prevalence values of overweight and obesity may differ in sub-populations and between countries – especially countries in the transitional phase report a heterogeneous picture – the entire distribution of BMI is shifted upwards in all countries. Moreover, in most countries the obesity epidemic is still growing perhaps with the exception of the United States, Australia and some European countries where the trend seems to have reached a plateau in recent years (Chapter 5; Olds et al. 2009; Stamatakis et al. 2009). In contrast some developing countries face the double burden of under- and overnutrition (Chapters 6, 8, 10–12).

Although a lot of research is going on in this field (see also Part II of this book) the growing obesity epidemic is not well understood. Further research is needed to explain and hopefully to reverse the global obesity burden. For this purpose, however, it would be more than desirable that national surveys are regularly conducted like NHANES in the US with a protocol that is standardized worldwide for measuring key health indicators and anthropometric parameters. Eventually, to make data comparable and to allow the assessments of time trends, the use of the same reference system to define cut-offs and the examination/reporting of the same age groups would be a major progress.

In Europe, studies like HELENA or the IDEFICS study, both funded within the 6th EU Framework Programme, tried to fulfill the above requirements. HELENA (Moreno et al. 2008a, b) focused on adolescents 12.5–17.5 years and investigated 3,000 adolescents in nine European countries following a standardized protocol. The IDEFICS study (Ahrens et al. 2006; Bammann et al. 2006) examined about 16,200 children in the age group from 2 to 10 years old in eight European countries also following a standardized protocol where the coordinators of both studies, Luis Moreno for HELENA and Wolfgang Ahrens for IDEFICS, exchanged the protocols and harmonized the measurement procedures as much as possible although the age groups of preschoolers, school children and adolescents all required special attention and thus tailored examination programs. Although the regions where data were collected in both studies may not in all cases be representative or typical for the whole country, both studies will yield valuable and comparable information on the distribution and on the etiology of overweight and obesity in children and adolescents.

References

Ahrens, W., Bammann, K., De Henauw, S., Halford, J., Palou, A., Pigeot, I., Siani, A., & Sjöström, M., on behalf of the European Consortium of the IDEFICS Project (2006). Understanding and preventing childhood obesity and related disorders – IDEFICS: a European multilevel epidemiological approach. *Nutrition, Metabolism and Cardiovascular Diseases, 16*, 302–308.

Bammann, K., Peplies, J., Sjöström, M., Lissner, L., De Henauw, S., Galli, C., Iacoviello, L., Krogh, V., Marild, S., Pigeot, I., Pitsiladis, Y., Pohlabeln, H., Reisch, L., Siani, A., & Ahrens, W., on behalf of the IDEFICS Consortium (2006). Assessment of diet, physical activity, biological, social and environmental factors in a multi-centre European project on diet- and lifestyle-related disorders in children (IDEFICS). *Journal of Public Health, 14*, 279–289.

Cole, T.J., Bellizzi, M.C., Flegal, K.M., & Dietz, W.H. (2000). Establishing a standard definition for child overweight and obesity worldwide: international survey. *British Medical Journal, 320(7244)*, 1240–1243.

de Onis, M., & Blössner, M. (2003). The World Health Organization Global Database on Child Growth and Malnutrition: methodology and applications. *International Journal of Epidemiology, 32(4)*, 518–526.

de Onis, M., Onyango, A.W., Borghi, E., Garza, C, & Yang, H., for the WHO Multicentre Growth Reference Study Group (2006). Comparison of the World Health Organization (WHO) Child Growth Standards and the National Center for Health Statistics/WHO international growth reference: implications for child health programmes. *Public Health Nutrition, 9*, 942–947.

de Onis, M., Onyango, A.W., Borghi, E., Siyam, A., Nishida, C., & Siekmann, J. (2007). Development of a WHO growth reference for school-aged children and adolescents. *Bulletin of the World Health Organization, 85*, 660–667.

Habicht, J.P., Martorell, R., Yarbrough, C., Malina, R.M., & Klein, R.E. (1974). Height and weight standards for preschool children; how relevant are ethnic differences in growth potential. *Lancet, 1*, 611–615.

Hamill, P.V., Drizd, T.A., Johnson, C.L., Reed, R.B., Roche, A.F., & Moore, W.M. (1979). Physical growth: National Center for Health Statistics percentiles. *American Journal of Clinical Nutrition, 32(3)*, 607–629.

Ji, C.Y., & Working Group on Obesity in China (WGOC) (2005). Report on childhood obesity in China (1): body mass index reference for screening overweight and obesity in Chinese school-age children. *Biomedical and Environmental Sciences, 18*, 390–400.

Kromeyer-Hauschild, K., Wabitsch, M., Kunze, D., Geller, F., Geiß, H.C., Hesse, V., von Hippel, A., Jaeger, U., Johnsen, D., Korte, W., Menner, K., Müller, G., Müller, J.M., Niemann-Pilatus, A., Remer, T., Schaefer, F., Wittchen, H.-U., Zabransky, S., Zellner, K., Ziegler, A., & Hebebrand, J. (2001). Perzentile für den Body-Mass-Index für das Kindes- und Jugendalter unter Heranziehung verschiedener deutscher Stichproben. *Monatsschrift für Kinderheilkunde, 149*, 807–818.

Kuczmarski, R.J., Ogden, C.L., Guo, S.S., Grummer-Strawn, L.M., Flegal, K.M., Mei, Z., Wei, R., Curtin, L.R., Roche, A.F., & Johnson, C.L. (2002). 2000 CDC Growth Charts for the United States: methods and development. *Vital and Health Statistics Series 11, 246*, 1–190.

Moreno, L.A., De Henauw, S., González-Gross, M.M., Kersting, M., Molnár, D., Gottrand, F., Barrios, L., Sjöström, M., Manios, Y., Gilbert, C.C., Leclercq, C., Widhalm, K., Kafatos, A., & Marcos, A., on behalf of the HELENA

Study Group (2008a). Design and implementation of the healthy lifestyle in Europe by nutrition in adolescence cross-sectional study. *International Journal of Obesity (London), 32 (Suppl 5)*, S4–S11.

Moreno, L.A., González-Gross, M., Kersting, M., Molnár, D., De Henauw, S., Beghin, L., Sjöström, M., Hagstromer, M., Manios, Y., Gilbert, C.C., Ortega, F.B., Dallongeville, J., Arcella, D., Wärnberg, J., Hallberg, M., Fredriksson, H., Maes, L., Widhalm, K., Kafatos, A.G., & Marcos, A., on behalf of the HELENA Study Group (2008b). Assessing, understanding and modifying nutritional status, eating habits and physical activity in European adolescents. The HELENA Study. *Public Health Nutrition, 11*, 288–299.

Must, A., Dallal, G.E., & Dietz, W.H. (1991). Reference data for obesity: 85th and 95th percentiles of body mass index (wt/ht2) and triceps skinfold thickness. *American Journal of Clinical Nutrition, 53(4)*, 839–846.

Olds, T.S., Tomkinson, G.R., Ferrar, K.E., & Maher, C.A. (2009). Trends in the prevalence of childhood overweight and obesity in Australia between 1985 and 2008. *International Journal of Obesity, 34*, 57–66.

Shrewsbury, V., & Wardle, J. (2008). Socioeconomic status and adiposity in childhood: a systematic review of cross-sectional studies 1990–2005. *Obesity, 16*, 275–284.

Stamatakis, E., Wardle, J., & Cole, T.J. (2009). Childhood obesity and overweight prevalence trends in England: evidence for growing socioeconomic disparities. *International Journal of Obesity, 34*, 41–47.

Waterlow, J.C., Buzina, R., Keller, W., Lane, J.M., Nichaman, M.Z., & Tanner, J.M. (1977). The presentation and use of height and weight data for comparing nutritional status of groups of children under the age of 10 years. *Bulletin of the World Health Organization, 55*, 489–498.

World Health Organization (WHO) (1995). *Physical status: the use and interpretation of anthropometry.* Report of a WHO Expert Committee. Technical Report Series No. 854. Geneva: World Health Organization.

World Health Organization (WHO) (2006). *WHO child growth standards: length/height-for-age, weight-for-age, weight-for-length, weight-for-height and body mass index-for-age: methods and development.* Geneva: WHO.

World Health Organization (WHO) (2009). *Global database on child growth and malnutrition.* Retrieved March 2009, http://www.who.int/nutgrowthdb/database/en/

World Health Organization (WHO) (2010). *WHO European Childhood Obesity Surveillance Initiative Protocol.* Copenhagen: WHO Regional Office for Europe.

Yang, H., & de Onis, M. (2008). Algorithms for converting estimates of child malnutrition based on the NCHS reference into estimates based on the WHO Child Growth Standards (World Health Organization) (National Center for Health Statistics) (Survey). *BMC Pediatrics, 8*, 19–25.

Part II
Etiological Factors

Chapter 14
Genetic Factors

Paola Russo, Fabio Lauria, and Alfonso Siani

Introduction

Obesity is a complex disease influenced by genetic and environmental factors and by their interaction. The most quoted theories attribute the current worldwide surge of obesity in both adults and children to the interaction between a genetic predisposition toward efficient energy storage, which is the legacy of the ancestral hunter-gatherer society, and a permissive (obesogenic) environment of readily available food and sedentary behaviors as it is the modern environment. This genetic predisposition, commonly described as "thrifty genotype" (Neel 1962), is nowadays maladaptive, increasing the individual predisposition to obesity and related metabolic disorders.

The "thrifty genotype" hypothesis postulates that certain genetic variants favored an efficient storage and utilization of energy stores during the frequent periods of starvation characterizing our ancestors' lives. While for this reason they underwent a positive selection, under the present condition of increased food availability and physical inactivity, these genetic variants confer a greater risk of metabolic derangement and finally body fat accumulation.

This theory, however, has been recently challenged with attractive arguments (Speakman 2006, 2007, 2008), but it still remains the most accepted, until alternative hypotheses will find confirmation. Moreover, in the last few years, the role of the complex interaction between genetic determinants and environmental factors in the rapid global increase of obesity has been further challenged by the entry of a new player, that is the epigenetic adaptation (Stoger 2008), fuelling the debate surrounding the etiology of obesity.

Obesity may be classified into three main categories on the basis of genetic etiology: monogenic, syndromic, and polygenic obesity (O'Rahilly and Farooqi 2006). This classification may be applied to both childhood and adult forms of human obesity, although monogenic and syndromic forms are most often evident very early in the life (Farooqi 2005a).

The study of the extreme human obesity phenotypes with Mendelian transmission pattern provided solid and consistent evidence in favor of the genetic origin of obesity and also offered clues for pharmacological treatment (Adan et al. 2006; Farooqi et al. 2002). The discussion of these severe and rare forms is beyond the objectives of this chapter, which is mainly devoted to the most relevant form of obesity in an epidemiological context, that is, polygenic obesity.

P. Russo, F. Lauria, and A. Siani (✉)
Unit of Epidemiology and Population Genetics, Institute of Food Sciences, CNR,
Via Roma 64-83100, Avellino, Italy
e-mail: asiani@isa.cnr.it

L.A. Moreno et al. (eds.), *Epidemiology of Obesity in Children and Adolescents*,
Springer Series on Epidemiology and Public Health 2, DOI 10.1007/978-1-4419-6039-9_14,
© Springer Science+Business Media, LLC 2011

Rather than providing a comprehensive overview of the current status of genetic research – which soon would be outdated – some questions and challenges of this new research field are brought into focus in this chapter.

It is important to note that the approach – both theoretical and methodological – to the study of the genetic basis of polygenic obesity is basically the same in the different stages of life. The situation becomes perhaps quite different when discussing the ethical issue in genetic research. Genetic testing of children and adolescents raises special concerns about the risks and benefits associated with this kind of research, particularly with regard to the informed consent, the use of genetic databases and the level of information to be delivered to both minors and parents. The benefits and consequences of genetic studies involving minors in relation to psychosocial risks have been exhaustively reviewed (Segal et al. 2004).

The purpose of this chapter is to review the evidence supporting the heritability of body weight, based on the results of classical genetic studies. The methodological problems and the different approaches to the study of polygenic obesity will be discussed, with focus on the results of recent genome-wide association (GWA) studies. The complex gene-environment interaction in the regulation of body weight and in the pathogenesis of obesity will be analyzed, taking into account the role of the epigenetic influences during pre-natal and peri-natal development.

Heritability of Body Weight

More than 100 years ago, Sir Francis Galton suggested for the first time the familial aggregation of the individual's growth (Galton 1889; Johnson et al. 1985). This initial observation – not specifically related to the issue of the heritability of body weight – was corroborated by studies in the first decades of the last century (Davemport 1923), showing a clear association between offspring and parental body weight. However, this observation could not dissect out the relative role of genetic and environmental factors in body weight determination, with parents and their progeny sharing the same environment. Thus, in the subsequent years, the work on the genetics of human obesity aimed to demonstrate that variation in obesity-related phenotypes could be attributable to varying degrees to the effect of genes, with the unambiguous result that obesity often tracks in families.

However, common forms of obesity are not transmitted in families according to a predictable pattern, like Mendelian diseases, but usually they follow complex patterns of segregation, involving the subtle influence of multiple genes (Comuzzie and Allison 1998).

The statistical definition of heritability *is the proportion of within-population phenotypic variance attributable to within-population genetic variance* (Falconer and Mackay 1996). Because heritability is a proportion, its numerical value will range from 0.0 (genes do not contribute at all to phenotypic differences between individuals) to 1.0 (genes are the only contributors to differences between individuals). The remaining variance of a phenotypic trait is attributable to the environmental effect (*environmentability*) that could be expressed as (1.0 – heritability). When discussing the relative influence of genes and environment on phenotypic variance, it should be clear that heritability and environmentability are abstract entities, particularly when complex traits, say, body weight, are to be explained. Heritability estimates indeed are unable to predict what specific genes contribute to a trait. Similarly, a numerical estimate of environmentability provides no information about the specific environmental factors that influence a trait. Heritability and environmentability are valid at the *population level*, thus not informative if considered on an individual basis. A heritability of 0.40 informs us that, on average, about 40% of the individual differences that we observe, e.g. in body weight, may in some way be attributable to genetic individual difference. It does not mean that 40% of any person's body weight is due to his/her genes and the other 60% is due to his/her environment. When considering the case of obesity, clearly heritability is not a fixed entity, as the proportion of the phenotype that can be explained by the genotype will depend on the exposure to obesogenic environmental factors that may profoundly vary in different individuals, families and populations as well.

Quantitative genetics analyses (studies of twins, siblings and families) provided strong evidence for the heritability of body weight (usually measured as body mass index, BMI). In particular, the classical twin studies, where monozygotic and dizygotic twin pairs were compared, yielded solid proofs in favor of the genetically determined aggregation of body weight. In different twin cohorts, the heritability coefficient derived by the intra-pair correlation for monozygotic twins was very high, ranging from 0.6 to 0.8 (Allison et al. 1996; Price and Gottesman 1991; Stunkard et al. 1990).

Data from controlled overfeeding studies in monozygotic twins showed that the tendency towards weight gain within each couple of twins was very similar, confirming the relevant role of genetic factors on body weight regulation, particularly evident when food intake and exercise are controlled to reduce the environmental variance (Bouchard and Tremblay 1990; Bouchard et al. 1990, 1996).

An alternative model to the twin study is the adoption study. This model allows to sort out the environmental influence inherent to the familial lifestyle. In fact, adoptive children share the environment with their adoptive parents while they share their genetic background only with their biological parents. The results of the adoption studies consistently showed that the adoptees present a highly statistically significant association of their BMI with that of their biological parents, but not with that of their adoptive parents (Chakraborty et al. 1986; Sorensen et al. 1989; Stunkard et al. 1986).

Methodological Approaches to the Study of Polygenic Obesity

The characterization of the relative role of gene–gene and gene–environment interaction in polygenic disorders such as obesity is extremely challenging. It seems conceivable that several gene products, each making a relatively small contribution, interact to build up the genetic component that, as described above, may explain a variable but significant proportion of the variance of obesity. The candidate-gene strategy has been the traditional approach for identifying the genes involved in complex diseases (Farooqi 2005b).

Candidate genes can be identified according to their biological function and/or by linkage studies, looking for significant differences in allele frequencies between carefully defined cases and controls. However, the identification of candidate genes represents a difficult task given the number of pathways involved and the subsequent huge number of potential candidate genes possibly involved. Genetic markers associated with obesity lie indeed on various biochemical and metabolic pathways, such as energy expenditure, appetite regulation, lipid metabolism, endothelial function, adrenergic activation, inflammation etc, raising the issue of multiple gene–gene, gene–nutrient and gene–nutrient- environment interactions in the pathogenesis of this complex disorder. In the case of rare monogenic diseases the molecular approach has proven extremely powerful in the identification of the genes responsible and in defining new syndromes (Farooqi 2007). Conversely, in common polygenic disorders like obesity most studies have claimed for genotype–phenotype associations without taking into account the fundamental influence of environmental factors (diet, sedentary lifestyle, socio-economic status, etc), so raising unwarranted enthusiasm, often followed by skepticism within the scientific community. Among the aspects hampering an integrated approach to the genetics of obesity are the limited study size and the inadequacy of available bio-computing tools. In fact, candidate gene studies are often statistically underpowered and give spurious results, unless they use large population samples (Colhoun et al. 2003), so raising the well-known need for replication studies (Redden and Allison 2003).

The issue of replication cannot be easily disregarded in this kind of study, because prior probabilities of true associations are low and, thus, all genetic associations demand a high level of proof (Hirschhorn and Altshuler 2002). In genetic association studies of complex diseases, it happens very often that the first report suggests a stronger genetic effect than is found by subsequent studies (Hirschhorn et al. 2002; Ioannidis et al. 2001). Important factors underlying inability to replicate previously reported associations are publication bias, failure to attribute results to chance and/or inadequate sample size and population stratification (Colhoun et al. 2003). While the first factors are quite obvious for epidemiologists, the latter deserves consideration, particularly when case–control models are adopted. In brief, population stratification may be defined as the presence of a systematic difference in allele frequencies between subgroups in the population of interest, possibly due to different ancestry. Population stratification is particularly relevant in case–control studies, because a systematic difference between cases and controls might be in fact due to differences in ancestry rather than to the association of a given gene variant with a given disease (Freedman et al. 2004). In this case, population stratification is a form of confounding where the gene under study shows marked variation in allele frequencies across subgroups of the population and where these subgroups also differ in their baseline risk of the disease. Not controlling for this factor may lead to false positive associations and has been advocated as a possible undermining cause of the lack of replication so often observed in genetic population studies. The strategies to overcome the possible bias related to population stratification in candidate gene association studies have been extensively reviewed (Thomas and Witte 2002; Wacholder et al. 2000). In summary, large studies, based on multicenter collections and done with standardized methods, may help to prevent replication failure (Colhoun et al. 2003).

Notwithstanding the above described difficulties and pitfalls, in recent years sizeable progress has been made toward the understanding of the genetic bases of polygenic obesity, although the different approaches used to define obesity add further complexity to this task. While most published studies regard the anthropometric characterization of the "obesity phenotype" – as measured by BMI, body circumferences and skinfold thicknesses –, there are other components of fat distribution and energy metabolism, such as body composition, resting metabolic rates, plasma levels of biomarkers (e.g. leptin, adiponectin etc) that were considered in the study of the genetic susceptibility of obesity. The level of complexity is witnessed by the continuous increase in the number of genetic markers possibly affecting the complex trait obesity.

From the first release of the Human Obesity Gene Map (Bouchard and Perusse 1996), the meritorious work of a group of researchers gave us the annual update of the state of art of the research on the genetics of obesity (Obesity Gene Map and http://obesitygene.pbrc.edu/, accessed on April 10, 2009). The last release (Rankinen et al. 2006) collated in 106 pages the scientific evidence available in this field up to October 2005. The impressive, though in some way discouraging, conclusion was that "The number of studies reporting associations between DNA sequence variation in specific genes and obesity phenotypes has also increased considerably, with 426 findings of positive associations with 127 candidate genes. A promising observation is that 22 genes are each supported by at least five positive studies. The obesity gene map shows putative loci on all chromosomes except Y." Unfortunately, in publishing the 12th update, the authors announced that it would be the last of the series, due to the lack of economical and human resources to collect and manage such enormous amount of information.

From that time on, thousands of researchers worldwide were challenged by the same question: among all the possibilities, what are the inherited genetic variants that really interact with environmental factors in shaping the susceptibility to common obesity? Different approaches were adopted to answer this question, including population-based or family-based genetic association studies, linkage disequilibrium mapping, haplotype tagging and the latest gene-finding strategy, that is the whole genome association scans. A discussion of the advantages/disadvantages of each of these techniques is beyond the objectives of this paper. Indeed, in spite of the difficulties, both the candidate single-nucleotide polymorphisms (SNPs) and the quantitative trait locus (QTL) strategies identified a large number of genetic markers potentially associated with the susceptibility to adult and childhood obesity on various chromosomes (Rankinen et al. 2006). However, many such associations failed to be replicated in subsequent studies, leading to calls to include documented replication of findings in reports of genetic association studies as a prerequisite for publication (Patterson and Cardon 2005; Todd 2006).

Many excellent papers, in which the various aspects of the genetic complexity underlying polygenic obesity have been reviewed, summarized progress and delusion on the way of the research of the genetic basis of obesity (Bell et al. 2005; Lyon and Hirschhorn 2005; Martínez-Hernandez et al. 2007; Mutch and Clément 2006; Walley et al. 2009). The scenario is rapidly changing. Large international collaborative studies allowed the researcher to access databases of well-defined phenotypes with related DNA and biological sample banks and more precise environmental information. For instance, the release of the haplotype map of the human genome by the HapMap Consortium (Altshuler et al. 2005) opened a new research avenue which in the future will improve the ability to deal with this complex disease. Combining "classical" genetic approaches with genomic, proteomic, metabolomic and eventually phenomic information will allow the integration of these different types of data.

Over the last few years, the immense progress in molecular biology tools, like microarrays and bioinformatics, has led to a dramatic increase in the identification of the genetic basis of complex, non-Mendelian diseases through the genome-wide association (GWA) approach. In short, high-throughput genotyping technologies were used to test hundreds of thousands of SNPs, each of them identified and assigned a unique reference number (rs) in the National Center for Biotechnology Information's dbSNP database (National Center for Biotechnology Information and National Library of Medicine. Database of Single Nucleotide Polymorphisms. http://www.ncbi.nlm.nih.gov/SNP/, accessed on April 10, 2009). The GWA approach represented a significant advance in gene-hunting strategies, because it is free from prior hypotheses regarding candidacy of genes, it permits to explore at the highest level of resolution the whole genome and it allows to associate hundreds of thousands of genetic variants with the phenotype (disease) of interest (Pearson and Manolio 2008). The GWA studies, driven by the completion of the Human Genome project (The International Human Genome Mapping Consortium 2001) and, more recently, by the International HapMap (Altshuler et al. 2005) updated in 2007 (The International HapMap Consortium 2007) and by the availability of the high-throughput technologies, are able, at least in part, to circumvent the obstacles encountered with both the candidate genes and the linkage approach.

Lessons from GWA Studies: The Case of *MC4R* and *FTO*

In the last years, an avalanche of results from GWA studies appeared in the scientific literature, linking common genetic variations to obesity and related metabolic traits. Apparently, these studies overcame the methodological problems that reduced the ability of earlier studies of candidate markers to detect true association with phenotypic traits. Here, we briefly comment on how the information gathered by these studies could help uncovering the genetic basis of obesity. Given that the list of obesity-associated loci is increasing day-by-day, we will focus on the role of two genes that recently emerged as being robustly associated to common obesity, that is the human melanocortin-4 receptor gene (*MC4R*) and the fat mass and obesity associated gene (*FTO*).

The Melanocortin-4 Receptor Gene (MC4R)

A large set of physiological and pharmacological studies strongly support the existence of a core neural network composed of hypothalamic "obesity neurons", controlling body weight through the regulation of central melanocortinergic systems. Along this pathway, the melanocortin (MC) family of receptors (*MC 1-5R*) has been implicated in the control of a wide variety of behavioral and physiological functions including the homeostatic control of food intake and body weight (Adan et al. 2006).

This hypothalamic regulation has been largely validated in rodent models. The first gene belonging to the MC family that was deleted in mice was *Mc4r*. Overall, disruption of *Mc4r* in mice results in an obese phenotype (Chen et al. 2000; Huszar et al. 1997), with intermediate degree of severity in heterozygotes. An indirect proof of the role of MC receptors in the control of appetite and body weight is that melanocortin agonists, including the non-selective peptide MTII, have been shown to decrease food intake and body weight (Adan et al. 2006). Following animal studies, inactivating mutations of the *MC4R* in humans have been identified. In particular, families with dominantly inherited heterozygous mutations in the MC4 receptor were first reported in 1998 (Vaisse et al. 1998; Yeo et al. 1998).

Since these first reports, several research groups identified multiple different mutations in *MC4R* in obese subjects from different ethnic groups (Dubern et al. 2001; Farooqi et al. 2000; Hinney et al. 1999; Kobayashi et al. 2002; Mergen et al. 2001; Vaisse et al. 2000).

Farooqi et al. (2003) made a systematic assessment of *MC4R* mutations in a series of 500 probands with severe childhood obesity. They found that the 5.8% of subjects with severe early onset obesity carried mutations in *MC4R*, with a common phenotype comparable to that reported in the *Mc4r* mutated mice. In particular, those subjects showed severe obesity, increased lean mass, increased linear growth, hyperphagia, severe hyperinsulinemia and increased bone mineral density and bone mineral content; homozygotes were more severely affected than heterozygotes. Interestingly, only 68% of heterozygotes were obese, thus suggesting that epigenetic and/or environmental factors could modify the penetrance of *MC4R* mutations in different pedigrees. The results of these studies indicated *MC4R*-linked obesity as the most frequent monogenic cause of early-onset severe obesity.

Very recent large-scale studies placed *MC4R* more firmly on the human obesity map. In 2008, two papers appeared in the same issue of Nature Genetics, reporting that common variants near the *MC4R* locus are associated with obesity-related phenotypes (Chambers et al. 2008; Loos et al. 2008). Loos et al. (2008) analyzed genome-wide association data from more than 67,000 adults and about 6,000 7–11 year old children of European descent. They found highly statistically significant associations of a signal (rs17782313) mapped 188 kb downstream of *MC4R* with BMI and obesity risk in these European population-based studies of both adults and children. Chambers et al. (2008) carried out a two-stage genome-wide association study (318,237 SNPs) for insulin resistance and related phenotypes, starting from 2,684 Indian Asians, with further testing in 11,955 individuals of Indian Asian or European ancestry. They found associations of rs12970134 near *MC4R* with waist circumference and, independently, with insulin resistance, measured as HOMA index, thus confirming the putative role of this genomic region in the susceptibility to obesity and related traits. These data are of uppermost interest since they provided a strong evidence of overlap in genetic factors associated with monogenic and polygenic forms of the same trait.

On the other end, although a strong biological plausibility links the results of the GWA studies on *MC4R* to that of the monogenic studies on severely obese individuals, a functional proof relating these newly discovered variants to altered expression of *MC4R* is still lacking. Moreover, it should be noted that in the study by Loos et al. (2008), the common rs17782313 variant near *MC4R* contributed only a minor fraction of the overall population variance of the traits examined (0.14% for adult BMI, and 0.26% for fat mass at age 9). Notwithstanding these limitations, the use of MC4R agonists as a promising pharmacological treatment of some forms of obesity is currently under development (Adan et al. 2006).

The Fat Mass and Obesity Associated Gene (FTO)

An even more impressive story is that of the fat mass and obesity associated gene (*FTO*). Almost simultaneously, three well-powered GWA studies published in 2007 identified a cluster of common SNPs in the first intron of *FTO* on chromosome 16 as unexpected but strong contributors to both childhood and adult obesity phenotypes (Dina et al. 2007; Frayling et al. 2007; Scuteri et al. 2007).

Human *FTO* is a gene of unknown function in an unknown pathway and presents high homology with the murine *Fto*, located on mouse chromosome 8 (Peters et al. 2002). It encodes for a member of the non-heme dioxygenase superfamily and it is ubiquitously expressed in fetal and adult tissues, particularly in the brain.

Interestingly, in the first published report by Frayling et al. (2007), the *FTO* locus was strongly associated with type 2 diabetes and secondarily with BMI in 1,924 U.K. type 2 diabetes patients and 2,938 U.K. population controls. The association with type 2 diabetes disappeared after adjustment for BMI, thus suggesting that BMI mediates the association with the risk of diabetes. In the same report, the association of the rs9939609 SNP of *FTO* with BMI was confirmed in 13 cohorts of adults and children with 38,759 participants of European origin. The 16% of adults who were homozygous for the risk allele weighed about 3 kilograms more and had 1.67-fold increased odds of obesity when compared with those not inheriting a risk allele. Effects of comparable magnitude were present in children. The association of a set of SNPs at this locus with BMI and obesity was unequivocally confirmed in the studies by Dina et al. (2007) in European adults and children and by Scuteri et al. (2007) in Sardinian adults, the latter study extending the analysis also to independent samples of European and Hispanic Americans. To date, several studies confirmed these initial observations, consistently linking SNPs at the *FTO* locus to other obesity-related phenotypes and markers, including body fat distribution, fat mass, and leptin levels (Loos and Bouchard 2008).

Of particular interest is the wide distribution of the risk-carrying *FTO* allele in European populations, with about 63% of the population being at least heterozygous and 16% homozygous for the risk allele. But data are not entirely consistent in some other ethnic groups, notably African American, Chinese and Japanese populations in which the *FTO* variants are not always associated with BMI or obesity phenotypes (Horikoshi et al. 2007; Li et al. 2008; Ohashi et al. 2007; Scuteri et al. 2007). In all these populations minor allele frequencies and linkage disequilibrium patterns are different form that reported for European populations. Despite the consistency of the association of *FTO* with BMI in people of European ancestry, the effect size is relatively small – as already observed for *MC4R* – explaining about 1% of the overall phenotypic variation of obesity observed in the general population (Bogardus 2009).

The relatively weak association of the *FTO* gene with metabolic factors and with obesity-associated conditions such as type 2 diabetes is in favor of a non-metabolic pathway of action of this gene. In February 2009, an elegant experimental study was published in Nature, providing clues towards possible mechanisms by which *FTO* acts on energy homeostasis and in turn on the regulation of body weight (Fischer et al. 2009). Fischer et al. (2009) generated an *Fto* knock-out mice strain and showed the absence of the *FTO* protein in the *Fto*$^{-/-}$ mutant. The loss of *Fto* was associated with post-natal growth retardation and significant reduction in both adipose tissue and lean body mass. The mechanisms advocated for these effects are increased energy expenditure and sympathetic activation. The results of this study provided the first translation of the human epidemiological data into functional evidence of the involvement of *Fto/FTO* in energy homeostasis and finally into body weight regulation.

In summary, the "agnostic" approach of the GWA studies opened a new research avenue to the study of the genetic roots of obesity and body weight regulation (Hofker and Wijmenga 2009). Nevertheless, the genetic variants of these "new" loci explain only a small fraction of the phenotypic variation observed in the general population. In fact, the combined effect of common variants in *FTO* and *MC4R* explains not more than 2% of the variance in BMI on the population level. It is conceivable that the remaining part of the BMI heritability may reside on a large number of very common genetic variants exerting small effects, each like the above described *FTO* and *MC4R*, and/ or on rare variants with large effects each (Bogardus 2009).

Gene–Environment Interaction and Obesity

Quantitative and molecular genetics studies clearly showed that a measurable proportion of body weight variance is attributable to genetic background. It should, however, be noted that the increasing prevalence of obesity and related disorders over the last half-century has been too rapid to be explained by large-scale changes in the genetic make-up of the population. Thus, there is no doubt that environmental factors play a fundamental role in the development of overweight and obesity (Papas et al. 2007). The unbalanced ratio between energy intake (diet) and energy expenditure (physical activity/sedentariness) results in a long term positive energy balance and finally in weight gain.

This positive energy balance is undoubtedly a major contributor to the current obesity epidemic in both developed and developing countries through the conditional effect of environmental factors on a receptive genetic background. Most descriptive studies showed that the increase in the average caloric intake, along with the decrease in physical activity is accompanied by rising rates of overweight and obesity (Astrup 1999; Rennie et al. 2006; Weinsier et al. 1998),.

Many researchers considered the worldwide increase in the prevalence of obesity a natural experiment exploring gene–environment interaction. A largely accepted hypothesis is that the genetic susceptibility to obesity is the result of an evolutionary process that favored the natural selection of a genetic background enabling energy storage through fat deposition in the body. This theory, commonly known as the "thrifty gene hypothesis", first proposed by Neel (1962), and supported by several authors (Chakravarthy and Booth 2004; Diamond 2003; Eaton et al. 1988; Prentice 2001, 2005a, b; Prentice et al. 2005; Ravussin 2002), provides a plausible explanation of the evolutionary impact of an environment characterized by repeated periods of food shortages. In fact, the selective advantage of the ability to cope with food shortages has become a disadvantage in the modern context, where food is abundantly available.

Further "experimental" proofs of this theory were provided by migration and urbanization studies showing a rapid increase in the prevalence of obesity and metabolic diseases in populations that migrated to affluent countries as compared to that observed in the countries of origin (Popkin and Udry 1998; Ravussin et al. 1994). A similar increase in the prevalence of these conditions is observed as a result of the so-called nutritional transition in developing countries (Amuna and Zotor 2008).

Consequently, the gene–environment interaction may be defined as the conditional effect of environmental exposure(s) acting through the individual genotype on the phenotype. A number of observational as well as intervention studies provided evidence on different aspects of this phenomenon (see Qi and Cho 2008 for review).

The validity of the "thrifty genotype" hypothesis has been recently questioned. In particular, John R. Speakman, in a series of intriguing papers (Speakman 2006, 2007, 2008), challenged the assumption that the ability to accumulate fat in periods of food abundance was evolutionary advantageous, suggesting rather that random mutations in obesity associated genes occurred over time. The author introduced the term *drifty genes* to indicate these mutant alleles whose propagation may casually increase the susceptibility to weight gain. It is well known indeed that the two most important mechanisms of evolution are natural selection and genetic drift. According to Speakman's theory, in the case of obesity a support in favor of the random drift selection, rather than the selective advantage, is that a large proportion of the population is not obese even in affluent societies.

The conceptual framework (albeit unproven) to support the thrifty genotype hypothesis has been disputed also on another basis. Some authors recently postulated that the rapid increase of the prevalence of obesity and diabetes mellitus in the last decades may not adequately be explained by the penetration of the thrifty genotype in the population. In particular, the epidemiological association between poor fetal and infant growth and excess body weight and metabolic derangement in adulthood suggests an important role of intra-uterine environment and early life nutrition in determining the metabolic fate later in the life (Dulloo 2006; Wells 2007). This concept is summarized under the definition of the "thrifty phenotype", that is the evolutionary adaptive consequence of the interaction between earlier reprogramming and exposure to the "toxic" environment of the affluent societies.

In 1989, Neel himself partially revised the "thrifty genotype" model in the light of the evidence suggesting that other players may intervene in shaping the interaction between non-genetic and genetic factors (Neel 1989). Among them, epigenetic factors are characterized by enough plasticity to enable a rapid adaptive response to changes in the environment, such as those underlying the current epidemic of obesity (James 2008).

Epigenetic Mechanisms in Obesity

In the previous sections, we documented that DNA sequence variants may influence an individual's susceptibility to obesity and related syndromes. Although gene hunters struggle to discover new obesity alleles, it is evident that the classical models to describe the gene–environment interaction do not provide satisfactory answers to the global obesity epidemic of the last five decades. In the past few years, epigenetics emerged as a complementary model to explain the rapid emergence of obesity and metabolic disorders (Stoger 2008). Epigenetics is defined as "the study of mitotically and/or meiotically heritable changes in gene function that cannot be explained by changes in DNA sequence" (Bird 2007; Russo et al. 1996).

These non-genetic alterations are under the tight regulation of two major epigenetic mechanisms acting at the transcriptional level: methylation of cytosine residues of DNA and modification of the histone proteins associated with DNA (chromatine remodeling). At the post-transcriptional level, a family of small, non-coding RNAs (MicroRNAs or siRNAs), completes the regulation of gene activity and expression during development or in response to environmental changes. Despite uncertainties about the mechanism(s) involved, epigenetic studies have opened new perspectives to the mechanistic explanation for the genome response under the influence of physiological and environmental factors. The scientific basis and the molecular mechanisms underlying epigenetics inheritance have been extensively reviewed (Jaenisch and Bird 2003).

While the knowledge of the role of epigenetic alterations in cancer is steeply increasing (Esteller 2008), epigenetic studies of obesity, type 2 diabetes and other related metabolic disorders are still in an early stage in humans (Gluckman and Hanson 2008; Junien and Nathanielsz 2007; Stoger 2008; Tremblay and Hamet 2008).

In particular, while there is no doubt that epigenetic modifications are heritable in somatic cells and have an important regulatory action in modifying gene expression in response to environmental stimuli, such as climate, famine, dietary changes etc, the possibility that they may remain stable and heritable from one generation to another is still not confirmed. However, a considerable evidence stems from animal models, showing that the environment can affect stable gene expression through methylation changes at different DNA level (Cavalli and Paro 1998; Morgan et al. 1999; Rakyan et al. 2003; Sutherland et al. 2000).

As a matter of fact, in certain parts of the genome, notably in the 5' region upstream of genes, there is an unusually high frequency of CpG dinucleotides, known as CpG islands in which the cytosines are unmethylated. About half of the human genes have CpG islands in their promoter regions and, for genes that are being transcribed, these islands are normally unmethylated. In association with chromatin modifications, promoter methylation prevents access by the transcription factors to specific DNA sequences and results in gene silencing. In effect, the epigenetic marks act as a switch alternatively silencing or inducing the expression of specific genes. Cell differentiation, X chromosome inactivation and genetic imprinting are all examples of epigenetic processes. Two studies (Wu et al. 1998, 1999) showed, in a rat model, that a maternal high-fat diet during intrauterine developmental stage may increase body-fat accumulation in the offspring, suggesting a role of maternal diet on the health of offspring through epigenetic inheritance mechanisms.

These and other observations suggest that some epigenetic modifications of the DNA sequence may persist in the next generations, thus influencing the epigenetic state of the genome and the activity of genes.

In summary, understanding the complex interplay between genetic susceptibility and epigenetic modulation will help not only to unravel the molecular causes underlying multifactorial diseases but also to provide a comprehensive explanation of the so called "gene–environment" interaction (Liu et al. 2008).

Conclusions

The phenotypic expression of polygenic obesity is mainly the result of a positive energy balance resulting from the changes in energy intake and energy expenditure in the modern environment. Nowadays, we are facing an obesity pandemic with devastating consequences on public health, due to the increased morbidity and mortality associated to obesity and its sequelae. The past decades of research yielded an immense progress in understanding of the genetic factors associated with body weight regulation in humans. In the post-genomic era, the advent of the GWA studies has changed the pace of gene discoveries in the field of complex diseases. The integration of different "omics" disciplines (transcriptomics, proteomics, metabolomics and nutrigenomics) will provide new tools to elucidate the molecular basis of obesity.

We should recognize that most of the recently identified obesity loci may not have a causal role, so that the prediction of the risk to develop obesity for individual patients is not straightforward. In addition, epigenetic studies suggested that the DNA sequence alone and its variation do not provide enough information to identify the molecular pathways modulating health and disease at the individual level. The interplay of several environmental factors such as nutrition, lifestyle, social influences, and fetal growth further limits the predictive value of genetic markers for complex diseases. Although the promise that genetic discoveries will have in the foreseeable future potential preventive and clinical application in obesity and related conditions remains a research endeavor, addressing current gaps in knowledge will ultimately lead to the identification of new mechanisms of disease and new options for treatments and prevention.

References

Adan, R.A.H., Tiesjema, B., Hillebrand, J.J.G., la Fleur, S.E., Kas, M.J.H., & de Krom, M. (2006). The MC4 receptor and control of appetite. *British Journal of Pharmacology, 149*, 815–827.

Allison, D.B., Kaprio, J., Korkeila, M., Koskenvuo, M., Neale, M.C., & Hayakawa, K. (1996). The heritability of body mass index among an international sample of monozygotic twins reared apart. *International Journal of Obesity and Related Metabolic Disorders, 20*, 501–506.

Altshuler, D., Brooks, L.D., Chakravarti, A., Collins, F.S., Daly, M.J., & Donnelly P. (2005). International HapMap Consortium. A haplotype map of the human genome. *Nature, 437*, 1299–1320.

Amuna, P., & Zotor, F.B. (2008). Epidemiological and nutrition transition in developing countries: impact on human health and development. *The Proceedings of the Nutrition Society, 67*, 82–90.

Astrup, A. (1999). Macronutrient balances and obesity: the role of diet and physical activity. *Public Health Nutrition, 2*, 341–347.

Bell, C.G., Walley, A.J., & Froguel, P. (2005). The genetics of human obesity. *Nature Reviews. Genetics, 6*, 221–234.

Bird, A. (2007). Perceptions of epigenetics. *Nature, 447*, 396–398.

Bogardus, C. (2009). Missing heritability and GWAS utility. *Obesity (Silver Spring, Md.)*, *17*, 209–210.

Bouchard, C., & Perusse, L. (1996). Current status of the human obesity gene map. *Obesity Research, 4*, 81–90.

Bouchard, C., & Tremblay, A. (1990). Genetic effects in human energy expenditure components. *International Journal of Obesity, 14*, 49–55.

Bouchard, C., Tremblay, A., Després, J.P., Nadeau, A., Lupien, P.J., Thériault, G., Dussault, J., Moorjani, S., Pinault, S., & Fournier, G. (1990). The response to long-term overfeeding in identical twins. *The New England Journal of Medicine, 322*, 1477–1482.

Bouchard, C., Tremblay, A., Després, J. P., Nadeau, A., Lupien, P.J., Moorjani, S., Theriault, G., & Kim, S.Y. (1996). Overfeeding in identical twins: 5-year postoverfeeding results. *Metabolism, 45*, 1042–1050.

Cavalli, G., & Paro, R. (1998). The Drosophila Fab-7 chromosomal element conveys epigenetic inheritance during mitosis and meiosis. *Cell, 93*, 505–518.

Chakraborty, R., Schull, W.J., & Schulsinger, F. (1986). An adoption study of human obesity. *The New England Journal of Medicine, 314*, 193–198.

Chakravarthy, M.V., & Booth, F.W. (2004). Eating, exercise, and "thrifty" genotypes:connecting the dots toward an evolutionary understanding of modern chronic diseases. *Journal of Applied Physiology, 96*, 3–10.

Chambers, J.C., Elliott, P., Zabaneh, D., Zhang, W., Li, Y., Froguel, P., Balding, D., Scott, J., & Kooner, J.S. (2008). Common genetic variation near MC4R is associated with waist circumference and insulin resistance. *Nature Genetics, 40*, 716–718.

Chen, A.S., Metzger, J.M., Trumbauer, M.E., Guan, X.M., Yu, H., Frazier, E.G., Marsh, D.J., Forrest, M.J., Gopal-Truter, S., Fisher, J., Camacho, R.E., Strack, A.M., Mellin, T.N., MacIntyre, D.E., Chen, H.Y., & Van der Ploeg, L.H. (2000). Role of the melanocortin-4 receptor in metabolic rate and food intake in mice. *Transgenic Research, 9*, 145–154.

Colhoun, H.M., McKeigue, P.M., & Davey Smith, G. (2003). Problems of reporting genetic associations with complex outcomes. *Lancet, 361*, 865–872.

Comuzzie, A.G., & Allison, D.B. (1998). The search for human obesity genes. *Science, 280*, 1374–1377.

Davemport, C.B. (1923). *Body built and its inheritance*. Washington DC: Carnegie Institution of Washington.

Diamond, J. (2003). The double puzzle of diabetes. *Nature*, *423*, 599–602.

Dina, C., Meyre, D., Gallina, S., Durand, E., Körner, A., Jacobson, P., Carlsson, L.M., Kiess, W., Vatin, V., Lecoeur, C., Delplanque, J., Vaillant, E., Pattou, F., Ruiz, J., Weill, J., Levy-Marchal, C., Horber, F., Potoczna, N., Hercberg, S., Le Stunff, C., Bougnères, P., Kovacs, P., Marre, M., Balkau, B., Cauchi, S., Chèvre, J.C., & Froguel, P. (2007). Variation in FTO contributes to childhood obesity and severe adult obesity. *Nature Genetics, 39*, 724–726.

Dubern, B., Clement, K., Pelloux, V., Froguel, P., Girardet, J.P., Guy-Grand, B., & Tounian, P. (2001). Mutational analysis of melanocortin-4 receptor, agouti-related protein, and α-melanocyte-stimulating hormone genes in severely obese children. *Journal of Pediatrics, 139*, 204–209.

Dulloo, A.G. (2006). Regulation of fat storage via suppressed thermogenesis: a thrifty phenotype that predisposes individuals with catch-up growth to insulin resistance and obesity. *Hormone Research, 65*, 90–97.

Eaton, S.B., Konner, M., Shostak, M. (1988). Stone agers in the fast lane: chronic degenerative diseases in evolutionary perspective. *American Journal of Medicine, 84*, 739–749.

Esteller, M. (2008). Epigenetics in cancer. *The New England Journal of Medicine, 358*, 1148–1159.

Falconer, D.S. & Mackay, T.F.C. (1996). *Introduction to quantitative genetics*. Fourth edition. Longman, Harlow, Essex, UK: Addison Wesley.

Farooqi, I.S. (2005a). Genetic and hereditary aspects of childhood obesity. *Best Practice & Research Clinical Endocrinology & Metabolism, 19*, 359–374.

Farooqi, I.S. (2005b). Candidate genes for obesity – how might they interact with environment and diet? *Advances in Experimental Medicine and Biology, 569*, 33–34.

Farooqi, I.S. (2007). Insights from the genetics of severe childhood obesity. *Hormone Research, 68*, 5–7.

Farooqi, I.S., Yeo, G.S., Keogh, J.M., Aminian, S., Jebb, S.A., Butler, G., Cheetham, T., & O'Rahilly, S. (2000). Dominant and recessive inheritance of morbid obesity associated with melanocortin 4 receptor deficiency. *The Journal of Clinical Investigation, 106*, 271–279.

Farooqi, I.S., Matarese, G., Lord, G.M., Keogh, J.M., Lawrence, E., Agwu, C., Sanna, V., Jebb, S.A., Perna, F., Fontana, S., Lechler, R.I., DePaoli, A.M., & O'Rahilly, S. (2002). Beneficial effects of leptin on obesity, T cell hyporesponsiveness, and neuroendocrine/metabolic dysfunction of human congenital leptin deficiency. *The Journal of Clinical Investigation, 110*, 1093–1103.

Farooqi, I.S., Keogh, J.M., Yeo, G.S., Lank, E.J., Cheetham, T., & O'Rahilly, S. (2003). Clinical spectrum of obesity and mutations in the melanocortin 4 receptor gene. *The New England Journal of Medicine, 348*, 1085–1095.

Fischer, J., Koch, L., Emmerling, C., Vierkotten, J., Peters, T., Brüning, J.C., & Rüther, U. (2009). Inactivation of the Fto gene protects from obesity. *Nature, 458*, 894–898.

Frayling, T.M., Timpson, N.J., Weedon, M.N., Zeggini, E., Freathy, R.M., Lindgren, C.M., Perry, J.R., Elliott, K.S., Lango, H., Rayner, N.W., Shields, B., Harries, L.W., Barrett, J.C., Ellard, S., Groves, C. J, Knight, B., Patch, A.M., Ness, A.R., Ebrahim, S., Lawlor, D.A., Ring, S.M., Ben-Shlomo, Y., Jarvelin, M.R., Sovio, U., Bennett, A.J.,

Melzer, D., Ferrucci, L., Loos, R.J., Barroso, I., Wareham, N.J., Karpe, F., Owen, K.R., Cardon, L.R., Walker, M., Hitman, G.A., Palmer, C.N., Doney, A.S., Morris, A.D., Smith, G.D., Hattersley, A.T., & McCarthy, M.I. (2007). A common variant in the FTO gene is associated with body mass index and predisposes to childhood and adult obesity. *Science, 316,* 889–894.

Freedman, M.L., Reich, D., Penney, K.L., McDonald, G.J., Mignault, A.A., Patterson, N., Gabriel, S.B., Topol, E.J., Smoller, J.W., Pato, C.N., Pato, M.T., Petryshen, T.L., Kolonel, LN., Lander, E.S., Sklar, P., Henderson, B., Hirschhorn, J.N., & Altshuler, D. (2004). Assessing the impact of population stratification on genetic association studies. *Nature Genetics, 36,* 388–393.

Galton, F. (1889). *Natural inheritance.* London: Macmillan.

Gluckman, P.D., & Hanson, M.A. (2008). Developmental and epigenetic pathways to obesity: an evolutionary-developmental perspective. *International Journal of Obesity (Lond), 32,* S62–S71.

Hinney, A., Schmidt, A., Nottebom, K., Heibult, O., Becker, I., Ziegler, A., Gerber, G., Sina, M., Gorg, T., Mayer, H., Siegfried, W., Fichter, M., Remschmidt, H., & Hebebrand, J. (1999). Several mutations in the melanocortin-4 receptor gene including a nonsense and a frameshift mutation associated with dominantly inherited obesity in humans. *The Journal of Clinical Endocrinology and Metabolism, 84,* 1483–1486.

Hirschhorn, J.N., & Altshuler, D. (2002). Once and again-issues surrounding replication in genetic association studies. *The Journal of Clinical Endocrinology and Metabolism, 87,* 4438–4441.

Hirschhorn, J.N., Lohmueller, K., Byrne, E., & Hirschhorn, K. (2002). A comprehensive review of genetic association studies. *Genetics in Medicine, 4,* 45–61.

Hofker, M., & Wijmenga, C. (2009). A supersized list of obesity genes. *Nature Genetics, 41,* 139–140.

Horikoshi, M., Hara, K., Ito, C., Shojima, N., Nagai, R., Ueki, K., Froguel, P., & Kadowaki, T. (2007). Variations in the HHEX gene are associated with increased risk of type 2 diabetes in the Japanese population. *Diabetologia, 50,* 2461–2466.

Huszar, D., Lynch, C.A., Fairchild-Huntress, V., Dunmore, J.H., Fang, Q., Berkemeier, L.R., Gu,W., Kesterson, R.A., Boston, B.A., Cone, R.D., Smith, F.J., Campfield, L.A., Burn, P., & Lee, F. (1997). Targeted disruption of the melanocortin-4 receptor results in obesity in mice. *Cell, 88,* 131–141.

Ioannidis, J.P., Ntzani, E.E., Trikalino, T.A., & Contopoulos- Ioannidis, D.G. (2001). Replication validity of genetic association studies. *Nature Genetics, 29,* 306–309.

Jaenisch, R., & Bird, A. (2003). Epigenetic regulation of gene expression: how the genome integrates intrinsic and environmental signals. *Nature Genetics, 33,* 245–254.

James, W.T.P. (2008). The epidemiology of obesity: the size of the problem. *Journal of Internal Medicine, 263,* 336–352.

Johnson, R.C., McClearn, G.E., Yuen, S., Nagoshi, C.T., Ahern, F.M., & Cole, R.E. (1985). Galton's data a century later. *The American Psychologist, 40,* 875–892.

Junien, C., & Nathanielsz, P. (2007). Report on the IASO Stock Conference 2006: early and lifelong environmental epigenomic programming of metabolic syndrome, obesity and type II diabetes. *Obesity Reviews, 8,* 487–502.

Kobayashi, H., Ogawa, Y., Shintani, M., Ebihara, K., Shimodahira, M., Iwakura, T., Hino, M., Ishihara, T., Ikekubo, K., Kurahachi, H., & Nakao, K. (2002). A novel homozygous missense mutation of melanocortin-4 receptor (MC4R) in a Japanese woman with severe obesity. *Diabetes, 51,* 243–246.

Li, H., Wu, Y., Loos, R.J., Hu, F.B., Liu, Y., Wang, J., Yu, Z., & Lin, X. (2008). Variants in the fatmass- and obesity-associated (FTO) gene are not associated with obesity in a Chinese Han population. *Diabetes, 57,* 264–268.

Liu, L., Li, Y., & Tollefsbol, T.O. (2008). Gene-environment interactions and epigenetic basis of human diseases. *Current Issues in Molecular Biology, 10,* 25–36.

Loos, R.J.F., & Bouchard C. (2008). *FTO*: the first gene contributing to common forms of human obesity. *Obesity Reviews, 9,* 246–250.

Loos, R.J., Lindgren, C.M., Li, S., Wheeler, E., Zhao, J.H., Prokopenko, I., Inouye, M., Freathy, R.M., Attwood, A.P., Beckmann, J.S., Berndt, S.I.; Prostate, Lung, Colorectal, and Ovarian (PLCO) Cancer Screening Trial, Jacobs, K.B., Chanock, S.J., Hayes, R.B., Bergmann, S., Bennett, A.J., Bingham, S.A., Bochud, M., Brown, M., Cauchi, S., Connell, J.M., Cooper, C., Smith, G.D., Day, I., Dina, C., De, S., Dermitzakis, E.T., Doney, A.S., Elliott, K.S., Elliott, P., Evans, D.M., Farooqi, I.S., Froguel, P., Ghori, J., Groves, C.J., Gwilliam, R., Hadley, D., Hall, A.S., Hattersley, A.T., Hebebrand, J., Heid, I.M.; KORA, Lamina, C., Gieger, C., Illig, T., Meitinger, T., Wichmann, H.E., Herrera, B., Hinney, A., Hunt, S.E., Jarvelin, M.R., Johnson, T., Jolley, J.D., Karpe, F., Keniry, A., Khaw, K.T., Luben, R.N., Mangino, M., Marchini, J., McArdle, W.L., McGinnis, R., Meyre, D., Munroe, P.B., Morris, A.D., Ness, A.R., Neville, M.J., Nica, A.C., Ong, K.K., O'Rahilly, S., Owen, K.R., Palmer, C.N., Papadakis, K., Potter, S., Pouta, A., Qi, L.; Nurses' Health Study, Randall, J.C., Rayner, N.W., Ring, S.M., Sandhu, M.S., Scherag, A., Sims, M.A., Song, .K, Soranzo, N., Speliotes, E.K.; Diabetes Genetics Initiative, Syddall, H.E., Teichmann, S.A., Timpson, N.J., Tobias, J.H., Uda, M.; SardiNIA Study, Vogel, C.I., Wallace, C., Waterworth, D.M., Weedon, M.N.; Wellcome Trust Case Control Consortium, Willer, C.J.; FUSION, Wraight, Yuan, X., Zeggini, E., Hirschhorn, J.N., Strachan, D.P., Ouwehand, W.H., Caulfield, M.J., Samani, N.J., Frayling, T.M., Vollenweider, P., Waeber, G., Mooser, V., Deloukas, P., McCarthy, M.I., Wareham, N.J., Barroso, I., Jacobs, K.B.,

Chanock, S.J., Hayes, R.B., Lamina, C., Gieger, C., Illig, T., Meitinger, T., Wichmann, H.E., Kraft, P., Hankinson, S. E., Hunter, D.J., Hu, F.B., Lyon, H.N., Voight, B.F., Ridderstrale, M., Groop, L., Scheet, P., Sanna, S., Abecasis, G.R., Albai, G., Nagaraja, R., Schlessinger, D., Jackson, A.U., Tuomilehto, J., Collins, F.S., Boehnke, M., & Mohlke, K.L. (2008). Common variants near MC4R are associated with fat mass, weight and risk of obesity. *Nature Genetics, 40,* 768–775.

Lyon, H.N., & Hirschhorn, J.N. (2005). Genetics of common forms of obesity: a brief overview. *The American Journal of Clinical Nutrition, 82,* 215S–217S.

Martínez-Hernandez, A., Enríquez, L., Moreno-Moreno, M.J., & Martí, A. (2007). Genetics of obesity. *Public Health Nutrition, 10,* 1138–1144.

Mergen, M., Mergen, H., Ozata, M., Oner, R., & Oner, C. (2001). A novel melanocortin 4 receptor (MC4R) gene mutation associated with morbid obesity. *The Journal of Clinical Endocrinology and Metabolism, 86,* 3448–3451.

Morgan, H.D., Sutherland, H.G., Martin, D.I., & Whitelaw, E. (1999). Epigenetic inheritance at the agouti locus in the mouse. *Nature Genetics, 23,* 314–318.

Mutch, D.M., & Clément, K. (2006). Unraveling the genetics of human obesity. *PLoS Genetics, 2,* 1956–1963.

National Center for Biotechnology Information, National Library of Medicine. Database of Single Nucleotide Polymorphisms. http://www.ncbi.nlm.nih.gov/SNP/, accessed on April 10, 2009.

Neel, J.V. (1962). Diabetes mellitus: a "thrifty" genotype rendered detrimental by "progress"? *American Journal of Human Genetics, 14,* 353–362.

Neel, J.V. (1989). Update to the study of natural selection in primitive and civilized human populations. *Human Biology, 61,* 811–823.

O'Rahilly, S., & Farooqi I.S. (2006). Genetics of obesity. *Philosophical Transactions of the Royal Society of London. Series B, Biological Sciences, 361,* 1095–1105.

Obesity Gene Map Database; http://obesitygene.pbrc.edu/, accessed on April 10, 2009.

Ohashi, J., Naka, I., Kimura, R., Natsuhara, K., Yamauchi, T., Furusawa, T., Nakazawa, M., Ataka, Y., Patarapotikul, J., Nuchnoi, P., Tokunaga, K., Ishida, T., Inaoka, T., Matsumura, Y., & Ohtsuka, R. (2007). FTO polymorphisms in oceanic populations. *Journal of Human Genetics, 52,* 1031–1035.

Papas, M.A., Alberg, A.J., Ewing, R., Helzlsouer, K.J., Gary, T.L., & Klassen, A.C. (2007). The built environment and obesity. *Epidemiologic Reviews, 29,* 129–143.

Patterson, M., & Cardon, L. (2005). Replication publication. *PLoS Biology, 3,* 1511.

Pearson, T.A., & Manolio, T.A. (2008). How to interpret a genome-wide association study. *Journal of the American Medical Association, 299,* 1335–1344.

Peters, T., Ausmeier, K., Dildrop, R., & Rüther, U. (2002). The mouse Fused toes (Ft) mutation is the result of a 1.6-Mb deletion including the entire Iroquois B gene cluster. *Mammalian Genome, 13,* 186–188.

Popkin, B.M., & Udry, J.R. (1998). Adolescent obesity increases significantly in second and third generation U.S. immigrants: the National Longitudinal Study of Adolescent Health. *The Journal of Nutrition, 128,* 701–706.

Prentice, A.M. (2001). Obesity and its potential mechanistic basis. *British Medical Bulletin, 60,* 51–67.

Prentice, A.M. (2005a). Starvation in humans: Evolutionary background and contemporary implications. *Mechanisms of Ageing and Development, 126,* 976–981.

Prentice, A.M. (2005b). Early influences on human energy regulation: Thrifty genotypes and thrifty phenotypes. *Physiology & Behavior, 86,* 640–645.

Prentice, A.M., Rayco-Solon, P., & Moore, S.E. (2005). Insights from the developing world: thrifty genotypes and thrifty phenotypes. *The Proceedings of the Nutrition Society, 64,* 153–161.

Price, R.A., & Gottesman, I.I. (1991). Body fat in identical twins reared apart: roles for genes and environment. *Behavior Genetics, 21,* 1–7.

Qi, L., & Cho, Y.A. (2008). Gene-environment interaction and obesity. *Nutrition Reviews, 66,* 684–694.

Rakyan, V.K., Chong, S., Champ, M.E., Cuthbert, P.C., Morgan, H.D., Luu, K.V., & Whitelaw, E. (2003). Transgenerational inheritance of epigenetic states at the murine Axin (Fu) allele occurs after maternal and paternal transmission. *Proceedings of the National Academy of Sciences of the United States of America, 100,* 2538–2543.

Rankinen, T., Zuberi, A., Chagnon, Y.C., Weisnagel, S.J., Argyropoulos, G., Walts, B., Pérusse, L., & Bouchard, C. (2006). The human obesity gene map: the 2005 update. *Obesity (Silver Spring), 14,* 529–644.

Ravussin, E. (2002). Cellular sensors of feast and famine. *Journal of Clinical Investigation, 109,* 1537–1540.

Ravussin, E., Valencia, M.E., Esparza, J., Bennett, P.H., & Schulz, L.O. (1994). Effects of a traditional lifestyle on obesity in Pima Indians. *Diabetes Care, 17,* 1067–1074.

Redden, D.T., & Allison D.B. (2003). Nonreplication in genetic association studies of obesity and diabetes research. *Journal of Nutrition, 133,* 3323–3326.

Rennie, K.L., Wells, J.C., McCaffrey, T.A., & Livingstone, M.B. (2006). The effect of physical activity on body fatness in children and adolescents. *The Proceedings of the Nutrition Society, 65,* 393–402.

Russo, V.E.A., Martienssen, R.A. & Riggs, A.D. (Eds) (1996). Epigenetic mechanisms of gene regulation. Woodbury: Cold Spring Harbor Laboratory Press.

Scuteri, A., Sanna, S., Chen, W.M., Uda, M., Albai, G., Strait, J., Najjar, S., Nagaraja, R., Orrú, M., Usala, G., Dei, M., Lai, S., Maschio, A., Busonero, F., Mulas, A., Ehret, G.B., Fink, A.A., Weder, A. B., Cooper, R.S., Galan, P., Chakravarti, A., Schlessinger, D., Cao, A., Lakatta, E., & Abecasis, G.R. (2007). Genome-wide association scan shows genetic variants in the FTO gene are associated with obesity-related traits. *PLoS Genetics, 3*, 1200–1210.

Segal, M.E., Sankar, P., & Reed D.R. (2004). Research issues in genetic testing of adolescents for obesity. *Nutrition Reviews, 62*, 307–320.

Sorensen, T.I., Price, R.A., Stunkard, A.J., & Schulsinger, F. (1989). Genetics of obesity in adult adoptees and their biological siblings. *British Medical Journal, 298*, 87–90.

Speakman, J.R. (2006). 'Thrifty genes' for obesity and the metabolic syndrome: time to call off the search? *Diabetes and Vascular Research, 3*, 7–11.

Speakman, J.R. (2007). A nonadaptive scenario explaining the genetic predisposition to obesity: the "predation release" hypothesis. *Cell Metabolism, 6*, 5–12.

Speakman, J.R. (2008). Thrifty genes for obesity, an attractive but flawed idea, and an alternative perspective: the 'drifty gene' hypothesis. *International Journal of Obesity (Lond), 32*, 1611–1617.

Stoger, R. (2008). Epigenetics and obesity. *Pharmacogenomics, 9*, 1851–1860.

Stunkard, A.J., Sorensen, T.I., Hanis, C., Teasdale, T.W., Chakraborty, R., Schull, W.J., & Schulsinger, F. (1986). An adoption study of human obesity. *The New England Journal of Medicine, 314*, 193–198.

Stunkard, A.J., Harris, J.R., Pedersen, N.L., & McClearn, G.E. (1990). The body-mass index of twins who have been reared apart. *The New England Journal of Medicine, 322*, 1483–1487.

Sutherland, H.G., Kearns, M., Morgan, H.D., Headley, A.P., Morris, C., Martin, D.I., & Whitelaw, E. (2000). Reactivation of heritably silenced gene expression in mice. *Mammalian Genome, 11*, 347–355.

The International HapMap Consortium (2007). A second generation human haplotype map of over 3.1 million SNPs. *Nature, 449*, 851–861.

The International Human Genome Mapping Consortium (2001). A physical map of the human genome. Nature, 409, 934–941.

Thomas, D.C., & Witte, J.S. (2002). Point: population stratification: a problem for case-control studies of candidate-gene associations? *Cancer Epidemiology, Biomarkers & Prevention, 11*, 505–512.

Todd, J.A. (2006). Statistical false positive or true disease pathway? *Nature Genetics, 38*, 731–733.

Tremblay, J., & Hamet, P. (2008). Impact of genetic and epigenetic factors from early life to later disease. *Metabolism, 57*, S27–31.

Vaisse, C., Clement, K., Guy-Grand, B., & Froguel, P. (1998). A frameshift mutation in human *MC4R* is associated with a dominant form of obesity. *Nature Genetics, 20*, 113–114.

Vaisse, C., Clement, K., Durand, E., Hercberg, S., Guy-Grand, B., & Froguel, P. (2000). Melanocortin-4 receptor mutations are a frequent and heterogeneous cause of morbid obesity. *Journal of Clinical Investigation, 106*, 253–262.

Wacholder, S., Rothman, N., & Caporaso, N. (2000). Population stratification in epidemiologic studies of common genetic variants and cancer: quantification of bias. *Journal of the National Cancer Institute, 92*, 1151–1158.

Walley, A.J., Asher, J.E., Froguel, P. (2009). The genetic contribution to non-syndromic human obesity. *Nature Review Genetics,10*, 431–442.

Weinsier, R.L., Hunter, G.R., Heini, A.F., Goran, M.I., & Sell, S.M. (1998). The etiology of obesity: relative contribution of metabolic factors, diet, and physical activity. *The American Journal of Medicine, 105*, 145–150.

Wells, J.C. (2007). The thrifty phenotype as an adaptive maternal effect. *Biological Reviews of the Cambridge Philosophical Society, 82*, 143–172.

Wu, Q., Mizushima, Y., Komiya, M., Matsuo, T., & Suzuki, M. (1998). Body fat accumulation in the male offspring of rats fed high-fat diet. *Journal of Clinical Biochemistry and Nutrition, 25*, 71–79.

Wu, Q., Mizushima, Y., Komiya, M., Matsuo, T., & Suzuki, M. (1999). The effects of high-fat diet feeding over generations on body fat accumulation associated with lipoprotein lipase and leptin in rat adipose tissues. *Asia Pacific Journal of Clinical Nutrition, 8*, 46–52.

Yeo, G.S., Farooqi, I.S., Aminian, S., Halsall, D.J., Stanhope, R.G., & O'Rahilly S. (1998). A frameshift mutation in MC4R associated with dominantly inherited human obesity. *Nature Genetics, 20*, 111–112.

Chapter 15
Genetics and Nutrigenomics of Obesity

Andreu Palou, M. Luisa Bonet, Francisca Serra, and Catalina Picó

Introduction

The prevalence of overweight and obesity is rapidly increasing in westernized countries, both in the general population and in children (see International Obesity Task Force 2009, http://www.iotf.org/). The increased availability of palatable, energy dense foods and the reduced requirement for physical exertion during working and domestic life as well as during leisure time contribute to a sustained state of positive energy balance and are, no doubt, critical factors underlying this obesity pandemic. Additional clues could relate to specific changes in diet composition, such as reduction of monounsaturated fat (Moussavi et al. 2008) or increment in the n-6/n-3 polyunsaturated fatty acid ratio (Ailhaud et al. 2006). Yet, as previously stated, "it will be unwise to view these environmental factors in isolation from the biological factors that normally control body weight and composition, and the compelling evidence that interindividual differences in susceptibility to obesity have strong genetic determinants" (O'Rahilly and Farooqi 2006).

Nowadays, substantive information has accumulated regarding the molecular constituents of physiological pathways controlling energy balance and body fat content in mammals. Analysis of these pathways has highlighted possible candidate genes whose variation – in terms of DNA sequence and/or epigenetic marks – might underlie the genetic basis of obesity and, more generally speaking, of variation in body fat mass and distribution. In turn, genetic studies can contribute significantly to understanding the physiology of weight regulation, mainly through the positional cloning of mutations that cause monogenic obesity syndromes in rodents and humans and the application of hypothesis-free approaches (such as genome-wide linkage and association studies) to reveal novel potential obesity-related genes for their subsequent physiological characterization. An overview of main genes whose variation has been implicated in human obesity is given in section on "Genetic influences in human obesity: A physiology-based overview".

Substantive information is also available regarding the effects of nutritional status and of specific nutrients and other dietary chemicals on the pathways controlling energy balance and adiposity in mammals. Nutrigenomics, a science at the interface between molecular nutrition and genomics, seeks to identify and understand the interrelationships between diet, genetic makeup and physiological responses which ultimately affect the individual's health status and/or predisposition to disease, at a genome-wide level. Nutrigenomics studies how nutrients and diets impact on gene expression and function and how the individual genetic makeup modifies or conditions diet effects, nutrient requirements and

---

A. Palou (✉), M.L. Bonet, F.S. Serra, and C. Picó
Laboratory of Molecular Biology, Nutrition and Biotechnology (Nutrigenomics), University of the Balearic Islands (UIB) and CIBER Fisiopatología de la Obesidad y Nutrición (CIBEROBN), Palma de Mallorca 07122, Spain
e-mail: andreu.palou@uib.es

L.A. Moreno et al. (eds.), *Epidemiology of Obesity in Children and Adolescents*,
Springer Series on Epidemiology and Public Health 2, DOI 10.1007/978-1-4419-6039-9_15,
© Springer Science+Business Media, LLC 2011

dietary preferences/habits. Core concepts of Nutrigenomics and selected examples in relation to obesity are addressed in section on "Gene-nutrient interactions: selected examples in connection with obesity and related disorders".

Environmental factors and lifestyle in adulthood are traditionally considered to contribute to many health problems in industrialized societies, including obesity and related metabolic disorders. This view, although true, should be extended, because environmental factors not only in adulthood but also in early life may have long-term consequences and be important in establishing the risk to disease, a concept that has been referred to as *programming* or *metabolic programming*. The impact of early life nutrition on later obesity is addressed in section on "Early life nutrition and later obesity".

Genetic Influences in Human Obesity: A Physiology-Based Overview

Obesity is usually defined as a body mass index – BMI, weight in kilograms divided by the square of the height in meters – greater than 30 kg/m^2. Monogenic obesity results from the mutation of a single gene, it is associated with morbid obesity in childhood and it is rare in humans (O'Rahilly and Farooqi 2006). Complex obesity is thought to depend on genetic variation at several susceptibility loci – each entailing usually only a modest effect per se – with a variable contribution from environmental factors such as diet and physical activity. This complex interplay of several genetic and environmental factors seems to underlie most cases of human obesity.

Many studies have examined the association of polymorphisms (usually single nucleotide polymorphisms, SNPs) or haplotypes (comprising specific combinations of polymorphisms in a single allele) in one or a few candidate genes with obesity and/or obesity-related phenotypes such as BMI as a continuous measure, skinfold thickness, waist circumference, waist-to-hip ratio, per cent body fat or abdominal fat, and others. More recently (since 2005), genome-wide association (GWA) studies have been implemented; these are hypothesis-free studies that screen the whole genome in very large cohorts of unrelated people, using SNP chips that can capture more than 80% of the registered common human genetic variation at HapMap. GWA studies already have allowed the identification of some novel candidate genes for complex human obesity (Li and Loos 2008).

In this section we present an overview of main genes whose variation has been related to monogenic and complex forms of obesity in humans (compiled in Table 15.1). We have adopted a physiology-based approach in which obesity-related genes are presented in connection with the biochemical process in which their encoded protein product(s) is (are) likely to be involved. Nevertheless, it should be kept in mind (and will be emphasized throughout the text) that many gene products have pleiotropic effects and that most, if not all, metabolic and regulatory pathways are closely interrelated.

Genes Related to the Central Regulation of Energy Balance

Central nervous system (CNS) control of feeding behavior and energy expenditure is critical to energy homeostasis and the control of body adiposity. To accomplish this control, the brain receives and integrates a continuous stream of neural and hormonal signals arising from the adipose tissue, gastrointestinal tract, liver, pancreas, and other organs/sites. These signals convey information on available energy, energetic needs or anticipated needs throughout the body and additional clues, including hedonic factors (reviewed in Woods et al. 2008).

Most identified monogenic defects that cause pure obesity syndromes in humans and rodents severely disrupt hypothalamic pathways involved in the central regulation of energy balance (reviewed in O'Rahilly and Farooqi 2006). The affected genes encode proteins of the *leptin system*:

Table 15.1 Genes reviewed herein whose variation has been related to variation in fat mass, monogenic obesity and complex forms of obesity in humans

Related to the central control of energy balance
  Leptin (LEP)
  Leptin receptor (LEPR)
  Pro-opiomelanocortin (POMC)
  Melanocortin-4 receptor (MC4R)
  Prohormone convertase 1/3 (PCSK1)
  Ghrelin (GHRL)
  Ghrelin receptor (GHSR)
  Fat mass and obesity associated (FTO) (*may also relate to lipolysis*)
Related to adipogenesis
  Peroxisome proliferator-activated receptor gamma (PPARG) (*also related to lipogenesis in adipose tissue*)
  Sterol regulatory element-binding protein 1 (SREBF1) (*also related to lipogenesis in liver*)
  Insulin induced protein 2(INSIG2)
  Lamins A and C (LMNA)
  Lipin 1 (LPIN1)
  Genes related to the Wnt/β-catenin signaling pathway (WNT10B, LRP5, CTNNBL1)
  Forkhead box C2 (FOXC2)
  Glucocorticoid receptor (NR3C1)
  11β-hydroxysteroid-dehydrogenase 1 (HSD11B1)
Related to lipid turnover (lipogenesis and lipolysis)
  Fatty acid synthase (FASN)
  Diacylglycerol acyltransferase 1 (DGAT1)
  Stearoyl-CoA desaturase (SCD)
  Platelet-type phosphofructokinase (PFKP)
  Beta-adrenoreceptor 1 (ADRB1) (*also related to adaptive thermogenesis*)
  Beta-adrenoreceptor 2 (ADRB2) (*also related to adaptive thermogenesis*)
  Beta-adrenoreceptor 3 (ADRB3) (*also related to adaptive thermogenesis*)
  Subunit beta 3 of G proteins (GNB3)
  G protein coupled receptor 74, also know as neuropeptide FF receptor 2 (NPFFR2)
  Hormone sensitive lipase (LIPE)
  Adiponutrin (PNPLA3)
  Perilipins (PLIN)
  Cell death-inducing DFFA-like effector a (CIDEA) (*may also relate to adaptive thermogenesis*)
  Aquaporin 7 (AQP7)
Related to adaptive thermogenesis/oxidative metabolism/fat oxidation
  Uncoupling protein 1 (UCP1)
  Uncoupling protein 2 (UCP2)
  Uncoupling protein 3 (UCP3)
  Peroxisome proliferator-activated receptor gamma coactivator 1alpha (PPARGC1A)
  Peroxisome proliferator-activated receptor gamma coactivator 1beta (PPARGC1B)
  Estrogen-related receptor alpha (ESRRA)
  Sirtuin 1 (SIRT1)
  Peroxisome proliferator-activated receptor delta (PPARD)
Related to insulin signaling
  Insulin (INS)
  Sorbin and SH3-domain-containing-1 gene (SORBS1)
  Alpha(2)-Heremans-Schmid glycoprotein (AHSG)
  Ectonucleotide pyrophosphatase/phosphodiesterase 1 (ENPP1)
  Protein tyrosine phosphatase-1B (PTPN1)
Related to other extracellular signals impinging on energy metabolism
  Adiponectin (ADIPOQ)

(continued)

Table 15.1 (continued)

Plasminogen activator inhibitor-1 (SERPINE1)
Interleukin 6 (IL6)
Interleukin 6 receptor (IL6R)
Tumor necrosis factor alpha (TNF)
Resistin (RETN)

The name of the encoded protein and the official human gene symbol (in brackets) is given

leptin itself, the leptin receptor, pro-opiomelanocortin (POMC), melanocortin 4 receptor (MC4R) and prohormone convertase 1/3. Leptin is an adiposity signal produced prominently (although not solely) by the adipocytes that circulates in blood at levels that fairly parallel body fat mass. Acting mainly in hypothalamic neurons via interaction with specific receptors, leptin modulates neuronal circuits leading to suppression of appetite and an increase in energy expenditure (reviewed in Ahima and Flier 2000) (see also section on "Early life nutrition and later obesity"). The functional form of the leptin receptor (long-form) is a cell-surface protein belonging to class I cytokine receptors. POMC is the protein precursor of a variety of bioactive peptides including the melanocortins mel-anocyte-stimulating hormones (αMSH, βMSH and γMSH), which are food intake suppressing (i.e., anorectic) neuropeptides whose expression and secretion is induced in response to leptin in defined subsets of hypothalamic neurons. MC4R is a G protein-coupled receptor highly expressed in the CNS that mediates central effects of melanocortins attenuating appetite and stimulating energy expenditure (reviewed in Fan et al. 2005). Prohormone convertase 1/3 is a serine endoprotease that cleaves POMC to generate the anorectic melanocortins as well as other prohormone protein sub-strates including proinsulin and proglucagon. Severe mutations in these genes of the leptin system are rare in humans, and all of them associate with early-onset hyperphagic obesity (O'Rahilly and Farooqi 2006). In particular, dominant mutations in the MC4R gene are the most common cause of monogenic, childhood-onset obesity described so far, accounting for 0.5–5% of the cases in various studies in different ethnic groups (O'Rahilly and Farooqi 2006). When lack of functional leptin is the problem, affected individuals benefit greatly from leptin replacement therapy (O'Rahilly and Farooqi 2006).

Interestingly, there is evidence that subtle variation in the same genes referred to above whose severe mutation causes monogenic obesity might be part of the polygenic influences in common human obesity. Thus, sequence variants in the 5′ flanking region (promoter region) of the leptin gene have been reported to be associated with low leptin levels, BMI, overweight (BMI >25 kg/m^2) or obesity (Hager et al. 1998; Jiang et al. 2004; Li et al. 1999; Mammes et al. 2000). Leptin receptor gene polymorphisms have also been associated with overweight and fat (especially abdominal fat) mass (Mammes et al. 2001; Quinton et al. 2001; Wauters et al. 2001), as well as with the response to low calorie diets (de Luis Roman et al. 2006; Mammes et al. 2001). However, negative results were reported for the same polymorphisms in the leptin and the leptin receptor gene in a meta-analysis (Paracchini et al. 2005). Interestingly, a missense polymorphism (Arg109Lys) in the leptin receptor gene associated with obesity along with a taste preference for sweet suggests that genetic variation in the leptin receptor gene can affect the development of obesity in part through effects on food preferences, possibly through the leptin-regulated ion channel activity of taste bud cells (Mizuta et al. 2008). Likewise, increased susceptibility to obesity has been described in humans heterozygous for a missense SNP (Arg236Gly) that disrupts a proteolytic processing site within POMC, giving rise to a fusion protein that still binds to the human MC4R, but has a markedly reduced ability to activate it (Challis et al. 2002). Common variants near the MC4R gene modestly but consistently influence fat mass, weight and obesity risk at the population level, according to a recent GWA study of 16,876 individuals of European descent (Loos et al. 2008). Finally, a recent large candidate gene study of 13,659 individuals of European ancestry found that common non-synonymous variants in the prohormone convertase 1/3 gene were consistently associated with obesity in adults and children, including one variant with significant impaired catalytic activity in functional studies (Benzinou et al. 2008).

Genetic variability in genes of the ghrelin system has also been related to common human obesity. Ghrelin is a peptide predominantly secreted by the stomach that functions as an orexigenic signal driving meal initiation, and that also fulfills established criteria for an adiposity signal, as circulating levels correlate inversely with measures of adiposity, rise with weight loss and fall with weight gain (reviewed in Cummings 2006). Ghrelin crosses the blood-brain barrier and most of its effects are thought to be centrally mediated after interaction with the growth hormone secretagogue receptor (GHSR, which can properly be re-named the ghrelin receptor). Some large studies sustain the concept that genetic variation in the ghrelin gene may have a modest impact on BMI (Ando et al. 2007; Chung et al. 2008; Ukkola et al. 2002), and association of SNPs and haplotypes within the ghrelin receptor gene (GHSR) and human obesity has also been reported (Baessler et al. 2005; Mager et al. 2008), although not in all concerned studies (Garcia et al. 2008).

Fat mass and obesity associated gene (FTO) is an obesity-susceptibility gene recently identified through GWA studies (see also Chapter 14). A cluster of variants in the first intron of FTO showed a strong and highly significant association with obesity-related traits in three independent GWA studies, a finding that has been replicated in several other studies including adults and children of European descent, but not in other ethnicities (reviewed in Loos and Bouchard 2008). Homozygotes for the risk allele weigh on average 3–4 kg more and have a 1.67-fold increased risk of obesity compared with those who did not inherit a risk allele. The physiological role of FTO is still unclear. Studies in humans and rodents have suggested a role in the central regulation of energy balance, as FTO is abundantly expressed in the hypothalamic nuclei involved, and its central expression seems to be dependent on the nutritional status (Loos and Bouchard 2008). Others have proposed a peripheral role of FTO through an effect on lipolytic activity in adipose tissue, with carriers of the risk allele having reduced lipolytic activity (Loos and Bouchard 2008).

Genes Related to Adipogenesis

Adipocyte number is a major determinant of fat mass in adult humans (Spalding et al. 2008). Adipocyte number depends on the balance among the processes of proliferation of precursor cells resident in the adipose tissue depots, adipose differentiation (adipogenesis) of the progeny, and apoptosis of adipocytes. Precursor cells contained in human fat depots retain the capacity to undergo adipogenesis throughout life (Hauner et al. 1989). Nevertheless, the number of adipocytes is set during childhood and adolescence in humans: in adults there is a remarkable turnover of adipocytes but its total number stays constant, even after marked weight loss (Spalding et al. 2008). This may contribute to explain why obese individuals have difficulties maintaining weight loss, and underscores the importance of understanding the mechanisms that control adipocyte number and of eventual intervention in the critical developmental periods in which adipocyte number is being set (Spalding et al. 2008).

The master regulator of adipogenesis is peroxisome proliferator-activated receptor γ (PPARγ), a fatty acid-activated transcription factor that induces the expression of key genes in fatty acid uptake and triacylglycerol synthesis in differentiating adipose cells, which is also crucial for lipogenesis in, and the survival of, mature adipocytes (reviewed in Tsai and Maeda 2005). PPARγ is implicated in whole-body insulin sensitivity, likely through its effects on adipocyte metabolism and secretory function. Quite paradoxically, however, both modest reductions in PPARγ activity and PPARγ activation (through binding of thiazolidinediones (TZDs), anti-diabetic drugs used to treat human type 2 diabetes though at the expense of subcutaneous fat gain) result in increased whole-body insulin sensitivity (Tsai and Maeda 2005). In humans, rare dominant loss-of-function mutations of PPARγ cause partial lipodystrophy and severe insulin resistance, which has been linked to the inability of adipose tissue to trap and store free fatty acids (reviewed in Meirhaeghe and Amouyel 2004). By contrast, a gain-of-function mutation in PPARγ was detected in four unrelated morbid obese individuals, although this mutation subsequently was shown to have no epidemiological impact on morbid obesity in large studies (Meirhaeghe and Amouyel 2004). In addition to these rare mutations, some common polymorphisms in the human PPARγ gene (PPARG) have been related to obesity and insulin sensitivity in humans, with conflicting results (Meirhaeghe and Amouyel 2004). The most prevalent is the Pro12Ala polymorphism in PPARγ2, the characteristic PPARγ isoform found in adipose tissue. In functional assays, the Ala12-PPARγ2 protein exhibits an impaired activity as a transcription factor (Meirhaeghe and Amouyel 2004). There is a significant body of data indicating that the Ala12 allele confers increased protection against the development of insulin resistance and type 2 diabetes (Meirhaeghe and Amouyel 2004). Impact on BMI is less clear, as association with higher BMI, lower BMI, and no association with BMI has been described for the Ala12 allele in different studies (Meirhaeghe and Amouyel 2004). A meta-analysis (comprising 30 independent studies and 19,136 subjects) concluded that the Ala12 allele associates with significantly higher BMI in the overweight and obese subjects (BMI > 27 kg/m^2), but that this association is not detected in lean subjects (Meirhaeghe and Amouyel 2004). Other authors favor the idea that the Ala12 allele confers subtle protection against obesity both in adults and children (Cecil et al. 2006). Interestingly, the effects of the Ala12 allele appear to be subject to modification by other genetic and dietary factors, which may, in part, explain apparently discordant results among studies examining its relationship with BMI/obesity (Meirhaeghe and Amouyel 2004) (see also section on "Gene-nutrient interactions: selected examples in connection with obesity and related disorders").

Another transcription factor involved in adipogenesis is sterol regulatory element-binding protein 1 (SREBP1), which is also involved in hepatic lipogenesis and encoded by the human gene SREBF1 (Horton et al. 2002, 2003; Kim and Spiegelman 1996). One SNP and one haplotype (corresponding to a specific combination of six SNPs) in SREBF1 were reported to associate with morbid obesity in French Caucasian cohorts (Eberle et al. 2004). Moreover, polymorphisms in genes encoding proteins that are likely to modulate SREBP1 activity in cells have been associated with obesity in humans. These include the gene encoding insulin induced protein 2 (INSIG2) and the gene encoding lamins A and B (LMNA). INSIG2 protein functions in cells to block proteolytic activation of the SREBPs, which are synthesized as inactive precursors and activated through a regulated cleavage process that releases the transcriptional active portion of the protein (Goldstein et al. 2006). A polymorphism (rs7566605) located 10 kb upstream of the INSIG2 gene was the first obesity-related gene variant identified through a GWA approach (Herbert et al. 2006). The association of rs7566605 with BMI has been reproduced in several but not all large cohorts subsequently examined (Andreasen et al. 2008, and references therein). Lamins A and C are components of the nuclear lamina. Rare mutations in their encoding gene (LMNA) leading to intracellular accumulation of the lamin A precursor (pre-lamin A) underlie some forms of familial partial lipodystrophy, indicating a role in human adipogenesis, and there is evidence that pre-lamin A can interact with and sequester SREBP1 at the nuclear rim, thus decreasing the pool of active SREBP1 that normally promotes preadipocyte differentiation (Capanni et al. 2005, and references therein). A common genetic variation in the LMNA gene has been associated with obesity-related traits in at least three different populations (Hegele et al. 2000, 2001; Wegner et al. 2007).

Lipin 1 is a protein that acts upstream of PPARγ in adipocyte differentiation and promotes fat storage and obesity in the mouse (Phan et al. 2004). Intragenic SNPs and corresponding allelic haplotypes in the human lipin 1 gene (LPIN1) exhibited associations with serum insulin levels and BMI in Finns (Suviolahti et al. 2006). Another recent study supports the hypothesis that sequence variation in LPIN1 contributes to variation in resting metabolic rate and obesity-related phenotypes potentially in an age-dependent manner (Loos et al. 2007a).

Forkhead box C2 (FOXC2) is a transcription factor with restricted expression in adipose tissues in both mice and humans for which animal and cell studies indicate a role opposing adipogenesis and the development of diet-induced obesity (Cederberg et al. 2001; Davis et al. 2004). One SNP in the putative FOXC2 human gene promoter (-512C>T) has been associated with obesity in two different populations (Carlsson et al. 2004; Kovacs et al. 2003).

The Wnt/β-catenin signaling pathway is an important negative regulator of adipogenesis. Preadipocytes produce and secrete specific Wnt proteins that, functioning in an autocrine/paracrine manner, repress their adipose conversion. The pathway begins with the interaction of the Wnt proteins with specific membrane receptors and coreceptors (including the low density lipoprotein receptor-related proteins, LRPs), followed by stabilization of β-catenin in the cytoplasm. Subsequently, β-catenin acts in the nucleus as a transcriptional coactivator that favors the expression of genes encoding proteins that inhibit adipogenesis (reviewed in Prestwich and Macdougald 2007). In response to an adipogenic stimulus, expression of the inhibitory Wnt signals declines, while the expression of β-catenin antagonists increases (Prestwich and Macdougald 2007). Polymorphisms in several genes encoding proteins related to this pathway have been associated with obesity in humans. In particular, polymorphisms of the WNT10B and LRP5 genes may be associated with obesity in populations of European origin (Christodoulides et al. 2006; Guo et al. 2006). Furthermore, recent GWA studies have identified CTNNBL1, which encodes a protein with structure homologous to that of β-catenin, as a novel candidate gene for obesity (Liu et al. 2008).

Glucocorticoids (GCs) are potent inducers of adipogenesis, besides having peripheral and central actions to enhance food intake and decrease thermogenesis (Vegiopoulos and Herzig 2007). GC excess, whether endogenous (Cushing's syndrome) or exogenous (GC therapy), promotes visceral obesity and obesity-associated clinical complications. Most actions of GCs are mediated by the intracellular glucocorticoid receptor (GR). At least three polymorphisms in the human GR gene appear to be associated with altered GC sensitivity and changes in body composition and metabolic parameters (reviewed in van Rossum and Lamberts 2004). GC action in target tissues greatly depends on tissue-specific intracellular GC metabolism by 11β-hydroxysteroid-dehydrogenases (11β-HSDs), which are enzymes that interconvert active GCs (cortisol in humans) and their inert 11-keto derivatives (cortisone) (reviewed in Wamil and Seckl 2007). Isoform 1 of 11β-HSD (11β-HSD1) is expressed primarily in GC target tissues such as liver, adipose tissue and the CNS, and predominantly regenerates active GCs, thus amplifying local GC action. A number of studies have shown increased adipose tissue expression and activity of 11β-HSD1 in human obesity (Wamil and Seckl 2007). Association of polymorphisms in the human 11β-HSD1 gene with obesity-related parameters such as BMI or waist-to hip ratio has been reported in some, but not all, studies concerned (Wamil and Seckl 2007).

Genes Related to Lipid Turnover

Alterations in the balance between lipogenesis (fatty acid and triacylglycerol synthesis in lipogenic tissues) and adipocyte lipolysis (triacylglycerol breakdown) can impact on obesity development and metabolism in distinct and complex ways. For instance, increased adipocyte lipolysis may favor leanness but also dyslipidemia and insulin resistance if not associated with the oxidation of the newly released fatty acids. Variability in genes encoding proteins involved in lipogenesis and lipolysis has been associated with obesity-related parameters in humans. The encoded proteins include: transcription factors that control tissue lipogenic capability (in particular SREBP-1c and PPARγ, which we have already presented in connection to adipogenesis as they also play an important role in this process, see above), enzymes directly or indirectly related to lipogenesis, and proteins related to lipolysis.

Genes Related to Lipogenesis

Fatty acid synthase (FAS) is necessary for the de novo synthesis of fatty acids from acetyl-CoA, malonyl-CoA and NADPH in lipogenic tissues (mainly liver and adipose tissue) and may also be important as part of energy sensory mechanisms in cells including neurons. Treatment of mice in vivo with FAS inhibitors reduces food intake, increases fatty acid oxidation in peripheral tissues, and induces a rapid decline in body fat stores (Loftus et al. 2000; Thupari et al. 2002). Anorexia after FAS inhibition has been related to results showing that malonyl-CoA, which accumulates upon FAS inhibition, can serve as an energy sensor in hypothalamic regulatory neurons, with increased levels indicating a good status and favoring suppression of food intake (Lane et al. 2008). These and other results strongly suggest a role for FAS in energy homeostasis. A genetic polymorphism that is predicted to result in the substitution of Val1483 by Ile in the FAS protein has been shown to associate with body fat content and substrate oxidation rate in Pima Indians (Kovacs et al. 2004). Subjects with the Ile/x genotype have a lower percentage of body fat and appear to preferentially oxidize lipids over carbohydrates compared with the Val/Val homozygotes (Kovacs et al. 2004). Evidence of a sex-specific protective effect of the Ile allele for obesity has also been reported in Caucasian boys (Korner et al. 2007). Interestingly, the Val1483Ile variant is positioned within a domain of the FAS monomer that may be important for active FAS dimer formation. Hence, substitution of Val by Ile at this site could potentially reduce FAS activity (Kovacs et al. 2004).

Diacylglycerol acyltransferase 1 (DGAT1) is one of the DGAT enzyme isoforms catalyzing the final step in triacylglycerol synthesis. The C allele of a common SNP near the DGAT1 transcriptional start site (T79C) is associated with increased promoter activity and higher BMI in Turkish women. However, this association has not been confirmed in a large French cohort (reviewed in Dahlman and Arner 2007).

Stearoyl-CoA desaturase (SCD) is the rate limiting enzyme in the biosynthesis of monounsaturated fats. It catalyzes the generation of palmitoleic (16:1) and oleic acid (18:1) from palmitic (16:0) and stearic acid (18:0), respectively (reviewed in Dobrzyn and Ntambi 2005). Studies in mice suggest that SCD1 (which is one of four characterized SCD genes in mice) is a key regulator of lipid partitioning, its activity favoring lipid synthesis over lipid oxidation (Dobrzyn and Ntambi 2005). Humans have a single characterized SCD gene that is highly homologous to murine SCD1. The rare alleles of certain SNPs in the human SCD gene have been reported to associate with reduced BMI, reduced waist circumference and increased insulin sensitivity in a Swedish population (Warensjo et al. 2007), although these findings await confirmation in other populations.

Lipogenesis strongly relies on glycolysis as a source of acetyl-CoA for the de novo fatty acid synthesis and of glycerol-3-phosphate for triacylglycerol synthesis. Phosphofructokinase (PFK) catalyzes a major rate-limiting step of glycolysis, the conversion of fructose 6-phosphate to fructose-1,6-bisphosphate. PFK acts as a homo- or hetero-tetramer of three types of subunits, encoded by different genes, which show partially overlapping patterns of expression in different cells and tissues. Platelet-type PFK (encoded by the human gene PFKP) is the most stringently regulated of these subunits (Hannemann et al. 2005). SNP rs6602024 in PFKP was identified in a GWA scan of obesity-related traits in 4,741 individuals from a genetically isolated population of Sardinia to associate strongly with BMI, body weight and hip circumference (Scuteri et al. 2007). It has been proposed that genetic variants of platelet-type PFK might alter the balance between glycolysis and glycogen production in cells, increasing glycolysis and thereby favoring lipogenesis – a possible step in the etiology of obesity (Scuteri et al. 2007). The association of rs6602024 in PFKP with obesity-related traits has, however, not been replicated in other populations (Andreasen et al. 2008; Scuteri et al. 2007).

Genes Related to Lipolysis

Catecholamines of neuronal and endocrine origin stimulate lipolysis in white and brown adipocytes and energy dissipation as heat (adaptive thermogenesis, see below) in brown adipocytes. This makes genes involved in the regulation of catecholamine function potential candidate genes for obesity. The pro-lipolytic and pro-thermogenic effect of catecholamines is dependent on their interaction with beta1-, beta2- and beta3-adrenoreceptors on the adipocyte cell membrane (encoded by the human genes ADRB1, ADRB2 and ADRB3, respectively). Non-synonymous polymorphisms in ADRB1 (Gly389Arg, Ser49Gly), ADRB2 (Arg16Gly, Gln27Glu) and ADRB3 (Trp64Arg) that might be of functional relevance were shown to associate with lipolysis rate, levels of circulating free fatty acids, obesity, weight gain over time and/or weight loss upon intervention in several human population studies, although the associations were not confirmed in all subsequent studies (reviewed in Dahlman and Arner 2007). More recently, specific ADRB2 haplotypes have been associated with receptor expression levels, sensitivity to catecholamine-stimulated lipolysis and obesity (Dahlman and Arner 2007). Beta-adrenoreceptors signal via G-stimulatory proteins. The rare T allele of polymorphism 825C>T in exon 10 of the gene coding isoform 3 of the β subunit of G proteins (Gβ3) has been reported to associate with reduced Gβ3 protein expression levels and impaired catecholamine-induced lipolysis in isolated subcutaneous adipocytes and in vivo, and with obesity in several, but not all, studied populations (Dahlman and Arner 2007; Ryden et al. 2002).

Specific membrane proteins are known that may interfere with beta-adrenoreceptor signaling. One of them is G protein coupled receptor 74 (GPR74), also known as neuropeptide FF receptor 2. GPR74 is a membrane receptor predominantly expressed in the brain, heart and adipose tissue in humans. Although its endogenous ligand is unknown, GPR74 has a high affinity for neuropeptide FF, a signal known to impact on food intake and on adipocyte lipolysis through interactions with the beta-adrenoreceptors (see Dahlman et al. 2007). A common haplotype in the human GPR74 gene associates with reduced BMI, smaller waist and increased lipolysis in Scandinavians (Dahlman et al. 2007). Studies in isolated human fat cells indicate that this haplotype improves the ability of catecholamines to stimulate lipolysis by weakening an intrinsic inhibitory effect of GPR74 on beta2-adrenoreceptor signaling (Dahlman et al. 2007).

Hormone sensitive lipase (HSL) is the primary intracellular triacylglycerol-hydolyzing enzyme in adipocytes and has traditionally been considered to be the rate-limiting enzyme in adipocyte lipolysis. Recent evidence points to the existence of additional intracellular lipases such as adiponutrin, which has both triacylglycerol lipase activity and a transacylase activity leading to triacylglycerol synthesis (Liu et al. 2004), and adipose triglyceride lipase (ATGL) (Raben and Baldassare 2005). These lipases are likely to participate in adipocyte lipolysis in both rodents and humans, although their roles are still poorly defined. Decreased adipocyte HSL activity and expression has been reported in human obese subjects, in keeping with reduced catecholamine-induced lipolysis in obesity (Langin et al. 2005; Ryden et al. 2007). A functional SNP in the HSL gene promoter (-60C>G) that results in reduced transcription associated with increased adiposity in some human population studies and with reduced adiposity in others. Furthermore, one allele of an intronic repeat in the HSL gene was reported to associate with impaired adipocyte lipolysis, obesity and type 2 diabetes (reviewed in Dahlman and Arner 2007). Several SNPs in the ATGL gene (PNPLA2) have been associated with the risk of type 2 diabetes and the levels of circulating lipids, but not so far with obesity in humans (Schoenborn et al. 2006). Finally, variation in the human adiponutrin gene may be associated with obesity, according to recent reports (Johansson et al. 2006, 2008). Thus, genetic variability in genes encoding different intracellular lipases has been related to human obesity.

Perilipins are a group of proteins that localize on the surface of intracellular lipid droplets. Perilipins contribute to modulate lipolysis by acting both as suppressors of basal lipolysis (in their unphosphorylated state) and as enhancers of catecholamine-stimulated lipolysis (in their phosphorylated state). Different perilipins are derived by alternative splicing from a single gene (PLIN in humans). Polymorphisms of PLIN have been associated with obesity (Qi et al. 2004a, b, 2005) and resistance to weight loss following low-energy diets (Corella et al. 2005).

Cell death-inducing DFFA-like effector a (Cidea) is a protein expressed predominantly in white adipose tissue (and specifically in the adipocytes) as compared with other tissues in humans (Gummesson et al. 2007). Available data are compatible with functions of Cidea in humans suppressing basal lipolysis in adipocytes (Nordstrom et al. 2005), promoting the enlargement of adipocyte intracellular lipid droplets (to which Cidea co-localizes) (Puri et al. 2008), and reducing basal metabolic rate through reduction of energy expenditure in adipose tissue (Gummesson et al. 2007). One non-synonymous SNP in the Cidea gene (predicting substitution of Val 115 by Phe), still of unknown functional significance, has been associated with obesity and phenotypes of the metabolic syndrome in Swedes and Japanese (Dahlman et al. 2005; Zhang et al. 2008).

Aquaporin 7 is a plasma membrane water and glycerol channel abundantly expressed in adipocytes, where it acts as a gateway molecule for the efficient release of lipolysis-derived glycerol (reviewed in Verkman 2005). Studies in mouse models have suggested that aquaporin 7 disruption, through defective glycerol exit and subsequent accumulation of glycerol and stimulation of glycerol kinase activity, can boost triacylglycerol synthesis in adipocytes thereby favoring obesity (Hara-Chikuma et al. 2005; Hibuse et al. 2005). In keeping, aquaporin 7 gene expression is downregulated in adipose depots of human obese subjects compared with lean controls (Marrades et al. 2006). One SNP in the human aquaporin 7 gene promoter (-953A>G) that leads to reduced expression in adipose tissues reportedly associates with obesity in humans (Prudente et al. 2007b).

Genes Related to Adaptive Thermogenesis and Oxidative Metabolism

Defects in (unconscious) energy expenditure and/or substrate oxidation can conceivably contribute to the development of obesity. This is supported by studies demonstrating that disruption of mechanisms of adaptive thermogenesis is a feature of many rodent models of obesity (Himms-Hagen 1989), and actually causes obesity in rodents (Lowell and Bachman 2003; Lowell et al. 1993). Adaptive thermogenesis is defined as energy dissipation as heat in response to environmental variables such as temperature and diet. In humans, there are important interindividual differences in the capacity to metabolize a fixed amount of ingested energy, with a strong genetic component according to classical twin studies (Bouchard et al. 1990). A low rate of 24-h energy expenditure (measured in respiratory chamber) has been shown to correlate with higher body weight gain over a 2-year follow-up period (Ravussin et al. 1988). Moreover, a reduced rate of fat oxidation appears to be a risk marker for future body weight gain independent of low energy expenditure (Treuth et al. 2003; Zurlo et al. 1990). Genetic variation in several genes encoding proteins related to adaptive thermogenesis, mitochondria oxidative metabolism and/or fat oxidation has been linked to human obesity. Main genes in this category other than the beta-adrenoreceptor genes – which are critical to the control of mechanisms of adaptive thermogenesis and of lipolysis, and which have already been presented in connection with lipolysis – are addressed next.

Uncoupling proteins (UCPs) are inner mitochondrial membrane proteins that behave functionally as regulated proton transporters. Their activity dissipates as heat part of the proton electrochemical gradient generated by the respiratory chain during substrate oxidation. The founder member of the UCP family, UCP1, is characteristically expressed in brown adipocytes and the molecular effector of thermogenesis in these specialized cells, which so far constitutes the best understood mechanism of adaptive thermogenesis in mammals (Palou et al. 1998). Thermogenesis in brown fat is under the control of sympathetic nervous system-derived catecholamines acting on beta-adrenoreceptors. In rodents, brown fat thermogenesis is critical for thermoregulation and it has also been implicated as a defense against obesity. The physiological significance of brown fat thermogenesis in humans is less clear, as it has been generally assumed that in humans brown fat atrophies after birth and is absent in adults (but see below). UCP2 and UCP3 are proteins highly homologous in sequence to UCP1. Both in rodents and humans, UCP2 is expressed in many tissues and UCP3 mainly in brown fat and skeletal muscle.

How important the contribution of the activity of the UCPs to energy balance might be in humans remains a matter of debate. Contrary to previous contentions, it is now recognized that defined brown fat depots are present and functional in adult humans (Nedergaard et al. 2007). In addition, UCP1 mRNA is detected at low levels in human white adipose tissue depots, likely reflecting the presence of some brown adipocytes interspersed among the white adipocytes (Oberkofler et al. 1997). Expression of UCP1 (Oberkofler et al. 1997) and UCP2 (Oberkofler et al. 1998) in visceral fat appears to be decreased in obese as compared to lean subjects. In addition, a low level of UCP3 expression in skeletal muscle reportedly correlates with resistance to weight loss on a low calorie diet (Harper et al. 2002). Polymorphisms in the genes encoding the different UCPs or their promoters have been shown to be associated with levels of uncoupling protein expression in fat depots, obesity, 24-h energy expenditure, respiratory quotient, or fat loss upon intervention in different studies, but their impact on these phenotypes in general is modest, and many of the associations have not been confirmed in subsequent studies (reviewed in Dalgaard and Pedersen 2001).

Peroxisome proliferator-activated receptor gamma coactivator 1α (PGC1α) and 1β (PGC1β) are two closely related transcriptional coactivators, encoded in separate genes, that promote the expression of genes involved in mitochondrial biogenesis and function (respiration) and fatty acid oxidation (reviewed in Handschin and Spiegelman 2006). PGC1α is also important for UCP1 expression. Expression of PGC1 isoforms at the mRNA level is reduced in white adipose tissue of morbidly obese humans (Semple et al. 2004). SNPs in the PGC1α gene have been reported to associate with obesity in Austrian women (Esterbauer et al. 2002), and one non-synonymous SNP in the PGC1β gene (Ala203Pro) to protect against obesity in a Danish population (Andersen et al. 2005).

Estrogen-related receptor alpha (ERRα) is an orphan nuclear receptor that positively controls genes involved in fatty acid oxidation and mitochondrial respiration (Huss et al. 2004; Sladek et al. 1997; Vega and Kelly 1997). It is highly expressed in tissues that preferentially metabolize fatty acids. ERRα induces cellular energy expenditure in the presence of PGC1α or PGC1β, both of which function as activating protein ligands of the ERRs (Kamei et al. 2003). Polymorphism in a 23-base microsatellite repeat in the 5′-flanking region of the human ERRα gene has been shown to associate with obesity in a Japanese population (Kamei et al. 2005), but the association was not reproduced in a Danish population (Larsen et al. 2007).

Sirtuins (SIRT1 to SIRT7) are a family of mammalian NAD^+-dependent protein deacetylases and ADP-ribosyltransferases involved in many cellular processes including the control of cellular energy metabolism (see Lagouge et al. 2006). In mice, pharmacological activation of sirtuins (through high oral doses of resveratrol) protects from diet-induced obesity and insulin resistance by triggering an increase in energy expenditure that is largely dependent on SIRT1 activation and subsequent deacetylation and activation of PGC1α (Lagouge et al. 2006). SNPs in the human SIRT1 gene associate with parameters of energy homeostasis (whole-body energy expenditure) in a Finnish population (Lagouge et al. 2006), and with visceral obesity in a case/control study in Belgians (Peeters et al. 2008).

PPARδ is a transcription factor coactivated by PGC1 isoforms that induces the expression of genes involved in fatty acid uptake, beta-oxidation and energy dissipation as heat (reviewed in Furnsinn et al. 2007). Its expression and function is particularly important in the skeletal muscle. PPARδ gene polymorphisms have been reported to associate with obesity and BMI in some studies (Aberle et al. 2006; Shin et al. 2004), but other studies have failed to find an association with adiposity-related phenotypes (Grarup et al. 2007; Lagou et al. 2008).

Genes Related to Insulin Signaling

Insulin has ying-yang effects on body fat content, as it stimulates the build-up of lipid stores in adipose tissue but also acts in the CNS to inhibit appetite and increase energy expenditure, thus providing a negative feedback in the control of energy stores (Niswender et al. 2004). Variability in several genes encoding proteins related to insulin signaling has been associated with the risk of obesity in humans. These genes are presented next.

The insulin gene has a polymorphic locus (named VNTR) that contains a variable number of tandem repeats. Class I VNTR alleles have been associated with higher insulin secretion and juvenile obesity (Le Stunff et al. 2000).

Sorbin and SH3-domain-containing-1 gene (SORBS1) is the human homologue of the mouse SH3P12 gene, which is highly expressed in adipocytes, is activated during adipogenesis, and encodes a protein involved in insulin-stimulated glucose uptake that interacts with the insulin receptor (Lin et al. 2001). A non-synonymous SNP, Thr228Ala, in exon 7 of SORBS1 has been associated with obesity and type 2 diabetes in Taiwanese, with the less common Ala allele being protective for both disorders (Lin et al. 2001). However, the functionality, if any, of this polymorphism remains unknown and no association with obesity was found in Caucasians (Nieters et al. 2002).

Alpha(2)-Heremans-Schmid glycoprotein (AHSG, also called fetuin) is a plasma protein synthesized predominantly in the liver that functions to attenuate insulin signaling by inhibiting insulin-induced insulin receptor autophosphorylation and tyrosine kinase activity. SNPs in the human AHSG gene have been reported to associate with sensitivity of adipocytes to insulin, obesity and type 2 diabetes (reviewed in Dahlman and Arner 2007). In particular, a three-marker haplotype comprising two SNPs previously shown to associate with a lower AHSG protein level was found to be more common among lean than obese and overweight subjects in a population of Swedish men (Lavebratt et al. 2005).

Ectonucleotide pyrophosphatase/phosphodiesterase 1 (ENPP1) is a membrane glycoprotein that attenuates insulin action by binding to the insulin receptor and inhibiting subsequent signaling. A non-synonymous SNP that changes one amino acid in the ENPP1 protein, K121Q (Lys to Gln), and a three-marker haplotype including the 121Q variant have been associated with type 2 diabetes and childhood and morbid obesity in some studies, but other studies have not confirmed these associations (reviewed in Dahlman and Arner 2007) or have reported the reverse association, i.e., that the 121Q variant is protective against weight excess (Matsuoka et al. 2006; Morandi et al. 2008; Prudente et al. 2007a). The 121Q variant binds to the insulin receptor with more affinity and inhibits insulin signaling more effectively than the 121K variant, which may lead to a diminished insulin-dependent fat accumulation at the adipose tissue level that could explain, at least in part, an association of this variant with leanness (Morandi et al. 2008; Prudente et al. 2007a). To reconcile seemingly contradictory results, it has been proposed that the 121Q allele of ENPP1 might have divergent modulation effects on BMI in lean and obese subjects, protecting against obesity in the lean and aggravating obesity in the obese (Morandi et al. 2008). Thus, in the case of severe obesity, where the multifactorial predisposition for adiposity is very strong, 121Q insulin inhibition may fail to be effective in hampering fat accumulation, while it may have a significant anti-anorecting effect at the brain level, thus being part of the complex risk of morbid adiposity (Morandi et al. 2008).

Protein tyrosine phosphatase 1B (PTP1B) down-regulates insulin signaling through dephosphorylation of the insulin receptor (Goldstein et al. 1998). In mouse models, whole-body and neuron-specific deficiency in PTP1B associates with leanness, improved glucose homeostasis and resistance to diet-induced obesity due to increased resting metabolic rate and total energy expenditure, whereas adipose tissue-specific deficiency in PTP1B associates with increased body weight gain on a high fat diet, conceivably by enhancing insulin action in adipocytes (Bence et al. 2006). Human genetic association studies support the hypothesis that genetic variability in PTP1B contributes to the polygenic basis of obesity, and that SNPs in the PTP1B gene may interact with environmental factors to induce more severe phenotypes, e.g. atherogenic dyslipidemia, in morbidly obese subjects (Cheyssac et al. 2006; Kipfer-Coudreau et al. 2004).

Genes Related to Other Extracellular Signals Impinging on Energy Metabolism

Besides the ones already addressed (leptin, glucocorticoids, catecholamines and insulin), there are many other extracellular protein signals that impact on energy metabolism. For some of them genetic variability has been linked to obesity-related traits in humans. Of note, many signals impinging on energy metabolism are produced in the adipose tissue. Adipose tissue-derived bioactive proteins (collectively termed adipokines) have local effects in this tissue and participate in the regulation of whole-body metabolism after they are released into the circulation.

One important protein signal predominantly expressed in differentiated adipocytes is adiponectin. This hormone has a well-established anti-diabetic and anti-inflammatory action, and may also impact on obesity development (reviewed in Kadowaki et al. 2008). Adiponectin expression is reduced in human obesity and insulin-resistant states, and upregulated following weight loss. Two SNPs in exon 2 of the human adiponectin gene (ADIPOQ), 45G>T and 276T>G, have been associated with obesity and insulin resistance, but with inconsistent results between different cohorts (Loos et al. 2007b) and references therein). Furthermore, SNPs in the ADIPOQ promoter (-11391G>A and -11377C>G) and specific haplotypes combining them have been associated with abdominal fat gain over a 7-year follow-up in a prospective study in French caucasians, suggesting a putative role of adiponectin in body fat gain in the general population (Dolley et al. 2008). Interestingly, the specific ADIPOQ promoter alleles and haplotypes linked to increased body fat gain associate with higher adiponectinemia in this latter study and other studies (Dolley et al. 2008, and references therein). It has been suggested that, even though adiponectin promotes fatty acid oxidation in liver and skeletal muscle, it may physiologically contribute to weight gain over time due to its insulin-sensitizing action in adipose tissue (Dolley et al. 2008, and references therein). Indeed, adiponectin has been shown to promote adipogenesis, lipid accumulation and insulin responsiveness in adipocytes (Fu et al. 2005). The overall adiponectin action is in keeping with the concept that efficient fat deposition in adipose tissue can have a beneficial effect in whole-body insulin sensitivity, possibly by preventing ectopic fat deposition in nonadipose tissues (Kim et al. 2007). Adiponectin acts through adiponectin receptors 1 and 2, encoded by the human genes ADIPOR1 and ADIPOR2, respectively. SNPs in these two genes have been associated with type 2 diabetes mellitus in a number of studies and, more recently, variability in their promoters has been reported to associate with measures of substrate oxidation (respiratory quotient) (Loos et al. 2007b).

Adipose tissue produces large amounts of plasminogen activator inhibitor-1 (PAI-1), and human obesity, especially abdominal obesity, associates with elevated circulating levels of PAI-1 and impaired fibrinolysis, which has been related to increased cardiovascular risk in obesity (Skurk and Hauner 2004). Besides its role in coagulation, PAI-1 and local activity of the fibrinolytic system might be involved in adipose tissue development through effects on interconnected aspects such as extracellular matrix remodeling, cell migration, angiogenesis, and adipocyte differentiation (Alessi et al. 2007). A functional polymorphism in the promoter region of the PAI-1 gene (-675 4G/5G) affecting transcription has been associated with obesity in humans (Hoffstedt et al. 2002), but this has not been confirmed by others (reviewed in Dahlman and Arner 2007).

Interleukin 6 (IL-6) is an immuno-modulating cytokine abundantly secreted by adipose tissue and skeletal muscle (during contraction) and also expressed together with its receptor in neurons of hypothalamic nuclei regulating energy homeostasis. Studies in rodents support an anti-obesity action of

IL-6 that appears to be largely dependent on central (CNS) action leading to the stimulation of the sympathetic nervous system and thereby to increased resting energy expenditure (Jansson et al. 2003). In addition, direct effects of IL-6 stimulating adipocyte lipolysis and activating fatty acid oxidation in skeletal muscle have been described in humans and human cells (Petersen et al. 2005). Several polymorphisms in the IL-6 gene have been reported to associate with obesity. The most studied one is polymorphism -174G>C in the IL-6 gene promoter. The -174C allele has been associated with lower IL-6 expression levels, lower energy expenditure, increased BMI, obesity and increased risk of type 2 diabetes in various studies (Dahlman and Arner 2007). However, a recent meta-analysis found no evidence for an association of this polymorphism with BMI (Huth et al. 2008; Qi et al. 2007) or circulating IL-6 levels (Huth et al. 2008) and concluded that carriers of the -174C allele are at decreased (rather than increased) risk of developing type 2 diabetes (Huth et al. 2008). Nevertheless, a particular haplotype (capturing the contribution of six different SNPs) of the IL-6 gene was consistently associated with increased adiposity in two independent healthy cohorts (Qi et al. 2007). Furthermore, polymorphisms in the gene encoding the IL-6 receptor have been reported to be associated with obesity in Pima Indians and a Spanish population (reviewed in Dahlman and Arner 2007).

Adipose tissue is a source of tumor necrosis factor α (TNFα), which in fat is expressed both in adipocytes and stromal-vascular macrophages. TNFα is a catabolic pro-inflammatory cytokine that might impact on lipid metabolism, adipocyte differentiation and (negatively) on insulin sensitivity (reviewed in Ryden and Arner 2007). Expression of TNFα in adipose tissue is elevated in many experimental rodent models of obesity and in morbid obese humans. In adipocytes, TNFα downregulates genes involved in insulin action, attenuates insulin receptor signaling, counteracts adipogenic transcription factors (including PPARγ) and stimulates lipolysis (Ryden and Arner 2007). Increased adipose TNFα expression in obesity might represent a compensatory response to limit further adipose tissue expansion, though at the expense of insulin resistance. A functional SNP (-308G>A) in the TNFα gene promoter that appears to influence the transcription rate has been found to associate with a modest increased risk of developing obesity, but strikingly not with BMI as a continuous variable, in a recent meta-analysis (Sookoian et al. 2005).

Resistin is a protein secreted by adipocytes in mice and by macrophages in humans that has been related to insulin resistance (a role well documented in mice, but not in humans), inflammation and the inhibition of adipogenesis (McTernan et al. 2006). Polymorphisms in the human resistin gene and its promoter have been associated with insulin resistance and obesity or BMI in humans, although not in all studied populations; in addition, for some of these polymorphisms association with opposite changes in BMI has been reported (Beckers et al. 2008, and references therein).

Summary

Variability in many genes has been associated with obesity and/or obesity-related phenotypes in humans (see the significant sample of them summarized in Table 15.1). The driver for these findings has been, in most cases, previous knowledge on the physiological role(s) of the encoded proteins, and the better this knowledge the better can be our understanding of observed associations. Nevertheless, complete understanding is often hampered by lack of data on the specific functional significance of the polymorphism(s) under investigation. Moreover, lack of replication of findings is more the rule than the exception in genetic association studies regarding complex human obesity (even results of GWA studies are not undebated). As a consequence, the majority of genes discussed above remain candidates of potential relevance. Lack of replication can be due to many factors, including poor study design (e.g., studies of small sample size), differences in the demographic parameters (sex, age, health status, ethnicity) or behavioral parameters (dietary intake behavior, fat intake, level of physical activity, drugs, alcohol, etc.) of the studied populations, and differences in the phenotype studied (for instance, recruiting subjects with mild or severe obesity). Control of environmental exposures has been addressed to date only in a minority of published studies in the field of the genetics of obesity, which represents a significant shortcoming. This situation is currently changing in parallel to the consolidation of the sciences of nutrigenomics and nutrigenetics.

Gene-Nutrient Interactions: Selected Examples in Connection with Obesity and Related Disorders

There is a complex and dynamic interaction between nutrition and the human genome. This interaction determines gene expression and the metabolic response, which ultimately affects an individual's health status and/or predisposition to disease. Nutrigenomics core concepts imply that the individual genetic background can influence nutrient status, metabolic response and predisposition to diet-related diseases; but also, that nutrients can have a direct effect on and may interact with transcription factors to regulate gene expression (Roche 2004).

In contrast to specific pharmacological ligands, nutrients and dietary components can affect directly and indirectly multiple cellular targets and co-ordinately modulate gene expression affecting simultaneously multiple pathways. Nutrients may directly interact with transcription factors modulating gene expression mainly at transcription level. Moreover, their central role as substrates in metabolic pathways conditions metabolic flux both through anabolic and catabolic processes. Furthermore, nutrient interaction with cellular receptors can alter cell signaling cascades which in turn affect gene expression (Fig. 15.1).

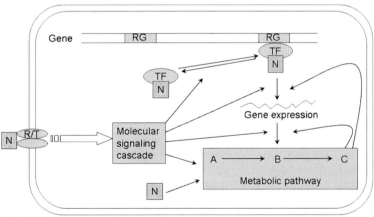

TF: Transcription factor
R/T: Cellular receptor/transporter
RG: Regulatory region
N: Nutrient

Fig. 15.1 Modulation of gene expression by dietary components. Dietary components can modulate gene expression by interaction with transcription factors modulating gene expression at transcriptional level or by direct and indirect effects on gene and regulatory regions. As substrates in metabolic pathways, nutrients condition metabolic flux either through anabolic or catabolic processes. Additionally, nutrient interaction with cellular proteins can alter signaling cascades which in turn affect gene expression

Obesity is a key etiological factor that predisposes to the development of metabolic syndrome and promotes insulin resistance. Insulin resistance in obesity is a reflection of a long-term nutrient excess and is manifested through complex, heterogeneous mechanisms that can involve increased fatty acid flux, nutrient overload, microhypoxia in adipose tissue, endoplasmic reticulum stress, secretion of adipocytes-derived cytokines, chronic tissue inflammation, genetic predisposition and CNS inputs.

Nutrigenomic Effects

Vitamin A-related compounds and specific fatty acids are good examples to analyze some of the effects on gene expression leading to certain obesity-linked phenotypes and to illustrate how this knowledge could be used as a potential target for the prevention of obesity.

The vitamin A vitamer retinoic acid, β-carotene and other naturally occurring carotenoids activate the expression of uncoupling proteins (UCPs) at the transcriptional level, which may play a role in the management of energy resources (Bonet et al. 2000; Puigserver et al. 1996; Serra et al. 1999). Furthermore, in rodents, treatment with retinoic acid causes a reduction of body adiposity that parallels a reduction in PPARγ levels in adipose tissue, associated with a reduced adipogenic/lipogenic potential. Furthermore, there is induction of UCP1 and UCP2 in brown adipocytes and of UCP3 in skeletal muscle which indicates increased thermogenic potential (Bonet et al. 2003). Similar metabolic adaptations are seen after chronic dietary supplementation with vitamin A, which appears to confer some resistance to the development of obesity under a high fat diet in obesity-prone mice (Felipe et al. 2003). Moreover, retinoic acid and vitamin A supplementation suppress the adipose expression of insulin resistance factors such as resistin (Felipe et al. 2004).

Obesity alters metabolic and endocrine function of adipose tissue and leads to an increased release of fatty acids, hormones and pro-inflammatory molecules that contribute to the associated complications of obesity. In obesity, adipose tissue contains an increased number of resident macrophages, which may constitute up to 40% of the cell population within adipose tissue depot (Weisberg et al. 2003; Xu et al. 2003). Adipocytes are able to synthesize and secrete the monocyte chemoattractant protein-1 (MCP-1), a recruiting factor for circulating monocytes (Christiansen et al. 2005). Accumulation of macrophages in adipose tissue may contribute to the enhanced systemic concentrations of pro-inflammatory cytokines in obesity such as TNFα, IL-6 and resistin. Specific fatty acids such as conjugated linoleic acid (CLA) may play a role in modulating inflammatory response in adipose tissue. A reduction in macrophage infiltration and down-regulation of several inflammatory markers in adipose tissue has been seen in mice fed a diet supplemented with cis-9, trans-11-CLA diet (Moloney et al. 2007). We have shown that feeding mice with equimolar mix of cis-9, trans-11- and trans-10, cis-12-CLA, in similar conditions to human CLA treatments, attenuates body fat deposition, without impairment of insulin sensitivity and of pro-inflammatory outcomes in adipose tissue (Parra et al. 2008).

Therefore, knowledge of nutrients with thermogenic, anti-adipogenic and/or anti-inflammatory properties could be useful in designing diets to help in control body fat content and body weight.

Nutrigenetic Interactions

The identification of gene variants associated with differential responses to diets/nutrients (both in terms of quantity and quality) is also very relevant, particularly in the obesity field, where a good number of candidate genes have been investigated for their potential involvement in the control of energy balance and the amount and distribution of body fat (see section on "Genetic influences in human obesity").

A good example of a nutrigenetic gene-diet interaction of relevance in the context of obesity is the finding that apolipoprotein A5 (ApoA5) gene variation can modulate the effects of dietary fat intake on BMI and obesity risk (Corella et al. 2007). In particular, an interaction was found between the -1131T>C polymorphism in the ApoA5 gene promoter and fat intake: individual homozygotes for the major allele (-1131T) show an increase in BMI associated with a higher fat intake, but this is not observed in the carriers of the -1131C minor allele (approximately 13% of the population) (Corella et al. 2007).

The Pro12Ala polymorphism in PPARγ (see section on "Genetic influences in human obesity") has also been associated with multiple gene-diet and environmental interactions (Meirhaeghe and Amouyel 2004; Memisoglu et al. 2003; Robitaille et al. 2003). For example, total dietary fat intake has been positively associated with BMI among ProPro individuals but not among Ala allele carriers (Memisoglu et al. 2003; Robitaille et al. 2003). Intake of monounsatured fat has been inversely associated with BMI among Ala carriers but not among ProPro women (Meirhaeghe and Amouyel 2004).

A number of interactions have been described involving dietary polyunsaturated fatty acids (PUFA), different gene variants, and plasma lipid profile as the outcome. For instance, a genetic polymorphism in PPARα (a PUFA-activated PPAR isoform relevant to the transcriptional control of hepatic fatty acid catabolism) may affect the response of plasma triacylglycerol levels to dietary PUFA intake. The gene for PPARα has a polymorphism at codon 162 that codifies for Leu or Val (Leu162Val). In men, the presence of the less common Val162 allele is associated with significantly higher serum concentrations of total cholesterol, LDL cholesterol, apo B, and apo C-III than in carriers of the Leu162 allele. In women, the trend is the same, but it is less pronounced (Tai et al. 2002). Increased intake of PUFAs had little effect on fasting triacylglycerol concentrations in persons with the common Leu162 allele, while in those with allele Val162, fasting triacylglycerol concentrations fell markedly with increasing PUFA intake (Dwyer et al. 2004). Thus, the well-known effect of PUFA in lowering plasma triacylglycerol levels in the general population is not found in carriers of a certain gene polymorphism.

Moreover, this is not the only genetic variant that is differently regulated by PUFA, which makes any attempt difficult to provide a simple dietary advice on genotype basis. For example, there are a number of genetic polymorphisms associated to apoA1, a key component of HDL. Both apoA1 and HDL cholesterol have been identified as protective factors for cardiovascular disease. Polymorphism -75G/A is located in the promoter of the ApoA1 gene and consists of a G/A substitution which is linked to a significant interaction in terms of HDL-cholesterol concentration and PUFA intake, particularly in women: HDL-cholesterol concentrations increase with increasing PUFA intake in carriers of the A allele, and the opposite effect is seen in women who are homozygous for the G allele in whom HDL-cholesterol concentrations decrease as PUFA intake increase (Ordovas et al. 2002).

Taking into account these two latter genetic combinations, in subjects who are homozygous for the Leu162 allele of PPARα and the -75G allele of Apo A1, an increased PUFA intake would decrease plasma HDL-cholesterol without affecting triacylglycerol concentration. Thus, the net effect would be an increase in cardiovascular risk, and a best dietary advice would be to consume less PUFA. On the contrary in view of these results, carriers of the variants Val162 of PPARα and -75A of Apo A1 should be advised to increase their PUFA intake (Ordovas 2006). This example illustrates the need to obtain sufficient information in order to make adequate dietary recommendations based on the impact of nutrients on gene expression and interaction with genotype combinations.

Nutrient Status Effects on Intracellular Signaling Pathways

Cells have several sensory systems that detect energy and metabolic status and adjust flux through metabolic pathways accordingly. Nutrients play a key role as signaling molecules and regulators of intermediary metabolism adjusting in an integrated manner nutrient availability and energy status at both the cellular and whole-body levels and then to coordinately regulate whole-body energy homeostasis. In fact, nutrients take on the attributes of hormones in that they circulate in the blood, bind to cell surface receptors and once internalized they alter signal transduction pathways and cellular metabolism (Marshall 2006).

Here we provide a functional and regulatory overview of the 5′ adenosine monophosphate-activated protein kinase (AMPK) and mammalian target of rapamycin (mTOR) signaling pathways to illustrate their crosstalk and connection between nutrients (glucose, amino acids) and insulin signaling and their potential role in the control of obesity.

AMPK is a central player in the maintenance of energy status. The adenosine monophosphate/adenosine-5′-triphosphate (AMP/ATP) ratio is a sensitive indicator of cellular energy status. Any metabolic stress, such as starvation, that raises the cellular AMP/ATP ratio (either by increasing the utilization of ATP or inhibiting its production) stimulates the AMPK pathway. When AMPK is activated, it stimulates fatty acid oxidation and glucose uptake and inhibits anabolic processes such as protein, fatty acid, glycogen and cholesterol synthesis. It functions both, acutely by directly phosphorylating enzymes involved in these pathways and long-term by regulating the expression of numerous genes (Lindsley and Rutter 2004).

Activated AMPK increases glucose transport into skeletal and cardiac muscle, independently of insulin action, increasing Glut4 and Glut1 translocation to the plasma membrane and increasing transcription of the gene Glut4. Following increased glucose uptake into cells, AMPK may increase flux through the glycolytic pathway while inhibiting glycogen synthesis. In liver, activation of AMPK reduces the expression of the genes for the gluconeogenic enzymes phosphoenolpyruvate carboxykinase (PEPCK) and glucose-6-phosphatase. Thus, it inhibits hepatic glucose output in an insulin-independent manner. Additionally, activation of AMPK results in the down-regulation of the Acetyl CoA carboxylase (ACC), which produces malonyl-CoA, an intermediate in the novo fatty acid synthesis and is also a potent inhibitor of carnitine-palmitoyl-CoA transferase (CPT1). Therefore, activated AMPK lowers malonyl-CoA levels, which simultaneously activates fatty acid oxidation and inhibits fatty acid synthesis. Cholesterol and triacylglycerol synthesis are also reduced via phosphorylation/inactivation of key enzymes. AMPK activation affects not only enzyme activity but also alters the expression of a number of genes at transcriptional and translational levels. In liver, AMPK activation causes the phosphorylation of the carbohydrate-response element-binding protein (ChREBP), thereby inhibiting the glucose-induced gene expression of pyruvate kinase, fatty acid synthase and ACC. It also suppresses expression of liver sterol-regulated-element binding protein-1 (SREBP-1), an important lipogenic transcription factor. AMPK has a global effect on protein synthesis, thus blocking the phosphorylation (activation) of the elongation factor 2 (eEF2) in the biosynthesis of proteins until ATP levels are restored and also inhibiting the mTOR signaling pathway (for a complete overview on the regulation of AMPK, see Lindsley and Rutter 2004; Towler and Hardie 2007).

It is already established that AMPK activation by pharmacological compounds (metformin, TZDs), adipokines (leptin, adiponectin) or physical activity causes many metabolic changes that would be beneficial for subjects with metabolic syndrome, such as increased glucose uptake and metabolism by muscle and other tissues, decreased glucose production by the liver and increased oxidation and decreased synthesis of fatty acids. Thus, the net effect of AMPK activation would be beneficial for the treatment of type 2 diabetes and insulin resistance. However, stimulation of the kinase signals nutrient starvation and its activation in pancreatic beta cells and hypothalamus may not result in fully beneficial effects for the treatment of obesity. For example, AMPK activation suppresses glucose-induced insulin secretion by inhibiting glucose metabolism and ATP production in pancreas and may stimulate appetite in the hypothalamus, therefore, contributing to obesity instead of counteracting it. AMPK activation is context specific and can be either beneficial or deleterious. Therefore, the widespread and diverse cellular functions of AMPK make its selective targeting difficult in therapeutics. Compounds that activate AMPK in peripheral tissues and inhibit it in hypothalamus would be ideal for obesity and glucose-insulin homeostasis (Viollet et al. 2007).

In contrast to AMPK, the mTOR (mammalian target of rapamycin) pathway is activated by nutrient-rich conditions, particularly by high levels of amino acids, being leucine the most effective stimulator, and by insulin. Interestingly, there is a cross talk between these two pathways and, for example, it has been shown that activated AMPK can inhibit mTOR function.

mTOR is a protein serine-threonine kinase that monitors intracellular amino acid availability and cellular energy status and links this information with external signals originating from cell surface receptors (such as insulin signaling). mTOR is an integral component of at least two multi-protein complexes (mTORC1 y mTORC2). mTORC1 contains the regulatory associated protein of mTOR (Raptor) and mTORC2 contains the rapamycin-insensitive companion of mTOR (Rictor) (Frias et al. 2006; Sarbassov et al. 2004). mTORC1 is the actual complex susceptible to rapamycin's action and is characterized by the classic features of mTOR by functioning as a sensor of nutrient and energy availability, redox status and controlling protein synthesis.

The most known function of mTOR is phosphorylation of proteins involved in the translation machinery of protein synthesis (Fig. 15.2) affecting both the initiation and elongation stages of mRNA translation.

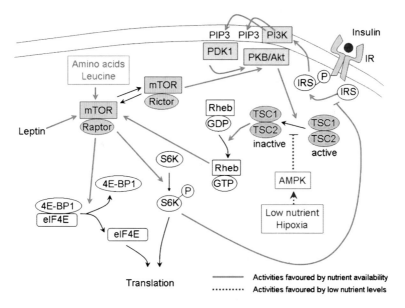

Fig. 15.2 A working model for the mTOR signaling pathway and its regulation by nutrients. mTOR is an integral component of at least two multi-protein complexes (mTORC1 and mTORC2). mTORC1 contains the regulatory associated protein of mTOR (Raptor) and mTORC2 contains the rapamycin-insensitive companion of mTOR (Rictor). Under nutrient availability, mTORC1 phosphorylates the ribosomal protein kinase S6K and the eukaryotic initiation factor 4E (eIF4E) binding protein 1 (4E-BP1) stimulating the initiation of protein synthesis. Additionally, mTORC1 phosphorylates 4E-BP1, which then releases eIF4E, allowing the formation of the initiation complex on the protein synthesis machinery. Therefore, mTORC1 affects both the initiation and elongation stages of mRNA translation. Insulin induces S6K activation through a signal transduction pathway that is initiated by insulin receptor (IR) autophosphorylation of IR substrates 1 and 2 (IRS) at multiple tyrosine residues. Then phosphoinositide 3-kinase (PI3K) leads to the production of PIP3 which recruits phosphoinositide-dependent protein kinase 1 (PDK1) and protein kinase B (Akt/PKB) to the plasma membrane. PDK1 can then phosphorylate and activate the kinase PKB. PKB is activated by the concerted action of the rapamycin insensitive Rictor-mTOR complex and PDK1, then subsequently phosphorylates the Tuberous Sclerosis Complex protein 2 (TSC2), inducing the degradation of the complex made by TSC2 and TSC1. In the active state, the GTPase-activating domain of TSC2 drives the small GTPase Ras homolog enriched in brain (Rheb) into the inactive GDP bound state. When inactive TSC2 leads to an increase in GTP bound Rheb which increases mTOR activity and further facilitates the phosphorylation of S6K1 and 4E-BP1. Under poor nutrient conditions, intracellular levels of AMP activate AMPK which phosphorylates and activates TSC2 then inhibiting mTORC1

Raptor might have roles in mTOR assembly, recruiting substrates to mTOR, and in regulating mTOR activity. The strength of the association between mTOR and raptor is regulated by nutrients (insulin and amino acids, particularly leucine) and other signals (Kim et al. 2002; Lian et al. 2008; Proud 2007). When stimulatory signals are sensed, such as high nutrient/energy levels, the mTOR-raptor interaction is weakened allowing mTOR kinase activity to be turned on. On the contrary, when stimulatory signals are withdrawn, such as low nutrient levels, the interaction is strengthened, essentially shutting off the kinase function of mTOR (Kim et al. 2002). In most cell types, the essential amino acid leucine appears to be the most important one for control of mTORC1 activity although other amino acids can also affect mTORC1 signaling (Beugnet et al. 2003). Interestingly, insulin signaling is confluent with the leucine-dependent activation of mTOR at the level of the ribosomal machinery for protein synthesis (Um et al. 2006) (see Fig. 15.2 for a more detailed description).

Under poor nutrient conditions, intracellular levels of AMP activate AMPK which phosphorylates and activates the Tuberous Sclerosis Complex protein 2 (TSC2), inhibiting mTORC1 (Huang and Manning 2008). mTOR signaling is also inhibited in conditions of hypoxia involving the participation of TSC1/2 complex. As oxygen is required for aerobic ATP production through mitochondrial oxidative phosphorylation, hypoxia causes energy stress and activates AMPK. Therefore, hypoxia, as found in obese adipocytes, can inhibit mTORC1 through AMPK-mediated phosphorylation and activation of the TSC1/2 complex (Huang and Manning 2008).

mTOR signaling plays an important role in the brain mechanisms to modulate food intake. Central administration of leucine increases hypothalamic mTOR signaling and decreases food intake. Leptin increases mTOR activity and rapamycin blunts leptin's anorectic effect (Cota et al. 2006). Consistent with this, rats fed on a low-protein diet show increased food intake and direct intracerebroventricular injection of leucine suppresses food intake, suggesting that leucine can act within the brain to inhibit food intake through mTOR signaling (Morrison et al. 2007). Interestingly, it has been shown that a high-protein diet is able to reduce body weight and fat deposition in both normal rats and *ob/ob* mice, which is associated to lower food intake but also to activation of the thermogenic capacity, decreased hypothalamic AMPK and increased mTOR activity and evidences that leucine would be the principal modulator (Ropelle et al. 2008).

Summary

Dietary compounds may act as regulators of gene expression at multiple levels, involving nutrigenomic effects, nutrigenetic interactions and modulation of intracellular signaling pathways. A better comprehension of the underlying mechanisms and their relationships would allow us to understand the phenotypes associated with obesity and get closer to potential targets for prevention and treatment of obesity.

Early Life Nutrition and Later Obesity

The notion that nutrition during early stages of life can predispose or program to suffer from certain diseases in adulthood, is becoming of increasingly significant interest, particularly since the last decade. In 1990, Barker proposed the hypothesis of "fetal origins of adult disease," which suggests that a poor fetal nutrition may cause adaptations that programs future propensity to obesity (Barker 1990). Since then, several epidemiological studies have shown that the nutritional conditions during critical stages of development, including the gestation and early postnatal period (primarily nursing) affect susceptibility to suffer from certain diseases in adulthood, including cardiovascular disease, obesity, type 2 diabetes, osteoporosis and other problems and alterations in health (see also Chapter17; Novak et al. 2006; Ong and Dunger 2004; Remacle et al. 2004; Valsamakis et al. 2006).

As it can be deduced from studies in animal models or in cultured cells, the differences are caused by the interaction between components of food or other environmental factors with our chromosomes, leading to an "imprinting" or programming of metabolic pathways in individuals that may confer a different susceptibility to suffer abnormalities in adulthood (Levin 2000). In this sense, the above referred concept of "programming" or "metabolic programming," is gaining importance in biomedical research, describing the processes whereby cells have a biological memory for external influences that can be passed on to daughter cells (Waterland and Garza 1999). It involves the concept that a stimulus or insult operating at a critical or sensitive period of development (the specific window of sensitivity) could result in a long-standing or life-long effect on the structure or function of the organism (Lucas 2000).

Metabolic imprinting on neural circuits and related processes involved in energy homeostasis during the perinatal period that can alter neuronal development may play an important role in setting the future patterns of body weight and fat gain in susceptible individuals (Levin 2000; Park 2005). Epigenetics refers to stable alterations in gene expression that do not involve mutations of the DNA itself while conferring stable maintenance of a particular gene expression pattern through mitotic cell division (Holliday and Pugh 1975). Because the pattern of DNA methylation is both stable and heritable, it has been considered that methylation is the main epigenetic basis for imprinting, and good evidence supports this connection (see Jirtle and Weidman 2007). Histone proteins also contribute and it has been suggested that DNA methylation is connected mechanically to histone modification (Jirtle and Weidman 2007).

According to Waterland and Garza (1999), metabolic imprinting encompasses adaptive responses to specific nutritional conditions early in life that are characterized by (1) susceptibility limited to a critical ontogenic period early in development (the critical window), (2) a persistent effect lasting into adulthood, (3) a specific and measurable outcome, and (4) a dose-response relationship between exposure and outcome.

Therefore, as subtle environmental influences during specific ontogenic periods can cause stable alterations in the mammalian epigenotype, early intervention in mothers and infants may be the way to prevent the formation of persistent neural connections that promote and perpetuate obesity in predisposed individuals. However, our knowledge of the biology underlying metabolic imprinting or programming is fairly limited.

Developmental Programming of Adulthood Obesity

Childhood and adult obesity are considered to be programmed by early life nutrition (Taylor and Poston 2007). First epidemiological studies in humans have focused on the relationship between low birth weight and the risk of obesity and metabolic syndrome in adulthood. However, there is also increasing evidence that excess weight and/or adiposity at birth is also associated with an increased risk of obesity in childhood and adulthood (Curhan et al. 1996). Thus, considering the relationship between early life nutrition and the incidence of obesity in later life, there are epidemiological studies that show an increased risk of obesity at both ends of the range of weights at birth. In particular, the following associations have been found (Martorell et al. 2001): (a) a poor nutrition during early stages of development increases the risk of obesity in adulthood, (b) at the other end, an overnutrition also increases the risk of obesity in adulthood, and (c) an optimal nutrition during infancy, represented by breastfeeding, is protective against later obesity. Several mechanisms have been proposed that may account for programming of adiposity, including disruptions in pancreatic structures and function, leading to alterations in insulin secretion and sensitivity, increases in the number and/or size of fat cell or alterations in adipose tissue function, and alterations in the development of the central nervous system, leading to an impairment in the feeding control (see Martorell et al. 2001).

Effects of Undernutrition in the Fetal Life on the Incidence of Obesity in Adulthood

Since 1990, when Barker proposed his hypothesis on the fetal origins of adult disease (Barker 1990), considerable epidemiological evidence has been published showing association between poor fetal growth with susceptibility to suffer from obesity and other diseases such as cardiovascular diseases, type 2 diabetes, and osteoporosis (see Langley-Evans 2004; Martorell et al. 2001).

An emblematic example is the Dutch famine that struck the western part of Holland during the Second World War. In a study involving 300,000 19 year-old men (when enlisted in the army) it was found that those who had been conceived during the last 6 months of the Second World War and whose mothers had experienced poor nutrition in the first and second quarter of their pregnancy were more prone to suffer from obesity than the children of those mothers who had not experienced hunger during this stage (Ravelli et al. 1999, 1976).

The most common and simple approach to estimate the importance of fetal nutrition on the incidence of obesity in adulthood has been to determine the weight at birth and their relationship with BMI in adulthood. Some of the studies in this area have found a J-shaped relationship between birth weight and later obesity, with values of BMI in adulthood higher for the highest weights of newborns and also for the lowest, compared with those born with a body weight around the mean.

An example of a study that shows these results is "The Nurses' Health Study I" (Curhan et al. 1996), that is based on 71,100 subjects aged 56 years. Other studies have failed to find such turning point for the values of low birth weight (Whitaker and Dietz 1998), so it is not clear that low birth weights are related to obesity in adulthood. However, other studies show that low birth weight can be predictive of other features of the metabolic syndrome, including type 2 diabetes, hypertension or hyperlipidemia (Barker et al. 1993; Hales et al. 1991). On the other hand, a high birth weight is generally associated with increased BMI in adulthood, but this increase can be explained in many cases by a greater accumulation of muscle mass (Singhal et al. 2003). Therefore, although birth weight is positively correlated with BMI in adulthood, it is also inversely associated with central obesity, insulin resistance, type 2 diabetes, cardiovascular disease, and in general with metabolic syndrome (Oken and Gillman 2003). Thus, we are faced with the seeming paradox of increased adiposity at both ends of the birth weight spectrum: higher BMI with higher birth weight and increased central obesity with lower birth weight (Oken and Gillman 2003).

The adverse effects of a poor fetal development on the incidence of cardiovascular disease and insulin resistance are exacerbated by a rapid catch-up growth (Ong et al. 2000; Taylor and Poston 2007). Some authors consider that catch-up growth in the first few weeks of postnatal life is particularly disadvantageous (Stettler et al. 2005), whereas other suggests that low birth weight children who grow excessively in later childhood are also at particular risk (Ong et al. 2000).

Effects of Overnutrition in the Fetal Life on the Incidence of Obesity in Adulthood. The Case of Gestational Diabetes

It is clear that the obesity prevalence is increasing significantly in developed countries, and it does not seem to be obvious that the reason or one of the reasons is due to undernutrition of the mother, but rather the opposite. In Europe and North America there is an increasingly high proportion of children born with high weight (4,500 g or higher) and this has been associated with an increased incidence of maternal obesity (see Surkan et al. 2004). Indeed, several studies have documented a clear relationship between maternal BMI and the incidence of high birth weight (see King 2006). For example, the increase from 25 to 36% in the incidence of overweight/obesity in mothers recorded in Sweden during the last decade has resulted in an approximately 25% increase in the incidence of high birth weight for gestational age (Surkan et al. 2004).

Many of the children with high weight at birth and suffering from obesity in adulthood are related to a gestational diabetes (Strauss 1997; Whitaker and Dietz 1998). Indeed the children of mothers with gestational diabetes have higher neonatal adiposity than children with same weight at birth whose mothers did not suffer from diabetes during pregnancy (Catalano et al. 2003). Insulin resistance that occurs with some frequency in the last stages of gestation is favored in obese women (King 2006). In fact, glucose intolerance, diabetes and gestational hyperlipidemia are much more common in obese women. They are associated with marked postprandial increases of glucose, lipids and amino acids in pregnant women. Therefore, the fetus is exposed to relatively high concentrations of these nutrients. Fetal hyperglycemia, in turn, leads to hyperinsulinemia and increased tissue and fat deposits. Consequently, babies of diabetic mothers are larger at birth compared to those born to nondiabetic mothers (Martorell et al. 2001). Of note, high birth weight associated with gestational diabetes seems to have different long term consequences compared to high birth weight not associated to gestational diabetes (Oken and Gillman 2003).

The association between maternal obesity with or without gestational diabetes and body composition of the developing child through adulthood requires further studies. Regardless of genetic factors, if pregnant women with high BMI deliver children with high birth weight that will also have a high BMI in adulthood, the worldwide increase in the prevalence of overweight and obesity in children and adolescents may perpetuate the problem.

Protective Effects of Breastfeeding Against Obesity

There is increasing epidemiological evidence suggesting that breastfeeding compared to infant formula confers protection against obesity later in life (Armstrong and Reilly 2002; Gillman et al. 2001; Harder et al. 2005; von Kries et al. 1999). A meta-analysis of the existing studies on duration of breastfeeding and risk of becoming overweight (Harder et al. 2005) strongly supports a dose-dependent association between a longer duration of breastfeeding and a decrease in the risk of becoming overweight.

A number of hypotheses can be raised as to the potential causes for the protective effect of breastfeeding, including differences in suckling patterns and in milk composition (Demmelmair et al. 2006). On the one hand, differences in mother-child-interaction between breast and formula fed infants as well as a different feeding behavior, with a higher suckling frequency in the case of breastfeeding, might play a role (Mathew and Bhatia 1989; Sievers et al. 2002). In addition, breastfeeding allows the infant to control intake based on internal satiety cues, thus helping infants to learn self-regulation of energy intake, whereas bottle-fed infants may be encouraged to finish bottle even if they are full (Dewey and Lonnerdal 1986; Sievers et al. 2002).

On the other hand, despite attempts by industry to produce breast milk-like infant formula, it is known that infant formula differs in composition with respect to mother's milk. Infant formula has, in general, increased caloric density than average values for breast milk (the energy supplied to children between 3 and 12 months of age has been estimated to be 10–18% higher in formula fed infants than in breastfed babies Heinig et al. 1993), and the difference is even greater in the protein content (the intake of protein per kg body weight is between 55 and 80% higher in formula than in breastfed infants until 6 months of age (Alexy et al. 1999). Such differences in milk composition could be significant. In fact, in rats, prenatal high protein exposure has been associated with a decrease in total energy expenditure and increased adiposity in the later life (Daenzer et al. 2002). During the postnatal period, a greater supply of protein and nutrients also results in increased deposition of fat and a higher body weight in adulthood (Kim et al. 1991). A high protein intake in excess of metabolic requirements may enhance the secretion of insulin and insulin like growth factor 1 (IGF1), increasing growth and adipogenic activity and adipocyte differentiation (see Demmelmair et al. 2006). In addition, high protein intakes may also decrease human growth hormone (hGH) secretion and lipolysis. These and other data support the hypothesis that a higher protein intake with infant formula than provided with breast milk and in excess of metabolic requirements may predispose an increased risk of obesity in adulthood (Koletzko et al. 2005).

In addition to the mentioned differences in the caloric content and macronutrients (mainly proteins) between breast milk and infant formula, it is possible that the protective effect of breast milk against the development of obesity in later life could be due to a particular component of the milk. Studies conducted in recent years in our laboratory have allowed us to discover a novel function for leptin during lactation – a protein that is naturally present in breast milk (Casabiell et al. 1997; Houseknecht et al. 1997) but is not present in infant formula (O'Connor et al. 2003) – to confer protection against the later development of overweight and other associated medical complications (see Palou et al. 2008; Palou and Pico 2009).

Leptin in the Regulation of Energy Balance. The Role of Breast Milk Leptin

Previously Known Functions of Leptin

Leptin is a hormone primarily produced and secreted by the adipose tissue, and its circulating levels correlate with the size of fat stores (Maffei et al. 1995; Ostlund et al. 1996). Leptin signals nutritional status and energy storage levels to feeding centers in the hypothalamus and other central areas, through its action on the expression and release of orexigenic and anorexigenic neuropeptides, including, respectively, neuropeptide Y (NPY) and pro-opiomelanocortin (POMC). In the arcuate nucleus, NPY and POMC neurons express the long form of leptin receptor (OB-Rb), which is functionally coupled to the Janus kinase-signal transducer and activator of transcription intracellular signaling cascade and produces an endogenous inhibitor (suppressor of cytokine signaling 3, SOCS-3) upon activation. This action prompts appropriate regulation of food intake and energy expenditure processes and, provided the system works well, helps our body to maintain the amount of fat stores within a certain range (Ahima and Flier 2000; Zhang et al. 1994). However, the vast majority of obese people have very high levels of circulating leptin in their blood and they appear to be resistant to the action of leptin. In fact, the administration of this hormone, while proven to be effective in reducing fat and normalizing metabolic disorders in leptin-deficient mice and humans, has not proven to be effective in most cases of obesity (Farooqi et al. 1999; Halaas et al. 1995; Pelleymounter et al. 1995).

Although leptin is mainly produced by the adipose tissue, this hormone is also produced by other tissues, such as stomach (Bado et al. 1998; Cinti et al. 2000, 2001), placenta (Masuzaki et al. 1997), skeletal muscle (Wang et al. 1998), and mammary epithelium (Smith-Kirwin et al. 1998) and it is naturally present in maternal milk (Casabiell et al. 1997; Houseknecht et al. 1997). While leptin produced by the adipose tissue is known to play a main role in the chronic control of energy balance, leptin produced by the stomach has been related to the short-term control of food intake, acting as a satiety signal (Cinti et al. 2001; Pico et al. 2002, 2003). There is evidence that feeding stimulates the secretion of leptin by the stomach in humans (Cinti et al. 2000, 2001) and in rats (Bado et al. 1998; Pico et al. 2002), and pepsinogen secretagogues such as cholecystokinin (CCK), gastrin or secretin also induce gastric leptin release in rats (Bado et al. 1998). Leptin receptors are present in the human stomach (Breidert et al. 1999) and in the mouse gastrointestinal tract (Morton et al. 1998). Additionally, leptin is capable of direct acute activation of vagal afferent neurons that originate in the gastric and intestinal walls and terminate in the nucleus tractus solitarius (Yuan et al. 1999), providing rapid information to the brain. These results suggest a role for gastric leptin in the short-term regulation of feeding, acting as a satiety signal (Cinti et al. 2001; Pico et al. 2002, 2003).

The New Function of Leptin in Breast Milk in the Prevention of Later Obesity

Leptin is produced by mammary epithelium (Smith-Kirwin et al. 1998) and is naturally present in breast milk (Casabiell et al. 1997; Houseknecht et al. 1997). Leptin concentrations in human milk vary significantly between people, and there is a positive correlation between leptin concentration in milk and maternal plasma leptin levels and adiposity (Houseknecht et al. 1997; Miralles et al. 2006; Uysal et al. 2002). Thus, breastfed infants nursed by severely obese mothers may be exposed to higher amounts of leptin than infants nursed by lean mothers, and much higher than those fed with infant formulas, which do not have leptin as an ingredient (O'Connor et al. 2003).

It was reported that leptin supplied by milk, or leptin supplied as a water solution, can be absorbed by the immature stomach of suckling rats (Casabiell et al. 1997; Oliver et al. 2002; Sanchez et al. 2005) and be transferred to the bloodstream (Casabiell et al. 1997; Sanchez et al. 2005). Of interest, this oral leptin in neonate rats could exert its physiological role, inhibiting food intake (Sanchez et al. 2005). This suggests that maternal milk leptin may control the amount of food intake of the offspring and probably plays other regulatory roles during development, at a time in which both the adipose tissue and appetite regulatory systems are immature (Sanchez et al. 2005).

Because (a) epidemiological evidence suggests that breastfeeding compared with infant formula provides protection against obesity later in life (Armstrong and Reilly 2002); (b) leptin is naturally present in the human breast milk (Casabiell et al. 1997) but not present in infant formula (O'Connor et al. 2003); and (c) our previous findings show that leptin orally administered to neonate rats can be absorbed by the immature stomach and inhibits food intake (Sanchez et al. 2005), we suggested the hypothesis that leptin could be the specific compound (or at least one of them) responsible of the beneficial effects of breast milk in providing protection against later obesity.

Concerning the role of breast milk leptin, a first indirect evidence was obtained in non-obese mothers and their children, showing an inverse association between leptin concentration in breast milk and body weight gain of their infants until the age of 2 years (Miralles et al. 2006). This evidence had been reinforced with the results obtained in rats supplemented with physiological doses of leptin during the suckling period, showing that the intake of leptin during this period prevents the development of overweight/obesity in adulthood (Pico et al. 2007; Sanchez et al. 2008), with an improvement of related parameters such as leptin and insulin sensitivity (Sanchez et al. 2008). Therefore, these results represent a direct cause-effect evidence of the role of leptin, as a component of breast milk, in the prevention of obesity in later life.

Interestingly, leptin supplementation of rats during lactation affected not only the amount of food intake in adulthood, which was lower than their controls, but also food preferences, in favor of a lower preference for fat-rich food than their controls (Sanchez et al. 2008). In humans, the failure to control obesity is generally associated with increased appetite and preference for highly caloric food, in addition to other factors such as reduced physical activity and increased lipogenic metabolism (Rissanen et al. 2002).

Thus, changes in food preferences in favor of less caloric food could be of interest to prevent obesity, particularly when energy-dense foods are widely available as in our developed societies. Other studies have also shown that changes during the perinatal period may influence long-term appetite and food preferences. In particular, exposure to a maternal low-protein diet during fetal life has been described to enhance fat preferences (Bellinger et al. 2004). Thus, maternal nutrition and nutrition during critical phases of development may promote changes in the systems involved in controlling appetite and the perception of palatability, and hence affect susceptibility to obesity.

The specific mechanisms involved in the programming effects of breast milk leptin remain to be further clarified but appear to be dependent on the leptin system. In fact, leptin seems to play a role during a critical window of development to ensure the normal development of hypothalamic pathways in the arcuate nucleus, which are important because they convey leptin signals to brain regions regulating body weight. An alteration in the development of these pathways may therefore alter the impact of leptin on energy homeostasis throughout life. In fact, it has been reported that neural projection pathways from the arcuate nucleus of the hypothalamus are permanently disrupted in leptin-deficient (Lepob/Lepob) mice (Bouret et al. 2004). Leptin treatment of leptin-deficient neonates with exogenous leptin has been shown to normalize the development of these neural projection pathways, but did not reverse these neuroanatomical defects when the treatment was made in adulthood (Bouret et al. 2004).

Thus, leptin seems to be an important factor that could explain, at least partially, the increased risk of obesity of formula-fed infants as compared to breastfed infants that is found in epidemiological studies. These findings open a new area of research on both the use of leptin in the design of more appropriate infant formula as well as the identification of potential factors influencing leptin levels in maternal milk, which are aspects of great relevance due to the increased prevalence of obesity and its associated health complications.

Summary

Environmental factors during perinatal life may be important determinants of the prevalence of obesity and their related pathologies in adulthood. The knowledge of the factors and the underlying mechanisms may be of interest to identify strategies to help prevention and treatment of these chronic pathologies.

Conclusions

In conclusion, considering that obesity is a chronic, multifactorial disease, new perspectives in obesity prevention and treatment are entailing the knowledge of candidate genes involved in body weight control, their variants and how they affect the propensity to develop obesity, the outcomes of gene-gene interactions, as well as how nutrients affect the expression of these genes. Moreover, individual characteristics, including adaptations during early development or exposure over long periods to particular diets or environmental factors, may also determine the propensity to adverse health outcomes in adult life, including obesity and its related metabolic pathologies. A better comprehension of these factors, the underlying mechanisms, and their interactions would allow us to perform more appropriate, personalized recommendations to curb obesity. This new focus to approach obesity is parallel to the consolidation of the relatively new sciences of nutrigenomics and nutrigenetics as well as the new omics disciplines transcriptomics, proteomics and metabolomics.

Acknowledgements European Commission (FP6-2004-FOOD-3-A 016181-2) and Spanish Government (grants AGL2006-04887/ALI, AGL2009-11277/ALI and AGL2006-27837-E). Our laboratory is a member of the European Research Network of Excellence NuGO (The European Nutrigenomics Organization, EU Contract: no. FP6-506360). The CIBER de Fisiopatología de la obesidad y nutrición is an initiative of the ISCIII

References

Aberle, J., Hopfer, I., Beil, F.U., & Seedorf, U. (2006). Association of peroxisome proliferator-activated receptor delta +294T/C with body mass index and interaction with peroxisome proliferator-activated receptor alpha L162V. *International Journal of Obesity (Lond), 30*, 1709–1713.

Ahima, R.S., & Flier, J.S. (2000). Leptin. *Annual Review of Physiology, 62*, 413–437.

Ailhaud, G., Massiera, F., Weill, P., Legrand, P., Alessandri, J.M., & Guesnet, P. (2006). Temporal changes in dietary fats: role of n-6 polyunsaturated fatty acids in excessive adipose tissue development and relationship to obesity. *Progress in Lipid Research, 45*, 203–236.

Alessi, M.C., Poggi, M., & Juhan-Vague, I. (2007). Plasminogen activator inhibitor-1, adipose tissue and insulin resistance. *Current Opinion in Lipidology, 18*, 240–245.

Alexy, U., Kersting, M., Sichert-Hellert, W., Manz, F., & Schoch, G. (1999). Macronutrient intake of 3- to 36-month-old German infants and children: results of the DONALD Study. Dortmund Nutritional and Anthropometric Longitudinally Designed Study. *Annals of Nutrition & Metabolism, 43*, 14–22.

Andersen, G., Wegner, L., Yanagisawa, K., Rose, C.S., Lin, J., Glumer, C., Drivsholm, T., Borch-Johnsen, K., Jorgensen, T., Hansen, T., Spiegelman, B.M., & Pedersen, O. (2005). Evidence of an association between genetic variation of the coactivator PGC-1beta and obesity. *Journal of Medical Genetics, 42*, 402–407.

Ando, T., Ichimaru, Y., Konjiki, F., Shoji, M., & Komaki, G. (2007). Variations in the preproghrelin gene correlate with higher body mass index, fat mass, and body dissatisfaction in young Japanese women. *American Journal of Clinical Nutrition, 86*, 25–32.

Andreasen, C.H., Mogensen, M.S., Borch-Johnsen, K., Sandbaek, A., Lauritzen, T., Sorensen, T.I., Hansen, L., Almind, K., Jorgensen, T., Pedersen, O., & Hansen, T. (2008). Non-replication of genome-wide based associations between common variants in INSIG2 and PFKP and obesity in studies of 18,014 Danes. *PLoS ONE, 3*, e2872.

Armstrong, J., & Reilly, J.J. (2002). Breastfeeding and lowering the risk of childhood obesity. *Lancet, 359*, 2003–2004.

Bado, A., Levasseur, S., Attoub, S., Kermorgant, S., Laigneau, J.P., Bortoluzzi, M.N., Moizo, L., Lehy, T., Guerre-Millo, M., Le Marchand-Brustel, Y., & Lewin, M.J. (1998). The stomach is a source of leptin. *Nature, 394*, 790–793.

Baessler, A., Hasinoff, M.J., Fischer, M., Reinhard, W., Sonnenberg, G.E., Olivier, M., Erdmann, J., Schunkert, H., Doering, A., Jacob, H.J., Comuzzie, A.G., Kissebah, A.H., & Kwitek, A.E. (2005). Genetic linkage and association of the growth hormone secretagogue receptor (ghrelin receptor) gene in human obesity. *Diabetes, 54*, 259–267.

Barker, D.J. (1990). The fetal and infant origins of adult disease. *British Medical Journal, 301*, 1111.

Barker, D.J., Hales, C.N., Fall, C.H., Osmond, C., Phipps, K., & Clark, P.M. (1993). Type 2 (non-insulin-dependent) diabetes mellitus, hypertension and hyperlipidaemia (syndrome X): relation to reduced fetal growth. *Diabetologia, 36*, 62–67.

Beckers, S., Peeters, A.V., Freitas, F., Mertens, I.L., Hendrickx, J.J., Van Gaal, L.F., & Van Hul, W. (2008). Analysis of genetic variations in the resistin gene shows no associations with obesity in women. *Obesity (Silver Spring), 16*, 905–907.

Bellinger, L., Lilley, C., & Langley-Evans, S.C. (2004). Prenatal exposure to a maternal low-protein diet programmes a preference for high-fat foods in the young adult rat. *The British Journal of Nutrition, 92*, 513–520.

Bence, K.K., Delibegovic, M., Xue, B., Gorgun, C.Z., Hotamisligil, G.S., Neel, B.G., & Kahn, B.B. (2006). Neuronal PTP1B regulates body weight, adiposity and leptin action. *Nature Medicine, 12*, 917–924.

Benzinou, M., Creemers, J.W., Choquet, H., Lobbens, S., Dina, C., Durand, E., Guerardel, A., Boutin, P., Jouret, B., Heude, B., Balkau, B., Tichet, J., Marre, M., Potoczna, N., Horber, F., Le Stunff, C., Czernichow, S., Sandbaek, A., Lauritzen, T., Borch-Johnsen, K., Andersen, G., Kiess, W., Korner, A., Kovacs, P., Jacobson, P., Carlsson, L.M., Walley, A.J., Jorgensen, T., Hansen, T., Pedersen, O., Meyre, D., & Froguel, P. (2008). Common nonsynonymous variants in PCSK1 confer risk of obesity. *Nature Genetics, 40*, 943–945.

Beugnet, A., Tee, A.R., Taylor, P.M., & Proud, C.G. (2003). Regulation of targets of mTOR (mammalian target of rapamycin) signalling by intracellular amino acid availability. *The Biochemical Journal, 372*, 555–566.

Bonet, M.L., Oliver, J., Pico, C., Felipe, F., Ribot, J., Cinti, S., & Palou, A. (2000). Opposite effects of feeding a vitamin A-deficient diet and retinoic acid treatment on brown adipose tissue uncoupling protein 1 (UCP1), UCP2 and leptin expression. *Journal of Endocrinology, 166*, 511–517.

Bonet, M.L., Ribot, J., Felipe, F., & Palou, A. (2003). Vitamin A and the regulation of fat reserves. *Cellular and Molecular Life Sciences, 60*, 1311–1321.

Bouchard, C., Tremblay, A., Despres, J. P., Nadeau, A., Lupien, P. J., Theriault, G., Dussault, J., Moorjani, S., Pinault, S., & Fournier, G. (1990). The response to long-term overfeeding in identical twins. *New England Journal of Medicine, 322*, 1477–1482.

Bouret, S.G., Draper, S.J., & Simerly, R.B. (2004). Trophic action of leptin on hypothalamic neurons that regulate feeding. *Science, 304*, 108–110.

Breidert, M., Miehlke, S., Glasow, A., Orban, Z., Stolte, M., Ehninger, G., Bayerdorffer, E., Nettesheim, O., Halm, U., Haidan, A., & Bornstein, S.R. (1999). Leptin and its receptor in normal human gastric mucosa and in Helicobacter pylori-associated gastritis. *Scandinavian Journal of Gastroenterology, 34*, 954–961.

Capanni, C., Mattioli, E., Columbaro, M., Lucarelli, E., Parnaik, V.K., Novelli, G., Wehnert, M., Cenni, V., Maraldi, N.M., Squarzoni, S., & Lattanzi, G. (2005). Altered pre-lamin A processing is a common mechanism leading to lipodystrophy. *Human Molecular Genetics, 14*, 1489–1502.

Carlsson, E., Almgren, P., Hoffstedt, J., Groop, L., & Ridderstrale, M. (2004). The FOXC2 C-512T polymorphism is associated with obesity and dyslipidemia. *Obesity Research, 12*, 1738–1743.

Casabiell, X., Pineiro, V., Tome, M.A., Peino, R., Dieguez, C., & Casanueva, F.F. (1997). Presence of leptin in colostrum and/or breast milk from lactating mothers: a potential role in the regulation of neonatal food intake. *The Journal of Clinical Endocrinology and Metabolism, 82*, 4270–4273.

Catalano, P.M., Thomas, A., Huston-Presley, L., & Amini, S.B. (2003). Increased fetal adiposity: a very sensitive marker of abnormal in utero development. *American Journal of Obstetrics and Gynecology, 189*, 1698–1704.

Cecil, J.E., Watt, P., Palmer, C.N., & Hetherington, M. (2006). Energy balance and food intake: the role of PPARgamma gene polymorphisms. *Physiology & Behavior, 88*, 227–233.

Cederberg, A., Gronning, L.M., Ahren, B., Tasken, K., Carlsson, P., & Enerback, S. (2001). FOXC2 is a winged helix gene that counteracts obesity, hypertriglyceridemia, and diet-induced insulin resistance. *Cell, 106*, 563–573.

Challis, B.G., Pritchard, L.E., Creemers, J.W., Delplanque, J., Keogh, J.M., Luan, J., Wareham, N.J., Yeo, G.S., Bhattacharyya, S., Froguel, P., White, A., Farooqi, I.S., & O'Rahilly, S. (2002). A missense mutation disrupting a dibasic prohormone processing site in pro-opiomelanocortin (POMC) increases susceptibility to early-onset obesity through a novel molecular mechanism. *Human Molecular Genetics, 11*, 1997–2004.

Cheyssac, C., Lecoeur, C., Dechaume, A., Bibi, A., Charpentier, G., Balkau, B., Marre, M., Froguel, P., Gibson, F., & Vaxillaire, M. (2006). Analysis of common PTPN1 gene variants in type 2 diabetes, obesity and associated phenotypes in the French population. *BMC Medical Genetics, 7*, 44.

Christiansen, T., Richelsen, B., & Bruun, J.M. (2005). Monocyte chemoattractant protein-1 is produced in isolated adipocytes, associated with adiposity and reduced after weight loss in morbid obese subjects. *International Journal of Obesity (Lond), 29*, 146–150.

Christodoulides, C., Scarda, A., Granzotto, M., Milan, G., Dalla Nora, E., Keogh, J., De Pergola, G., Stirling, H., Pannacciulli, N., Sethi, J.K., Federspil, G., Vidal-Puig, A., Farooqi, I.S., O'Rahilly, S., & Vettor, R. (2006). WNT10B mutations in human obesity. *Diabetologia, 49*, 678–684.

Chung, W.K., Patki, A., Matsuoka, N., Boyer, B.B., Liu, N., Musani, S.K., Goropashnaya, A.V., Tan, P.L., Katsanis, N., Johnson, S.B., Gregersen, P.K., Allison, D.B., Leibel, R.L., & Tiwari, H.K. (2008). Analysis of 30 genes (355 SNPS) related to energy homeostasis for association with adiposity in European-American and Yup'ik Eskimo populations. *Human Heredity, 67*, 193–205.

Cinti, S., De Matteis, R., Pico, C., Ceresi, E., Obrador, A., Maffeis, C., Oliver, J., & Palou, A. (2000). Secretory granules of endocrine and chief cells of human stomach mucosa contain leptin. *International Journal of Obesity and Related Metabolic Disorders, 24*, 789–793.

Cinti, S., De Matteis, R., Ceresi, E., Pico, C., Oliver, J., Oliver, P., Palou, A., Obrador, A., & Maffeis, C. (2001). Leptin in the human stomach. *Gut, 49*, 155.

Corella, D., Qi, L., Sorli, J.V., Godoy, D., Portoles, O., Coltell, O., Greenberg, A.S., & Ordovas, J.M. (2005). Obese subjects carrying the 11482G>A polymorphism at the perilipin locus are resistant to weight loss after dietary energy restriction. *The Journal of Clinical Endocrinology and Metabolism, 90*, 5121–5126.

Corella, D., Lai, C.Q., Demissie, S., Cupples, L.A., Manning, A.K., Tucker, K.L., & Ordovas, J.M. (2007). APOA5 gene variation modulates the effects of dietary fat intake on body mass index and obesity risk in the Framingham Heart Study. *Journal of Molecular Medicine, 85*, 119–128.

Cota, D., Proulx, K., Smith, K.A., Kozma, S.C., Thomas, G., Woods, S.C., & Seeley, R.J. (2006). Hypothalamic mTOR signaling regulates food intake. *Science, 312*, 927–930.

Cummings, D.E. (2006). Ghrelin and the short- and long-term regulation of appetite and body weight. *Physiology & Behavior, 89*, 71–84.

Curhan, G.C., Chertow, G.M., Willett, W.C., Spiegelman, D., Colditz, G.A., Manson, J.E., Speizer, F.E., & Stampfer, M.J. (1996). Birth weight and adult hypertension and obesity in women. *Circulation, 94*, 1310–1315.

Daenzer, M., Ortmann, S., Klaus, S., & Metges, C.C. (2002). Prenatal high protein exposure decreases energy expenditure and increases adiposity in young rats. *The Journal of Nutrition, 132*, 142–144.

Dahlman, I., & Arner, P. (2007). Obesity and polymorphisms in genes regulating human adipose tissue. *International Journal of Obesity (Lond), 31*, 1629–1641.

Dahlman, I., Kaaman, M., Jiao, H., Kere, J., Laakso, M., & Arner, P. (2005). The CIDEA gene V115F polymorphism is associated with obesity in Swedish subjects. *Diabetes, 54*, 3032–3034.

Dahlman, I., Dicker, A., Jiao, H., Kere, J., Blomqvist, L., van Harmelen, V., Hoffstedt, J., Borch-Johnsen, K., Jorgensen, T., Hansen, T., Pedersen, O., Laakso, M., & Arner, P. (2007). A common haplotype in the G-protein-coupled receptor gene GPR74 is associated with leanness and increased lipolysis. *American Journal of Human Genetics, 80*, 1115–1124.

Dalgaard, L.T., & Pedersen, O. (2001). Uncoupling proteins: functional characteristics and role in the pathogenesis of obesity and Type II diabetes. *Diabetologia, 44*, 946–965.

Davis, K.E., Moldes, M., & Farmer, S.R. (2004). The forkhead transcription factor FoxC2 inhibits white adipocyte differentiation. *The Journal of Biological Chemistry, 279*, 42453–42461.

de Luis Roman, D., de la Fuente, R.A., Sagrado, M.G., Izaola, O., & Vicente, R.C. (2006). Leptin receptor Lys656Asn polymorphism is associated with decreased leptin response and weight loss secondary to a lifestyle modification in obese patients. *Archives of Medical Research, 37*, 854–859.

Demmelmair, H., von Rosen, J., & Koletzko, B. (2006). Long-term consequences of early nutrition. *Early Human Development, 82*, 567–574.

Dewey, K.G., & Lonnerdal, B. (1986). Infant self-regulation of breast milk intake. *Acta Paediatrica Scandinavica, 75*, 893–898.

Dobrzyn, A., & Ntambi, J.M. (2005). The role of stearoyl-CoA desaturase in the control of metabolism. *Prostaglandins, Leukotrienes, and Essential Fatty Acids, 73*, 35–41.

Dolley, G., Bertrais, S., Frochot, V., Bebel, J.F., Guerre-Millo, M., Tores, F., Rousseau, F., Hager, J., Basdevant, A., Hercberg, S., Galan, P., Oppert, J.M., Lacorte, J.M., & Clement, K. (2008). Promoter adiponectin polymorphisms and waist/hip ratio variation in a prospective French adults study. *International Journal of Obesity (Lond), 32*, 669–675.

Dwyer, J.H., Allayee, H., Dwyer, K.M., Fan, J., Wu, H., Mar, R., Lusis, A.J., & Mehrabian, M. (2004). Arachidonate 5-lipoxygenase promoter genotype, dietary arachidonic acid, and atherosclerosis. *New England Journal of Medicine, 350*, 29–37.

Eberle, D., Clement, K., Meyre, D., Sahbatou, M., Vaxillaire, M., Le Gall, A., Ferre, P., Basdevant, A., Froguel, P., & Foufelle, F. (2004). SREBF-1 gene polymorphisms are associated with obesity and type 2 diabetes in French obese and diabetic cohorts. *Diabetes, 53*, 2153–2157.

Esterbauer, H., Oberkofler, H., Linnemayr, V., Iglseder, B., Hedegger, M., Wolfsgruber, P., Paulweber, B., Fastner, G., Krempler, F., & Patsch, W. (2002). Peroxisome proliferator-activated receptor-gamma coactivator-1 gene locus: associations with obesity indices in middle-aged women. *Diabetes, 51*, 1281–1286.

Fan, W., Voss-Andreae, A., Cao, W.H., & Morrison, S.F. (2005). Regulation of thermogenesis by the central melanocortin system. *Peptides, 26*, 1800–1813.

Farooqi, I.S., Jebb, S.A., Langmack, G., Lawrence, E., Cheetham, C.H., Prentice, A.M., Hughes, I.A., McCamish, M.A., & O'Rahilly, S. (1999). Effects of recombinant leptin therapy in a child with congenital leptin deficiency. *New England Journal of Medicine, 341*, 879–884.

Felipe, F., Bonet, M.L., Ribot, J., & Palou, A. (2003). Up-regulation of muscle uncoupling protein 3 gene expression in mice following high fat diet, dietary vitamin A supplementation and acute retinoic acid-treatment. *International Journal of Obesity and Related Metabolic Disorders, 27*, 60–69.

Felipe, F., Bonet, M.L., Ribot, J., & Palou, A. (2004). Modulation of resistin expression by retinoic acid and vitamin A status. *Diabetes, 53*, 882–889.

Frias, M.A., Thoreen, C.C., Jaffe, J.D., Schroder, W., Sculley, T., Carr, S.A., & Sabatini, D.M. (2006). mSin1 is necessary for Akt/PKB phosphorylation, and its isoforms define three distinct mTORC2s. *Current Biology, 16*, 1865–1870.

Fu, Y., Luo, N., Klein, R.L., & Garvey, W.T. (2005). Adiponectin promotes adipocyte differentiation, insulin sensitivity, and lipid accumulation. *Journal of Lipid Research, 46*, 1369–1379.

Furnsinn, C., Willson, T.M., & Brunmair, B. (2007). Peroxisome proliferator-activated receptor-delta, a regulator of oxidative capacity, fuel switching and cholesterol transport. *Diabetologia, 50*, 8–17.

Garcia, E.A., Heude, B., Petry, C.J., Gueorguiev, M., Hassan-Smith, Z.K., Spanou, A., Ring, S.M., Dunger, D.B., Wareham, N., Sandhu, M.S., Ong, K.K., & Korbonits, M. (2008). Ghrelin receptor gene polymorphisms and body size in children and adults. *The Journal of Clinical Endocrinology and Metabolism, 93*, 4158–4161.

Gillman, M.W., Rifas-Shiman, S.L., Camargo, C.A., Jr., Berkey, C.S., Frazier, A.L., Rockett, H.R., Field, A.E., & Colditz, G.A. (2001). Risk of overweight among adolescents who were breastfed as infants. *The Journal of the American Medical Association, 285*, 2461–2467.

Goldstein, B.J., Ahmad, F., Ding, W., Li, P.M., & Zhang, W.R. (1998). Regulation of the insulin signalling pathway by cellular protein-tyrosine phosphatases. *Molecular and Cellular Biochemistry, 182*, 91–99.

Goldstein, J.L., DeBose-Boyd, R.A., & Brown, M.S. (2006). Protein sensors for membrane sterols. *Cell, 124*, 35–46.

Grarup, N., Albrechtsen, A., Ek, J., Borch-Johnsen, K., Jorgensen, T., Schmitz, O., Hansen, T., & Pedersen, O. (2007). Variation in the peroxisome proliferator-activated receptor delta gene in relation to common metabolic traits in 7,495 middle-aged white people. *Diabetologia, 50*, 1201–1208.

Gummesson, A., Jernas, M., Svensson, P.A., Larsson, I., Glad, C.A., Schele, E., Gripeteg, L., Sjoholm, K., Lystig, T.C., Sjostrom, L., Carlsson, B., Fagerberg, B., & Carlsson, L.M. (2007). Relations of adipose tissue CIDEA gene expression to basal metabolic rate, energy restriction, and obesity: population-based and dietary intervention studies. *The Journal of Clinical Endocrinology and Metabolism, 92*, 4759–4765.

Guo, Y.F., Xiong, D.H., Shen, H., Zhao, L.J., Xiao, P., Guo, Y., Wang, W., Yang, T.L., Recker, R.R., & Deng, H.W. (2006). Polymorphisms of the low-density lipoprotein receptor-related protein 5 (LRP5) gene are associated with obesity phenotypes in a large family-based association study. *Journal of Medical Genetics, 43*, 798–803.

Hager, J., Clement, K., Francke, S., Dina, C., Raison, J., Lahlou, N., Rich, N., Pelloux, V., Basdevant, A., Guy-Grand, B., North, M., & Froguel, P. (1998). A polymorphism in the 5' untranslated region of the human ob gene is associated with low leptin levels. *International Journal of Obesity and Related Metabolic Disorders, 22*, 200–205.

Halaas, J.L., Gajiwala, K.S., Maffei, M., Cohen, S.L., Chait, B.T., Rabinowitz, D., Lallone, R.L., Burley, S.K., & Friedman, J.M. (1995). Weight-reducing effects of the plasma protein encoded by the obese gene. *Science, 269*, 543–546.

Hales, C.N., Barker, D.J., Clark, P.M., Cox, L.J., Fall, C., Osmond, C., & Winter, P.D. (1991). Fetal and infant growth and impaired glucose tolerance at age 64. *British Medical Journal, 303*, 1019–1022.

Handschin, C., & Spiegelman, B.M. (2006). Peroxisome proliferator-activated receptor gamma coactivator 1 coactivators, energy homeostasis, and metabolism. *Endocrine Reviews, 27*, 728–735.

Hannemann, A., Jandrig, B., Gaunitz, F., Eschrich, K., & Bigl, M. (2005). Characterization of the human P-type 6-phosphofructo-1-kinase gene promoter in neural cell lines. *Gene, 345*, 237–247.

Hara-Chikuma, M., Sohara, E., Rai, T., Ikawa, M., Okabe, M., Sasaki, S., Uchida, S., & Verkman, A.S. (2005). Progressive adipocyte hypertrophy in aquaporin-7-deficient mice: adipocyte glycerol permeability as a novel regulator of fat accumulation. *The Journal of Biological Chemistry, 280*, 15493–15496.

Harder, T., Bergmann, R., Kallischnigg, G., & Plagemann, A. (2005). Duration of breastfeeding and risk of overweight: a meta-analysis. *American Journal of Epidemiology, 162*, 397–403.

Harper, M.E., Dent, R., Monemdjou, S., Bezaire, V., Van Wyck, L., Wells, G., Kavaslar, G.N., Gauthier, A., Tesson, F., & McPherson, R. (2002). Decreased mitochondrial proton leak and reduced expression of uncoupling protein 3 in skeletal muscle of obese diet-resistant women. *Diabetes, 51*, 2459–2466.

Hauner, H., Entenmann, G., Wabitsch, M., Gaillard, D., Ailhaud, G., Negrel, R., & Pfeiffer, E.F. (1989). Promoting effect of glucocorticoids on the differentiation of human adipocyte precursor cells cultured in a chemically defined medium. *The Journal of Clinical Investigation, 84*, 1663–1670.

Hegele, R.A., Cao, H., Harris, S.B., Zinman, B., Hanley, A.J., & Anderson, C.M. (2000). Genetic variation in LMNA modulates plasma leptin and indices of obesity in aboriginal Canadians. *Physiological Genomics, 3*, 39–44.

Hegele, R.A., Huff, M.W., & Young, T.K. (2001). Common genomic variation in LMNA modulates indexes of obesity in Inuit. *The Journal of Clinical Endocrinology and Metabolism, 86*, 2747–2751.

Heinig, M.J., Nommsen, L.A., Peerson, J.M., Lonnerdal, B., & Dewey, K.G. (1993). Energy and protein intakes of breast-fed and formula-fed infants during the first year of life and their association with growth velocity: the DARLING Study. *American Journal of Clinical Nutrition, 58*, 152–161.

Herbert, A., Gerry, N.P., McQueen, M.B., Heid, I.M., Pfeufer, A., Illig, T., Wichmann, H.E., Meitinger, T., Hunter, D., Hu, F.B., Colditz, G., Hinney, A., Hebebrand, J., Koberwitz, K., Zhu, X., Cooper, R., Ardlie, K., Lyon, H., Hirschhorn, J.N., Laird, N.M., Lenburg, M.E., Lange, C., & Christman, M.F. (2006). A common genetic variant is associated with adult and childhood obesity. *Science, 312*, 279–283.

Hibuse, T., Maeda, N., Funahashi, T., Yamamoto, K., Nagasawa, A., Mizunoya, W., Kishida, K., Inoue, K., Kuriyama, H., Nakamura, T., Fushiki, T., Kihara, S., & Shimomura, I. (2005). Aquaporin 7 deficiency is associated with development of obesity through activation of adipose glycerol kinase. *Proceedings of the National Academy of Sciences of the United States of America, 102*, 10993–10998.

Himms-Hagen, J. (1989). Brown adipose tissue thermogenesis and obesity. *Progress in Lipid Research, 28*, 67–115.

Hoffstedt, J., Andersson, I.L., Persson, L., Isaksson, B., & Arner, P. (2002). The common -675 4G/5G polymorphism in the plasminogen activator inhibitor-1 gene is strongly associated with obesity. *Diabetologia, 45*, 584–587.

Holliday, R., & Pugh, J.E. (1975). DNA modification mechanisms and gene activity during development. *Science, 187*, 226–232.

Horton, J.D., Goldstein, J.L., & Brown, M.S. (2002). SREBPs: activators of the complete program of cholesterol and fatty acid synthesis in the liver. *The Journal of Clinical Investigation, 109*, 1125–1131.

Horton, J.D., Shimomura, I., Ikemoto, S., Bashmakov, Y., & Hammer, R.E. (2003). Overexpression of sterol regulatory element-binding protein-1a in mouse adipose tissue produces adipocyte hypertrophy, increased fatty acid secretion, and fatty liver. *The Journal of Biological Chemistry, 278*, 36652–36660.

Houseknecht, K.L., McGuire, M.K., Portocarrero, C.P., McGuire, M.A., & Beerman, K. (1997). Leptin is present in human milk and is related to maternal plasma leptin concentration and adiposity. *Biochemical and Biophysical Research Communications, 240*, 742–747.

Huang, J., & Manning, B.D. (2008). The TSC1-TSC2 complex: a molecular switchboard controlling cell growth. *The Biochemical Journal, 412*, 179–190.

Huss, J.M., Torra, I.P., Staels, B., Giguere, V., & Kelly, D.P. (2004). Estrogen-related receptor alpha directs peroxisome proliferator-activated receptor alpha signaling in the transcriptional control of energy metabolism in cardiac and skeletal muscle. *Molecular and Cellular Biology, 24*, 9079–9091.

Huth, C., Illig, T., Herder, C., Gieger, C., Grallert, H., Vollmert, C., Rathmann, W., Hamid, Y.H., Pedersen, O., Hansen, T., Thorand, B., Meisinger, C., Doring, A., Klopp, N., Gohlke, H., Lieb, W., Hengstenberg, C., Lyssenko, V., Groop, L., Ireland, H., Stephens, J.W., Wernstedt Asterholm, I., Jansson, J.O., Boeing, H., Mohlig, M., Stringham, H M., Boehnke, M., Tuomilehto, J., Fernandez-Real, J.M., Lopez-Bermejo, A., Gallart, L., Vendrell, J., Humphries, S.E., Kronenberg, F., Wichmann, H.E., & Heid, I.M. (2008). Joint analysis of individual participants' data from 17 studies on the association of the IL6 variant -174G >C with circulating glucose levels, interleukin-6 levels, and body mass index. *Annals of Medicine, 27*, 1–21.

International Obesity Task Force (2009). London (February 1, 2009); http://www.iotf.org

Jansson, J.O., Wallenius, K., Wernstedt, I., Ohlsson, C., Dickson, S.L., & Wallenius, V. (2003). On the site and mechanism of action of the anti-obesity effects of interleukin-6. *Growth Hormone & IGF Research, 13 Suppl A*, S28–S32.

Jiang, Y., Wilk, J.B., Borecki, I., Williamson, S., DeStefano, A.L., Xu, G., Liu, J., Ellison, R.C., Province, M., & Myers, R.H. (2004). Common variants in the 5′ region of the leptin gene are associated with body mass index in men from the National Heart, Lung, and Blood Institute Family Heart Study. *American Journal of Human Genetics, 75*, 220–230.

Jirtle, R.L., & Weidman, J.R. (2007). Imprinted and more equal. *American Scientist, 95*, 143–149.

Johansson, L.E., Hoffstedt, J., Parikh, H., Carlsson, E., Wabitsch, M., Bondeson, A.G., Hedenbro, J., Tornqvist, H., Groop, L., & Ridderstrale, M. (2006). Variation in the adiponutrin gene influences its expression and associates with obesity. *Diabetes, 55*, 826–833.

Johansson, L.E., Lindblad, U., Larsson, C.A., Rastam, L., & Ridderstrale, M. (2008). Polymorphisms in the adiponutrin gene are associated with increased insulin secretion and obesity. *European Journal of Endocrinology, 159*, 577–583.

Kadowaki, T., Yamauchi, T., & Kubota, N. (2008). The physiological and pathophysiological role of adiponectin and adiponectin receptors in the peripheral tissues and CNS. *FEBS Letters, 582*, 74–80.

Kamei, Y., Ohizumi, H., Fujitani, Y., Nemoto, T., Tanaka, T., Takahashi, N., Kawada, T., Miyoshi, M., Ezaki, O., & Kakizuka, A. (2003). PPARgamma coactivator 1beta/ERR ligand 1 is an ERR protein ligand, whose expression induces a high-energy expenditure and antagonizes obesity. *Proceedings of the National Academy of Sciences of the United States of America, 100*, 12378–12383.

Kamei, Y., Lwin, H., Saito, K., Yokoyama, T., Yoshiike, N., Ezaki, O., & Tanaka, H. (2005). The 2.3 genotype of ESRRA23 of the ERR alpha gene is associated with a higher BMI than the 2.2 genotype. *Obesity Research, 13*, 1843–1844.

Kim, J.B., & Spiegelman, B.M. (1996). ADD1/SREBP1 promotes adipocyte differentiation and gene expression linked to fatty acid metabolism. *Genes & Development, 10*, 1096–1107.

Kim, S.H., Mauron, J., Gleason, R., & Wurtman, R. (1991). Selection of carbohydrate to protein ratio and correlations with weight gain and body fat in rats allowed three dietary choices. *International Journal for Vitamin and Nutrition Research, 61*, 166–179.

Kim, D.H., Sarbassov, D.D., Ali, S.M., King, J.E., Latek, R.R., Erdjument-Bromage, H., Tempst, P., & Sabatini, D.M. (2002). mTOR interacts with raptor to form a nutrient-sensitive complex that signals to the cell growth machinery. *Cell, 110*, 163–175.

Kim, J.Y., van de Wall, E., Laplante, M., Azzara, A., Trujillo, M.E., Hofmann, S.M., Schraw, T., Durand, J.L., Li, H., Li, G., Jelicks, L.A., Mehler, M.F., Hui, D.Y., Deshaies, Y., Shulman, G.I., Schwartz, G.J., & Scherer, P.E. (2007). Obesity-associated improvements in metabolic profile through expansion of adipose tissue. *The Journal of Clinical Investigation, 117*, 2621–2637.

King, J.C. (2006). Maternal obesity, metabolism, and pregnancy outcomes. *Annual Review of Nutrition, 26*, 271–291.

Kipfer-Coudreau, S., Eberle, D., Sahbatou, M., Bonhomme, A., Guy-Grand, B., Froguel, P., Galan, P., Basdevant, A., & Clement, K. (2004). Single nucleotide polymorphisms of protein tyrosine phosphatase 1B gene are associated with obesity in morbidly obese French subjects. *Diabetologia, 47*, 1278–1284.

Koletzko, B., Broekaert, I., Demmelmair, H., Franke, J., Hannibal, I., Oberle, D., Schiess, S., Baumann, B.T., & Verwied-Jorky, S. (2005). Protein intake in the first year of life: a risk factor for later obesity? The E.U. childhood obesity project. *Advances in Experimental Medicine and Biology, 569*, 69–79.

Korner, A., Ma, L., Franks, P.W., Kiess, W., Baier, L.J., Stumvoll, M., & Kovacs, P. (2007). Sex-specific effect of the Val1483Ile polymorphism in the fatty acid synthase gene (FAS) on body mass index and lipid profile in Caucasian children. *International Journal of Obesity (Lond), 31*, 353–358.

Kovacs, P., Lehn-Stefan, A., Stumvoll, M., Bogardus, C., & Baier, L.J. (2003). Genetic variation in the human winged helix/forkhead transcription factor gene FOXC2 in Pima Indians. *Diabetes, 52*, 1292–1295.

Kovacs, P., Harper, I., Hanson, R.L., Infante, A.M., Bogardus, C., Tataranni, P.A., & Baier, L.J. (2004). A novel missense substitution (Val1483Ile) in the fatty acid synthase gene (FAS) is associated with percentage of body fat and substrate oxidation rates in nondiabetic Pima Indians. *Diabetes, 53,* 1915–1919.

Lagou, V., Scott, R.A., Manios, Y., Chen, T.L., Wang, G., Grammatikaki, E., Kortsalioudaki, C., Liarigkovinos, T., Moschonis, G., Roma-Giannikou, E., & Pitsiladis, Y.P. (2008). Impact of peroxisome proliferator-activated receptors gamma and delta on adiposity in toddlers and preschoolers in the GENESIS Study. *Obesity (Silver Spring), 16,* 913–918.

Lagouge, M., Argmann, C., Gerhart-Hines, Z., Meziane, H., Lerin, C., Daussin, F., Messadeq, N., Milne, J., Lambert, P., Elliott, P., Geny, B., Laakso, M., Puigserver, P., & Auwerx, J. (2006). Resveratrol improves mitochondrial function and protects against metabolic disease by activating SIRT1 and PGC-1alpha. *Cell, 127,* 1109–1122.

Lane, M.D., Wolfgang, M., Cha, S.H., & Dai, Y. (2008). Regulation of food intake and energy expenditure by hypothalamic malonyl-CoA. *International Journal of Obesity (Lond), 32 Suppl 4,* S49–S54.

Langin, D., Dicker, A., Tavernier, G., Hoffstedt, J., Mairal, A., Ryden, M., Arner, E., Sicard, A., Jenkins, C.M., Viguerie, N., van Harmelen, V., Gross, R.W., Holm, C., & Arner, P. (2005). Adipocyte lipases and defect of lipolysis in human obesity. *Diabetes, 54,* 3190–3197.

Langley-Evans, S.C. (2004). *Fetal nutrition and adult disease. Programming of chronic disease through fetal exposure to undernutrition.* Oxfordshire: CABI Publishing.

Larsen, L.H., Rose, C.S., Sparso, T., Overgaard, J., Torekov, S.S., Grarup, N., Jensen, D.P., Albrechtsen, A., Andersen, G., Ek, J., Glumer, C., Borch-Johnsen, K., Jorgensen, T., Hansen, T., & Pedersen, O. (2007). Genetic analysis of the estrogen-related receptor alpha and studies of association with obesity and type 2 diabetes. *International Journal of Obesity (Lond), 31,* 365–370.

Lavebratt, C., Wahlqvist, S., Nordfors, L., Hoffstedt, J., & Arner, P. (2005). AHSG gene variant is associated with leanness among Swedish men. *Human Genetics, 117,* 54–60.

Le Stunff, C., Fallin, D., Schork, N.J., & Bougneres, P. (2000). The insulin gene VNTR is associated with fasting insulin levels and development of juvenile obesity. *Nature Genetics, 26,* 444–446.

Levin, B.E. (2000). The obesity epidemic: metabolic imprinting on genetically susceptible neural circuits. *Obesity Research, 8,* 342–347.

Li, S., & Loos, R.J. (2008). Progress in the genetics of common obesity: size matters. *Current Opinion in Lipidology, 19,* 113–121.

Li, W.D., Reed, D.R., Lee, J.H., Xu, W., Kilker, R.L., Sodam, B.R., & Price, R.A. (1999). Sequence variants in the 5′ flanking region of the leptin gene are associated with obesity in women. *Annals of Human Genetics, 63,* 227–234.

Lian, J., Yan, X.H., Peng, J., & Jiang, S.W. (2008). The mammalian target of rapamycin pathway and its role in molecular nutrition regulation. *Molecular Nutrition and Food Research, 52,* 393–399.

Lin, W.H., Chiu, K.C., Chang, H.M., Lee, K.C., Tai, T.Y., & Chuang, L.M. (2001). Molecular scanning of the human sorbin and SH3-domain-containing-1 (SORBS1) gene: positive association of the T228A polymorphism with obesity and type 2 diabetes. *Human Molecular Genetics, 10,* 1753–1760.

Lindsley, J.E., & Rutter, J. (2004). Nutrient sensing and metabolic decisions. *Comparative Biochemistry and Physiology. Part B, Biochemistry and Molecular Biology, 139,* 543–559.

Liu, Y.M., Moldes, M., Bastard, J.P., Bruckert, E., Viguerie, N., Hainque, B., Basdevant, A., Langin, D., Pairault, J., & Clement, K. (2004). Adiponutrin: a new gene regulated by energy balance in human adipose tissue. *The Journal of Clinical Endocrinology and Metabolism, 89,* 2684–2689.

Liu, Y.J., Liu, X.G., Wang, L., Dina, C., Yan, H., Liu, J.F., Levy, S., Papasian, C.J., Drees, B.M., Hamilton, J.J., Meyre, D., Delplanque, J., Pei, Y.F., Zhang, L., Recker, R.R., Froguel, P., & Deng, H.W. (2008). Genome-wide association scans identified CTNNBL1 as a novel gene for obesity. *Human Molecular Genetics, 17,* 1803–1813.

Loftus, T.M., Jaworsky, D.E., Frehywot, G.L., Townsend, C.A., Ronnett, G.V., Lane, M.D., & Kuhajda, F.P. (2000). Reduced food intake and body weight in mice treated with fatty acid synthase inhibitors. *Science, 288,* 2379–2381.

Loos, R.J., & Bouchard, C. (2008). FTO: the first gene contributing to common forms of human obesity. *Obesity Reviews, 9,* 246–250.

Loos, R.J., Rankinen, T., Perusse, L., Tremblay, A., Despres, J.P., & Bouchard, C. (2007a). Association of lipin 1 gene polymorphisms with measures of energy and glucose metabolism. *Obesity (Silver Spring), 15,* 2723–2732.

Loos, R.J., Ruchat, S., Rankinen, T., Tremblay, A., Perusse, L., & Bouchard, C. (2007b). Adiponectin and adiponectin receptor gene variants in relation to resting metabolic rate, respiratory quotient, and adiposity-related phenotypes in the Quebec Family Study. *American Journal of Clinical Nutrition, 85,* 26–34.

Loos, R.J., Lindgren, C.M., Li, S., Wheeler, E., Zhao, J.H., Prokopenko, I., Inouye, M., Freathy, R.M., Attwood, A.P., Beckmann, J.S., Berndt, S.I., Jacobs, K.B., Chanock, S.J., Hayes, R.B., Bergmann, S., Bennett, A.J., Bingham, S.A., Bochud, M., Brown, M., Cauchi, S., Connell, J.M., Cooper, C., Smith, G.D., Day, I., Dina, C., De, S., Dermitzakis, E.T., Doney, A.S., Elliott, K.S., Elliott, P., Evans, D.M., Farooqi, I.S., Froguel, P., Ghori, J., Groves, C.J., Gwilliam, R., Hadley, D., Hall, A.S., Hattersley, A.T., Hebebrand, J., Heid, I.M., Lamina, C., Gieger, C., Illig, T., Meitinger, T., Wichmann, H.E., Herrera, B., Hinney, A., Hunt, S.E., Jarvelin, M.R., Johnson, T., Jolley, J.D., Karpe, F., Keniry, A., Khaw, K.T., Luben, R.N., Mangino, M., Marchini, J., McArdle, W.L., McGinnis, R., Meyre, D., Munroe, P.B.,

Morris, A.D., Ness, A.R., Neville, M.J., Nica, A.C., Ong, K.K., O'Rahilly, S., Owen, K.R., Palmer, C.N., Papadakis, K., Potter, S., Pouta, A., Qi, L., Randall, J.C., Rayner, N.W., Ring, S.M., Sandhu, M.S., Scherag, A., Sims, M.A., Song, K., Soranzo, N., Speliotes, E.K., Syddall, H.E., Teichmann, S.A., Timpson, N.J., Tobias, J.H., Uda, M., Vogel, C.I., Wallace, C., Waterworth, D.M., Weedon, M.N., Willer, C.J., Wraight, Y.X., Zeggini, E., Hirschhorn, J.N., Strachan, D.P., Ouwehand, W.H., Caulfield, M.J., Samani, N.J., Frayling, T.M., Vollenweider, P., Waeber, G., Mooser, V., Deloukas, P., McCarthy, M.I., Wareham, N.J., Barroso, I., Jacobs, K.B., Chanock, S.J., Hayes, R.B., Lamina, C., Gieger, C., Illig, T., Meitinger, T., Wichmann, H.E., Kraft, P., Hankinson, S.E., Hunter, D.J., Hu, F.B., Lyon, H.N., Voight, B.F., Ridderstrale, M., Groop, L., Scheet, P., Sanna, S., Abecasis, G.R., Albai, G., Nagaraja, R., Schlessinger, D., Jackson, A.U., Tuomilehto, J., Collins, F.S., Boehnke, M., & Mohlke, K.L. (2008). Common variants near MC4R are associated with fat mass, weight and risk of obesity. *Nature Genetics, 40*, 768–775.

Lowell, B.B., & Bachman, E.S. (2003). Beta-adrenergic receptors, diet-induced thermogenesis, and obesity. *The Journal of Biological Chemistry, 278*, 29385–29388.

Lowell, B.B., S-Susulic, V., Hamann, A., Lawitts, J.A., Himms-Hagen, J., Boyer, B.B., Kozak, L.P., & Flier, J.S. (1993). Development of obesity in transgenic mice after genetic ablation of brown adipose tissue. *Nature, 366*, 740–742.

Lucas, A. (2000). Programming not metabolic imprinting. *American Journal of Clinical Nutrition, 71*, 602.

Maffei, M., Halaas, J., Ravussin, E., Pratley, R.E., Lee, G.H., Zhang, Y., Fei, H., Kim, S., Lallone, R., Ranganathan, S., Kern, P.A., & Friedman, J.M. (1995). Leptin levels in human and rodent: measurement of plasma leptin and ob RNA in obese and weight-reduced subjects. *Nature Medicine, 1*, 1155–1161.

Mager, U., Degenhardt, T., Pulkkinen, L., Kolehmainen, M., Tolppanen, A.M., Lindstrom, J., Eriksson, J.G., Carlberg, C., Tuomilehto, J., & Uusitupa, M. (2008). Variations in the ghrelin receptor gene associate with obesity and glucose metabolism in individuals with impaired glucose tolerance. *PLoS ONE, 3*, e2941.

Mammes, O., Betoulle, D., Aubert, R., Herbeth, B., Siest, G., & Fumeron, F. (2000). Association of the G-2548A polymorphism in the 5' region of the LEP gene with overweight. *Annals of Human Genetics, 64*, 391–394.

Mammes, O., Aubert, R., Betoulle, D., Pean, F., Herbeth, B., Visvikis, S., Siest, G., & Fumeron, F. (2001). LEPR gene polymorphisms: associations with overweight, fat mass and response to diet in women. *European Journal of Clinical Investigation, 31*, 398–404.

Marrades, M.P., Milagro, F.I., Martinez, J.A., & Moreno-Aliaga, M.J. (2006). Differential expression of aquaporin 7 in adipose tissue of lean and obese high fat consumers. *Biochemical and Biophysical Research Communications, 339*, 785–789.

Marshall, S. (2006). Role of insulin, adipocyte hormones, and nutrient-sensing pathways in regulating fuel metabolism and energy homeostasis: a nutritional perspective of diabetes, obesity, and cancer. *Science's STKE: Signal Transduction Knowledge Environment, 2006*, re7.

Martorell, R., Stein, A.D., & Schroeder, D.G. (2001). Early nutrition and later adiposity. *The Journal of Nutrition, 131*, 874S–880S.

Masuzaki, H., Ogawa, Y., Sagawa, N., Hosoda, K., Matsumoto, T., Mise, H., Nishimura, H., Yoshimasa, Y., Tanaka, I., Mori, T., & Nakao, K. (1997). Nonadipose tissue production of leptin: leptin as a novel placenta-derived hormone in humans. *Nature Medicine, 3*, 1029–1033.

Mathew, O.P., & Bhatia, J. (1989). Sucking and breathing patterns during breast- and bottle-feeding in term neonates. Effects of nutrient delivery and composition. *American Journal of Diseases of Children, 143*, 588–592.

Matsuoka, N., Patki, A., Tiwari, H.K., Allison, D.B., Johnson, S.B., Gregersen, P.K., Leibel, R.L., & Chung, W.K. (2006). Association of K121Q polymorphism in ENPP1 (PC-1) with BMI in Caucasian and African-American adults. *International Journal of Obesity (Lond), 30*, 233–237.

McTernan, P.G., Kusminski, C.M., & Kumar, S. (2006). Resistin. *Current Opinion in Lipidology, 17*, 170–175.

Meirhaeghe, A., & Amouyel, P. (2004). Impact of genetic variation of PPARgamma in humans. *Molecular Genetics and Metabolism, 83*, 93–102.

Memisoglu, A., Hu, F.B., Hankinson, S.E., Manson, J.E., De Vivo, I., Willett, W.C., & Hunter, D.J. (2003). Interaction between a peroxisome proliferator-activated receptor gamma gene polymorphism and dietary fat intake in relation to body mass. *Human Molecular Genetics, 12*, 2923–2929.

Miralles, O., Sanchez, J., Palou, A., & Pico, C. (2006). A physiological role of breast milk leptin in body weight control in developing infants. *Obesity (Silver Spring), 14*, 1371–1377.

Mizuta, E., Kokubo, Y., Yamanaka, I., Miyamoto, Y., Okayama, A., Yoshimasa, Y., Tomoike, H., Morisaki, H., & Morisaki, T. (2008). Leptin gene and leptin receptor gene polymorphisms are associated with sweet preference and obesity. *Hypertension Research, 31*, 1069–1077.

Moloney, F., Toomey, S., Noone, E., Nugent, A., Allan, B., Loscher, C.E., & Roche, H.M. (2007). Antidiabetic effects of cis-9, trans-11-conjugated linoleic acid may be mediated via anti-inflammatory effects in white adipose tissue. *Diabetes, 56*, 574–582.

Morandi, A., Pinelli, L., Petrone, A., Vatin, V., Buzzetti, R., Froguel, P., & Meyre, D. (2008). The Q121 variant of ENPP1 may protect from childhood overweight/obesity in the Italian population. *Obesity (Silver Spring), 17*(1), 202–206.

Morrison, C.D., Xi, X., White, C.L., Ye, J., & Martin, R.J. (2007). Amino acids inhibit Agrp gene expression via an mTOR-dependent mechanism. *American Journal of Physiology, Endocrinology and Metabolism, 293*, E165–E171.

Morton, N.M., Emilsson, V., Liu, Y.L., & Cawthorne, M.A. (1998). Leptin action in intestinal cells. *The Journal of Biological Chemistry, 273*, 26194–26201.

Moussavi, N., Gavino, V., & Receveur, O. (2008). Is obesity related to the type of dietary fatty acids? An ecological study. *Public Health Nutrition, 11*, 1149–1155.

Nedergaard, J., Bengtsson, T., & Cannon, B. (2007). Unexpected evidence for active brown adipose tissue in adult humans. *American Journal of Physiology, Endocrinology and Metabolism, 293*, E444–E452.

Nieters, A., Becker, N., & Linseisen, J. (2002). Polymorphisms in candidate obesity genes and their interaction with dietary intake of n-6 polyunsaturated fatty acids affect obesity risk in a sub-sample of the EPIC-Heidelberg cohort. *European Journal of Nutrition, 41*, 210–221.

Niswender, K.D., Baskin, D.G., & Schwartz, M.W. (2004). Insulin and its evolving partnership with leptin in the hypothalamic control of energy homeostasis. *Trends in Endocrinology and Metabolism, 15*, 362–369.

Nordstrom, E.A., Ryden, M., Backlund, E.C., Dahlman, I., Kaaman, M., Blomqvist, L., Cannon, B., Nedergaard, J., & Arner, P. (2005). A human-specific role of cell death-inducing DFFA (DNA fragmentation factor-alpha)-like effector A (CIDEA) in adipocyte lipolysis and obesity. *Diabetes, 54*, 1726–1734.

Novak, D.A., Desai, M., & Ross, M.G. (2006). Gestational programming of offspring obesity/hypertension. *The Journal of Maternal-Fetal & Neonatal Medicine, 19*, 591–599.

O'Connor, D., Funanage, V., Locke, R., Spear, M., & Leef, K. (2003). Leptin is not present in infant formulas. *The Journal of Endocrinological Investigation, 26*, 490.

O'Rahilly, S., & Farooqi, I.S. (2006). Genetics of obesity. *Philosophical Transactions of the Royal Society of London, Series B, Biological Sciences, 361*, 1095–1105.

Oberkofler, H., Dallinger, G., Liu, Y.M., Hell, E., Krempler, F., & Patsch, W. (1997). Uncoupling protein gene: quantification of expression levels in adipose tissues of obese and non-obese humans. *Journal of Lipid Research, 38*, 2125–2133.

Oberkofler, H., Liu, Y.M., Esterbauer, H., Hell, E., Krempler, F., & Patsch, W. (1998). Uncoupling protein-2 gene: reduced mRNA expression in intraperitoneal adipose tissue of obese humans. *Diabetologia, 41*, 940–946.

Oken, E., & Gillman, M.W. (2003). Fetal origins of obesity. *Obesity Research, 11*, 496–506.

Oliver, P., Pico, C., De Matteis, R., Cinti, S., & Palou, A. (2002). Perinatal expression of leptin in rat stomach. *Developmental Dynamics, 223*, 148–154.

Ong, K.K., & Dunger, D.B. (2004). Birth weight, infant growth and insulin resistance. *European Journal of Endocrinology, 151 Suppl 3*, U131–U139.

Ong, K.K., Ahmed, M.L., Emmett, P.M., Preece, M.A., & Dunger, D.B. (2000). Association between postnatal catch-up growth and obesity in childhood: prospective cohort study. *British Medical Journal, 320*, 967–971.

Ordovas, J.M. (2006). Genetic interactions with diet influence the risk of cardiovascular disease. *American Journal of Clinical Nutrition, 83*, 443S–446S.

Ordovas, J.M., Corella, D., Cupples, L.A., Demissie, S., Kelleher, A., Coltell, O., Wilson, P.W., Schaefer, E.J., & Tucker, K. (2002). Polyunsaturated fatty acids modulate the effects of the APOA1 G-A polymorphism on HDL-cholesterol concentrations in a sex-specific manner: the Framingham Study. *American Journal of Clinical Nutrition, 75*, 38–46.

Ostlund, R.E., Jr., Yang, J.W., Klein, S., & Gingerich, R. (1996). Relation between plasma leptin concentration and body fat, gender, diet, age, and metabolic covariates. *The Journal of Clinical Endocrinology and Metabolism, 81*, 3909–3913.

Palou, A., & Pico, C. (2009). Leptin intake during lactation prevents obesity and affects food intake and food preferences in later life. *Appetite, 52*, 249–252.

Palou, A., Pico, C., Bonet, M.L., & Oliver, P. (1998). The uncoupling protein, thermogenin. *The International Journal of Biochemistry & Cell Biology, 30*, 7–11.

Palou, A., Oliver, P., Sanchez, J., Priego, T., & Pico, C. (2008). The role of breast milk leptin in the prevention of obesity and related medical complications in later life. In M. Cerf (Ed.), *Developmental programming of diabetes and metabolic syndrome* (pp. 39–49). India: Transworld Research network.

Paracchini, V., Pedotti, P., & Taioli, E. (2005). Genetics of leptin and obesity: a HuGE review. *American Journal of Epidemiology, 162*, 101–114.

Park, C.S. (2005). Role of compensatory mammary growth in epigenetic control of gene expression. *The FASEB Journal, 19*, 1586–1591.

Parra, P., Serra, F., & Palou, A. (2008). Moderate doses of conjugated linoleic acid isomers-mix contribute to lower body fat content maintaining insulin sensitivity and a non-inflammatory pattern in adipose tissue in mice. *Journal of Nutritional Biochemistry*, doi:10.1016/j.jnutbio.2008.10010.

Peeters, A.V., Beckers, S., Verrijken, A., Mertens, I., Roevens, P., Peeters, P.J., Van Hul, W., & Van Gaal, L.F. (2008). Association of SIRT1 gene variation with visceral obesity. *Human Genetics, 124*, 431–436.

Pelleymounter, M.A., Cullen, M.J., Baker, M.B., Hecht, R., Winters, D., Boone, T., & Collins, F. (1995). Effects of the obese gene product on body weight regulation in ob/ob mice. *Science, 269*, 540–543.

Petersen, E.W., Carey, A.L., Sacchetti, M., Steinberg, G.R., Macaulay, S.L., Febbraio, M.A., & Pedersen, B.K. (2005). Acute IL-6 treatment increases fatty acid turnover in elderly humans in vivo and in tissue culture in vitro. *American Journal of Physiology, Endocrinology and Metabolism, 288*, E155–E162.

Phan, J., Peterfy, M., & Reue, K. (2004). Lipin expression preceding peroxisome proliferator-activated receptor-gamma is critical for adipogenesis in vivo and in vitro. *The Journal of Biological Chemistry, 279*, 29558–29564.

Pico, C., Sanchez, J., Oliver, P., & Palou, A. (2002). Leptin production by the stomach is up-regulated in obese (fa/fa) zucker rats. *Obesity Research, 10*, 932–938.

Pico, C., Oliver, P., Sanchez, J., & Palou, A. (2003). Gastric leptin: a putative role in the short-term regulation of food intake. *British Journal of Nutrition, 90*, 735–741.

Pico, C., Oliver, P., Sanchez, J., Miralles, O., Caimari, A., Priego, T., & Palou, A. (2007). The intake of physiological doses of leptin during lactation in rats prevents obesity in later life. *International Journal of Obesity (Lond), 31*, 1199–1209.

Prestwich, T.C., & Macdougald, O.A. (2007). Wnt/beta-catenin signaling in adipogenesis and metabolism. *Current Opinion in Cell Biology, 19*, 612–617.

Proud, C.G. (2007). Amino acids and mTOR signalling in anabolic function. *Biochemical Society Transactions, 35*, 1187–1190.

Prudente, S., Chandalia, M., Morini, E., Baratta, R., Dallapiccola, B., Abate, N., Frittitta, L., & Trischitta, V. (2007a). The Q121/Q121 genotype of ENPP1/PC-1 is associated with lower BMI in non-diabetic whites. *Obesity (Silver Spring), 15*, 1–4.

Prudente, S., Flex, E., Morini, E., Turchi, F., Capponi, D., De Cosmo, S., Tassi, V., Guida, V., Avogaro, A., Folli, F., Maiani, F., Frittitta, L., Dallapiccola, B., & Trischitta, V. (2007b). A functional variant of the adipocyte glycerol channel Aquaporin 7 gene is associated with obesity and related metabolic abnormalities. *Diabetes, 56*(5), 1468–1474.

Puigserver, P., Vazquez, F., Bonet, M.L., Pico, C., & Palou, A. (1996). In vitro and in vivo induction of brown adipocyte uncoupling protein (thermogenin) by retinoic acid. *The Biochemical Journal, 317*(Pt 3), 827–833.

Puri, V., Ranjit, S., Konda, S., Nicoloro, S.M., Straubhaar, J., Chawla, A., Chouinard, M., Lin, C., Burkart, A., Corvera, S., Perugini, R.A., & Czech, M.P. (2008). Cidea is associated with lipid droplets and insulin sensitivity in humans. *Proceedings of the National Academy of Sciences of the United States of America, 105*, 7833–7838.

Qi, L., Corella, D., Sorli, J.V., Portoles, O., Shen, H., Coltell, O., Godoy, D., Greenberg, A.S., & Ordovas, J.M. (2004a). Genetic variation at the perilipin (PLIN) locus is associated with obesity-related phenotypes in White women. *Clinical Genetics, 66*, 299–310.

Qi, L., Shen, H., Larson, I., Schaefer, E.J., Greenberg, A.S., Tregouet, D.A., Corella, D., & Ordovas, J.M. (2004b). Gender-specific association of a perilipin gene haplotype with obesity risk in a white population. *Obesity Research, 12*, 1758–1765.

Qi, L., Tai, E.S., Tan, C.E., Shen, H., Chew, S.K., Greenberg, A.S., Corella, D., & Ordovas, J.M. (2005). Intragenic linkage disequilibrium structure of the human perilipin gene (PLIN) and haplotype association with increased obesity risk in a multiethnic Asian population. *Journal of Molecular Medicine, 83*, 448–456.

Qi, L., Zhang, C., van Dam, R.M., & Hu, F.B. (2007). Interleukin-6 genetic variability and adiposity: associations in two prospective cohorts and systematic review in 26,944 individuals. *The Journal of Clinical Endocrinology and Metabolism, 92*, 3618–3625.

Quinton, N.D., Lee, A.J., Ross, R.J., Eastell, R., & Blakemore, A.I. (2001). A single nucleotide polymorphism (SNP) in the leptin receptor is associated with BMI, fat mass and leptin levels in postmenopausal Caucasian women. *Human Genetics, 108*, 233–236.

Raben, D.M., & Baldassare, J.J. (2005). A new lipase in regulating lipid mobilization: hormone-sensitive lipase is not alone. *Trends in Endocrinology and Metabolism, 16*, 35–36.

Ravelli, G.P., Stein, Z.A., & Susser, M.W. (1976). Obesity in young men after famine exposure in utero and early infancy. *New England Journal of Medicine, 295*, 349–353.

Ravelli, A.C., van Der Meulen, J.H., Osmond, C., Barker, D.J., & Bleker, O.P. (1999). Obesity at the age of 50 y in men and women exposed to famine prenatally. *American Journal of Clinical Nutrition, 70*, 811–816.

Ravussin, E., Lillioja, S., Knowler, W.C., Christin, L., Freymond, D., Abbott, W.G., Boyce, V., Howard, B.V., & Bogardus, C. (1988). Reduced rate of energy expenditure as a risk factor for body-weight gain. *New England Journal of Medicine, 318*, 467–472.

Remacle, C., Bieswal, F., & Reusens, B. (2004). Programming of obesity and cardiovascular disease. *International Journal of Obesity and Related Metabolic Disorders, 28 Suppl 3*, S46–S53.

Rissanen, A., Hakala, P., Lissner, L., Mattlar, C.E., Koskenvuo, M., & Ronnemaa, T. (2002). Acquired preference especially for dietary fat and obesity: a study of weight-discordant monozygotic twin pairs. *International Journal of Obesity and Related Metabolic Disorders, 26*, 973–977.

Robitaille, J., Despres, J.P., Perusse, L., & Vohl, M.C. (2003). The PPAR-gamma P12A polymorphism modulates the relationship between dietary fat intake and components of the metabolic syndrome: results from the Quebec Family Study. *Clinical Genetics, 63*, 109–116.

Roche, H.M. (2004). Dietary lipids and gene expression. *Biochemical Society Transactions, 32*, 999–1002.

Ropelle, E.R., Pauli, J.R., Fernandes, M.F., Rocco, S.A., Marin, R.M., Morari, J., Souza, K.K., Dias, M.M., Gomes-Marcondes, M.C., Gontijo, J.A., Franchini, K.G., Velloso, L.A., Saad, M.J., & Carvalheira, J.B. (2008). A central role for neuronal AMP-activated protein kinase (AMPK) and mammalian target of rapamycin (mTOR) in high-protein diet-induced weight loss. *Diabetes, 57*, 594–605.

Ryden, M., & Arner, P. (2007). Tumour necrosis factor-alpha in human adipose tissue – from signalling mechanisms to clinical implications. *Journal of Internal Medicine, 262*, 431–438.

Ryden, M., Faulds, G., Hoffstedt, J., Wennlund, A., & Arner, P. (2002). Effect of the (C825T) Gbeta(3) polymorphism on adrenoceptor-mediated lipolysis in human fat cells. *Diabetes, 51*, 1601–1608.

Ryden, M., Jocken, J., van Harmelen, V., Dicker, A., Hoffstedt, J., Wiren, M., Blomqvist, L., Mairal, A., Langin, D., Blaak, E., & Arner, P. (2007). Comparative studies of the role of hormone-sensitive lipase and adipose triglyceride lipase in human fat cell lipolysis. *American Journal of Physiology, Endocrinology and Metabolism, 292*, E1847–E1855.

Sanchez, J., Oliver, P., Miralles, O., Ceresi, E., Pico, C., & Palou, A. (2005). Leptin orally supplied to neonate rats is directly uptaken by the immature stomach and may regulate short-term feeding. *Endocrinology, 146*, 2575–2582.

Sanchez, J., Priego, T., Palou, M., Tobaruela, A., Palou, A., & Pico, C. (2008). Oral supplementation with physiological doses of leptin during lactation in rats improves insulin sensitivity and affects food preferences later in life. *Endocrinology, 149*, 733–740.

Sarbassov, D.D., Ali, S.M., Kim, D.H., Guertin, D.A., Latek, R.R., Erdjument-Bromage, H., Tempst, P., & Sabatini, D.M. (2004). Rictor, a novel binding partner of mTOR, defines a rapamycin-insensitive and raptor-independent pathway that regulates the cytoskeleton. *Current Biology, 14*, 1296–1302.

Schoenborn, V., Heid, I.M., Vollmert, C., Lingenhel, A., Adams, T.D., Hopkins, P.N., Illig, T., Zimmermann, R., Zechner, R., Hunt, S.C., & Kronenberg, F. (2006). The ATGL gene is associated with free fatty acids, triglycerides, and type 2 diabetes. *Diabetes, 55*, 1270–1275.

Scuteri, A., Sanna, S., Chen, W.M., Uda, M., Albai, G., Strait, J., Najjar, S., Nagaraja, R., Orru, M., Usala, G., Dei, M., Lai, S., Maschio, A., Busonero, F., Mulas, A., Ehret, G.B., Fink, A.A., Weder, A.B., Cooper, R.S., Galan, P., Chakravarti, A., Schlessinger, D., Cao, A., Lakatta, E., & Abecasis, G.R. (2007). Genome-wide association scan shows genetic variants in the FTO gene are associated with obesity-related traits. *PLoS Genetics, 3*, e115.

Semple, R.K., Crowley, V.C., Sewter, C.P., Laudes, M., Christodoulides, C., Considine, R.V., Vidal-Puig, A., & O'Rahilly, S. (2004). Expression of the thermogenic nuclear hormone receptor coactivator PGC-1alpha is reduced in the adipose tissue of morbidly obese subjects. *International Journal of Obesity and Related Metabolic Disorders, 28*, 176–179.

Serra, F., Bonet, M.L., Puigserver, P., Oliver, J., & Palou, A. (1999). Stimulation of uncoupling protein 1 expression in brown adipocytes by naturally occurring carotenoids. *International Journal of Obesity and Related Metabolic Disorders, 23*, 650–655.

Shin, H.D., Park, B.L., Kim, L.H., Jung, H.S., Cho, Y.M., Moon, M.K., Park, Y.J., Lee, H.K., & Park, K.S. (2004). Genetic polymorphisms in peroxisome proliferator-activated receptor delta associated with obesity. *Diabetes, 53*, 847–851.

Sievers, E., Oldigs, H.D., Santer, R., & Schaub, J. (2002). Feeding patterns in breast-fed and formula-fed infants. *Annals of Nutrition & Metabolism, 46*, 243–248.

Singhal, A., Wells, J., Cole, T.J., Fewtrell, M., & Lucas, A. (2003). Programming of lean body mass: a link between birth weight, obesity, and cardiovascular disease? *American Journal of Clinical Nutrition, 77*, 726–730.

Skurk, T., & Hauner, H. (2004). Obesity and impaired fibrinolysis: role of adipose production of plasminogen activator inhibitor-1. *International Journal of Obesity and Related Metabolic Disorders, 28*, 1357–1364.

Sladek, R., Bader, J.A., & Giguere, V. (1997). The orphan nuclear receptor estrogen-related receptor alpha is a transcriptional regulator of the human medium-chain acyl coenzyme A dehydrogenase gene. *Molecular and Cellular Biology, 17*, 5400–5409.

Smith-Kirwin, S.M., O'Connor, D.M., De Johnston, J., Lancey, E.D., Hassink, S.G., & Funanage, V.L. (1998). Leptin expression in human mammary epithelial cells and breast milk. *The Journal of Clinical Endocrinology and Metabolism, 83*, 1810–1813.

Sookoian, S.C., Gonzalez, C., & Pirola, C.J. (2005). Meta-analysis on the G-308A tumor necrosis factor alpha gene variant and phenotypes associated with the metabolic syndrome. *Obesity Research, 13*, 2122–2131.

Spalding, K.L., Arner, E., Westermark, P.O., Bernard, S., Buchholz, B.A., Bergmann, O., Blomqvist, L., Hoffstedt, J., Naslund, E., Britton, T., Concha, H., Hassan, M., Ryden, M., Frisen, J., & Arner, P. (2008). Dynamics of fat cell turnover in humans. *Nature, 453*, 783–787.

Stettler, N., Stallings, V.A., Troxel, A.B., Zhao, J., Schinnar, R., Nelson, S.E., Ziegler, E.E., & Strom, B.L. (2005). Weight gain in the first week of life and overweight in adulthood: a cohort study of European American subjects fed infant formula. *Circulation, 111*, 1897–1903.

Strauss, R.S. (1997). Effects of the intrauterine environment on childhood growth. *British Medical Bulletin, 53*, 81–95.

Surkan, P.J., Hsieh, C.C., Johansson, A.L., Dickman, P.W., & Cnattingius, S. (2004). Reasons for increasing trends in large for gestational age births. *Obstetrics and Gynecology, 104*, 720–726.

Suviolahti, E., Reue, K., Cantor, R.M., Phan, J., Gentile, M., Naukkarinen, J., Soro-Paavonen, A., Oksanen, L., Kaprio, J., Rissanen, A., Salomaa, V., Kontula, K., Taskinen, M.R., Pajukanta, P., & Peltonen, L. (2006). Cross-species analyses implicate Lipin 1 involvement in human glucose metabolism. *Human Molecular Genetics, 15*, 377–386.

Tai, E.S., Demissie, S., Cupples, L.A., Corella, D., Wilson, P.W., Schaefer, E.J., & Ordovas, J.M. (2002). Association between the PPARA L162V polymorphism and plasma lipid levels: the Framingham Offspring Study. *Arteriosclerosis, Thrombosis, and Vascular Biology, 22*, 805–810.

Taylor, P.D., & Poston, L. (2007). Developmental programming of obesity in mammals. *Experimental Physiology, 92*, 287–298.

Thupari, J.N., Landree, L.E., Ronnett, G.V., & Kuhajda, F.P. (2002). C75 increases peripheral energy utilization and fatty acid oxidation in diet-induced obesity. *Proceedings of the National Academy of Sciences of the United States of America, 99*, 9498–9502.

Towler, M.C., & Hardie, D.G. (2007). AMP-activated protein kinase in metabolic control and insulin signaling. *Circulation Research, 100*, 328–341.

Treuth, M.S., Butte, N.F., & Sorkin, J.D. (2003). Predictors of body fat gain in nonobese girls with a familial predisposition to obesity. *American Journal of Clinical Nutrition, 78*, 1212–1218.

Tsai, Y.S., & Maeda, N. (2005). PPARgamma: a critical determinant of body fat distribution in humans and mice. *Trends in Cardiovascular Medicine, 15*, 81–85.

Ukkola, O., Ravussin, E., Jacobson, P., Perusse, L., Rankinen, T., Tschop, M., Heiman, M.L., Leon, A.S., Rao, D.C., Skinner, J.S., Wilmore, J.H., Sjostrom, L., & Bouchard, C. (2002). Role of ghrelin polymorphisms in obesity based on three different studies. *Obesity Research, 10*, 782–791.

Um, S.H., D'Alessio, D., & Thomas, G. (2006). Nutrient overload, insulin resistance, and ribosomal protein S6 kinase 1, S6K1. *Cell Metabolism, 3*, 393–402.

Uysal, F.K., Onal, E.E., Aral, Y.Z., Adam, B., Dilmen, U., & Ardicolu, Y. (2002). Breast milk leptin: its relationship to maternal and infant adiposity. *Clinical Nutrition, 21*, 157–160.

Valsamakis, G., Kanaka-Gantenbein, C., Malamitsi-Puchner, A., & Mastorakos, G. (2006). Causes of intrauterine growth restriction and the postnatal development of the metabolic syndrome. *Annals of the New York Academy of Sciences, 1092*, 138–147.

van Rossum, E.F., & Lamberts, S.W. (2004). Polymorphisms in the glucocorticoid receptor gene and their associations with metabolic parameters and body composition. *Recent Progress in Hormone Research, 59*, 333–357.

Vega, R.B., & Kelly, D.P. (1997). A role for estrogen-related receptor alpha in the control of mitochondrial fatty acid beta-oxidation during brown adipocyte differentiation. *The Journal of Biological Chemistry, 272*, 31693–31699.

Vegiopoulos, A., & Herzig, S. (2007). Glucocorticoids, metabolism and metabolic diseases. *Molecular and Cellular Endocrinology, 275*, 43–61.

Verkman, A.S. (2005). More than just water channels: unexpected cellular roles of aquaporins. *Journal of Cell Science, 118*, 3225–3232.

Viollet, B., Mounier, R., Leclerc, J., Yazigi, A., Foretz, M., & Andreelli, F. (2007). Targeting AMP-activated protein kinase as a novel therapeutic approach for the treatment of metabolic disorders. *Diabetes & Metabolism, 33*, 395–402.

von Kries, R., Koletzko, B., Sauerwald, T., von Mutius, E., Barnert, D., Grunert, V., & von Voss, H. (1999). Breast feeding and obesity: cross sectional study. *British Medical Journal, 319*, 147–150.

Wamil, M., & Seckl, J.R. (2007). Inhibition of 11beta-hydroxysteroid dehydrogenase type 1 as a promising therapeutic target. *Drug Discovery Today, 12*, 504–520.

Wang, J., Liu, R., Hawkins, M., Barzilai, N., & Rossetti, L. (1998). A nutrient-sensing pathway regulates leptin gene expression in muscle and fat. *Nature, 393*, 684–688.

Warensjo, E., Ingelsson, E., Lundmark, P., Lannfelt, L., Syvanen, A.C., Vessby, B., & Riserus, U. (2007). Polymorphisms in the SCD1 gene: associations with body fat distribution and insulin sensitivity. *Obesity (Silver Spring), 15*, 1732–1740.

Waterland, R.A., & Garza, C. (1999). Potential mechanisms of metabolic imprinting that lead to chronic disease. *American Journal of Clinical Nutrition, 69*, 179–197.

Wauters, M., Mertens, I., Chagnon, M., Rankinen, T., Considine, R.V., Chagnon, Y.C., Van Gaal, L.F., & Bouchard, C. (2001). Polymorphisms in the leptin receptor gene, body composition and fat distribution in overweight and obese women. *International Journal of Obesity and Related Metabolic Disorders, 25*, 714–720.

Wegner, L., Andersen, G., Sparso, T., Grarup, N., Glumer, C., Borch-Johnsen, K., Jorgensen, T., Hansen, T., & Pedersen, O. (2007). Common variation in LMNA increases susceptibility to type 2 diabetes and associates with elevated fasting glycemia and estimates of body fat and height in the general population: studies of 7,495 Danish whites. *Diabetes, 56*, 694–698.

Weisberg, S.P., McCann, D., Desai, M., Rosenbaum, M., Leibel, R.L., & Ferrante, A.W., Jr. (2003). Obesity is associated with macrophage accumulation in adipose tissue. *The Journal of Clinical Investigation, 112*, 1796–1808.

Whitaker, R.C., & Dietz, W.H. (1998). Role of the prenatal environment in the development of obesity. *The Journal of Pediatrics, 132*, 768–776.

Woods, S.C., Seeley, R.J., & Cota, D. (2008). Regulation of food intake through hypothalamic signaling networks involving mTOR. *Annual Review of Nutrition, 28*, 295–311.

Xu, H., Barnes, G.T., Yang, Q., Tan, G., Yang, D., Chou, C.J., Sole, J., Nichols, A., Ross, J.S., Tartaglia, L.A., & Chen, H. (2003). Chronic inflammation in fat plays a crucial role in the development of obesity-related insulin resistance. *The Journal of Clinical Investigation, 112*, 1821–1830.

Yuan, C.S., Attele, A.S., Wu, J.A., Zhang, L., & Shi, Z.Q. (1999). Peripheral gastric leptin modulates brain stem neuronal activity in neonates. *The American Journal of Physiology, 277*, G626–G630.

Zhang, Y., Proenca, R., Maffei, M., Barone, M., Leopold, L., & Friedman, J.M. (1994). Positional cloning of the mouse obese gene and its human homologue. *Nature, 372*, 425–432.

Zhang, L., Miyaki, K., Nakayama, T., & Muramatsu, M. (2008). Cell death-inducing DNA fragmentation factor alpha-like effector A (CIDEA) gene V115F (G-->T) polymorphism is associated with phenotypes of metabolic syndrome in Japanese men. *Metabolism, 57*, 502–505.

Zurlo, F., Lillioja, S., Esposito-Del Puente, A., Nyomba, B.L., Raz, I., Saad, M.F., Swinburn, B.A., Knowler, W.C., Bogardus, C., & Ravussin, E. (1990). Low ratio of fat to carbohydrate oxidation as predictor of weight gain: study of 24-h RQ. *The American Journal of Physiology, 259*, E650–E657.

Chapter 16
Neuroendocrine Regulation

Vicente Barrios, Gabriel Ángel Martos-Moreno, Laura M. Frago, Julie A. Chowen, and Jesús Argente

Introduction

Obesity is a major problem in developed countries and the development of an effective treatment is an important area of research. In order to reach this goal, we must first know how metabolism and appetite are controlled, both in the periphery, as well as in the central nervous system. Due to the increased interest in this area of research, our understanding of the neuroendocrine control of food intake and energy expenditure has increased dramatically in recent years. New neuropeptides have been identified and new metabolic roles of previously known neuropeptides and neurotransmissors have been demonstrated. This chapter will briefly describe the various brain areas involved in metabolic control, concentrating on the hypothalamus and the specific nuclei of this brain area most intimately involved in the control of appetite and metabolism. Special attention will be paid to the hypothalamic neuronal populations that produce neuropeptide Y (NPY)/agouti-related protein (AgRP) and proopiomelanortin (POMC)/cocaine- and amphetamine-regulated transcript (CART). These two neuronal populations are central to metabolic and have been the subject of much investigation.

How other neuropeptides and neurotransmitters as well as circulating metabolic signals affect these two neuronal populations to modulate appetite and energy expenditure is briefly described. Nutrients, such as fatty acids and glucose, have specific feed-back effects at the level of the hypothalamus to control appetite and metabolism. In addition, the effects of hormones produced by fat tissue, such as leptin, adiponectin and other cytokines, and those synthesized by the digestive tract, such as insulin, ghrelin, amongst others, on metabolism are also described briefly. As exogenous obesity is normally associated with a decrease in the sensitivity to leptin and insulin signaling, the intracellular signaling mechanisms activated in the central nervous system in response to leptin and

V. Barrios, G.Á. Martos-Moreno, J.A. Chowen, and J. Argente (✉)
Department of Endocrinology, Hospital Infantil Universitario Niño Jesús, Madrid, Spain
and CIBER Fisiopatología de la Obesidad y Nutrición (CIBEROBN),
Instituto Carlos III, Madrid, Spain
and
Department of Pediatrics, Hospital Infantil Universitario Niño Jesús,
Avda. Menéndez Pelayo, 65, E-28009 Madrid, Spain
e-mail: argentefen@terra.es

L.M. Frago and J. Argente
Department of Pediatrics, Universidad Autónoma de Madrid, Madrid, Spain

L.A. Moreno et al. (eds.), *Epidemiology of Obesity in Children and Adolescents*,
Springer Series on Epidemiology and Public Health 2, DOI 10.1007/978-1-4419-6039-9_16,
© Springer Science+Business Media, LLC 2011

insulin are discussed in detail. How some of these mechanisms may be changed during obesity is briefly discussed. As the reader will appreciate, the central control of metabolism is quite complex with many factors, both central and peripheral, involved. This chapter attempts to introduce the reader to some of the main factors involved in this process.

Central Neuroendocrine System

Despite the almost daily variation in food intake and energy expenditure, body weight remains relatively constant. Only when small differences in energy expenditure/intake are integrated over long periods of time is an increase in adiposity produced. During the last decade, a complex network of hormones, neuropeptides and metabolites involved in the regulation of appetite and metabolism has been identified. Moreover, compelling evidence suggests that the primary cause of peripheral fat accumulation could involve modifications at the level of the central nervous system (CNS) (Schwartz et al. 2000).

It has been more than 60 years since the hypothalamus was first shown to be involved in body weight control (Heatherington and Ranson 1940). These pioneering studies demonstrated that lesions in the ventromedial hypothalamus provoked hyperphagia and obesity, while a few years later lesions in the lateral hypothalamus were shown to decrease appetite (Anand and Brobeck 1951). Indeed, it is now accepted that the hypothalamus is a primary target for metabolic signals and plays a fundamental role in the integration of these inputs; however, other brain areas, in particular the brainstem, are also intimately involved in the control of food intake and body weight (Morton et al. 2006). Furthermore, the list of neuropeptides, neurotransmitters and peripheral signals modulating metabolic control has increased rapidly during the past decade, increasing our understanding of this phenomenon, but also adding to its complexity.

The Hypothalamus

The hypothalamic nuclei most closely associated with food intake and body weight include the arcuate, paraventricular and dorsomedial nuclei, as well as the ventromedial and lateral hypothalamus (Arch 2005). The arcuate nucleus contains two neuronal populations fundamental for metabolic control. One neuronal population stimulates food intake and decreases energy expenditure through the release of neuropeptide Y (NPY) and agouti-related peptide (AgRP) (Hahn et al. 1998), whereas the other population, which produces proopiomelanocortin (POMC) and cocaine- and amphetamine-regulated transcript (CART), inhibits food intake and increases energy expenditure (Ellacott and Cone 2004). Figure 16.1 shows a schematic representation of how these two neuronal populations integrate metabolic signals received from the periphery, as well as their interaction. Both neuronal systems are direct targets for peripheral metabolic and hormonal signals as the arcuate nucleus is in close proximity to the median eminence, a region outside of the blood-brain barrier (BBB) allowing signals to reach these neurons in an efficient manner (Gross 1992). However, specific transport systems exist for some of these signals to cross the BBB, such as leptin and ghrelin, with this transport also being regulated by metabolic signals (Banks 2006).

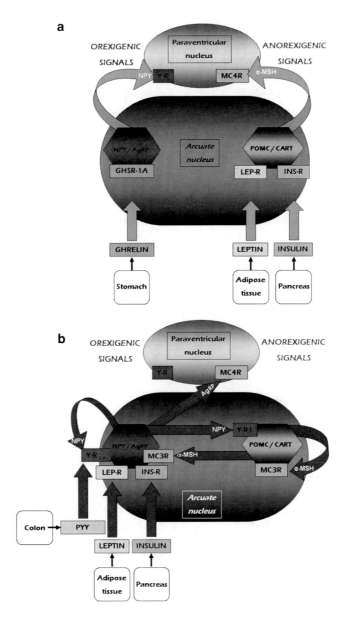

Fig. 16.1 Schematic representation of the excitatory (*arrows in Figure* **a**) and inhibitory (*arrows in Figure* **b**) stimuli in NPY/AgRP and POMC/CART producing neurons in the hypothalamus. When activated, NPY/AgRP neurons send out orexigenic signals, while POMC/CART neurons relay anorexigenic signals. These neuronal groups reciprocally inhibit each other, through direct signaling, and limit their own activity by acting on presynaptic receptors (*curved arrows*). When NPY/AgRP producing neurons are activated, AgRP prevents α-MSH signaling by blocking MC4R, whereas NPY directly decreases POMC release. Conversely, α-MSH is able to interfere with NPY/AgRP release by acting on MC3R. In addition, the effect of peripherally produced leptin, insulin, ghrelin and PYY on these two neuron populations are shown. Ghrelin stimulates food intake and decreases energy expenditure through activation of NPY/AgRP neurons. Leptin and insulin inhibit food intake and increase energy expenditure through activation of POMC/CART neurons and inhibition of NPY/AgRP neurons. *AgRP* agouti protein related peptide; *CART* cocaine and amphetamine related transcript; *GHSR-1A* growth hormone secretagogue receptor type 1A; *INS-R* insulin receptor; *LEP-R* leptin receptor; *MC3R* melanocortin receptor number 3; *MC4R* melanocortin receptor number 4; *NPY* neuropeptide Y; *POMC* proopiomelanocortin; *PYY* peptide YY; *Y-R* Y receptor (numbers indicate subtype); *α-MSH* alpha melanocyte stimulating hormone

Hypothalamic POMC neurons increase energy expenditure and decrease body weight by production of α-melanocyte-stimulating hormone (α-MSH), a cleavage product of the POMC precursor protein. This peptide binds to a family of melanocortin receptors, including melanocortin receptor number 4 (MC4R), which is highly expressed in the paraventricular nucleus to control metabolism (Sindelar et al. 2002). Many POMC neurons in the arcuate nucleus also produce CART, which acts as a neurotransmitter both centrally and peripherally and is implicated in feeding, stress, and reward processes (Vicentic and Jones 2007). Indeed, CART is a strong inhibitor of appetite and synthesis of this protein is modulated in response to food intake (Dunbar et al. 2005). It is also co-expressed with other neuropeptides in other feeding-associated brain regions such as in thyrotropin-releasing hormone (Broberger 1999) and corticotropin-releasing hormone neurons (Sarkar et al. 2004) in the paraventricular nucleus and MCH neurons in the dorsomedial nucleus and lateral hypothalamus (Vrang et al. 1999).

Neuropeptide Y is the most potent endogenous orexigenic signal known in mammals. Hypothalamic NPY levels increase with fasting and decrease after food intake (Swart et al. 2002). Intracerebroventricular (*i.c.v.*) administration of NPY reduces energy expenditure and increases insulin levels, independently of food intake (Zarjevski et al. 1993). Many NPY neurons in the arcuate nucleus coexpress AgRP. Increased AgRP levels lead to obesity, most likely through AgRP's actions as an MC4R antagonist. A unidirectional anatomical interaction between NPY/AgRP and POMC perikarya results in tonic inhibition of the POMC cells whenever NPY/AgRP neurons are active and may help to explain why the feeding circuit is more likely to promote feeding than satiety.

The hypothalamic POMC and NPY systems are sexually dimorphic, with males having significantly more NPY producing cells in the arcuate nucleus than do females (Urban et al. 1993) and the synthesis of NPY and POMC is modulated by gonadal steroids (Chowen et al. 1989; Urban et al. 1993). Thus, gonadal steroids have a direct effect on the hypothalamic neurons controlling metabolism which could explain the differential effects seen between the sexes in response to some metabolic signals.

The hypothalamic NPY/AgRP and POMC/CART neurons innervate neurons of the lateral hypothalamus and perifornical area that produce other orexigenic neuropeptides. One such neuropeptide is melanin-concentrating hormone (MCH), which stimulates food intake and is modulated by fasting and refeeding (Ludwig et al. 2001).

Corticotropin-releasing hormone (CRH), produced by neurons of the paraventricular nucleus (Cone 2000) not only orchestrates the hypothalamic-pituitary-adrenal axis in response to stress, but also participates in regulation of food intake and energy expenditure, with central administration of CRH inhibiting food intake (Krahn et al. 1988). Leptin mediates part of its satiety effects through increasing CRH synthesis and release (Huang et al. 1998).

Orexin and galanin producing neurons exhibit reciprocal changes in their activities in response to fasting and refeeding (Leibowitz 1998; Mondal et al. 1999). Galanin-positive neurons are present in the paraventricular nucleus, lateral hypothalamus and arcuate nucleus (Ceccatelli et al. 1989). Neurons producing orexin A and B (also called hypocretin 1 and 2) are found in the dorsal and lateral hypothalamus, and perifornical area and exert their actions through projections to the arcuate nucleus, paraventricular nucleus, thalamus, brainstem and cerebral cortex (de Lecea et al. 1998; Takenoya et al. 2003). Both galanin and orexin neurons express leptin receptors (Hakansson et al. 1998, 1999), suggesting that they are direct targets for metabolic hormones. Indeed, hypothalamic orexin release is inhibited by leptin and glucose and increased by ghrelin. Orexin stimulates appetite, at least partially through activation of NPY neurons (Ganjavi and Shapiro 2007). The orexin, or hypocretin, system also regulates sleep and reward or pleasure seeking (Ganjavi and Shapiro 2007) and represents an important link between these behaviors.

Galanin-like peptide (GALP) is expressed in the arcuate nucleus, median eminence, and neurohypophysis (Juréus et al. 2001), with the majority (85%) of these neurons expressing the leptin receptor (Cunningham et al. 2002; Krasnow et al. 2003). Administration of GALP increases food intake and body weight (Hensen et al. 2003). Furthermore, GALP is co-expressed with α-MSH (Takenoya et al. 2002) and orexin receptor-1 (Takenoya et al. 2003) in some arcuate nucleus neurons, suggesting that it may have a multifunctional role in metabolic control.

The continuous discovery of new appetite-modulating proteins indicates that our current knowledge of appetite regulation is incomplete. Nesfatin, discovered in 2006, is expressed in several hypothalamic nuclei implicated in appetite control (Oh-I et al. 2006). This peptide is co-expressed with oxytocin and vasopressin in the paraventricular and supraoptic nuclei (Kohno et al. 2008) and with MCH in tuberal hypothalamic neurons (Fort et al. 2008). This peptide is also produced in gastric endocrine cells (Stengel et al. 2008) and can cross the BBB (Pan et al. 2007). Injection of nesfatin-1, an amino-terminal fragment of this molecule, diminishes appetite and administration of a blocking antibody increases food intake. Furthermore, central administration of MSH increases nesfatin expression, whereas antagonists of MC4R abolish nesfatin-1 induced satiety, suggesting that this protein modulates melanocortin signaling (Oh-I et al. 2006).

Some classical neurotransmitters such as serotonin and acetylcholine may act on feeding through modulation of NPY and/or POMC neurons. Serotonin stimulated hypophagia is most likely mediated through activation of MC4R (Xu et al. 2003) as the serotonin analog fenfluramine suppresses appetite, by activating the melatonin pathway in the arcuate nucleus (Kim et al. 2000). Acetylcholine may also modulate MCH signaling through the M3 muscarinic receptor (Kim et al. 2002) and mice deficient in this receptor have a reduction in food intake and body weight (Chen et al. 2004).

Cannabinoids have long been known to be associated with appetite stimulation, although it was only in recent years that scientific evidence has been generated to support this hypothesis. In 1992, the first endogenous cannabinoid anandamide, or AEA, was identified (Devane et al. 1992). After that 2-arachidonoyl glycerol (2-AG) was discovered (Mechoulam et al. 1995). Both of these compounds are derivatives of arachidonic acid and bind CB1 and CB2 receptors, although with different affinities and activation efficacies (Howlett 2002). Endocannabinoids stimulate appetite in a dose-dependent manner through the CB1 receptor and are believed to be involved in increasing the motivation to eat. The CB1 receptor is expressed in key hypothalamic peptidergic systems, such as those producing CRH in the paraventricular nucleus, CART in the dorsal medial hypothalamus, and MCH and orexins in the lateral hypothalamic-perifornical area (Cota et al. 2003) indicating the possibility of direct actions on metabolic control. Indeed, this receptor is modified in a temporal and site-specific pattern in response to a high fat diet (South and Huang 2008). However, the NPY/AgRP system in the arcuate nculeus does not seem to be directly targeted by endocannabinoid action (Cota et al. 2003; Di Marzo et al. 2001).

Endocannabinoids gradually increase during inter-meal intervals and the greater the time interval between meals, the greater the activity of the endocannabinoid circuits and as a consequence, the motivation to eat. Leptin is a strong inhibitor of hypothalamic endocannabinoid levels (Di Marzo et al. 2001). Ghrelin may act on neurons of the arcuate nucleus by increasing endocannabinoids (Tucci et al. 2004). It has been suggested that obesity is associated with a chronic hypothalamic over-activation of the endocannabinoid system. Antagonists to the CB1 receptor as appetite inhibitors are an intense area of pharmaceutical investigation; however, the currently available agents have been removed from clinical trials due to various side-effects including depression and impairment of the ACTH-cortisol axis.

Brain Circuitry Involved in Appetite, Metabolism and Satiety

Although the hypothalamus plays a key role in the integration of signals and orchestrating the response to the diverse inputs, it is clear that the central control of energy homeostasis is much more widely distributed. Within the hypothalamus, the paraventricular nucleus receives innervation from both NPY/AgRP and POMC/CART neurons of the arcuate nucleus. The interplay between AgRP and α-MSH fibers on MC4R-expressing neurons in this nucleus is thought to be one of the most crucial for metabolic regulation. From the paraventricular nucleus, efferents are sent to the brainstem, spinal cord, cortex and thalamus, as well as to the portal vasculature whereby signals can reach the anterior pituitary. Neuropeptide Y and POMC neurons of the arcuate nucleus also send projections to the ventralmedial hypothalamus. As mentioned above, this nucleus expresses MC4R receptors that respond to α-MSH released by arcuate neurons, which inhibits food intake.

The brainstem is interconnected to several neural networks involved in the regulation of food intake and energy balance. Initial indications of the importance of the brainstem in the control of energy homeostasis came from experiments performed in decerebrated animals. These studies demonstrated that the brainstem alone is sufficient to integrate oropharyngeal and digestive tract signals to establish the size of meals during a short-time period, although decerebrated animals cannot act in response to food deprivation (Grill and Kaplan 2002). Later studies showed that caudal brainstem mechanisms integrated gut-derived satiety signals to determine the level of satiety (Berthoud et al. 2006).

The hypothalamus and brainstem have reciprocal connections that are involved in appetite and metabolism (Ter Horst et al. 1989). Descending efferents from the hypothalamus, including melanocortinergic and orexinergic projections, reach the nucleus tractus solitarius, which contains POMC neurons and NPY neurons and MC4R and NPY receptors (Kishi et al. 2003) and responds to food intake with an increase in NPY levels.

The nucleus tractus solitarius also sends projections to the hypothalamus, especially to the paraventricular nucleus, where both autonomic and neuroendocrine information is integrated (Williams et al. 2000). The nucleus tractus solitarius, which is close to the area postrema a structure with an incomplete BBB, responds efficiently to peripheral signals, such as leptin and adiponectin (Huo et al. 2006), similar to the arcuate nucleus Figure 16.1.

Peripheral Hormone Feedback at the Hypothalamus

Adipose Tissue Signals

Leptin is the most important adipokine in energy homeostasis control, with its circulating levels being directly correlated with body fat content (Argente et al. 1997); thus leptin is considered an adiposity, rather than satiety, signal. It is mainly produced by differentiated adipocytes, although several other tissues also produce this peptide (Meier and Gressner 2004). The highest density of the leptin receptor isoform most implicated in metabolism is found in the hypothalamus. Specific receptors for transporting leptin across the BBB, as well as a soluble isoform that apparently modulates leptin activities, are also important for metabolic control (Korner et al. 2005).

Leptin uptake into the brain decreases during fasting, concomitantly with the fall in circulating leptin levels, whereas after food intake there is a parallel increase in serum leptin levels and brain transport (Kastin and Pan 2000). Leptin modulates neurons, especially in the brainstem and hypothalamus, where its receptors are most highly expressed in the arcuate nucleus, paraventricular nucleus and dorsomedial hypothalamus (Sone and Osamura 2001), and present in lower levels in other hypothalamic nuclei and different areas of the brainstem, including the nucleus tractus solitarius (Grill and Kaplan 2002). Other proteins secreted by adipose tissue, such as *adiponectin*, resistin or interleukin 6 (IL-6), appear to be more closely related with modulation of insulin's actions than with a direct effect on the CNS. However, a central effect of these adipokines cannot be ruled out. Although whether *adiponectin* crosses the BBB is still controversial, its trimers and low molecular weight forms have been detected in cerebral spinal fluid CSF, its specific receptors are widely distributed in the brain and its CSF levels increase after *i.v.* injection (Ahima and Lazar 2008). Adiponectin *i.c.v.* injection decreases body weight through stimulation of energy expenditure, decreases serum glucose, triglycerides and non esterified fatty acids, and increases CRH expression in the paraventricular nucleus (Ahima et al. 2006). Adiponectin might act through the melanocortin pathway or by inhibiting central IL-6 release (Spranger et al. 2006). Furthermore, adiponectin has recently been shown to directly depolarize parvocellular neurons in the paraventricular nucleus, thus controlling neuroendocrine and autonomic functions (Hoyda et al. 2009).

Some reports describe inhibition of food intake and generation of hepatic insulin resistance after *resistin* administration (*i.c.v.*) in mice (Ahima et al. 2006; Tovar et al. 2005). In a similar fashion, *i.c.v.* infusion of the ubiquituosly expressed *IL-6* has been shown to increase energy expenditure and decrease body fat in rats (Ahima 2005; Wallenius et al. 2002), although their real pathophysiological role in energy homeostasis is far from being understood.

Digestive System Signals

The gastrointestinal (GI) tract and the pancreas produce several peptides related to satiation (the feeling of fullness which terminates eating) and satiety (the prolongation of the interval between meals), with the exception of gastric derived ghrelin, which is known to be a powerful orexigenic signal (Woods and D´Alessio 2008).

Signals from GI tract

Ghrelin is mainly produced by the oxyntic cells in the gastric mucosa and derived from pre-pro-ghrelin, whose posttranslational modifications can also lead to the expression of *obestatin* with postulated antagonistic activities to ghrelin (Zhang et al. 2005) that have been challenged (Chartrel et al. 2007). Ghrelin was first described as the endogenous ligand for the GH secretagogue receptor (GHS-R), and undergoes acylation in its serine residue at position 3 by a molecule of *n*-octanoid acid (Kojima et al. 1999). This acylation allows it to cross the BBB and to bind the 1a subtype of the GHS-R. However, des-acyl ghrelin is the most abundant form in plasma and is thought to bind other GHS-R isoforms, although its specific receptor remains unknown. In addition, *i.c.v.* but not peripheral administration of des-acyl ghrelin increases appetite through GHS-R independent activation of hypothalamic orexin producing neurons (Murphy et al. 2006; Toshinai et al. 2006; Wynne et al. 2005a).

Ghrelin modulates energy homeostasis by stimulating NPY/AgRP neurons in the arcuate nucleus, thus activating the orexigenic pathway (Wynne et al. 2005a) (Fig. 16.1). Serum ghrelin levels are influenced by both short and long term changes in energy homeostasis, increasing during fasting and decreasing in the postprandial period (Murphy et al. 2006; Wynne et al. 2005b). A long term decrease or increase in the body's energy stores (i.e., anorexia or obesity) lead to hyper- and hypoghrelinemia, respectively; with a trend towards normalization after weight gain or weight loss, respectively (Soriano-Guillén et al. 2004).

As previously stated, most of the signals derived from the GI tract and involved in energy homeostasis, with the exception of ghrelin, are satiation or satiety signals. These include cholecystokinin (CCK), peptide YY (PYY), glicentin, glucagon-like peptide (GLP) 1 and 2, the bombesin family (bombesin, glucagon related peptide [GRP] and neuromedin B [NMB]), oxyntomodulin, enterostatin and apo A-IV. Moreover, the majority of these peptides (CCK, GLP-1 and 2, PYY, GRP, NMB, oxyntomodulin and apo A-IV) are also synthesized in the brain.

Cholecystokinin is rapidly secreted to the bloodstream by the I cells in the small intestine in response to dietary fats and proteins entering the duodenum and has a paracrine effect by activating its specific G-protein coupled receptors (mainly CCK_A) in the afferent branches of the vagus nerve (Woods and D´Alessio 2008). CCK suppresses food intake during meals, although its short half life does not prevent the occurrence of a second meal (Jayasena and Bloom 2008).

PYY is secreted by the L cells in the distal ileum and colon as PYY_{1-36} and then transformed into PYY_{3-36} by the enzyme dipeptyl peptidase IV (DPP-IV). Both PYY_{1-36} and PYY_{3-36} can be found in peripheral blood, but the latter is more abundant. PYY secretion is stimulated by food intake and the presence of nutrients (mainly lipids) in the GI lumen in proportion to caloric intake (Woods and D´Alessio 2008). PYY locally decreases GI motility, can freely cross the BBB (Nonaka et al. 2003) and has high affinity for the Y_2 presynaptic receptor, inhibiting NPY release in the hypothalamic arcuate nucleus, thus decreasing appetite.

GLP-1 is produced from proglucagon by the L cells in the distal small intestine and colon in response to ingested nutrients, mainly carbohydrates and lipids. There are two main circulating bioactive forms, GLP_{7-36} amide and GLP_{7-37}, that are rapidly inactivated by DPP-IV. It has been shown to slow GI motility and to decrease food intake in both lean and obese humans (Gutzwiller et al. 1999; Näslund et al. 1999). Its anorexigenic activity is mediated by a GLP-1 specific receptor, which is expressed in the gut, brainstem and hypothalamus among other locations (Baggio et al. 2004).

Oxyntomodulin, another proglucagon product, is also secreted by the L cells in the distal intestine, where it colocalizes with PYY and GLP-1. Oxyntomodulin is secreted postprandially in proportion to the amount of calories in a meal and slows gastric emptying and gut motility and has been shown to decrease food intake in humans, with weight loss associated with its chronic administration (Wynne et al. 2005b), possibly through stimulation of the GLP-1 receptor in neurons of the arcuate nucleus (Wynne and Bloom 2006).

Signals from the pancreas

Fasting serum *insulin* levels increase in parallel with adiposity, as does leptin. Insulin fulfills the criteria to be considered as both a satiation and an adiposity signal, as it chronically increases with adiposity and quickly rises after meals (Gerozissis 2008). Insulin and its receptor are widely distributed in the CNS with high concentrations in the hypothalamus, especially the arcuate nucleus, and *i.c.v.* insulin administration results in powerful anorectic effects. Eating increases and fasting decreases the amount of insulin in the CSF and brain (Orosco et al. 1995), with insulin inducing both short and long term effects on feeding behavior and body weight. It acts by down-regulating the production of orexigenic peptides such as NPY and AgRP in the arcuate nucleus and, in collaboration with serotonin, by enhancing POMC production and release (Gerozissis 2008).

Pancreatic polypeptide (*PP*) is produced post-prandially by F cells under vagal control in proportion to the calories ingested and its blood levels remain elevated for approximately 6 h post-prandially (Katsuura et al. 2002). This peptide binds and activates mainly Y_4, but also Y_5 receptors and its peripheral injection inhibits food intake (Jayasena and Bloom 2008); however, centrally injected PP increases food intake (Asakawa et al. 1999). *Amylin* (islet amyloid polypeptide) is cosecreted postprandially with insulin by the β cells. It signals through the calcitonin receptor, once it has been modified by receptor activity modifying proteins (Martínez et al. 2000). Amylin appears to inhibit food intake by acting directly on the area postrema, without interacting with the visceral nerves, thus behaving as a true hormone. Both peripheral and central administration of amylin decrease meal size in a dose-dependent fashion, whereas antagonism of its actions increases body weight (Lutz 2006). Moreover, amylin has synergistic actions with other digestive signals, having a more intense anorexigenic effect when brain insulin levels are elevated and also being necessary for correct CCK and bombesin signaling (Woods and D´Alessio 2008).

Nutrient Effects on Hypothalamic Signaling

Hypothalamic neurons respond to circulating free fatty acids and glucose in cooperation with appetite-modulating hormones to regulate feeding behavior.

Free Fatty Acids

Central administration of long-chain fatty acids (LCFA) inhibits food intake via NPY neurons in the arcuate nucleus, involving accumulation of LCFA-CoA (Obici et al. 2002a). Since FFAs access the brain in proportion to their plasma levels, LCFAs may regulate energy homeostasis by acting as an abundance signal (Lam et al. 2005). Their effects are related to a reduction in NPY and an increase in POMC expression (Shimokawa et al. 2002). Central production of enzymes involved in fatty acid synthesis, such as acetyl-CoA carboxylase and fatty acid synthase (FAS), may indicate that de novo lipogenesis could be involved in feeding behavior (López et al. 2006).

Glucose

Glucose is a modulatory signal that activates neurons in both the peripheral and central nervous systems. Two glucose responsive populations of neurons have been identified in hypothalamic nuclei. The first group, called glucose-responsive (excited) neurons, enhance their firing rate in response to a rise in glucose concentrations and the second, glucose-sensitive (inhibited), are activated by a decrease in glucose (Yang et al. 2004). The glucose sensing mechanism used by hypothalamic cells is similar to that found in pancreatic β-cells. In this regard, glucose uptake by glucose transporter 2 (GLUT2) is essential, with subsequent phosphorylation in the cell and metabolism by glycolysis to increase the ATP/ADP ratio. This results in the closing of ATP-dependent potassium channels with membrane depolarization and calcium influx (Marty et al. 2007). In glucose-inhibited neurons, the mechanism appears to involve the opening of potassium and possibly chloride channels. These glucose-sensing neurons activate NPY and AgRP neurons in the arcuate nulceus, promoting food intake. Factors affecting glucose sensing such as GLUT2 require functional coupling between glial cells and neurons (Marty et al. 2005). This coupling may be dependent on uptake of glucose by astrocytes through GLUT2, catabolizing it to lactate and shuttling this metabolite to neurons via specific transporters in order to produce ATP (Marty et al. 2007).

Intracellular Signaling in Hypothalamic Neurons

Leptin and insulin have overlapping effects in the arcuate nucleus, with defects in their signaling resulting in disordered energy homeostasis (Niswender and Schwartz 2003).

Insulin Signaling

As shown in Fig. 16.2, after binding of insulin to its receptor, the receptor is autophosphorylated (Morton et al. 2006). This phosphorylation produces a binding site for insulin-receptor-substrate

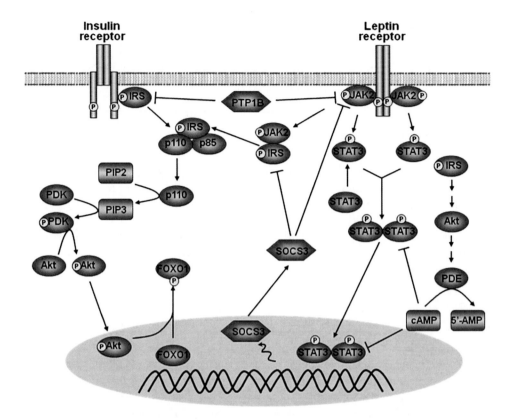

Fig. 16.2 Insulin and leptin signaling in the hypothalamus. Insulin receptor activation induces tyrosine kinase activity, resulting in receptor autophosphorylation and subsequently in the phosphorylation of insulin receptor substrate (IRS) proteins. This event activates a regulatory subunit (p85) of phosphatidyl inositol 3-kinase (PI3K) and the catalytic subunit (p110) phosphorylates phosphatidylinositol-4',5'-biphosphatate (PIP2) on position 3', producing PIP3, which activates the phosphoinositide-dependent protein kinase (PDK). This kinase phosphorylates the protein kinase B (Akt) that enters the nucleus, where it phosphorylates forkhead-O transcription factor (FOXO1). This results in FOXO1 exiting the nucleus and its inactivation. Leptin binds to its receptor and induces activation of Janus kinase-2 (JAK2), followed by phosphorylation and activation of signal transducer and activator of transcription-3 (STAT3). Activated STAT3 dimerizes, translocates to the nucleus and activates target genes, including the suppressor of cytokine signaling-3 (SOCS3), which feedbacks to inhibit JAK2 and IRS. Thus, SOCS3 can modulate signaling by insulin and leptin receptors. In addition, leptin can activate the IRS-PI3K cascade, probably due to tyrosine phosphorylation of IRS proteins by JAK2. The tyrosine phosphatase PTP1B is involved in termination of signals generated by insulin and leptin through its actions on JAK2 and IRS proteins, similar to SOCS3. Thus, there are different steps by which leptin and insulin signaling can interact

(IRS) proteins. IRS proteins bind and activate the enzyme phosphatidylinositol-3-OH kinase (PI3K) that catalyzes the phosphorylation of phosphatidylinositol (PI)-4,5-biphosphate (PIP2) to PI-3,4,5-triphosphate (PIP3). This product mediates the activation of phosphoinositide-dependent kinase 1 (PDK1) and the enzyme cascade that includes protein kinase B (PKB, also known as Akt) and forkhead-O transcription factor 1 (FOXO1) that is inhibited by Akt-mediated phosphorylation.

Leptin Signaling

Leptin receptors act on and activate signal transducers and activators of transcription (STATs). Binding of leptin to the long form of its receptor induces the phosphorylation and activation of

JAK2 and mediates cytokine receptor-like signals, including those mediated by STAT-3 (Myers 2004). Phosphorylated STAT-3 is translocated to the nucleus where it modulates the expression of target promoters (Sahu 2004) (Fig. 16.2). The JAK/STAT pathway is under negative feedback control by different suppressor of cytokine signaling (SOCS) proteins (Cooney 2002). Leptin induces SOCS3 mRNA levels and activates SOCS3 expression in NPY and POMC neurons (Higuchi et al. 2005). Leptin stimulates the insulin-like signaling pathway through PI3K-activation of phosphodiesterase 3B (PDE3B) and reduction of cAMP levels (Zhao et al. 2000).

Ghrelin Signaling

Although several intracellular pathways have been implicated in ghrelin signaling, none has been shown to be directly involved with regulation of food intake or production of neuropeptides in the arcuate nucleus in response to ghrelin (Andersson et al. 2004; Baldanzi et al. 2002; Murata et al. 2002).

Hypothalamic-Pituitary-Adipose Axis: "Adipotropins"

Schäffler and coworkers proposed the term "*adipotropins*" to categorize hormones and factors produced in the pituitary or hypothalamus with known effects on adipocytes (Schäffler et al. 2006). Among these, prolactin, GH, thyrotropin (TSH) and ACTH are the most widely studied *adipotropins*.

Functional *prolactin* receptors are expressed in human adipocytes (Viengchareun et al. 2004). Prolactin may play a role in adipose tissue development and remodeling (Flint et al. 2003). It also has been shown to reduce adiponectin production, as well as insulin binding and glucose transport into the adipocyte (Flint et al. 2003).

Adipose tissue is one of the main target sites for direct *GH* action, with mature functional GH receptors existing in both preadipocytes and adipocytes. GH plays a major role in adipose tissue accumulation and distribution, as well as in metabolic regulation by enhancing protein synthesis and lipolysis (Flint et al. 2003) and displaying direct insulin antagonistic effects on adipocytes (del Rincon et al. 2007).

Human preadipocytes and adipocytes also have functional thyrotropin (*TSH*) receptors (Sorisky et al. 2000), with TSH apparently acting as a survival factor by reducing apoptosis in preadipocytes (Bell et al. 2002). TSH displays species specific effects on leptin secretion, down-regulating it in mice (Shintani et al. 1999) and enhancing it in human adipocytes (Menéndez et al. 2003), whereas IL-6 expression is enhanced in adipocytes from both species (Antunes et al. 2005).

There are limited reports about the direct effect of *ACTH* on adipocytes, although ACTH receptors are present in mouse brown and white adipocytes and in the mouse 3T3-L1 lineage, and their expression increases during differentiation (Boston and Cone 1996; Iwen et al. 2008). Chronic ACTH stimulation induces major metabolic effects in white adipocytes by reducing insulin-induced glucose uptake (Iwen et al. 2008) and increasing lipolysis (Cho et al. 2005). ACTH also influences the endocrine function of adipose tissue by down-regulating 11-β-hydroxysteroid dehydrogenase (11β-HSD) activity (Friedberg et al. 2003). In addition, in response to ACTH visfatin and adiponectin gene expression and leptin mRNA levels and secretion are reduced, while monocyte chemoattractant protein-1 (MCP-1) and interleukin-6 (IL-6) mRNA levels and secretion are increased (Iwen et al. 2008; Norman et al. 2003).

Hypothalamic Changes in Obesity

The hypothalamus regulates energy homeostasis by integrating numerous input signals. Thus, obesity may result in changes at the hypothalamic level or the loss of homeostatic processes at this level may result in obesity.

Neuropeptide Changes

Although leptin resistance seems to be a result of obesity, it cannot be discarded that the lack of leptin sensitivity may contribute to the development of obesity. Rats with reduced leptin sensitivity are prone to develop obesity in the presence of a high-energy diet (Scarpace and Zhang 2009). These rats have increased NPY mRNA levels in the arcuate nucleus; however, after a prolonged period of obesity, these levels decrease. One possible mechanism against becoming obese is the increase in POMC synthesis after increased caloric intake (Ziotopoulou et al. 2000).

In-Put Signals

Hypothalamic alterations in leptin and/or insulin signaling cause increased body weight (Pelleymounter et al. 1995). Obese humans have increased serum leptin levels and are not responsive to leptin administration, supporting the theory of leptin resistance in exogenous obesity (Ahima 2005). Indeed, mutations resulting in the loss of leptin signaling are associated with early-onset morbid obesity (Clement et al. 1998).

Impaired brain insulin signaling, a link coupling obesity to diabetes, may be related to environmental factors such as stress, over-feeding and an unbalanced diet. Mice with neuron-specific insulin receptor deletions have increased body weight and restoration of the insulin receptor in the brain maintains energy homeostasis (Okamoto et al. 2004). Moreover, central injection of an insulin mimetic reduces food intake and body weight in rats and alters the expression of hypothalamic genes regulating food intake and body weight (Air et al. 2002), with NPY most likely mediating some of these actions.

Leptin Signaling Down-Regulation

In most situations, obesity cannot be attributed to defects in leptin or its receptor, and as obese humans are hyperleptinemic (Argente et al. 1997), it is suggested that these patients are leptin-resistant (Sahu 2004), which is characterized as a lower activation of STAT3. Leptin resistance involves at least two mediators, SOCS3 and protein tyrosine phosphatase 1B (PTP1B). Neuron-specific conditional SOCS-3 knockout mice are resistant to diet-induced obesity (Mori et al. 2004) and mice genetically deficient for PTP1B are lean and hypersensitive to leptin (Xue et al. 2007). Chronic central leptin infusion induces leptin resistance involving the PDE3B-cAMP pathway. An increase in PDE3B activity together with a reduction in cAMP concentrations were detected in the hypothalamus of leptin-infused rats, with no changes in JAK-2/STAT-3 signaling (Pal and Sahu 2003).

Insulin Signaling Down-Regulation

The high concordance of obesity and type 2 diabetes insinuates at least a partially common pathophysiological mechanism between leptin and insulin resistance. Mice with neuron-specific deletion of the insulin receptor in the brain are obese, with increased peripheral levels of insulin (Bruning et al. 2000; Obici et al. 2002b). High fat feeding of animals causes insulin resistance by impairing the ability of this hormone to activate the PI3K pathway. The mechanism appears to involve inactivation of phosphorylation of IRS proteins, and subsequently a reduced capacity to activate PI3K and finally, a reduction in glucose transporter translocation (Perseghin et al. 2003; Wynne et al. 2005a).

Conclusions

It is clear that our understanding of the neuroendocrine control of appetite and metabolism has increased rapidly in recent years. However, it is also clear that this system is very complex, with numerous factors and hormones involved. Indeed, there are many redundancies, including more than one hormone with very similar functions, within this control system that have made development of rapid and easy treatment of excess body weight to date impossible. We now know that the main central control of metabolism occurs in the hypothalamus. In this brain region, NPY/AgRP neurons integrate multiple signals to then send out signals to increase food intake and decrease metabolism. In contrast, POMC/CART neurons within the hypothalamic arcuate nucleus have the opposite function, decreasing appetite and increasing metabolic out-put. Many circulating hormones reach these neuronal populations, either by active or passive transport into the brain, to modulate their output signals and control eating behavior and metabolic rate. Amongst these signals, leptin and insulin have been the most highly studied appetite suppressing signals. These two hormones feed-back at the hypothalamus to inform the control system of the systemic fat content and the short-term nutritional status. Ghrelin, produced in the gastrointestinal tract, stimulates appetite and reduces energy expenditure. Both leptin and ghrelin have been and continue to be major targets for the development of effective obesity treatments. Exogenous obesity, however, is usually associated with increased circulating leptin levels, indicating a situation of leptin insensitivity and decreasing the effectiveness of leptin as a treatment. Indeed, we now know that in exogenous obesity the central control system is modulated such that the perception of these signals is changed, resulting in a shift in the set-point of the system, allowing increased weight gain. These changes in sensitivity to metabolic signals can include changes in the number of receptors for the specific signal and/or modifications in their intracellular signaling mechanisms.

In addition, the fact that the metabolic and hormonal environment during early development can impact on the wiring of the neuroendocrine hypothalamus increasing or decreasing its capacity to induce fat accumulation indicates that in order to curtail the rapid rise in obesity in many countries, prenatal care and early postnatal care must also be taken into consideration.

References

Ahima, R.S. (2005). Central actions of adipocyte hormones. *Trends in Endocrinology and Metabolism, 16,* 307–313.

Ahima, R.S. & Lazar, M.A. (2008). Adipokines and the peripheral and neural control of energy balance. *Molecular Endocrinology, 22,* 1023–1031.

Ahima, R.S., Qi, Y., Singhal, N.S., Jackson, M.B., & Scherer, P.E. (2006). Brain adipocytokine action and metabolic regulation. *Diabetes, 55,* S145–S154.

Air, E.L., Strowski, M.Z., Benoit, S.C., Conarello, S.L., Salituro, G.M., Guan, X.M., Liu, K., Woods, S.C., & Zhang, B.B. (2002). Small molecule insulin mimetics reduce food intake and body weight and prevent development of obesity. *Nature Medicine, 8,* 179–183.

Anand, B.K., & Brobeck, J.R. (1951). Localization of feeding center in the hypothalamus of the rat. *Proceedings of the Society for Experimental Biology and Medicine, 11,* 323–324.

Andersson, U., Filipsson, K., Abbott, C.R., Woods, A., Smith, K., Bloom, S.R., Carling D., & Small, C.J. (2004). AMP-activated protein kinase plays a role in the control of food intake. *The Journal of Biological Chemistry, 279,* 12005–12008.

Antunes, T.T., Gagnon, A., Bell, A., & Sorisky, A. (2005). Thyroid-stimulating hormone stimulates interleukin-6 release from 3T3-L1 adipocytes through a cAMP-protein kinase A pathway. *Obesity Research, 13,* 2066–2071.

Arch, J.R. (2005). Central regulation of energy balance: inputs, outputs and leptin resistance. *Proceedings of the Nutrition Society, 64,* 39–46.

Argente, J., Barrios, V., Chowen, J.A., Sinha, M.K., & Considine, R.V. (1997). Leptin plasma levels in healthy Spanish children and adolescents, children with obesity, and adolescents with anorexia nervosa and bulimia nervosa. *The Journal of Pediatrics, 131,* 833–838.

Asakawa, A., Inui, A., Ueno, N., Fujimiya, M., Fujino, M.A., & Kasuga, M. (1999). Mouse pancreatic polypeptide modulates food intake, while not influencing anxiety in mice. *Peptides, 20,* 1445–1448.

Baggio, L.L., Huang, Q., Brown, T.J., & Drucker, D.J. (2004). Oxyntomodulin and glucagon-like peptide-1 differentially regulate murine food intake and energy expenditure. *Gastroenterology, 127,* 546–558.

Baldanzi, G., Filigheddu, N., Cutrupi, S., Catapano, F., Bonissoni, S., Fubini, A., Malan, D., Baj, G., Granata, R., Broglio, F., Papotti, M., Surico, N., Bussolino, F., Isgaard, J., Deghenghi, R., Sinigaglia, F., Prat, M., Muccioli, G., Ghigo, E., & Graziani, A. (2002). Ghrelin and des-acyl ghrelin inhibit cell death in cardiomyocytes and endothelial cells through ERK1/2 and PI 3-kinase/AKT. *The Journal of Cell Biology, 159,* 1029–1037.

Banks, W.A. (2006). The blood-brain barrier as a regulatory interface in the gut-brain axes. *Physiology & Behavior, 89,* 472–476.

Bell, A., Gagnon, A., Dods, P., Papineau, D., Tiberi, M., & Sorisky, A. (2002). TSH signaling and cell survival in 3T3-L1 preadipocytes. *American Journal of Physiology. Cell Physiology, 283,* C1056–C1064.

Berthoud, H.R., Sutton, G.M., Townsend, R.L., Patterson, L.M., & Zheng, H. (2006). Brainstem mechanisms integrating gut-derived satiety signals and descending forebrain information in the control of meal size. *Physiology & Behavior, 89,* 517–524.

Boston, B.A., & Cone, R.D. (1996). Characterization of melanocortin receptor subtype expression in murine adipose tissues and in the 3T3-L1 cell line. *Endocrinology, 137,* 2043–2050.

Broberger, C. (1999). Hypothalamic cocaine-and amphetamine-regulated transcript (CART) neurons: histochemical relationship to thyrotropin-releasing hormone, melanin-concentrating hormone, orexin/hypocretin and neuropeptide Y. *Brain Research, 289,* 101–113.

Bruning, J.C., Gautam, D., Burks, D.J., Gillette, J., Schubert, M., Orban, P.C., Klein, R., Krone, W., Muller-Wieland, D., & Kahn, C.R. (2000). Role of brain insulin receptor in control of body weight and reproduction. *Science, 289,* 2122–2125.

Ceccatelli, S., Eriksson, M., & Hokfelt, T. (1989). Distribution and coexistence of corticotropin-releasing factor-, neurotensin-, enkephalin-, cholecystokinin-, galanin- and vasoactive intestinal polypeptide/peptide histidine isoleucine-like peptides in the parvocellular part of the paraventricular nucleus. *Neuroendocrinology, 49,* 309–323.

Chartrel, N., Alvear-Perez, R., Leprince, J., Iturrioz, X., Reaux-Le Goazigo, A., Audinot, V., Chomarat, P., Coge, N., Nosjean, O., Rodriguez, M., Galizzi, J.P., Boutin, J.A., Vaudry, H., & Llorens-Cortes, C. (2007). Comment on "Obestatin, a peptide encoded by the ghrelin gene, opposes ghrelin's effects on food intake". *Science, 315,* 766.

Chen, P., Williams, S.M., Grove, K.L., & Smith, M.S. (2004). Melanocortin 4 receptor-mediated hyperphagia and activation of neuropeptide Y expression in the dorsomedial hypothalamus during lactation. *The Journal of Neuroscience, 24,* 5091–5100.

Cho, K.J., Shim, J.H., Cho, M.C., Choe, Y.K., Hong, J.T., Moon, D.C., Kim, J.W., & Yoon, D.Y. (2005). Signaling pathways implicated in alpha-melanocyte stimulating hormone-induced lipolysis in 3T3-L1 adipocytes. *The Journal of Cell Biochemistry, 96,* 869–878.

Chowen, J., Fraser, H.M., Vician, L., Damassa, D.A., Clifton, D.K., & Steiner, R.A. (1989). Testosterone regulation of proopiomelanocortin messenger ribonucleicacid in the arcuate nucleus of the male rat. *Endocrinology, 124,* 1697–1702.

Clement, K., Vaisse, C., Lahlou, N., Cabrol, S., Pelloux, V., Cassuto, D., Gourmelen, M., Dina, C., Chambaz, J., Lacorte, J.M., Basdevant, A., Bougneres, P., Lebouc, Y., Froguel, P., & Guy-Grand, B. (1998). A mutation in the human leptin receptor gene causes obesity and pituitary dysfunction. *Nature, 392,* 398–401.

Cone, R.D. (2000). The corticotropin-releasing hormone system and feeding behavior – a complex web begins to unravel. *Endocrinology, 141,* 2713–2714.

Cooney, R.N. (2002). Suppressors of cytokine signaling (SOCS): inhibitors of the JAK/STAT pathway. *Shock, 17,* 83–90.

Cota, D., Marsicano, G., Tschoep, M., Gruebler, Y., Flachskamm, C., Schubert, M., Auer, D., Yassouridis, A., Thöne-Reineke, C., Ortmann, S., Tomassoni, F., Cervino, C., Nisoli, E., Linthorst, A.C., Pasquali, R., Lutz, B., Stalla, G.K., & Pagotto, U. (2003). The endogenous cannabinoid system affects energy balance via central orexigenic drive and peripheral lipogenesis. *The Journal of Clinical Investigation, 112*, 423–431.

Cunningham, M.J., Scarlett, J.M., & Steiner, R.A. (2002). Cloning and distribution of galaninlike peptide mRNA in the hypothalamus and pituitary of the macaque. *Endocrinology, 143*, 755–776.

de Lecea, L., Kilduff, T.S., Peyron, C., Gao, X., Foye, P.E., Danielson, P.E., Fukuhara, C., Battenberg, E.L., Gautvik, VT., Bartlett, F.S. II, Frankel, W.N., van der Pol, A.N., Bloom, F.E., Gautvik, K.M., & Sutcliffe, J.G. (1998). The hypocretins: hypothalamus-specific peptides with neuroexcitatory activity. *Proceedings of the National Academy of Science of the United States of America, 95*, 322–327.

del Rincon, J.P., Iida, K., Gaylinn, B.D., McCurdy, C.E., Leitner, J.W., Barbour, L.A., Kopchick, J.J., Friedman, J.E., Draznin, B., & Thorner, M.O. (2007). Growth hormone regulation of p85alpha expression and phosphoinositide 3-kinase activity in adipose tissue: mechanism for growth hormone-mediated insulin resistance. *Diabetes, 56*, 1638–1646.

Devane, W.A., Hanus, L., Breuer, A., Pertwee, R.G., Stevenson, L.A., Griffin, G., Gibson, D., Mandelbaum, A., Etinger, A., & Mechoulam, R. (1992). Isolation and structure of a brain constituent that binds to the cannabinoid receptor. *Science, 258*, 1946–1949.

Di Marzo, V., Goparaju, S.K., Wang, L., Liu, J., Batkai, S., Jarai, Z., Fezza, F., Miura, G.I., Palmiter, R.D., Sugiura, T., & Kunos, G. (2001). Leptin regulated endocannabinoids are involved in maintaining food intake. *Nature, 410*, 822–825.

Dunbar, J., Lapanowski, K., Barnes, M., & Rafols, J. (2005). Hypothalamic agouti-related protein immunoreactivity in food-restricted, obese, and insulin-treated animals: evidence for glia cell localization. *Experimental Neurology, 191*, 184–192.

Ellacott, K.L., & Cone, R.D. (2004). The central melanocortin system and the integration of short- and long-term regulators of energy homeostasis. *Recent Progress in Hormone Research, 59*, 395–408.

Flint, D.J., Binart, N., Kopchick, J., & Kelly, P. (2003). Effects of growth hormone and prolactin on adipose tissue development and function. *Pituitary, 6*, 97–102.

Fort, P., Salvert, D., Hanriot, L., Jego, S., Shimizu, H., Hashimoto, K., Mori, M., & Luppi, P.H. (2008). The satiety molecule nesfatin-1 is co-expressed with melanin concentrating hormone in tuberal hypothalamic neurons of the rat. *Neuroscience, 155*, 174–181.

Friedberg, M., Zoumakis, E., Hiroi, N., Bader, T., Chrousos, G.P., & Hochberg, Z. (2003). Modulation of 11 beta-hydroxysteroid dehydrogenase type 1 in mature human subcutaneous adipocytes by hypothalamic messengers. *The Journal of Clinical Endocrinology and Metabolism, 88*, 385–393.

Ganjavi, H., & Shapiro, C.M. (2007). Hypocritin/Orexin: a molecular link between sleep, energy regulation and pleasure. *Journal of Neuropsychiatry and Clinical Neuroscience, 19*, 413–419.

Gerozissis, K. (2008). Brain insulin, energy and glucose homeostasis: genes, environment and metabolic pathologies. *European Journal of Pharmacology, 585*, 38–49.

Grill, H.J., & Kaplan, J.M. (2002). The neuroanatomical axis for control of energy balance. *Frontiers in Neuroendocrinology, 23*, 2–40.

Gross, P.M. (1992). Circumventricular organ capillaries. *Progress in Brain Research, 91*, 219–233.

Gutzwiller, J.P., Göke, B., Drewe, J., Hildebrand, P., Ketterer, S., Handschin, D., Winterhalder, R., Conen, D., & Beglinger, C. (1999). Glucagon-like peptide-1: a potent regulator of food intake in humans. *Gut, 44*, 81–86.

Hahn, T.M., Breininger, J.F., Baskin, D.G., & Schwartz, M.W. (1998). Coexpression of Agrp and NPY in fasting-activated hypothalamic neurons. *Nature Neuroscience, 1*, 271–272.

Hakansson, M.L., Brown, H., Ghilardi, N., Skoda, R.C., & Meister, B. (1998). Leptin receptor immunoreactivity in chemically defined target neurons of the hypothalamus. *The Journal of Neuroscience, 18*, 559–572.

Hakansson, M., de Lecea, L., Sutcliffe, J.G., Yanagisawa, M., & Meister, B. (1999). Leptin receptor- and STAT3-immunoreactivities in hypocretin/orexin neurones of the lateral hypothalamus. *Journal of Neuroendocrinology, 11*, 653–663.

Heatherington, A.W., & Ranson, S.W. (1940). Hypothalamic lesions and adiposity in the rat. *Anatomical Records, 78*, 149–172.

Hensen, K.R., Krasnow, S.M., Nolan, M.A., Fraley, G.S., Baumgartner, J.W., Clifton, D.K., & Steiner, R.A. (2003). Activation of the sympathetic nervous system by galanin-like peptide--a possible link between leptin and metabolism. *Endocrinology, 144*, 4709–4717.

Higuchi, H., Hasegawa, A., & Yamaguchi, T. (2005). Transcriptional regulation of neuronal genes and its effect on neural functions: transcriptional regulation of neuropeptide Y gene by leptin and its effect on feeding. *Journal of Pharmacological Sciences, 98*, 225–231.

Howlett, A.C. (2002). The cannabinoid receptors. *Prostaglandins Other Lipid Mediators, 68–69*, 619–631.

Hoyda, T.D., Samson, W.K., & Ferguson, A.V. (2009). Adiponectin depolarizes parvocellular paraventricular nucleus neurons controlling neuroendocrine and autonomic function. *Endocrinology, 150*, 832–840.

Huang, Q., Rivest, R., & Richard, D. (1998). Effects of leptin on corticotropin-releasing factor (CRF) synthesis and CRF neuron activation in the paraventricular hypothalamic nucleus of obese (ob/ob) mice. *Endocrinology, 139*, 1524–1532.

Huo, L., Grill, H.J., & Bjorbaek, C. (2006). Divergent regulation of proopiomelanocortin neurons by leptin in the nucleus of the solitary tract and in the arcuate hypothalamic nucleus. *Diabetes, 55*, 567–573.

Iwen, K.A., Senyaman, O., Schwartz, A., Drenckhan, M., Meier, B., Hadaschik, D., & Klein J. (2008). Melanocortin crosstalk with adipose functions: ACTH directly induces insulin resistance, promotes a pro-inflammatory adipokine profile and stimulates UCP-1 in adipocytes. *Journal of Endocrinology, 196*, 465–472.

Jayasena, C.N., & Bloom, S.R. (2008). Role of gut hormones in obesity. *Endocrinology Metabolism Clinics of North America, 37*, 769–787.

Juréus, A., Cunningham, M.J., Li, D., Johnson, J.L., Krasnow, S.M., Teklemichael, D.N., Clifton, D.K., & Steiner, R.A. (2001). Distribution and regulation of galanin-like peptide (GALP) in the hypothalamus of the mouse. *Endocrinology, 142*, 5140–5144.

Kastin, A.J., & Pan, W. (2000). Dynamic regulation of leptin entry into brain by the blood-brain barrier. *Regulatory Peptides, 92*, 37–43.

Katsuura, G., Asakawa, A., & Inui, A. (2002). Roles of pancreatic polypeptide in regulation of food intake. *Peptides, 23*, 323–329.

Kim, M.S., Rossi, M., Abusnana, S., Sunter, D., Morgan, D.G., Small, C.J., Edwards, C.M., Heath, M.M., Stanley, S.A., Seal, L.J., Bhatti, J.R., Smith, D.M., Ghatei, M.A., & Bloom, S.R. (2000). Hypothalamic localization of the feeding effect of agouti-related peptide and alpha-melanocyte-stimulating hormone. *Diabetes, 49*, 177–182.

Kim, E.M., Grace, M.K., O'Hare, E., Billington, C.J. & Levine A.S. (2002). Injection of alpha-MSH, but not beta-endorphin, into the PVN decreases POMC gene expression in the ARC. *NeuroReport, 13*, 497–500.

Kishi, T., Aschkenasi, C.J., Lee, C.E., Mountjoy, K.G., Saper, C.B. & Elmquist, J.K. (2003). Expression of melano-cortin 4 receptor mRNA in the central nervous system of the rat. *Journal of Comparative Neurology, 457*, 213–235.

Kohno, D., Nakata, M., Maejima, Y., Shimizu, H., Sedbazar, U., Yoshida, N., Dezaki, K., Onaka, T., Mori, M., & Yada, T. (2008). Nesfatin-1 neurons in paraventricular and supraoptic nuclei of the rat hypothalamus coexpress oxytocin and vasopressin and are activated by refeeding. *Endocrinology, 149*, 1295–1301.

Kojima, M., Hosoda, H., Date, Y., Nakazato, M., Matsuo, H., & Kangawa, K. (1999). Ghrelin is a growth-hormone-releasing acylated peptide from stomach. *Nature, 402*, 656–660.

Korner, A., Kratzsch, J., & Kiess, W. (2005). Adipocytokines: leptin–the classical, resistin–the controversial, adiponectin–the promising, and more to come. *Best Practice & Research Clinical Endocrinology & Metabolism, 19*, 525–546.

Krahn, D.D., Gosnell, B.A., Levine, A.S., & Morley, J.E. (1988). Behavioral effects of corticotropin-releasing factor: localization and characterization of central effects. *Brain Research, 443*, 63–69.

Krasnow, S.M., Fraley, G.S., Schuh, S.M., Baumgartner, J.W., Clifton, D.K., & Steiner, R.S. (2003). A role for galanin-like peptide in the integration of feeding, body weight regulation, and reproduction in the mouse. *Endocrinology, 144*, 813–822.

Lam, T.K., Schwartz, G.J., & Rossetti, L. (2005). Hypothalamic sensing of fatty acids. *Nature Neuroscience, 8*, 579–584.

Leibowitz, S.F. (1998). Differential functions of hypothalamic galanin cell grows in the regulation of eating and body weight. *Annals of the New York Academy of Science, 863*, 206–220.

López, M., Lelliott, C.J., Tovar, S., Kimber, W., Gallego, R., Virtue, S., Blount, M., Vázquez, M.J., Finer, N., Powles, T.J., O'Rahilly, S., Saha, A.K., Diéguez, C., & Vidal-Puig A.J. (2006). Tamoxifen-induced anorexia is associated with fatty acid synthase inhibition in the ventromedial nucleus of the hypothalamus and accumulation of malonyl-CoA. *Diabetes, 55*, 1327–1336.

Ludwig, D.S., Tritos, N.A., Mastaitis, J.W., Kulkarni, R., Kokkotou, E., Elmquist, J., Lowell, B., Flier, J.S. & Maratos-Flier, E. (2001). Melanin-concentrating hormone overexpression in transgenic mice leads to obesity and insulin resistance. *The Journal of Clinical Investigation, 107*, 379–386.

Lutz, T.A. (2006). Amylinergic control of food intake. *Physiology & Behavior, 89*, 465–471.

Martínez, A., Kapas, S., Miller, M.J., Ward, Y., & Cuttitta, F. (2000). Coexpression of receptors for adrenomedullin, calcitonin gene-related peptide, and amylin in pancreatic beta-cells. *Endocrinology, 141*, 406–411.

Marty, N., Dallaporta, M., Foretz, M., Emery, M., Tarussio, D., Bady, I., Binnert, C., Beermann, F., & Thorens, B. (2005). Regulation of glucagon secretion by glucose transporter type 2 (glut2) and astrocyte-dependent glucose sensors. *The Journal of Clinical Investigation, 115*, 3545–3553.

Marty, N., Dallaporta, M., & Thorens, B. (2007). Brain glucose sensing, counterregulation, and energy homeostasis. *Physiology (Bethesda), 22*, 241–251.

Mechoulam, R., Ben-Shabat, S., Hanus, L., Ligumsky, M., Kaminski, N.E., Schatz, A.R., Gopher, A., Almog, S., Martin, B.R., & Compton, D.R. (1995). Identification of an endogenous 2-monoglyceride, present in canine gut, that binds to cannabinoid receptors. *Biochemical Pharmacology, 50*, 83–90.

Meier, U., & Gressner, A.M. (2004). Endocrine regulation of energy metabolism: review of pathobiochemical and clinical chemical aspects of leptin, ghrelin, adiponectin, and resistin. *Clinical Chemistry, 50,* 1511–1525.

Menéndez, C., Baldelli, R., Camiña, J.P., Escudero, B., Peino, R, Diéguez, C., & Casanueva, F.F (2003). TSH stimulates leptin secretion by a direct effect on adipocytes. *Journal of Endocrinology, 176,* 7–12.

Mondal, M.S., Nakazato, M., Date, Y., Murakami, N., Yanagisawa, M., & Matsukura, S. (1999). Widespread distribution of orexin in rat brain and its regulation upon fasting. *Biochemical and Biophysical Research Communications, 256,* 495–499.

Mori, H., Hanada, R., Hanada, T., Aki, D., Mashima, R., Nishinakamura, H., Torisu, T., Chien, K.R., Yasukawa, H., & Yoshimura, A. (2004). Socs3 deficiency in the brain elevates leptin sensitivity and confers resistance to diet-induced obesity. *Nature Medicine, 10,* 739–743.

Morton, G.J., Cummings, D.E., Baskin, D.G., Barsh, G.S., & Schwartz, M.W. (2006). Central nervous system control of food intake and body weight. *Nature, 443,* 289–295.

Murata, M., Okimura, Y., Iida, K., Matsumoto, M., Sowa, H., Kaji, H., Kojima, M., Kangawa, K., & Chihara, K. (2002). Ghrelin modulates the downstream molecules of insulin signaling in hepatoma cells. *The Journal of Biological Chemistry, 277,* 5667–5674.

Murphy, K.G., Dhillo, W.S., & Bloom, S.R. (2006). Gut peptides in the regulation of food intake and energy homeostasis. *Endocrine Reviews, 27,* 719–727.

Myers, M.G. Jr. (2004). Leptin receptor signaling and the regulation of mammalian physiology. *Recent Progress in Hormone Research, 59,* 287–304.

Näslund, E., Barkeling, B., King, N., Gutniak, M., Blundell, J.E., Holst, J.J., Rössner S., & Hellström, P.M. (1999). Energy intake and appetite are suppressed by glucagon-like peptide-1 (GLP-1) in obese men. *International Journal of Obesity and Related Metabolic Disorders, 23,* 304–311.

Niswender, K.D., & Schwartz, M.W. (2003). Insulin and leptin revisited: adiposity signals with overlapping physiological and intracellular signaling capabilities. *Frontiers in Neuroendocrinology, 24,* 1–10.

Nonaka, N., Shioda, S., Niehoff, M.L., & Banks, W.A. (2003). Characterization of blood-brain barrier permeability to PYY3-36 in the mouse. *Journal of Pharmacology and Experimental Therapeutics, 306,* 948–953.

Norman, D., Isidori, A.M., Frajese, V., Caprio, M., Chew, S.L., Grossman, A.B., Clark, A.J., Michael Besser, G., & Fabbri, A. (2003). ACTH and alpha-MSH inhibit leptin expression and secretion in 3T3-L1 adipocytes: model for a central-peripheral melanocortin-leptin pathway. *Molecular and Cellular Endocrinology, 200,* 99–109.

Obici, S., Feng, Z., Morgan, K., Stein, D., Karkanias, G., & Rossetti L. (2002a). Central administration of oleic acid inhibits glucose production and food intake. *Diabetes, 51,* 271–275.

Obici, S., Feng, Z., Karkanias, G., Baskin, D.G., & Rossetti, L. (2002b). Decreasing hypothalamic insulin receptors causes hyperphagia and insulin resistance in rats. *Nature Neuroscience, 5,* 566–572.

Oh-I, S., Shimizu, H., Satoh, T., Okada, S., Adachi, S., Inoue, K., Eguchi, H., Yamamoto, M., Imaki, T., Hashimoto, K., Tsuchiya, T., Monden, T., Horiguchi, K., Yamada, M., & Mori, M. (2006). Identification of nesfatin-1 as a satiety molecule in the hypothalamus. *Nature, 443,* 709–712.

Okamoto, H., Nakae, J., Kitamura, T., Park, B.C., Dragatsis, I., & Accili, D. (2004). Transgenic rescue of insulin receptor-deficient mice. *Journal of Clinical Investigation, 114,* 214–223.

Orosco, M., Gerozissis, K., Rouch, C., & Nicolaïdis, S. (1995). Feeding-related immunoreactive insulin changes in the PVN-VMH revealed by microdialysis. *Brain Research, 671,* 149–158.

Pal, R., & Sahu, A. (2003). Leptin signaling in the hypothalamus during chronic central leptin infusion. *Endocrinology, 144,* 3789–3798.

Pan, W., Hsuchou, H., & Kastin, A.J. (2007). Nesfatin-1 crosses the blood-brain barrier without saturation. *Peptides, 28,* 2223–2228.

Pelleymounter, M.A., Cullen, M.J., Baker, M.B., Hecht, R., Winters, D., Boone, T., & Collins, F. (1995). Effects of the obese gene product on body weight regulation in ob/ob mice. *Science, 269,* 540–543.

Perseghin, G., Petersen, K., & Shulman, G.I. (2003). Cellular mechanism of insulin resistance: potential links with inflammation. *International Journal of Obesity and Related Metabolic Disorders, 27 (Suppl 3),* S6–S11.

Sahu, A. (2004). Minireview: a hypothalamic role in energy balance with special emphasis on leptin. *Endocrinology, 145,* 2613–2620.

Sarkar, S., Wittmann, G., Fekete, C., & Lechan, R.M. (2004). Central administration of cocaine-and amphetamine-regulated transcript increases phosphorylation of cAMP response element binding protein in corticotrophin-releasing hormone-producing neurons but not in protyrotropin-releasing hormone-producing neurons in the hypothalamic paraventricular nucleus. *Brain Research, 999,* 181–192.

Scarpace, P.J. & Zhang, Y. (2009). Leptin resistance: a predisposing factor for diet-induced obesity. *American Journal of Regulatory and Integrative Comparative Physiology, 296,* R493–R500.

Schäffler, A., Schölmerich, J., & Buechler, C. (2006). The role of 'adipotropins' and the clinical importance of a potential hypothalamic-pituitary-adipose axis. *Nature Clinical Practice Endocrinology & Metabolism, 2,* 374–383.

Schwartz, M.W., Woods, S.C., Porte, D. Jr., Seeley, R.J., & Baskin, D.G. (2000). Central nervous system control of food intake. *Nature, 404,* 661–671.

Shimokawa, T., Kumar, M.V., & Lane, M.D. (2002). Effect of a fatty acid synthase inhibitor on food intake and expression of hypothalamic neuropeptides. *Proceedings of the National Academy of Sciences of the United States of America, 99,* 66–71.

Shintani, M., Nishimura, H., Akamizu, T., Yonemitsu, S., Masuzaki, H., Ogawa, Y., Hosoda, K., Inoue, G., Yoshimasa, Y., & Nakao, K. (1999). Thyrotropin decreases leptin production in rat adipocytes. *Metabolism, 48,* 1570–1574.

Sindelar, D.K., Mystkowski, P., Marsh, D.J., Palmiter, R.D., & Schwartz, M.W. (2002). Attenuation of diabetic hyperphagia in neuropeptide Y-deficient mice. *Diabetes, 51,* 778–783.

Sone, M., & Osamura, R.Y. (2001). Leptin and the pituitary. *Pituitary, 4,* 15–23.

Soriano-Guillén, L., Barrios, V., Campos-Barros, A., & Argente, J. (2004). Ghrelin levels in obesity and anorexia nervosa: effect of weight reduction or recuperation. *The Journal of Pediatrics, 144,* 36–42.

Sorisky, A., Bell, A., & Gagnon, A. (2000). TSH receptor in adipose cells. *Hormone and Metabolic Research, 32,* 468–474.

South, T., & Huang, X.F. (2008). Temporal and site-specific brain alterations in CB1 receptor binding in high fat diet-induced obesity in C57Bl/6 mice. *Journal of Neuroendocrinology, 20,* 1288–1294.

Spranger, J., Verma, S., Göhring, I., Bobbert, T., Seifert, J., Sindler, A.L., Pfeiffer, A., Hileman, S.M., Tschöp, M., & Banks, W.A. (2006). Adiponectin does not cross the blood-brain barrier but modifies cytokine expression of brain endothelial cells. *Diabetes, 55,* 141–147.

Stengel, A., Goebel, M., Yakubov, I., Wang, L., Witcher, D., Coskun, T., Taché, Y., Sachs, G., & Lambrecht, N.W. (2008). Identification and characterization of nesfatin-1 immunoreactivity in endocrine cell types of the rat gastric oxyntic mucosa. *Endocrinology* [doi: 10.1210/en.2008-00747].

Swart, I., Jahng, J.W., Overton, J.M., & Houpt, T.A. (2002). Hypothalamic NPY, AGRP, and POMC mRNA responses to leptin and refeeding in mice. *American Journal of Physiology. Regulatory, Integrative and Comparative Physiology, 283,* R1020–R1026.

Takenoya, F., Funahashi, H., Matsumoto, H., Ohtaki, T., Katoh, S., Kageyama, H., Suzuki, R., Takeuchi, M., & Shioda, S. (2002). Galanin-like peptide is co-localized with alpha-melanocyte stimulating hormone but not with neuropeptide Y in the rat brain. *Neuroscience Letters, 331,* 119–122.

Takenoya, F., Aihara, K., Funahashi, H., Matsumoto, H., Ohtaki, T., Tsurugano, S., Yamada, S., Katoh, S., Kageyama, H., Takeuchi, M., & Shioda, S. (2003). Galanin-like peptide is target for regulation by orexin in the rat hypothalamus. *Neuroscience Letters, 340,* 209–212.

Ter Horst, G.J., de Boer, P., Luiten, P.G., & van Willigen, J.D. (1989). Ascending projections from the solitary tract nucleus to the hypothalamus. A Phaseolus vulgaris lectin tracing study in the rat. *Neuroscience, 31,* 785–797.

Toshinai, K., Yamaguchi, H., Sun, Y., Smith, R.G., Yamanaka, A., Sakurai, T., Date, Y., Mondal, M.S., Shimbara, T., Kawagoe, T., Murakami, N., Miyazato, M., Kangawa, K., & Nakazato, M. (2006). Des-acyl ghrelin induces food intake by a mechanism independent of the growth hormone secretagogue receptor. *Endocrinology, 147,* 2306–2314.

Tovar, S., Nogueiras, R., Tung, L.Y., Castañeda, T.R., Vázquez, M.J., Morris, A., Williams, L.M., Dickson, S.L., & Diéguez, C. (2005). Central administration of resistin promotes short-term satiety in rats. *European Journal of Endocrinology, 153,* R1–R5.

Tucci, S.A., Rogers, E.K., Korbonits, M., & Kirkham, T.C. (2004). The cannabinoid CB1 receptor antagonist SR141716 blocks the orexigeneic effects of intrahypothalamic ghrelin. *British Journal of Pharmacology, 143,* 520–523.

Urban, J.H., Bauer-Dantoin, A.C., & Levine, J.E. (1993). Neuropeptide Y gene expression in the arcuate nucleus: sexual dimorphism and modulation by testosterone. *Endocrinology, 132,* 139–145.

Vicentic, A., & Jones, D.C. (2007). The CART (cocaine-and amphetamine-regulated transcript) system in appetite and drug addiction. *Journal of Pharmacology and Experimental Therapeutics, 320,* 499–506.

Viengchareun, S., Bouzinba-Segard, H., Laigneau, J.P., Zennaro, M.C., Kelly, P.A., Bado, A., Bado, A., Lombès, M., & Binart, N. (2004). Prolactin potentiates insulin-stimulated leptin expression and release from differentiated brown adipocytes. *Journal of Molecular Endocrinology, 33,* 679–691.

Vrang, N., Larsen, P.J., Clausen, J.T., & Kristensen, P. (1999). Neurochemical characterization of the hypothalamic cocaine-amphetamine-regulated transcript neurons. *The Journal of Neuroscience, 19,* RC5: 1–8.

Wallenius, K., Wallenius, V., Sunter, D., Dickson, S.L., & Jansson, J.O. (2002). Intracerebroventricular interleukin-6 treatment decreases body fat in rats. *Biochemical and Biophysical Research Communication, 293,* 560–565.

Williams, D.L., Kaplan, J.M., & Grill, H.J. (2000). The role of the dorsal vagal complex and the vagus nerve in feeding effects of melanocortin-3/4 receptor stimulation. *Endocrinology, 141,* 1332–1337.

Woods, S.C., & D'Alessio, D.A. (2008). Central control of body weight and appetite. *The Journal of Clinical Endocrinology and Metabolism, 93,* S37–S50.

Wynne, K., & Bloom, S.R. (2006). The role of oxyntomodulin and peptide tyrosine-tyrosine (PYY) in appetite control. *Nature Clinical Practice Endocrinology and Metabolism, 2,* 612–620.

Wynne, K., Stanley S., McGowan, B., & Bloom, S. (2005a). Appetite control. *The Journal of Endocrinology, 184,* 291–318.

Wynne, K., Park, A.J., Small, C.J., Patterson, M., Ellis, S.M., Murphy, K.G., Wren, A.M., Frost, G.S., Meeran, K., Ghatei, M.A., & Bloom, S.R. (2005b). Subcutaneous oxyntomodulin reduces body weight in overweight and obese subjects: a double-blind, randomized, controlled trial. *Diabetes, 54,* 2390–2395.

Xu, B., Goulding, E.H., Zang, K., Cepoi, D., Cone, R.D., Jones, K.R., Tecott, L.H., & Reichardt, L.F. (2003). Brain-derived neurotrophic factor regulates energy balance downstream of melanocortin-4 receptor. *Nature Neuroscience, 6,* 736–742.

Xue, B., Kim, Y.B., Lee, A., Toschi, E., Bonner-Weir, S., Kahn, C.R., Neel, B.G., & Kahn, B.B. (2007). Protein-tyrosine phosphatase 1B deficiency reduces insulin resistance and the diabetic phenotype in mice with polygenic insulin resistance. *The Journal of Biological Chemistry, 282,* 23829–23840.

Yang, X.J., Kow, L.M., Pfaff, D.W., & Mobbs, C.V. (2004). Metabolic pathways that mediate inhibition of hypothalamic neurons by glucose. *Diabetes, 53,* 67–73.

Zarjevski, N., Cusin, I., Vettor, R., Rohner-Jeanrenaud, F., & Jeanrenaud, B. (1993). Chronic intracerebroventricular neuropeptide-Y administration to normal rats mimics hormonal and metabolic changes of obesity. *Endocrinology, 133,* 1753–1758.

Zhang, J.V., Ren, P.G., Avsian-Kretchmer, O., Luo, C.W., Rauch, R., Klein, C., & Hsueh, A.J. (2005). Obestatin, a peptide encoded by the ghrelin gene, opposes ghrelin's effects on food intake. *Science, 310,* 996–999.

Zhao, A.Z., Shinohara, M.M., Huang, D., Shimizu, M., Eldar-Finkelman, H., Krebs, E.G., Beavo, J.A., & Bornfeldt, K.E. (2000). Leptin induces insulin-like signaling that antagonizes cAMP elevation by glucagon in hepatocytes. *The Journal of Biological Chemistry, 275,* 11348–11354.

Ziotopoulou, M., Mantzoros, C.S., Hileman, S.M., & Flier, J.S. (2000). Differential expression of hypothalamic neuropeptides in the early phase of diet-induced obesity in mice. *American Journal of Physiology, Endocrinology and Metabolism, 279,* E838–E845.

Chapter 17
Perinatal and Infant Determinants of Obesity

Debbie A. Lawlor, George Davey Smith, and Richard Martin

Introduction

Both professionals and the public view obesity as one of, if not *the*, most important public health problem of our times and concerns are increasingly focused on childhood obesity. Obesity has been included in the international classification of diseases since 1948, since when we have seen an epidemic develop internationally affecting all age groups, including children and adolescents (Kipping et al. 2008). Whilst, repeat cross-sectional surveys such as the Health Survey for England in the UK and the USA National Health and Nutrition Examination Survey show year on year increases in the prevalence of overweight and obesity in children aged 2–15 for at least the last 2–3 decades, it is unclear whether these represent period or cohort effects (Kipping et al. 2008). A recent study comparing two birth cohorts from the UK (one born in 1946 and the other in 1958) found that mean birth weight and body mass index (BMI) from childhood to age 20 years were similar, but that by mid-adulthood the cohort born in 1958 had on average a greater BMI (1–2 kg/m^2 greater), waist circumference (6–7 cm) and hip circumference (5 cm) and also a higher prevalence of obesity (25 vs. 11%) than those born in 1946 (Li et al. 2008). The obesity epidemic in the UK began around the late 1970s to early 1980s and the separation of obesity prevalence in the 1958 birth cohort compared to those born in 1946 from their early 20s corresponds to a period effect – starting to affect both cohorts in the late 70s/early 80s when they were aged mid-20s (1958 cohort) and mid-30s (1946 cohort) respectively. The large difference in obesity prevalence for these cohorts born just 12 years apart illustrates the likely effect on contemporary children who will have higher prevalences of obesity from earlier in childhood and potentially more marked differences in adulthood.

Obese children often become obese adults. Childhood obesity increased the risk of adult obesity fourfold in men, and 3.2-fold in women in the British 1958 birth cohort, although child to adult BMI correlations across the range were modest (Power et al. 1997). Among contemporary children and adolescents, obesity is associated with elevated blood pressure, dyslipidemia, glucose intolerance, hyperinsulinemia and greater left ventricular mass (Berenson et al. 1998; Forrester et al. 1996; Law et al. 1995; Lawlor et al. 2004; Owen et al. 2003). In a recent large prospective study greater BMI, waist circumference and DXA determined fat mass assessed at age 9–12 were all found to be associated

D.A. Lawlor (✉) and G.D. Smith
MRC Centre for Causal Analyses in Translational Epidemiology, Department of Social Medicine, University of Bristol, Oakfield House, Oakfield Grove, BS8 2BN, Bristol, UK
e-mail: d.a.lawlor@bristol.ac.uk

R. Martin
Department of Social Medicine, University of Bristol, Canynge Hall, Whiteladies Road, Bristol BS8 2PR, UK

L.A. Moreno et al. (eds.), *Epidemiology of Obesity in Children and Adolescents*,   311
Springer Series on Epidemiology and Public Health 2, DOI 10.1007/978-1-4419-6039-9_17,
© Springer Science+Business Media, LLC 2011

with adverse cardiovascular risk factors at age 15–16, with the magnitudes of association for these three measurements of adiposity being very similar. These results suggest that in childhood BMI is as good a measure of adiposity related future adverse cardiovascular risk factors as is total fat mass or a measure of centrally distributed fat (waist circumference) (Lawlor et al. 2010a). Type 2 diabetes, which just 10 years ago was believed to be a disease of adults only (hence its previous name of "adult onset diabetes") is now increasingly diagnosed in obese children and adolescents (Ehtisham et al. 2000; Fagot-Campagna et al. 2000). Furthermore, higher BMI in childhood and adolescence, from age 7–10 years and above, is associated with increased future risk of all-cause mortality, cardiovascular disease, respiratory disease and some cancers (Baker et al. 2007; Bjorge et al. 2008; Owen et al. 2007). Given the evidence that obesity in childhood and adolescence is already associated with adverse metabolic and vascular risk factors and is associated with future cardiovascular risk and other adverse outcomes, understanding the determinants of childhood obesity is essential to future prevention of these diseases.

This chapter explores current evidence for prenatal and infant determinants of childhood obesity. Specifically, we examine the evidence for risk factors that have been proposed to act only or to a greater extent during intrauterine development or infancy (defined as the first year of life).

Prenatal Risk Factors for Obesity

Gestational Diabetes or Hyperglycemia and Offspring Obesity Risk

The Diabetic and Hyperglycemic Intrauterine Environment and Infant Adiposity

Maternal diabetes (either existing type 1 or 2 diabetes or gestational diabetes) during pregnancy is associated with higher birth weight and greater fetal adiposity (Catalano et al. 2003; Jovanovic and Pettitt 2001; Kjos and Buchanan 1999). The effects of maternal hyperglycemia on fetal growth and adiposity are not limited to women with diagnosed diabetes. Among non-diabetic mothers there is a linear or "J" shaped association between fasting and post-challenge glucose levels during pregnancy and greater birth size and other adverse perinatal outcomes (Metzger et al. 2008; Scholl et al. 2001; Sermer et al. 1995). For example, the recent Hyperglycemia and Adverse Pregnancy Outcomes (HAPO) study with more than 20,000 mothers and babies noted a strong, continuous association of maternal glucose levels below those diagnostic of diabetes with increased birth weight and cord-blood serum C-peptide (a marker of insulin resistance) (Metzger et al. 2008). However, whether these more subtle changes in maternal glycemia (at levels lower than those seen for diagnosed gestational diabetes) are associated with increased offspring obesity risk in later life remains unclear.

The Diabetic and Hyperglycemic Intrauterine Environment and Later Obesity Risk

In addition to the association with greater adiposity at birth, there is increasing evidence that the offspring of women with pregnancy diabetes are at increased risk of obesity (Dabelea 2007; Kostalova et al. 2001; Pettitt et al. 1983, 1987, 1993; Pribylova and Dvorakova 1996; Silverman et al. 1991), impaired glucose tolerance (Dabelea 2007; Dabelea and Pettitt 2001; Kostalova et al. 2001; Pettitt et al. 1993; Pribylova and Dvorakova 1996; Silverman et al. 1995), hyperinsulinemia (Pribylova and Dvorakova 1996), dyslipidemia (Manderson et al. 2002) and high blood pressure (Pribylova and Dvorakova 1996) in later life. However, a recent review of the long-term effects of exposure to an intrauterine diabetes environment on offspring obesity and glucose metabolism concluded that the strongest evidence (largest and most consistent studies) for these associations comes from studies of Pima Indians, a population in whom obesity and type 2 diabetes risk is particularly high (Dabelea 2007). Further studies in general populations that are not at particularly high risk for these outcomes are needed to understand the likely impact of maternal pregnancy diabetes on future offspring obesity risk.

Several mechanisms that are not mutually exclusive may explain the associations of maternal diabetes during pregnancy with obesity and related outcomes in offspring later in life. These include genetic predisposition, shared familial socioeconomic and lifestyle factors, as well as specific intrauterine effects. Work from the Pima Indian population suggests that the effect of maternal pregnancy diabetes on offspring obesity risk is not fully explained by genetic and shared familial lifestyle factors. In studies amongst Pima Indians a marked excess in the risk of obesity was found in offspring (assessed up to age 20 years) born to mothers who had diabetes during their pregnancy compared to either the offspring of mothers who developed diabetes later in their lives (but were non-diabetic in pregnancy) or those who never developed diabetes (risk of offspring obesity was similar in these two latter groups) (Pettitt et al. 1983, 1987). In a nuclear family study (52 families, 182 siblings), also conducted in the Pima Indian population, obesity was greater among offspring born after the mother had been diagnosed with diabetes (i.e. exposure to increased intrauterine glucose levels) than in their sibs born before their mother's diagnosis (i.e. exposed to lower intrauterine glucose levels) (Dabelea et al. 2000). These siblings will have experienced similar familial socioeconomic position and behaviors and on average 50% of their genetic variation, making these characteristics unlikely to fully explain the differences. Furthermore, the offspring of fathers with type 2 diabetes, but whose mothers are free of diabetes, in the Pima Indian population are no more at risk of future obesity than those whose fathers did not have diabetes, whereas for genetic variation to explain the maternal-offspring associations one would also expect a paternal-offspring association (Pettitt and Knowler 1998). Thus, these studies provide some evidence for an intrauterine mechanism, at least in the specific population of Pima Indians.

In a small French study the offspring of mothers with type 1 diabetes during pregnancy ($N = 15$) were compared to a control group of offspring of fathers with type 1 diabetes ($N = 16$) (Sobngwi et al. 2003). The group whose mothers had type 1 diabetes during pregnancy (offspring exposed to intrauterine diabetic environment) had similar mean BMI, waist-to-hip ratio, total fat mass and truncal fat mass to those whose father's had type 1 diabetes (and hence were exposed to genetically increased risk but not an intrauterine exposure) (Sobngwi et al. 2003). Most parameters from an oral glucose tolerance test conducted in the offspring in later life were also similar, though early insulin secretion was lower and 120 min mean glucose levels were higher in those whose mothers had had type 1 diabetes during their pregnancy than the control group of offspring of fathers with type 1 diabetes. The small sample size and multiple comparisons in this study make firm conclusions difficult. In a more recent study of Danish individuals four groups were compared: (a) offspring of women with a genetic predisposition to type 2 diabetes (defined on the basis of existing risk factors such as family history) and with oral glucose tolerance test diagnosed and diet treated gestational diabetes – i.e. defined as genetic and intrauterine risk ($N = 168$); (b) offspring of women with a genetic predisposition to type 2 diabetes and with a normal oral glucose tolerance test during pregnancy – i.e. genetic but no intrauterine risk ($N = 141$); (c) offspring of women with no genetic predisposition to type 2 diabetes and with oral glucose tolerance test diagnosed and diet treated gestational diabetes – i.e. no genetic but positive intrauterine risk ($N = 160$) and (d) offspring of women with no genetic predisposition to type 2 diabetes and a normal pregnancy oral glucose tolerance test – i.e. no genetic or intrauterine risk ($N = 128$) (Clausen et al. 2008). In a large UK prospective study gestational diabetes and glycosuria in pregnancy were associated with increased BMI, waist circumference and DXA determined fat mass at age 9–12 in offspring (Lawlor et al. 2010b). Furthermore, in a recent very large sibling study, which used a similar approach to that used previously in the Pima Indians but which included over 130,000 siblings, offspring of mothers who were exposed to diabetes during pregnancy had greater mean BMI at mean age 18 years than their older siblings born before their mother was diagnosed with diabetes (Lawlor et al. 2010c). This suggests that in Western populations, as with the Pima, that intrauterine mechanisms explain at least some of the association of pregnancy diabetes with later offspring adiposity. Mean BMI, fasting and 2-h postload glucose were all higher in groups (a)–(c) compared to individuals in group (e), leading the authors to conclude that both genetic predisposition to type 2 diabetes and intrauterine exposure to gestational diabetes increase the risk of future obesity and glucose intolerance (Clausen et al. 2008).

The long-term follow-up of the offspring of mothers who have been involved in randomized trials of the effectiveness of strict glycemic control during pregnancy will provide particularly valuable insights into the potential of intervening during this period to improve obesity risk and related outcomes in the offspring. In the short term, improved perinatal outcomes have been observed amongst those women with gestational diabetes randomized to intensive glycemic control vs. those on standard care (Crowther et al. 2005). There were fewer large for gestational age infants amongst those in the intervention group (13 vs. 22%, $P<0.001$) and fewer infants with macrosomia (10 vs. 21%, $P<0.001$). However, these differences may have been largely driven by the shorter period of gestation among the intensively treated group, due mainly to the greater rate of inductions of labor in that group (Crowther et al. 2005). Nevertheless, long-term follow-up of these infants to determine whether a brief intervention during the intrauterine period has long-term beneficial effects on the offspring in terms of the development of obesity and its associated diseases is important for testing the developmental overnutrition hypothesis (see below) and determining whether a brief intervention during the intrauterine period among this high risk group has a lasting effect.

Developmental Overnutrition

The developmental overnutrition hypothesis (also known as fetal teratogenesis) provides a possible intrauterine mechanism for the association of maternal pregnancy diabetes/hyperglycemia with offspring adiposity (Dabelea 2007). This hypothesis was first proposed in the 1950s by Pederson to explain the association between maternal diabetes in pregnancy and excessive growth in the developing fetus (Pederson 1954). According to this hypothesis the greater delivery of glucose to the fetus in the diabetic pregnancy results in fetal hyperinsulinemia (a necessary response to prevent fetal hyperglycemia) and as a consequence increased insulin-mediated fetal growth. In the 1980s this hypothesis was broadened to include the possibility that other fuels, in addition to glucose but also related to maternal hyperglycemia/diabetes, such as free fatty acids, ketone bodies and amino acids also contributed to fetal hyperinsulinemia and increased fetal growth (Freinkel 1980). The original hypothesis was specific to intrauterine growth. However, birth weight is positively correlated with later weight and BMI, and a further expansion of the original hypothesis has been the suggestion that developmental overnutrition resulting from a diabetic intrauterine environment may program offspring to life-long increased adiposity (Whitaker and Dietz 1998).

In support of the developmental overnutrition hypothesis, high concentrations of maternal glucose among those with gestational diabetes has been shown to increase nutrient (glucose, amino acids, free fatty acids) transfer to the fetus and result in fetal hyperinsulinemia and increased fetal growth (Freinkel 1980; Pederson 1954). In studies of humans, fetal hyperinsulinemia has been detected in the offspring of diabetic mothers both in utero (assessed in samples of amniotic fluid) (Persson et al. 1982; Silverman et al. 1993, 1995; Weiss et al. 2000) and immediately after birth (assessed in samples of cord blood) (Dornhorst et al. 1994). Furthermore, this hyperinsulinemia is associated, not just with increased fetal growth, but with later obesity and glucose intolerance in the offspring (Metzger et al. 1990; Silverman et al. 1993, 1995; Weiss et al. 2000). Offspring of female rats with diet-induced obesity during pregnancy have been found to be heavier than the offspring of rats with the same genotype, but without the diet-induced maternal obesity (Levin and Govek 1998). In vitro, animal and human studies have also demonstrated that fetal pancreatic development and fat stores are influenced by the availability of fetal fuels – in particular glucose, lipids and amino-acids – which are in turn determined by maternal adiposity, insulin secretion and responsiveness, plasma levels of glucose, free fatty acids and inflammatory signals (Dahlgren et al. 2001; Freinkel and

Metzger 1979; Ramsay et al. 2002). As noted above, evidence from sibling studies in Pima Indians and a European population, support an intrauterine mechanism for the association of pregnancy diabetes with later offspring greater adiposity.

Maternal Adiposity During Pregnancy and Future Offspring Obesity Risk

Obesity is a major risk factor for diabetes and several studies have shown an independent (of pregnancy diabetes) association of maternal obesity with excessive fetal growth and adiposity (Baeten et al. 2001; Guillaume et al. 1995; Okun et al. 1997; Sebire et al. 2001). Thus, there is increasing interest in the hypothesis that maternal obesity, and also "excessive" weight gain during pregnancy, in healthy non-diabetic women, are associated with life long obesity and related metabolic and vascular abnormalities in offspring (Ebbeling et al. 2002; Freinkel and Metzger 1979; Whitaker and Dietz 1998). It has been suggested that the consequences of this hypothesis, if true, are formidable: "the obesity epidemic could accelerate through successive generations independent of further genetic or environmental factors" (Catalano 2003; Ebbeling et al. 2002). In this respect the developmental overnutrition hypothesis has been expanded to include not only hyperglycemia/diabetes in pregnancy but also greater maternal adiposity during pregnancy as a key risk factor for future offspring obesity risk.

Epidemiological support for this hypothesis is provided by studies finding a positive association between maternal pre-pregnancy or early pregnancy BMI and offspring BMI or obesity in later life (Laitinen et al. 2001; Li et al. 2005; Parsons et al. 2001; Stettler et al. 2000; Whitaker 2004). For example, a record linkage study of families in the Special Supplemental Nutrition Program for Women, Infants, and Children in Ohio, which included over 5,000 children, found strong and linear associations between maternal BMI in the first trimester of pregnancy and the risk of childhood obesity up to age 4 years: the adjusted odds ratio of obesity at age 4 comparing the highest fifth of maternal BMI to the lowest fifth was 4.31 (95% confidence interval (CI): 3.17, 5.87) (Whitaker 2004). This association was independent of a range of covariables including birth weight, socioeconomic position, maternal smoking in pregnancy and weight gain during pregnancy. However, an association between maternal BMI and offspring obesity may be explained by shared genetic risk factors or familial lifestyle characteristics for obesity.

One proposed mechanism for distinguishing intrauterine mechanisms is to compare the association of maternal BMI, assessed pre-pregnancy or in early pregnancy, with offspring adiposity to the association of paternal BMI assessed at the same time with offspring adiposity, the assumption being that a stronger maternal-offspring, than paternal-offspring association would support specific maternal effects, of which intrauterine mechanisms would be a candidate. By contrast a similar maternal-offspring to paternal-offspring association would support shared genetic, socioeconomic or lifestyle characteristics which would be likely to be similar for both parents. Several studies have made such comparisons with varying results that may be explained by chance, differences in how parental BMI was obtained and different measurements of offspring adiposity (Davey Smith et al. 2007; Kivimaki et al. 2007; Lake et al. 1997; Lawlor et al. 2007).

In the Avon Longitudinal Study of Parents and Children (ALSPAC) the associations of maternal and paternal pre-pregnancy BMI with offspring DXA determined fat mass measured at 9 and 11 (4,091 parent-offspring trios) were compared. Both maternal and paternal BMI were positively associated with offspring fat mass, but the size of the maternal association was larger than that of the paternal association in all models: mean difference in offspring sex- and age-standardized fat mass z-score per 1 standard deviation (SD) BMI were 0.24 (95% CI: 0.22, 0.26) for maternal BMI vs. 0.13 (95% CI: 0.11, 0.15) for paternal BMI (P-value for difference in effect <0.001) (Lawlor et al. 2008b). The stronger maternal association was robust to sensitivity analyses assuming levels of non-paternity up to 20%. A plausible explanation for the stronger maternal association is provided by the developmental overnutrition hypothesis. However, in the same study, maternal *FTO* genotype, controlling for offspring *FTO*, was used as an instrument for maternal adiposity, and these analyses did not provide strong support for the developmental overnutrition hypothesis (Lawlor et al. 2008b).

An instrumental variable is one that is associated with the exposure/risk factor of interest (in this case maternal BMI) but is not associated with the outcome (here offspring fat mass) of interest by any mechanism other than through its association with the exposure of interest (Lawlor et al. 2008a). If these assumptions hold, the instrumental variable can be used to provide an estimate of the causal association of exposure with outcome that will not be biased by confounding or reverse causality (Lawlor et al. 2008a). It has been suggested that a genetic variant that is robustly associated with an exposure of interest provides a powerful instrumental variable for that exposure (Davey Smith and Ebrahim 2003). This is because the random allocation of genetic variants from parents to offspring results in them rarely being associated with any of the environmental and lifestyle characteristics that commonly confound conventional epidemiological associations (Davey Smith and Ebrahim 2003; Davey Smith et al. 2008). Furthermore, genetic variation is determined at conception and cannot be influenced by later outcomes and hence associations of genetic variants with outcomes cannot be explained by reverse causation.

Variation in *FTO* predisposes to greater BMI and fat mass (Frayling et al. 2007; see also Chapters 14 and 15). Mothers with one or two A alleles of *FTO* will on average have greater fat mass than those with two T alleles. This association with adiposity will be present throughout life, including during pregnancy. When maternal *FTO*, controlling for offspring *FTO*, was used as an instrumental variable to determine the causal association of maternal adiposity with offspring adiposity it was found that the mean difference in offspring fat mass z-score per 1 SD maternal BMI was −0.08 (95% CI: −0.56, 0.41) (Lawlor et al. 2008b). The point estimate (−0.08 SD) for this instrumental variable analysis suggests that greater maternal adiposity during pregnancy does not result in greater fat mass in later life in her offspring. However, the confidence interval is wide and statistically this finding is not different from that found for the parental comparison. Thus, these analyses cannot rule out a small intrauterine effect of greater maternal adiposity on offspring future risk of greater adiposity.

One of the strongest pieces of evidence for an effect of maternal obesity during pregnancy on future obesity risk comes from a study of obesity surgery (Kral et al. 2006). In that study the prevalence of obesity was compared between 172 children (aged 2–18 years) born to 113 women who had been morbidly obese (mean BMI 48 kg/m^2) and who had experienced substantial weight loss following biliopancreatic bypass surgery prior to their pregnancy with 45 of their siblings who were born prior to their mother's surgery (i.e. exposed to extreme maternal obesity during pregnancy) and were assessed at a similar age to their younger siblings. Compared to their siblings born prior to their mothers' surgery-related weight loss, those conceived after mother's surgery had a reduced prevalence of obesity (relative reduction 52%) and severe obesity (relative reduction 45%) (Kral et al. 2006). This study suggests that extreme obesity during pregnancy is causally (and through intrauterine mechanisms) related to future offspring obesity risk, but whether less extremes of maternal overweight or obesity that do not warrant surgical intervention are associated with future offspring obesity are unclear. If the effect of maternal obesity is only seen at these extreme levels then it will have limited public health impact and will not have been a major driver of the obesity epidemic.

Maternal Weight Gain During Pregnancy

A number of studies have also examined the association between maternal weight gain during pregnancy (as opposed to BMI at the start of pregnancy) and later BMI or obesity in offspring, with all but one of these (Whitaker 2004), finding an association between greater weight gain during pregnancy and greater mean BMI or increased risk of obesity in offspring (Fisch et al. 1975; Mamun et al. 2009; Moreira et al. 2007; Okens et al. 2005; Schack-Nielsen et al. 2005; Sharma et al. 2005; Seidman et al. 1996). This association appears to be robust to adjustment for indicators of socioeconomic position, maternal pre-pregnancy or early pregnancy BMI and infant birth size. In a recent study from Australia the association remained up to age 21 years in the offspring and was also associated with an increase in systolic blood pressure of the magnitude predicted by the association of maternal pregnancy weight gain with offspring BMI at age 21 and the association of offspring BMI with their systolic blood pressure (Mamun et al. 2009). In a second large study (N=5154) greater gestational weight gain up to 36 weeks gestation was associated with greater offspring BMI, waist circumference, fat mass and a wide range of adverse cardiovascular risk factors at age 9–10 years (Fraser et al. 2010).

Maternal Diet During Pregnancy

The developmental overnutrition hypothesis might imply that high fat and high energy diets during pregnancy will be associated with future offspring obesity risk. Results from a study of mice presented at the Society for Neuroscience's 38th annual conference support this assertion (naturenews 2009; http://www.nature.com/news/2008/081120/full/news.2008.1240.html). The offspring of mice fed a high-fat diet throughout their pregnancies and suckling were more obese than the offspring of mice fed a normal diet during pregnancy and sucking. Furthermore, the greater risk of obesity was transmitted into the next generation (the original experimented upon mother's grand-children), without any further manipulation of their mother's diet. However, whether these findings would translate into similar results in humans is unclear. Parental-offspring association comparisons, suggest that mother's diet during pregnancy is more strongly associated with offspring diet than in father's diet, which may represent an intrauterine effect or the greater impact of mothers on family diet in general (Brion et al. 2010a). Randomized controlled trials of different dietary intakes in pregnancy with long-term follow-up would be expensive and potentially difficult to undertake, as pregnant women are unlikely to be happy to be randomized to different dietary intake. In the future it may be possible to use genetic variants that have been shown to be robustly associated with clear differences in dietary intake as instrumental variables to assess these associations (Davey Smith and Ebrahim 2003; Lawlor et al. 2008a).

Maternal Smoking During Pregnancy

Several studies have found an association of maternal smoking during pregnancy with greater offspring BMI or obesity risk in later life (Mamun et al. 2006; Power and Jefferis 2002; Toschke et al. 2003; von Kries et al. 2002). It has been suggested that exposing the developing fetus to nicotine might adversely affect development of hypothalamic function and through this mechanism impact appetite control over the life course and hence increase the risk of future obesity (Kane et al. 2000; Slotkin 1998). However, there are many confounding factors that could generate noncausal links between maternal smoking and the later offspring adiposity. As noted above, one approach to this issue is to compare the strength of associations between an exposure among mothers and offspring outcomes and the same exposure among fathers and the offspring outcomes. If there were a direct biological effect of intrauterine exposure to maternal smoking on offspring obesity, then the link with offspring obesity should be much stronger for exposure among mothers than for exposure among fathers (Davey Smith 2008). This can be illustrated with respect to birth weight where there is strong evidence of a causal influence of maternal smoking during pregnancy. Figure 17.1 demonstrates that, in ALSPAC, maternal smoking during pregnancy is associated with lower offspring birth weight (with a magnitude, 162 g lower weight in those whose mothers smoked during pregnancy compared to those who did not, consistent with other studies), whereas partner smoking during pregnancy is only weakly associated with birth weight (Davey Smith 2008). When both maternal and partner smoking during pregnancy are taken into account in the same multivariable statistical model, the former shows a robust association that is little attenuated, whereas the latter association is essentially abolished. These results suggest that the weak association of paternal smoking with offspring birth weight is explained by the association of paternal smoking with maternal smoking and provides very little evidence of any effect of second hand smoking on birth weight.

If we now apply the same logic to offspring adiposity in later life the results are notably different to those seen for birth weight. In ALSPAC, data show that the average BMI at age 7 of children whose mothers smoked during pregnancy is raised compared to those whose mothers did not smoke, with the magnitude of this effect being similar to findings of previous epidemiological studies (Leary et al. 2006). However a similar sized association is seen with partner smoking, and including both maternal and partner smoking behavior in the same model leaves residual effects of similar magnitude (Leary et al. 2006). Furthermore, when a more direct measure of adiposity – DXA scan determined fat mass – was used as the outcome the findings were similar (Fig. 17.2) (Leary et al. 2006). These results suggest that in the case of offspring adiposity, maternal smoking during pregnancy does not have a direct intrauterine effect, rather confounding factors associated with parental smoking and offspring adiposity generate an association between both maternal and paternal smoking and greater offspring adiposity. Similar findings are seen with respect to parental smoking and offspring blood pressure (Brion et al. 2007).

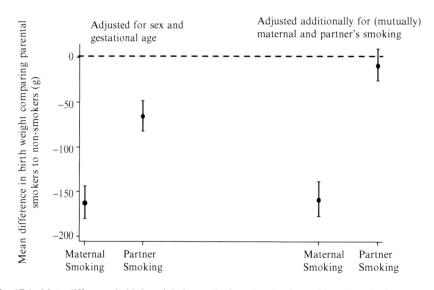

The analyses are restricted to singleton births and all results are adjusted for infant sex and gestational age; the results on the right are additionally mutually adjusted for mother's and partner's smoking status during pregnancy. Partner's were described as being biological fathers by the mothers

Fig. 17.1 Mean difference in birth weight by mother's and partner's smoking status during pregnancy

The analyses are restricted to singleton births and all results are adjusted for sex, age, height and height squared; the results on the right are additionally mutually adjusted for mother's and partner's smoking status during pregnancy. Fat mass was determined by DXA scan at mean age 9.9 years

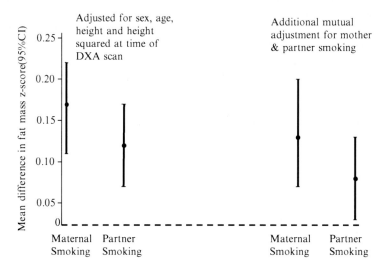

Fig. 17.2 Mean difference in total fat mass *z*-score at 9.9 years by mother's and partner's smoking status during pregnancy

Intrauterine Growth and Later Risk of Obesity

A large number of studies have demonstrated inverse associations (sometimes "reverse-J" shaped) between birth size (most commonly birth weight or birth weight standardized for gestational age) and coronary heart disease (Barker 1995; Huxley et al. 2007), type 2 diabetes (Whincup et al. 2008) and a wide-range of cardiovascular risk factors that are all thought to be influenced by obesity, including blood pressure (Whincup et al. 2004), fasting glucose (Forouhi et al. 2004), insulin (Forouhi et al. 2004), total cholesterol and triglycerides (Gluckman and Hanson 2004; Owen et al. 2003). Low levels of high density lipoprotein cholesterol (HDLc) is associated with increased risk of cardiovascular disease and is more commonly seen in obese compared with lean individuals and for this risk factor birth weight is positively associated with HDLc (i.e. lower birth weight is associated with lower HDLc which is an adverse cardiovascular risk factor and consequence of obesity) (Gluckman and Hanson 1995). Despite these associations with adverse consequences of obesity, birth weight and ponderal index (birth weight relative to height) have been found to be positively associated with mean infant, childhood and adulthood BMI and overweight/obesity in a large number of studies (Binkin et al. 1988; Duran-Tauleria et al. 1995; Fisch et al. 1975; Hediger et al. 1999; Kramer et al. 1985; Pietilainen et al. 2001; Rasmussen and Johansson 1998; Seidman et al. 1991; Strauss 1997).

Despite the positive associations of childhood BMI with cardiovascular risk factors in childhood (Berenson et al. 1998; Forrester et al. 1996; Law et al. 1995; Lawlor et al. 2004; Owen et al. 2003; Lawlor et al. 2010a) and with adult cardiovascular mortality (Baker et al. 2007; Bjorge et al. 2008; Owen et al. 2007), investigators have criticized the examination of birth size with BMI or overweight/obesity based on BMI suggesting that birth size may be differentially associated with fat and lean mass, and with fat distribution, and that these differential associations may mediate the association between lower birth weight and higher later cardiovascular disease risk. That is to say, it is suggested that individuals with lower birth weight (a marker for poorer intrauterine nutrition) will be programmed to greater fat mass and in particular greater central/visceral fat in later life and that this will increase their risk of adverse cardiovascular and metabolic outcomes (Law et al. 1992).

Studies examining the associations of birth size with fat mass and fat distribution have reported inconsistent conclusions. In by far the largest study to date ($N = 6,086$) birth weight was positively associated with both DXA determined lean and fat mass in males and females, with a 1 SD greater birth weight being associated with a 4.3% greater fat mass at age 9–10 years in models that adjusted for height, age, sex, pubertal stage, gestational age, family socioeconomic position, maternal parity, age and smoking during pregnancy (Rogers et al. 2006). Ponderal index in that study was also positively associated with DXA determined fat and lean mass (Rogers et al. 2006). In a smaller study of 78 adolescents (mean age 15 years) and 86 children (mean age 7 years) birth weight was positively associated with fat-free (lean) mass, but there was no association with fat mass (Singhal et al. 2003a, b). The latter may reflect a type 2 error given the small study size. In a third small study ($N = 32$), 16 men aged 64–72 years at time of assessment, whose birth weight was below the 25th centile (mean birth weight 2.76 kg) had a higher DXA assessed fat mass than 16 age matched men whose birth weight was above the 75th percentile (mean 4.23 kg): 29.3 vs. 25.3%, $P = 0.03$ after adjustment for BMI (Kensara et al. 2005). A smaller difference was found without adjustment for BMI (28.7 vs. 26.0%, $P = 0.15$) and the very small sample size of this study make it difficult to make valid inferences.

Inverse associations of birth weight with measurements of central adiposity (based on subscapular skinfold thickness, subscapular to triceps skinfold ratio, waist circumference or waist-to-hip ratio) in children, adolescents and adults have been reported (Labayen et al. 2006; Law et al. 1992; te Velde et al. 2003; Walker et al. 2002). However, most studies to date have had small sample sizes (three with fewer than 250 participants and one with 1,084). The largest study, to date, relied on adjustment for BMI to unmask associations with central adiposity (Law et al. 1992) and two of the three small studies reported sex differences that were inconsistent between studies. Thus, in one there was an inverse association of birth weight with central adiposity in boys only (Labayen et al. 2006) and in the other an inverse association only in females (te Velde et al. 2003). Thus, evidence to date suggests that birth weight is positively associated with BMI and total fat and lean mass, but whether there is an inverse association with central adiposity remains unclear due to a paucity of large well-conducted studies of this association.

Infant Risk Factors of Obesity

Accelerated Infant Growth

Amongst preterm infants in a UK study rapid weight gain in very early infancy (first 2 weeks after birth) has been shown to be associated with greater insulin resistance (Singhal et al. 2003a, b) and this has led to the suggestion that rapid weight gain in early infancy might predispose to obesity and cardiovascular disease risk (Singhal and Lucas 2004). However, results from preterm infants may not be generalizable to the majority of the population born at term. Three general population cohort studies, two from the UK (McCarthy et al. 2007; Ong et al. 2009; Howe et al. 2010) and one from Delhi in India (Sachdev et al. 2005), have examined detailed growth trajectories from birth to childhood and their relationship to later obesity. One of the UK studies, based on a cohort of men only from Wales ($N = 679$) found positive associations between weight velocity (rate of weight gain) in the immediate infancy period (between birth and 5 months) and greater BMI and waist-to-hip ratio in early adulthood (mean age 25 years) (McCarthy et al. 2007). This association was independent of a range of potential confounding factors and weight velocity in childhood (rate of weight gain between 1.75 and 5 years), though the latter was more strongly associated with adult BMI and waist-to-hip ratio than weight velocity in infancy. The second UK study, based on a cohort of girls only from South West England ($N = 2,715$) found that faster weight gain between the three time points with measurements – 0–2; 2–9 and 9–19 months – were all positively associated with BMI at 9–10 years (Ong et al. 2009). However, only faster early infancy weight gain (0–2 and 2–9 months) were positively associated with DXA determined fat mass, with later faster growth (9–19 months) being positively associated with fat free mass, but not fat mass at age 9–10 years. However, a more detailed assessment in that same study, with longer follow-up, found that later childhood rapid BMI gain (more so that gain in infancy) was more strongly associated with fat mass and adverse cardiovascular risk factors at age 15–16 years, with no evidence that infancy was a particularly sensitive period (Howe et al. 2010). By contrast, in the Delhi study, where many participants were stunted and underweight in infancy, weight velocity in infancy was associated with adult lean mass, with little association with general or central adiposity (Sachdev et al. 2005). Taken together these findings suggest that the impact of rate of weight gain in early infancy on later risk of adiposity and its associated adverse cardiovascular and metabolic outcomes may vary depending upon the underlying nutritional status of the infants being studied. The UK studies also suggest that rate of weight gain in later childhood is more important than that in infancy with respect to later adiposity and associated cardiovascular risk factors (McCarthy et al. 2007; Howe et al. 2010).

Infant Nutrition

During the last two decades there have been numerous and rapidly increasing claims about potential long-term beneficial effects of having been breastfed, including papers suggesting protection against the development of obesity in childhood and adulthood. Breastfeeding is known to be associated with multiple social, behavioral and biological exposures that are themselves correlated with obesity. The evidence-base, however, for long-term protective effects of breastfeeding on obesity is largely observational and not experimental (i.e. randomized controlled trials). A major challenge, therefore, in understanding the current epidemiological literature is that it is difficult to disentangle breastfeeding effects from the influence of factors correlated with maternal choice to breastfed.

Owen et al. published a systematic review of breastfeeding and mean levels of BMI in 2005 (Owen et al. 2005b). The meta-analysis was based on a systematic search that identified 36 individual effect-estimates. Those who were breastfed had a BMI that was, on average, 0.04 kg/m² less (95% CI: −0.05, −0.02) than those who were bottle-fed. This was conventionally "statistically significant," but is a very small effect. For example, a reduction of 2 kg/m² (a 50-fold greater effect than the observed effect of breastfeeding) is needed to reduce the incidence of coronary heart disease and type 2 diabetes by 10%. Arguing against causality for the association of breastfeeding and BMI in this systematic review, were the observations that the difference in BMI by type of infant feeding was less in those studies that defined breastfeeding as exclusive, the absence of any association in the pooled estimate of the 11 studies that controlled for maternal smoking, social class and parental BMI, and that there was convincing evidence of small study bias, suggesting the possibility of publication bias.

It has been suggested that the lack of any important association with mean BMI is because breastfeeding only affects the upper and lower tails of the distribution. There have been at least three quantitative systematic reviews of the effect of breastfeeding on risk of obesity, defined in most studies by cut-offs at the 95th or 97th percentile (Arenz et al. 2004; Harder et al. 2005; Owen et al. 2005a). The largest and most recent meta-analysis included 28 studies with almost 300,000 participants (Owen et al. 2005a). Breastfeeding was associated with a reduction in risk of obesity of 13% compared to formula-feeding (pooled odds ratio (OR) = 0.87; 95% CI: 0.85, 0.89) and the effect was greater in studies that defined breastfeeding as exclusive (OR = 0.76; 95% CI: 0.70,

0.83) or those breastfed for 2 months or more (OR = 0.81; 95% CI: 0.77, 0.84). However, the association was strongest amongst the smallest studies indicating possible publication bias, i.e. small studies being more likely to be published if they showed a large effect (pooled OR in studies of <500 participants = 0.43; OR in studies of >2,500 participants = 0.88). The effect of adjustment for potentially important confounders could only be examined in six studies. In these six studies, the pooled odds ratio before adjustment was 0.86, but after controlling for parental obesity, maternal smoking and social class, this was reduced to 0.93. Thus, as with the systematic review of mean BMI, this review does not provide strong evidence for a causal protective effect of breastfeeding on future obesity risk.

Kramer et al. have illustrated that reverse causality is a major concern in observational studies of the association of breastfeeding duration with adiposity (Kramer et al. 2002). It may be that breast milk output is sufficient for slower-growing infants, destined to remain relatively thin; such infants are satisfied by continued exclusive breastfeeding. In contrast, faster growing infants, destined to become obese, may be switched to formula to meet their higher energy demands and satisfy more frequent hunger. An association of exclusive or prolonged duration of breastfeeding compared with lesser degrees of breastfeeding with adiposity may reflect the fact that the faster-growing infant "causes" supplementation with formula feeding, rather than the formula feeding causing the faster growth.

Well conducted randomized controlled trials remove problems of confounding, reverse causality and selection bias that afflict observational studies, but randomization to breast- vs. formula-feeding is not feasible and may be unethical. However, randomization to a breastfeeding promotion intervention is ethical and feasible, particularly if mothers who intend to breastfeed are randomized to an intervention that promotes breastfeeding duration and exclusivity. A large randomized controlled trial of an intervention to promote breastfeeding exclusivity and duration, with analysis by "intention to treat" has been conducted, involving over 17,000 term and normal weight children in the Republic of Belarus who are now aged 11.5 years (Promotion of Breastfeeding Intervention Trial, PROBIT) (Kramer et al. 2001). Infants from the intervention sites were 7 times more likely to be exclusively breastfed at 3 months (43.3 vs. 6.4%) and 13 times more likely at 6 months (7.9 vs. 0.6%), and were breastfed to any degree at higher rates throughout infancy. Thus, the PROBIT trial resulted in two cohorts that differed substantially in the exclusivity and duration of breastfeeding. These cohorts were created by randomization, not the choice of the mother, enabling strong causal inferences with respect to breastfeeding effects on long-term outcomes. Despite the fact that the breastfeeding promotion intervention resulted in considerable increases in the duration and exclusivity of breastfeeding, it did not reduce measures of adiposity at age 6.5 years (Table 17.1) (Kramer et al. 2007). Neither was any important effect of the experimental intervention observed on the risk of overweight or obesity defined, respectively, by the BMI ≥ 85th percentile (cluster-adjusted OR = 1.1; 95% CI: 0.8, 1.4) or ≥95th percentile [cluster-adjusted OR = 1.2 (0.8, 1.6)] (Kramer et al. 2007). These findings are also supported by a recent cross cohort comparison study in which breast feeding was not found to be associated with offspring BMI in a cohort from Brazil where socioeconomic position (a likely key confounder in the association) is not related to breast feeding (Brion et al. 2010b).

Table 17.1 Cluster-adjusted differences in adiposity comparing the breastfeeding promotion intervention (experimental) arm with the control arm of PROBIT

Outcome	Experimental	Control	Difference (95% CI)
BMI (kg/m²)	15.6	15.6	+0.1 (−0.2, 0.3)
Waist circumference (cm)	54.6	54.2	+0.3 (−0.8, 1.4)
Triceps skinfold (mm)	9.9	10.0	−0.4 (−1.8, 1.0)
Subscapular skinfolds (mm)	5.9	5.8	0.0 (−0.4, 0.5)

Adapted from Kramer et al. (2007)

Conclusions

Evidence to date suggests an association between maternal hyperglycemia/diabetes during pregnancy and future risk of greater offspring adiposity, with some evidence that this is at least in part explained by intrauterine mechanisms that are consistent with developmental overnutrition. Evidence for an effect of greater maternal BMI or weight gain during pregnancy is less clear. Extreme obesity during pregnancy (even in the absence of diagnosed diabetes) might, via an intrauterine mechanism, result in increased offspring obesity, but further research is required to determine whether less extreme levels of maternal overweight/obesity and weight gain during pregnancy are causally related to future offspring obesity risk. Comparisons of maternal and paternal associations suggest that exposure to maternal tobacco smoking during pregnancy is not causally (via intrauterine mechanisms) associated with future offspring obesity, although the clear adverse health consequences of smoking during pregnancy on the developing fetus (intrauterine growth retardation) and on the mother's own health warrant advice and interventions to reduce smoking in women of reproductive age.

Recent systematic reviews of observational studies, and the PROBIT randomized controlled trial of breast feeding promotion, suggest that previous reports of protective effects of breastfeeding against the later development of obesity may reflect uncontrolled confounding and bias. The continued follow-up of PROBIT will help unpick whether any effects emerge later in life as adiposity rates increase.

The exact mechanisms underlying prenatal and infant exposures that do appear to be causal are unclear. Epigenetic effects are frequently invoked as potentially important mechanisms for associations of prenatal risk factors with a range of later life outcomes. However, as yet there is insufficient research in humans to make clear conclusions about the nature and importance of these effects. Whilst there is strong evidence for causal effects of some prenatal and infant exposures (maternal hyperglycemia and extreme obesity during pregnancy and rapid weight gain in early infancy), there is no clear evidence that interventions during this period of the life course are effective at reducing childhood or later life obesity.

References

Arenz, S., Ruckerl, R.., Koletzko, B., & von Kries, R. (2004). Breast-feeding and childhood obesity – a systematic review. *International Journal of Obesity and Related Metabolic Disorders, 28*, 1247–1256.
Baeten, J.M., Bukusi, E.A., & Lambe, M. (2001). Pregnancy complications and outcomes among overweight and obese nulliparous women. *American Journal of Public Health, 91*, 436–440.
Baker, J.L., Olsen, L.W., & Sorensen T.I. (2007). Childhood body-mass index and the risk of coronary heart disease in adulthood. *New England Journal of Medicine, 357*, 2329–2337.
Barker, D.J. (1995). Fetal origins of coronary heart disease. *British Medical Journal, 311*, 171–174.
Berenson, G.S., Srinivasan, S.R., & Nicola, N.A. (1998). Atherosclerosis: a nutritional disease of childhood. *The American Journal of Cardiology, 82*, 22–29.
Binkin, N.J., Yip, R., Fleshood, L., & Trowbridge, F.L. (1988). Birth weight and childhood growth. *Pediatrics, 82*, 828–834.
Bjorge, T., Engeland, A., Tverdal, A., & Smith, G.D. (2008). Body mass index in adolescence in relation to cause-specific mortality: a follow-up of 230,000 Norwegian adolescents. *American Journal of Epidemiology, 168*, 30–37.
Brion, M.J., Leary, S.D., Davey Smith, G., & Ness, A.R. (2007). Similar associations of parental prenatal smoking suggest child blood pressure is not influenced by intrauterine effects. *Hypertension, 49*, 1422–1428.
Brion, M.-J.A., Ness, A.R., Rogers, I., Emmett, P., Cribb, V., Davey Smith, G., & Lawlor, D.A. (2009). Maternal diet in pregnancy and offspring diet at ten years: exploring parental comparisons and prenatal effects, submitted.
Brion, M.-J.A., Ness, A.R., Rogers, I., Emmett, P., Cribb, V., Davey Smith, G., & Lawlor, D.A. (2010a). Maternal macronutrient and energy intake in pregnancy and offspring intake at 10 years: exploring parental comparisons and prenatal effects. *American Journal of Clinical Nutrition, 91*:748–756.

Brion, M.-J. A., Lawlor, D.A., Matijasevich, A., Horta, B., Anselmi, L., Araújo, C.L., Menezes, A.M.B., Victora, C.G., & Davey, Smith, G. (2010b). What are the causal effects of breastfeeding on IQ, obesity and blood pressure? Evidence from comparing high-income and middle-income cohorts. International Journal of Epidemiology, in press (accepted November 2010).

Catalano, P.M. (2003). Obesity and pregnancy – the propagation of a viscous cycle? The Journal of Clinical Endocrinology and Metabolism, 88, 3505–3506.

Catalano, P.M., Thomas, A., Huston-Presley, L., & Amini, S.B. (2003). Increased fetal adiposity: a very sensitive marker of abnormal in utero development. American Journal of Obstetrics and Gynecology, 189, 1698–1704.

Clausen, T.D., Mathiesen, E.R., Hansen, T., Pedersen, O., Jensen, D.M., Lauenborg, J., & Damm, P. (2008). High prevalence of type 2 diabetes and pre-diabetes in adult offspring of women with gestational diabetes mellitus or type 1 diabetes: the role of intrauterine hyperglycemia. Diabetes Care, 31, 340–346.

Crowther, C.A., Hiller, J.E., Moss, J.R., McPhee, A.J., Jeffries, W.S., & Robinson, J.S. (2005). Effect of treatment of gestational diabetes mellitus on pregnancy outcomes. New England Journal of Medicine, 352, 2477–2486.

Dabelea, D. (2007). The predisposition to obesity and diabetes in offspring of diabetic mothers. Diabetes Care, 30, 169–174.

Dabelea, D., & Pettitt, D.J. (2001). Intrauterine diabetic environment confers risks for type 2 diabetes mellitus and obesity in the offspring, in addition to genetic susceptibility. Journal of Pediatric Endocrinology & Metabolism, 14, 1085–1091.

Dabelea, D., Hanson, R.L., Lindsay, R.S., Pettitt, D.J., Imperatore, G., Gabir, M.M., Roumain, J., Bennett, P.H., & Knowler, W.C. (2000). Intrauterine exposure to diabetes conveys risks for type 2 diabetes and obesity: a study of discordant sibships. Diabetes, 49, 2208–2211.

Dahlgren, J., Nilsson, C., Jennische, E., Ho, H.P., Eriksson, E., Niklasson, A., Björntorp, P., Wikland, K.A., & Holmäng, A. (2001). Prenatal cytokine exposure results in obesity and gender-specific programming. American Journal of Physiology, Endocrinology and Metabolism, 281, 326–334.

Davey Smith, G. (2008). Assessing intrauterine influences on offspring health outcomes: can epidemiological studies yield robust findings? Basic & Clinical Pharmacology & Toxicology, 102, 245–256.

Davey Smith, G., & Ebrahim, S. (2003). "Mendelian randomisation": can genetic epidemiology contribute to understanding environmental determinants of disease? International Journal of Epidemiology, 32, 1–22.

Davey Smith, G., Steer, C., Leary, S., & Ness, A. (2007). Is there an intra-uterine influence on obesity? Evidence from parent-child associations in the Avon Longitudinal Study of Parents and Children (ALSPAC). Archives of Disease in Childhood, 92, 876–880.

Davey Smith, G., Lawlor, D.A., Harbord, R., Timpson, N., Day, I.N.M., & Ebrahim, S. (2008). Clustered environments and randomized genes: a fundamental distinction between conventional and genetic epidemiology. PLoS Medicine, 4, e352.

Dornhorst, A., Nicholls, J.S., Ali, K., Andres, C., Adamson, D.L., Kelly, L.F., Niththyananthan, R., Beard, R.W., & Gray, I.P. (1994). Fetal proinsulin and birth weight. Diabetic Medicine: A Journal of the British Diabetic Association, 11, 177–181.

Duran-Tauleria, E., Rona, R.J., & Chinn, S. (1995). Factors associated with weight for height and skinfold thickness in British children. Journal of Epidemiology and Community Health, 49, 466–473.

Ebbeling, C.B., Pawlak, D.B., & Ludwig, D.S. (2002). Childhood obesity: public-health crisis, common sense cure. Lancet, 360, 473–481.

Ehtisham, S., Barrett, T.G., & Shaw, N.J. (2000). Type 2 diabetes mellitus in UK children – an emerging problem. Diabetic Medicine: A Journal of the British Diabetic Association, 17, 867–871.

Fagot-Campagna, A., Pettitt, D.J., Engelgau, M.M., Burrows, N.R., Geiss, L.S., Valdez, R., Beckles, G.L., Saaddine, J., Gregg, E.W., Williamson, D.F., & Narayan, K.M. (2000). Type 2 diabetes among North American children and adolescents: an epidemiologic review and a public health perspective. The Journal of Pediatrics, 136, 664–672.

Fisch, R.O., Bilek, M.K., & Ulstrom, R. (1975). Obesity and leanness at birth and their relationship to body habitus in later childhood. Pediatrics, 56, 521–528.

Forouhi, N., Hall, E., & McKeigue, P. (2004). A life course approach to diabetes. In D. Kuh & Y. Ben-Shlomo (Eds.), A life course approach to chronic disease epidemiology (pp. 165–188). Second ed. Oxford: University Press.

Forrester, T.E., Wilks, R.J., Bennett, F.I., Simeon, D., Osmond, C., & Allen, M. (1996). Fetal growth and cardiovascular risk factors in Jamaican school children. British Medical Journal, 312, 156–160.

Fraser, A., Tilling, K., Macdonald-Wallis, C., Sattar, N., Brion, M.-J., Benfield, L., Ness, A., Deanfield, J., Hingorani, A., Nelson, S.M., Davey Smith, G., & Lawlor, D.A. (2010). Association of maternal weight gain in pregnancy with offspring obesity and metabolic and vascular traits in childhood. Circulation, 121:2557–2564.

Frayling, T.M., Timpson, N.J., Weedon, M.N., Zeggini, E., Freathy, R.M., Lindgren, C.M., Perry, J.R.B., Eilliot, K.S., Lango, H., Rayner, N.W., Sheilds, B., Harries, L.W., Barrett, J.C., Ellard, S., Groves, C.J., Knight, B., Patch, A.-M., Ness, A.R., Ebrahim, S., Lawlor, D.A., Ring, S.M., Ben-Shlomo, Y., Javelin, M.-R., Sovio, U., Bennett, A.J., Meltzer, D., Ferrucci, L., Loos, R.J.F., Wareham, N.J., Karpe, F., Owen, K.R., Cardon, L.R., Walker, M., Hitman, G.A., Palmer, C.N.A., Doney, A.S.F., Morris, A.D., Davey Smith, G., The Wellcome Trust Case Control

Consortium, Hattersley, A.T., & McCarthy, M.I. (2007). A common variant in the FTO gene is associated with body mass index and predisposes to childhood and adult obesity. *Science, 316*, 889–894.

Freinkel, N. (1980). Of pregnancy and progeny. *Diabetes, 29*, 1023–1035.

Freinkel, N., & Metzger, B.E. (1979). Pregnancy as a tissue culture experience, the critical implications of maternal metabolism for fetal development. In Ciba Foundation (Eds.), *Pregnancy metabolism, diabetes and the fetus (Ciba Foundation Symposium No. 63)* (pp. 3–23). Amsterdam: Excerpta Medica.

Gluckman, P.D., & Hanson, M.A. (2004). The developmental origins of the metabolic syndrome. *Trends in Endocrinol Metab, 15*, 183–187.

Guillaume, M., Lapidus, L., Beckers, F., Lambert, A., & Bjorntorp, P. (1995). Familial trends of obesity through three generations: the Belgian-Luxembourg child study. *International Journal of Obesity and Related Metabolic Disorders, 19, Suppl 3*, 5–9.

Harder, T., Bergmann, R., Kallischnigg, G., & Plagemann, A. (2005). Duration of breastfeeding and risk of overweight: a meta-analysis. *American Journal of Epidemiology, 162*, 397–403.

Hediger, M.L., Overpeck, M.D., McGlynn, A., Kuczmarski, R.J., Maurer, K.R., & Davis, W.W. (1999). Growth and fatness at three to six years of age of children born small- or large-for-gestational age. *Pediatrics, 104*, e33.

Howe, L.D., Tilling, K., Benfield, L., Sattar, N., Ness, A.R., Davey Smith, G., & Lawlor, D.A. (2010). Changes in ponderal index and body mass index across childhood and their association with fat mass and cardiovascular risk factors at age 15. PLoS One, (accepted October 2010)

Huxley, R., Owen, C.G., Whincup, P.H., Cook, D.G., Rich-Edwards, J., & Davey Smith, G. (2007). Is birth weight a risk factor for ischemic heart disease in later life? *American Journal of Clinical Nutrition, 85*, 1244–1250.

Jovanovic, L., & Pettitt, D.J. (2001). Gestational diabetes mellitus. *Journal of the American Medical Association, 286*, 2516–2518.

Kane, J.K., Parker, S.L., Matta, S.G., Fu, Y., Sharp, B.M., & Li, M.D. (2000). Nicotine up-regulates expression of orexin and its receptors in rat brain. *Endocrinology, 141*, 3623–3629.

Kensara, O.A., Wootton, S.A., Phillips, D.I., Patel, M., Jackson, A.A., Elia, M., & Hertfordshire Study Group (2005). Fetal programming of body composition: relation between birth weight and body composition measured with dual-energy X-ray absorptiometry and anthropometric methods in older Englishmen. *American Journal of Clinical Nutrition, 82*, 980–987.

Kipping, R.R., Jago, R., & Lawlor, D.A. (2008). Obesity in children. Part 1: epidemiology, measurement, risk factors, and screening. *British Medical Journal, 337*, a1824.

Kivimaki, M., Lawlor, D.A., Smith, G.D., Elovainio, M., Jokela, M., Keltikangas-Jarvinen, L., Viikari, J.S., & Raitakari, O.T. (2007). Substantial intergenerational increases in body mass index are not explained by the fetal overnutrition hypothesis: the Cardiovascular Risk in Young Finns Study. *American Journal of Clinical Nutrition, 86*, 1509–1514.

Kjos, S.L., & Buchanan, T.A. (1999). Gestational diabetes mellitus. *New England Journal of Medicine, 341*, 1749–1756.

Kostalova, L., Leskova, L., Kapellerova, A., & Strbak, V. (2001). Body mass, plasma leptin, glucose, insulin and C-peptide in offspring of diabetic and non-diabetic mothers. *European Journal of Endocrinology, 145*, 53–58.

Kral, J.G., Biron, S., Simard, S., Hould, F.S., Lebel, S., Marceau, S., & Marceau, P. (2006). Large maternal weight loss from obesity surgery prevents transmission of obesity to children who were followed for 2 to 18 years. *Pediatrics, 118*, 1644–1649.

Kramer, M.S., Barr, R.G., Leduc, D.G., Boisjoly, C., McVey-White, L., & Pless, I.B. (1985). Determinants of weight and adiposity in the first year of life. *The Journal of Pediatrics, 106*, 10–14.

Kramer, M.S., Chalmers, B., Hodnett, E.D., Sevkovskaya, Z., Dzikovich, I., Shapiro, S., Collet, J.P., Vanilovich, I., Mezen, I., Ducruet, T., Shishko, G., Zubovich, V., Mknuik, D., Gluchanina, E., Dombrovskiy, V., Ustinovitch, A., Kot, T., Bogdanovich, N., Ovchinikova, L., Helsing, E., & PROBIT Study Group (Promotion of Breastfeeding Intervention Trial) (2001). Promotion of Breastfeeding Intervention Trial (PROBIT): a randomized trial in the Republic of Belarus. *Journal of the American Medical Association, 285*, 413–420.

Kramer, M.S., Guo, T., Platt, R.W., Shapiro, S., Collet, J.P., Chalmers, B., Hodnett, E., Sevkovskaya, Z., Dzikovich, I., Vanilovich, I., & PROBIT Study Group (2002). Breastfeeding and infant growth: biology or bias? *Pediatrics, 110*, 343–347.

Kramer, M.S., Matush, L., Vanilovich, I., Platt, R., Bogdanovich, N., Sevkosvkaya, Z., Dzikovich, I., Shishko, G., Collet, J.P., Martin, R.M., Davey Smith, G., Gillman, M.W., Chalmers, B., Hodnett, E., Shapiro, S., & Promotion of Breastfeeding Intervention Trial (PROBIT) Study Group (2007). Effects of prolonged and exclusive breastfeeding on child height, weight, adiposity, and blood pressure at age 6.5y: evidence from a large randomized trial. *American Journal of Clinical Nutrition, 86*, 1717–1721.

Labayen, I., Moreno, L.A., Blay, M.G., Blay, V.A., Mesana, M.I., Gonzalez-Gross, M., Bueno, G., Sarria, A., & Bueno, M. (2006). Early programming of body composition and fat distribution in adolescents. *Journal of Nutrition, 136*, 147–152.

Laitinen, J., Power, C., & Jarvelin, M.R. (2001). Family social class, maternal body mass index, childhood body mass index, and age at menarche as predictors of adult obesity. *American Journal of Clinical Nutrition, 74*, 287–294.

Lake, J.K., Power, C., & Cole, T.J. (1997). Child to adult body mass index in the 1958 British birth cohort: associations with parental obesity. *Archives of Disease in Childhood, 77*, 376–381.

Law, C.M., Barker, D.J., Osmond, C., Fall, C.H., & Simmonds, S.J. (1992). Early growth and abdominal fatness in adult life. *Journal of Epidemiology and Community Health, 46*, 184–186.

Law, C.M., Gordon, G.S., Shiell, A.W., Barker, D.J., & Hales, C.N. (1995). Thinness at birth and glucose tolerance in seven-year-old children. *Diabetic Medicine, 12*, 24–29.

Lawlor, D.A., Riddoch, C.J., Page, A.S., Anderssen, S.A., Froberg, K., & Harro, M. (2004). The association of birth weight and contemporary size with insulin resistance among children from Estonia and Denmark: findings from the European Heart Study. *Diabetic Medicine, 22*, 921–930.

Lawlor, D.A., Davey Smith, G., O'Callaghan, M., Alati, R., Mamun, A.A., Williams, G.M., & Najman, J.M. (2007). Epidemiologic evidence for the fetal overnutrition hypothesis: findings from the mater-university study of pregnancy and its outcomes. *American Journal of Epidemiology, 165*, 418–424.

Lawlor, D.A., Harbord, R.M., Sterne, J.A.C., Timpson, N.J., & Davey Smith, G. (2008a). Mendelian randomization and instrumental variables. *Statistics in Medicine, 27*, 1133–1163.

Lawlor, D.A., Timpson, N., Harbord, R., Leary, S., Ness, A., McCarthy, M.I., Frayling, T.M., Hattersley, A.T., & Davey Smith, G. (2008b). Exploring the developmental overnutrition hypothesis using parental-offspring associations and the *FTO* gene as an instrumental variable for maternal adiposity: findings from the Avon Longitudinal Study of Parents and Children (ALSPAC). *PLoS Medicine, 5*, e33.

Lawlor, D.A., Benfield, L., Logue, J., Tilling, K., Howe, L.D., Fraser, A., Cherry, L., Watt, P., Ness, A.R., Davey Smith, G., & Sattar, N. (2010a). The association of general and central adiposity, and change in these with cardiovascular risk factors in adolescence: A prospective cohort study. *BMJ*, in press (accepted September 2010)

Lawlor, D.A., Fraser, A., Lindsay, R.S., Ness, A., Dabelea, D., Catalano, P., Davey Smith, G., Sattar, N., & Nelson, S.M. (2010b). The association of existing diabetes, gestational diabetes and glycosuria in pregnancy with macrosomia and offspring body mass index, waist and fat mass in later childhood: findings from a prospective pregnancy cohort. *Diabetologia, 53*, 89–97

Lawlor, D.A., Lichtenstein, P., & Långström, N. (2010c). Maternal diabetes in pregnancy programmes greater offspring adiposity into early adulthood: Sibling study in a prospective cohort of 280,866 men from 248,293 families. *Circulation*, in press (accepted October 2010)

Leary, S.D., Davey Smith, G., Rogers, I.S., Reilly, J.J., Wells, J.C., & Ness, A.R. (2006). Smoking during pregnancy and offspring fat and lean mass in childhood. *Obesity, 14*, 2284–2293.

Levin, B.E., & Govek, E. (1998). Gestational obesity accentuates obesity in obesity-prone progeny. *American Journal of Physiology, 275*, 1374–1379.

Li, C., Kaur, H., Choi, W.S., Huang, T.T., Lee, R.E., & Ahluwalia, J.S. (2005). Additive interactions of maternal prepregnancy BMI and breast-feeding on childhood overweight. *Obesity Research, 13*, 362–371.

Li, L., Hardy, R., Kuh, D., Lo, C.R., & Power, C. (2008). Child-to-adult body mass index and height trajectories: a comparison of 2 British birth cohorts. *American Journal of Epidemiology, 168*, 1008–1015.

Mamun, A.A., Lawlor, D.A., Alati, R., O'Callaghan, M.J., Williams, G.M., & Najman, J.M. (2006). Does maternal smoking during pregnancy have a direct effect on future offspring obesity? Evidence from a prospective birth cohort study. *American Journal of Epidemiology, 164*, 317–325.

Mamun, A.A., O'Callaghan, M., Callaway, L., Williams, G., Najman, J., & Lawlor, D.A. (2009). Associations of gestational weight gains with offspring body mass index and blood pressure at 21 years: evidence from a birth cohort study. *Circulation, 119*, 1720–1727.

Manderson, J.G., Mullan, B., Patterson, C.C., Hadden, D.R., Traub, A.I., & McCance, D.R. (2002). Cardiovascular and metabolic abnormalities in the offspring of diabetic pregnancy. *Diabetologia, 45*, 991–996.

McCarthy, A., Hughes, R., Tilling, K., Davies, D., Davey Smith, G., & Ben-Shlomo, Y. (2007). Birth weight; post-natal, infant, and childhood growth; and obesity in young adulthood: evidence from the Barry Caerphilly Growth Study. *American Journal of Clinical Nutrition, 86*, 907–913.

Metzger, B.E., Silverman, B.L., Freinkel, N., Dooley, S.L., Ogata, E.S., & Green, O.C. (1990). Amniotic fluid insulin concentration as a predictor of obesity. *Archives of Disease in Childhood, 65*, 1050–1052.

Metzger, B.E., Lowe, L.P., Dyer, A.R., Trimble, E.R., Chaovarindr, U., Coustanm, D.R., Hadden, D.R., McCance, D.R., Hod, M., McIntyre, H.D., Oats, J.J.N., Persson, B., Rogers, M.S., & Sacks, D.A. (2008). Hyperglycemia and adverse pregnancy outcomes. *New England Journal of Medicine, 358*, 1991–2002.

Moreira, P., Padez, C., Mourao-Carvalhal, I., & Rosado, V. (2007). Maternal weight gain during pregnancy and over-weight in Portuguese children. *International Journal of Obesity (London), 31*, 608–614.

Naturenews. (2009). http://www.nature.com/news/2008/081120/full/news.2008.1240.html, accessed on April 14, 2009.

Okens, K., Taveras, E.M., Kleinman, K.P., Rich-Edwards, J.W., & Gillman, M.W. (2005). Maternal weight gain during pregnancy and child adiposity at age 3 years. *Pediatric Research, 58*, 1127.

Okun, N., Verma, A., Mitchell, B.F., & Flowerdew, G. (1997). Relative importance of maternal constitutional factors and glucose intolerance of pregnancy in the development of newborn macrosomia. *The Journal of Maternal-Fetal Medicine, 6*, 285–290.

Ong, K.K., Emmett, P., Northstone, K., Golding, J., Rogers, I., Ness, A.R., Wells, J.C., & Dunger, D.B. (2009). Infancy weight gain predicts childhood body fat and age at menarche in girls. *Journal of Clinical Endocrinology and Metabolism*, doi:10.1210/jc.2008-2489.

Owen, C.G., Whincup, P.H., Odoki, K., Gilg, J.A., & Cook, D.G. (2003). Birth weight and blood cholesterol level: a study in adolescents and systematic review. *Pediatrics, 111*, 1081–1089.

Owen, C.G., Martin, R.M., Whincup, P.H., Davey Smith, G., & Cook, D.G. (2005a). Effect of infant feeding on the risk of obesity across the life course: a quantitative review of published evidence. *Pediatrics, 115*, 1367–1377.

Owen, C.G., Martin, R.M., Whincup, P.H., Davey Smith, G., Gillman, M.W., & Cook, D.G. (2005b). The effect of breast feeding on mean body mass index throughout the lifecourse; a quantitative review of published and unpublished observational evidence. *American Journal of Clinical Nutrition, 82*, 1298–1307.

Owen, C.G., Whincup, P.H., Orfei, L., Chou, Q., Eriksson, J., & Osmond, C. (2007). Body mass index and risk of coronary heart disease: a lifecourse approach. *Early Human Development, 83*, 78.

Parsons, T.J., Power, C., & Manor, O. (2001). Fetal and early life growth and body mass index from birth to early adulthood in 1958 British cohort: longitudinal study. *British Medical Journal, 323*, 1331–1335.

Pederson, J. (1954). Weight and length at birth of infants of diabetic mothers. *Acta Endocrinologica, 16*, 330–342.

Persson, B., Heding, L.G., Lunell, N.O., Pschera, H., Stangenberg, M., & Wager, J. (1982). Fetal beta cell function in diabetic pregnancy. Amniotic fluid concentrations of proinsulin, insulin, and C-peptide during the last trimester of pregnancy. *American Journal of Obstetrics and Gynecology, 144*, 455–459.

Pettitt, D.J., & Knowler, W.C. (1998). Long-term effects of the intrauterine environment, birthweight, and breast-feeding in Pima Indians. *Diabetes Care, 21*, 138–141.

Pettitt, D.J., Baird, H.R., Aleck, K.A., Bennett, P.H., & Knowler, W.C. (1983). Excessive obesity in offspring of Pima Indian women with diabetes during pregnancy. *New England Journal of Medicine, 308*, 242–245.

Pettitt, D.J., Knowler, W.C., Bennett, P.H., Aleck, K.A., & Baird, H.R. (1987). Obesity in offspring of diabetic Pima Indian women despite normal birth weight. *Diabetes Care, 10*, 76–80.

Pettitt, D.J., Nelson, R.G., Saad, M.F., Bennett, P.H., & Knowler, W.C. (1993). Diabetes and obesity in the offspring of Pima Indian women with diabetes during pregnancy. *Diabetes Care, 16*, 310–314.

Pietilainen, K.H., Kaprio, J., Rasanen, M., Winter, T., Rissanen, A., & Rose, R.J. (2001). Tracking of body size from birth to late adolescence: contributions of birth length, birth weight, duration of gestation, parents' body size and twinship. *American Journal of Epidemiology, 154*, 21–29.

Power, C., & Jefferis, B.J. (2002). Fetal environment and subsequent obesity: a study of maternal smoking. *International Journal of Epidemiology, 31*, 413–419.

Power, C., Lake, J.K., & Cole, T.J. (1997). Body mass index and height from childhood to adulthood in the 1958 British born cohort. *American Journal of Clinical Nutrition, 66*, 1094–1101.

Pribylova, H., & Dvorakova, L. (1996). Long-term prognosis of infants of diabetic mothers. Relationship between metabolic disorders in newborns and adult offspring. *Acta Diabetologica, 33*, 30–34.

Ramsay, J.E., Ferrell, W.R., Crawford, L., Wallace, A.M., Greer, I.A., & Sattar, N. (2002). Maternal obesity is associated with dysregulation of metabolic, vascular, and inflammatory pathways. *The Journal of Clinical Endocrinology and Metabolism, 87*, 4231–4237.

Rasmussen, F., & Johansson, M. (1998). The relation of weight, length and ponderal index at birth to body mass index and overweight among 18-year-old males in Sweden. *European Journal of Epidemiology, 14*, 373–380.

Rogers, I.S., Ness, A.R., Steer, C.D., Wells, J.C.K., Emmett, P.M., Reilly, J.R., Tobias, J., & Davey Smith, G. (2006). Associations of size at birth and dual-energy X-rat absorptiometry measures of lean and fat mass at 9 to 10 years of age. *American Journal of Clinical Nutrition, 84*, 739–747.

Sachdev, H.S., Fall, C.H, Osmond, C., Lakshmy, R., Dey Biswas, S.K., Leary, S.D., Reddy, K.S., Barker, D.J.P., & Bhargava, S.K. (2005). Anthropometric indicators of body composition in young adults: relation to size at birth and serial measurements of body mass index in childhood in the New Delhi birth cohort. *American Journal of Clinical Nutrition, 82*, 456–466.

Schack-Nielsen, L., Mortensen, E.L., Michaelsen, K.F., & Ti, S. (2005). High maternal pregnancy weight gain is associated with an increased risk of obesity in childhood and adulthood independent of maternal BMI. *Pediatric Research, 58*, 1020.

Scholl, T.O., Sowers, M., Chen, X., & Lenders, C. (2001). Maternal glucose concentration influences fetal growth, gestation, and pregnancy complications. *American Journal of Epidemiology, 154*, 514–520.

Sebire, N.J., Jolly, M., Harris, J.P., Wadsworth, J., Joffe, M., Beard, R.W., Regan, L., & Robinson, S. (2001). Maternal obesity and pregnancy outcome: a study of 287,213 pregnancies in London. *International Journal of Obesity and Related Metabolic Disorders, 25*, 1175–1182.

Seidman, D.S., Laor, A., Gale, R., Stevenson, D.K., & Danon, Y.L. (1991). A longitudinal study of birth weight and being overweight in late adolescence. *American Journal of Diseases in Children, 145*, 782–785.

Seidman, D.S., Laor, A., Shemer, J., Gale, R., & Stevenson, D.K. (1996). Excessive maternal weight gain during pregnancy and being overweight at 17 years of age. *Pediatric Research, 39*, 112A.

Sermer, M., Naylor, C.D., Gare, D.J., Kenshole, A.B., Ritchie, J.W., Farine, D., Cohen, H.R., McArthur, K., Holzapfel, S., Biringer, A., Chen, E., & Toronto Tri-Hospital Gestational Diabetes Investigators (1995). Impact of increasing carbohydrate intolerance on maternal-fetal outcomes in 3637 women without gestational diabetes. The Toronto Tri-Hospital Gestational Diabetes Project. *American Journal of Obstetrics and Gynecology, 173*, 146–156.

Sharma, A.J., Cogswell, M.E., & Grummer-Strawn, L.M. (2005). The association between pregnancy weight gain and childhood overweight is modified by mother's pre-pregnancy BMI. *Pediatric Research, 58*, 1038.

Silverman, B.L., Rizzo, T., Green, O.C., Cho, N.H., Winter, R.J., Ogata, E.S., Richards, G.E., & Metzger, B.E. (1991). Long-term prospective evaluation of offspring of diabetic mothers. *Diabetes, 40, Suppl 2*, 121–125.

Silverman, B.L., Landsberg, L., & Metzger, B.E. (1993). Fetal hyperinsulinism in offspring of diabetic mothers. Association with the subsequent development of childhood obesity. *Annals of the New York Academy of Sciences, 699*, 36–45.

Silverman, B.L., Metzger, B.E., Cho, N.H., & Loeb, C.A. (1995). Impaired glucose tolerance in adolescent offspring of diabetic mothers. Relationship to fetal hyperinsulinism. *Diabetes Care, 18*, 611–617.

Singhal, A., & Lucas, A. (2004). Early origins of cardiovascular disease: is there a unifying hypothesis? *Lancet, 363*, 1642–1645.

Singhal, A., Fewtrell, M., Cole, T.J., & Lucas, A. (2003a). Low nutrient intake and early growth for later insulin resistance in adolescents born preterm. *Lancet, 361*, 1089–1097.

Singhal, A., Wells, J., Cole, T.J., Fewtrell, M., & Lucas, A. (2003b). Programming of lean body mass: a link between birth weight, obesity and cardiovascular disease? *American Journal of Clinical Nutrition, 77*, 726–730.

Slotkin, T.A. (1998). Fetal nicotine or cocaine exposure: which one is worse? *The Journal of Pharmacology and Experimental Therapeutics, 285*, 931–945.

Sobngwi, E., Boudou, P., Mauvais-Jarvis, F., Leblanc, H., Velho, G., Vexiau, P., Porcher, R., Hadjadj, S., Pratley, R., Tataranni, P.A., Calvo, F., & Gautier, J.F. (2003). Effect of a diabetic environment in utero on predisposition to type 2 diabetes. *Lancet, 361*, 1861–1865.

Stettler, N., Tershakovec, A.M., Zemel, B.S., Leonard, M.B., Boston, R.C., Katz, S.H., & Stallings, V.A. (2000). Early risk factors for increased adiposity: a cohort study of African American subjects followed from birth to young adulthood. *American Journal of Clinical Nutrition, 72*, 378–383.

Strauss, R.S. (1997). Effects of the intrauterine environment on childhood growth. *British Medical Bulletin, 53*, 81–95.

Te Velde, S.J., Twisk, J.W.E., Van Mechelan, W., & Kemper, H.C.G. (2003). Birth weight, adult body composition, and subcutaneous fat distribution. *Obesity Research, 11*, 202–208.

Toschke, A.M., Montgomery, S.M., Pfeiffer, U., & von Kries, R. (2003). Early intrauterine exposure to tobacco-inhaled products and obesity. *American Journal of Epidemiology, 158*, 1068–1074.

Von Kries, R., Toschke, A.M., Koletzko, B., & Slikker, W., Jr. (2002). Maternal smoking during pregnancy and childhood obesity. *American Journal of Epidemiology, 156*, 954–961.

Walker, S.P., Gaskin, P.S., Powell, C.A., & Bennett, F.I. (2002). The effects of birth weight and postnatal linear growth retardation on body mass index, fatness and fat distribution in mid and late childhood. *Public Health Nutrition, 5*, 391–396.

Weiss, P.A., Scholz, H.S., Haas, J., Tamussino, K.F., Seissler, J., & Borkenstein, M.H. (2000). Long-term follow-up of infants of mothers with type 1 diabetes: evidence for hereditary and nonhereditary transmission of diabetes and precursors. *Diabetes Care, 23*, 905–911.

Whincup, P.H., Cook, D.G., & Geleijnse, J.M. (2004). A life course approach to blood pressure. In D. Kuh & Y. Ben-Shlomo (Eds.), *A life course approach to chronic disease epidemiology* (pp. 218–239). Second ed. Oxford: University Press.

Whincup, P.H., Kaye, S.J., Owen, C.G., Huxley, R., Cook, D.G., Anazawa, S., Barrett-Connor, E., Bhargava, S.K., Birgisdottir, B., Carlsson, S., De Rooij, S., Dyck, R., Eriksson, J.G., Falkner, B., Fall, C., Forsen, T., Grill, V., Gudnason, V., Hulman, S., Hypponen, E., Jeffreys, M., Lawlor, D.A., Leon, D.A., Mi, J., Minami, J., Mishra, G., Osmond, C., Power, C., Rich-Edwards, J., Roseboom, T.J., Sachdev, H.P.S., Suzuki, T., Syddall, H., Thorsdottir, I., Vanhala, M., Wadsworth, M., & Yarbrough, D.E. (2008). Birthweight and risk of type 2 diabetes: a quantitative systematic review of published evidence. *Journal of the American Medical Association, 300*, 2886–2897.

Whitaker, R.C. (2004). Predicting preschooler obesity at birth: the role of maternal obesity in early pregnancy. *Pediatrics, 114*, 29–36.

Whitaker, R.C., & Dietz, W.H. (1998). Role of the prenatal environment in the development of obesity. *The Journal of Pediatrics, 132*, 768–776.

Chapter 18
Food Patterns and Nutrient Intake in Relation to Childhood Obesity

Gerardo Rodríguez, Agneta Sjöberg, Lauren Lissner, and Luis A. Moreno

Introduction

Childhood and adolescence are pivotal periods in human life characterized, among others by intense metabolic rate, continuous body growth and development, physical and psychological changes, and the onset of habits that will probably continue in later ages. All these characteristics may confer high vulnerability in relation to the risk of obesity development in predisposed subjects. Body composition and psycho-social changes determine nutritional requirements as well as dietary and physical activity behavior variability but, at the same time, these latter and other environmental and behavioral factors could also influence the former (Rodríguez et al. 2004). Among all risk factors that are known to modulate obesity development and its persistence into adulthood, diet composition and food patterns are among the main environmental determinants of energy balance along different periods of life (Rodríguez and Moreno 2006) (Fig. 18.1).

Although energy imbalance has to be a constant and basic cause of overweight, fat deposition does not always occur in the case of excess energy availability. Energy balance homeostasis and body composition maintenance are both regulated by a complex net of neuro-hormonal and metabolic processes which strongly preserve an individual resilience in maintaining weight. Variations in any component or physiological determinant of this balance are compensated with other changes that modify energy expenditure or energy intake in order to re-establish energy equilibrium. Exogenous obesity develops when energy intake exceeds energy expenditure during long periods of time, leading to slow accumulation of body fat. Even a small maintained daily energy imbalance can result in significant weight gain. The "energy gap" is the small positive energy imbalance that causes body fat increase after compensating energy changes have failed attempting to maintain body weight. Metabolically, it is very easy to achieve a continuous positive energy balance in our "obesogenic" environment (abundant food supply and sedentary lifestyle), especially after negative energy balance

G. Rodríguez (✉)
Departamento de Pediatría, Universidad de Zaragoza, Zaragoza. Instituto Aragonés
de Ciencias de la Salud, Zaragoza, Spain
e-mail: gereva@comz.org

A. Sjöberg and L. Lissner
Department of Public Health and Community Medicine/EPI, University of Gothenburg, Gothenburg, Sweden

L.A. Moreno
GENUD (Growth, Exercise, Nutrition and Developement) Research Group, Universitaria de Ciencias de la Salud, Universidad de Zaragoza, Zaragoza, Spain

L.A. Moreno et al. (eds.), *Epidemiology of Obesity in Children and Adolescents*,
Springer Series on Epidemiology and Public Health 2, DOI 10.1007/978-1-4419-6039-9_18,
© Springer Science+Business Media, LLC 2011

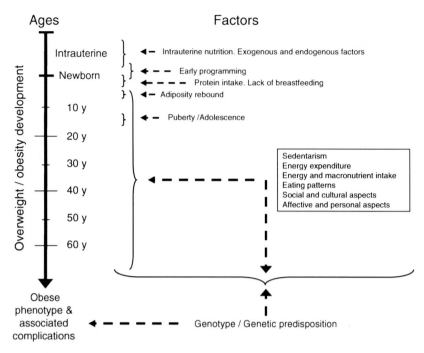

Fig. 18.1 Potential factors influencing obesity development along different periods of life. Adapted from Rodríguez and Moreno (2008)

periods due to human predisposition to store energy. Longer-term neuro-endocrine signals depend on the magnitude of energy stores and, when adipose tissue mass has decreased, hunger is activated to restore the loss by stimulating food intake and inhibiting thermogenesis. In contrast, the response to energy excess is relatively weak and compensatory food intake decreases are not complete.

In spite of simple theoretical relations between positive energy balance and obesity development, no consistent information exists about which is the strongest environmental factor influencing body fatness in children and adolescents (Gibson and Neate 2007; Gillis et al. 2002; Guillaume et al. 1998; Moreno and Rodríguez 2007; Rodríguez and Moreno 2006, 2008; Veugelers and Fitzgerald 2005). Excessive global energy intake due to easy and continuous food accessibility, consumption of energy-dense foods (Alexy et al. 2004; Atkin and Davies 2000; Berkey et al. 2000; Bogaert et al. 2003; Gazanniga and Burns 1993; Hassapidou et al. 2006; McGloin et al. 2002; Ong et al. 2006; Parizkova and Rolland-Cachera 1997; Scaglioni et al. 2000; Skinner et al. 2004), excessive percentage of energy intake from fats (Alexy et al. 2004; McGloin et al. 2002) or high macronutrient consumption (for example, excessive protein intake) (Parizkova and Rolland-Cachera 1997; Scaglioni et al. 2000), contemporary eating patterns (Berkey et al. 2004; Bowman et al. 2004; Bray et al. 2004; Colapinto et al. 2007; Ello-Martin et al. 2005; Field et al. 2004; Fisher et al. 2007; Francis et al. 2003; Gillman et al. 2000; James et al. 2004; Kral et al. 2007; Ludwig et al. 2001; Moreno et al. 2005; Niemeier et al. 2006; Orlet Fisher et al. 2003; Phillips et al. 2004; Rolls et al. 2000; Sen 2006; Serra et al. 2003; Toschke et al. 2005; Welsh et al. 2005) (elevated consumption of bakery foods, sweetened beverages, sweets or low-quality foods, the low consumption of fruit and vegetables, big portion size intake, daily meal patterns and daily energy intake distribution) are all considered potential contributors of the "obesity epidemic". Nowadays, diet aspects and eating behaviors are also strongly influenced by environmental, socio-cultural, economic, affective and marketing factors (food advertising and promotion). People eat frequently away from home (French et al. 2001; Schmidt et al. 2005), there are time limitations with respect to eating and meal preparation (Bowman et al. 2004;

Rolls et al. 2000), children eat alone without family supervision (Gillman et al. 2000; Sen 2006) (sometimes watching television) and children with both parents at work eat in school dining halls. The food industry has responded to this social demand by increasing convenience foods and prepared meals that could also be associated with the increase in the prevalence of overweight (Berkey et al. 2004; Bowman et al. 2004; Bray et al. 2004; Field et al. 2004; French et al. 2001; James et al. 2004; Ludwig et al. 2001; Orlet Fisher et al. 2003; Phillips et al. 2004; Rolls et al. 2000; Schmidt et al. 2005; Welsh et al. 2005). In this context, this chapter reviews the potential contribution of energy, nutrient intake, eating patterns and other dietary intake factors on overweight prevalence.

Methodological Challenges in Studying Children's Diets

Instrumentation Issues in Measuring Children's Diets

Accurate assessment of dietary intake in obese children is of major concern in population-based nutrition research, given the dramatically increased prevalence of childhood obesity together with the growing list of obesity-related comorbidities as well as psychological consequences. This issue is also of obvious relevance within clinical settings where dietary intakes of children are being monitored. Potential methodological problems that are most clearly documented in adults include obesity-related underreporting, selective underreporting of undesirable foods, and biased reporting associated with other psychosocial characteristics of individuals. Surprisingly little is known on how to obtain accurate measures of dietary intake in obese and normal weight children. Thus dietary instrumentation in obese children is a topic that urgently requires attention by researchers in nutrition.

Assessment of diet in normal- and overweight children, either directly or by adult proxy, introduces some special methodological challenges, in addition to some of the well-known ones. For instance, the average age at which children develop cognitive skills required for self-reporting of diet differs cross-culturally and between individuals, and the minimal age at which children are able to conceptualize time frames used in dietary instruments (e.g. 24 h, 1 week, 1 month) is not well established. The ability of children under 10 years to give valid responses to food frequency questionnaires covering periods of more than a day is questionable because of difficulties in estimating frequences and averages. The need for adult assistance in dietary reporting is also driven by the limited scope of the child's experience and knowledge of recipes and food composition (e.g. fat content of milk). It may be safely assumed that adults reporting their young children's intakes are likely to be affected by social desirability biases as the desire to report that their children consume healthy diets (USDA 2005). Finally, it should be pointed out that in countries where most children attend after-school care and daycare centers that provide one or more meals, parental proxy reports are likely to be inadequate. For instance, in Swedish pre-schools children may have as many as three meals a day at the daycare center (breakfast, lunch and mid-day snack). In such settings, it is unlikely that valid data can be collected without the support of the personnel at the daycare.

Adolescents, on the other hand, are frequently asked to report their own diets by recall or questionnaire. Challenges in dietary assessment of adolescents include: rapidly changing eating habits due to growth; unstructured consumption of snacks and skipping meals, eating away from home frequently; and high prevalence of dietary restraint, particularly among girls. In addition, similar to the situation among adults, overweight and obesity in adolescents has been associated with underreporting of intake: up to 40% of energy may not be reported in obese adolescents (Bandini et al. 1990). Energy underreporting also increases with age across adolescence (Livingstone and Robson 2000). Obesity-related underreporting by food record has also been documented in Swedish adolescents (Bratteby et al. 1998).

Food frequency questionnaires (FFQs) have been developed for adolescents (Rockett et al. 1997; Vereecken et al. 2005) and in the near future electronic and web-based tools will have increasing appeal within this age group. Research in school settings has many advantages in terms of data collection (Rockett et al. 1997; Vereecken et al. 2005). However, there are difficulties within the school setting, including competing time constraints from school curricula resulting in limited time for recruitment, adequate explanation of study forms and procedures, and data collection. Alternative approaches and settings that appeal to young people are needed (Coufopoulos et al. 2001; Frank 1994). It is unclear which methods may minimize or avoid some of the biased reporting related to overweight and restrained eating that are known to exist in this age group (Frank 1994).

Summary

In summary, while a general underreporting bias exists in free-living subjects describing their diets, regardless of weight status, all evidence points to this problem being magnified in the obese, including children and adolescents. Although existing data suggest that it is possible to obtain valid intake data from sufficiently motivated obese adults (Lindroos et al. 1999), obesity-related underreporting biases have been reported for most of the commonly used dietary assessment instruments, and relatively little focus has been placed on how to solve this problem. Given the known importance of obesity for a number of health outcomes, it is critical to develop instruments that can rank and differentiate obese and non-obese individuals of all ages with respect to dietary intakes.

Other Methodological Challenges

Problems of instrumentation are accompanied by other methodological concerns when studying potentially etiological roles of diet in childhood obesity. One problem is that the importance of food choice may be obscured when studying diets at the macronutrient and micronutrient levels. It may be easier to communicate advice about healthy foods than giving recommendations about nutrients. A second problem is that many confounding factors may be present, which bias observed associations between nutrients and obesity. These include age, physical activity, socio-economic status, and other socio-cultural factors such as gender and ethnicity. To give an example, failure to consider physical activity when studying associations between energy intake and body mass index (BMI) might result in an underestimation of the association due to influence of lean, athletic subgroups of children. Similarly, poorer reporting accuracy and more underreporting in less educated or socially disadvantaged groups might obscure an association between energy intake and obesity.

Finally it should be pointed out that study design is a key factor when interpreting associations between dietary intake and obesity. Cross-sectional survey data, in which anthropometric measures and dietary assessments are conducted simultaneously, cannot be assumed to reflect causal associations and may be affected by problems of reversed causality, where diets have already changed as a consequence of obesity or weight gain. Prospective designs are often assumed to alleviate this problem by observing diet at one point in time in relation to subsequent weight gain or incidence of obesity. However, this design does not take into account the fact that diet may change over time. Studies of concurrent change in both diet and obesity are frequently undertaken in efforts to address these design issues. The next two sections will offer an overview of different types of studies that have been used to describe associations between dietary intake and obesity in children. We will start with examples from the literature describing energy and nutrient composition of diets in relation to obesity and continue to describe studies of dietary patterns. Because some of the individual publications describe both nutrients and diet patterns, we have combined a summary of all cited studies in Table 18.1.

Table 18.1 Characteristics of cross-sectional and prospective studies relating food patterns and nutrients with body composition

Age group/sample size	Methods	Dietary and energy expenditure variables studied	Reference
	Cross-sectional		
7–12 y/2,440	Diet history	EI, g and E% protein, carb and fat, animal protein, foods	Rolland-Cachera and Bellisle (1986)
15–17 y/64	5-d food record (child)	EI, g + E% protein, carb, fat, fatty acids, micronutrients, foods	Ortega et al. (1995)
1.5–4.5 y/1,444	4-d weighed record	EI, E% fat, protein and carb	Davies (1997)
15 y/50	7-d record/DLW (child)	EI	Bratteby et al. (1998)
6–12 y/955	3-d record	EI, fat, SFA, cholesterol, protein and fiber in g and g/kcal	Guillaume et al. (1998)
1.5–4.5 y/77	4-d weighed record, DLW (parents)	TEE, BMR, PAL, EI, E% fat, protein and Carb	Atkin and Davies (2000)
7–11 y/530	Diet history	EI, EI/BMR, E% protein, carb, fat, E% meals	Maffeis et al. (2000)
4–16 y/181	Diet history	EI, fat in g, E% and RNI%, SFA in g and RNI%	Gillis et al. (2002)
5–8 y/114	7-d weighed record, DLW	EI, TEE, E%+g fat, carb, protein	McGloin et al. (2002)
15–16 y/37	Diet history, DLW	EI, EI/TEE	Sjöberg et al. (2003)
8th grade + 4th grade/3,000	FFQ, self reported weight and height	EI, E% fat and sugar, sweetened soft drinks, sweets, breakfast	Andersen et al. (2005)
11–14 y/512	3-d weighed record	EI, g, E% and g/kg body weight of protein, carb and fat, g of starch, intake of micronutrients and foods	Hassapidou et al. (2006)
6–14 y/142	2x24-h recall + 1d record	EI, g and E% of fat, atty acids, proetin, carb. and intake of fiber and micronutrients, foods	Aeberli et al. (2007)
4 y/153	7-d recod	E% fat, carb, sucrose, n-3 fatty acids	Garemo et al. (2007)
4 y/1,780	3-d record		Jouret et al. (2007)
10–11 y/4,289	Diet history	SES. Dietary intake and habits, meal behaviors (with family, watching TV, fast food restaurants)	Veugelers and Fitzgerald (2005)
7–18 y/1,294	7-d weighed record, BMI, 7-d physical activity diaries	Nutrient intake, non-milk sugars, soft drinks. PAL	Gibson and Neate (2007)
3–11 y/748	7-d food portion record, physical activity questionnaire	Portion size, foods (energy-dense, nutrient-poor)	Lioret et al. (2009)
5–6 y/4,370	Diet history. BMI	Meal frequency. Foods, macro- and micronutrients	Toschke et al. (2005)
9–14 y/16,202	Semiquantitative food frequency questionnaire. Self reported weight and height	Frequency of family dinners. Foods	Gillman et al. (2000)
12–15 y/5,014	Diet history. Self reported weight and height	Frequency of family dinners.	Sen (2006)

(continued)

Table 18.1 (continued)

Age group/sample size	Methods	Dietary and energy expenditure variables studied	Reference
7–12 y/4,746	Semiquantitative food frequency questionnaire. Measured weight and height	Frequency of fast food restaurant use. Energy and food intake. Demographic and behavioral data	French et al. (2001)
8–9 y/137 and 13–15 y/243	Location of major fast food outlets. Measured weight and height	Presence and distance of fast food outlets	Crawford et al. (2008)
2–5 y/1,160	24-h recall	Demographic descriptors. Food comsumption (including beverage). Physical activity	O'Connor et al. (2006)
5–14 y/3,049	24-h recall Prospective	Energy intake. Sucrose intake. Beverages	Parnell et al. (2008)
8 y, follow-up at 12 y/112	Diet history	EI, protein, carb, fat in g and E%, simple carb in g	Maffeis et al. (1998)
Birth, 1 y, 5y171 newborn, 147 at 5-y follow-up	Infant feeding practice retrosp. 1 y, FFQ+24-h recall	EI, EI/kg, weigt and BMI at birth, 1 y and 5 y, E% protein, carb, fats, SFA, monounsaturated, polyunsaturated FA	Scaglioni et al. (2000)
9–14 y/>10,0001 y follow-up	FFQ	EI, g of fat, fiber	Berkey et al. (2000)
Birth to 15 y/150 (of 500)	3 d weighed rec. At2, 4, 6 y and 4-d rec at 8, 11, 13 and 15 y	EI, g and E% protein, carb, fat, skinfolds, E% SFA	Magarey et al. (2001)
6–9 y / 41 children in 12-month follow-up	3-day food record	EI, E% protein, fat, carb+fatty acids	Bogaert et al. (2003)
5, 7–9 y	Repeated 3-d records at 5 y, 7 y, questionnaire at 4.5 y	Diet at 5 and 7 y: food groups from which dietary pattern scores were derived	Johnson et al. (2008)
6–8 to 13–17 y/50	7-d record	Energy density ED by total diet and excluding different fractions of diet	McCaffrey et al. (2008)
From birth to 7 y/8,234	Food frequency cuestionnaire at 30 and 38 months. Infant feeding at 6 months. Weight and BMI increases	Social and family characteristics. Intrauterine and perinatal factors. Behavioral patterns	Reilly et al. (2005)
Non-hispanic white girls 5–9 y/137	Three 24-h recalls within a 2–3-week period. Especific snacking and TV viewing questionnaires. Increase in BMI	Snacking frequency, TV viewing patterns, snacking while watching TV. Fat intake from energy-dense snacks	Francis et al. (2003)
2–8 y/70	24-h recall 3-d record and food records. BMI changes and adiposity rebound	%E from macronutrient. Energy density intake. Food group intakes	Skinner et al. (2004)
3–6 y/49	3-d record in children born at low or high risk for obesity based on maternal pregnancy BMI. Children BMI and abdominal circumference changes	Beverage (milk, fruit juice and drinks, sodas, soft drinks) consumption patterns	Kral et al. (2007)
2–18 y (at least 10 years of long-term participation)/228	Weighed dietary records. BMI changes	Fat intake patterns. %E from macronutrient. Energy density intake. Food group intakes	Alexy et al. (2004)

(continued)

Table 18.1   (continued)

Age group/sample size	Methods	Dietary and energy expenditure variables studied	Reference
11.7 y until 19 months later/548	Frequency questionnaire. BMI	Sugar-sweetened drinks	Ludwig et al. (2001)
11–21 to 18–27 y/9,919	Food intake questionnaire. BMI and weight gain	Fast food consumption. Breakfast skipping	Niemeier et al. (2006)
8–12 y non-obese premenarcheal girls until 4 y after menarche/196	Annual controls. Food intake questionnaire. BMI and percentage of body fat	Foods. Energy dense snacks	Phillips et al. (2004)
9–14 y between 1996 and 1998/14,977	Food frequency questionnaire. BMI	Snacks	Field et al. (2004)
9 y black and white girls to 19 y/2,379	3-day food record and food-patterns questionnaire; annually in the first 5 years and then in years 7, 8, and 10	Food consumption (including fast food) and nutrient intake	Schmidt et al. (2005)
7–11 y during one school year/644	Three 3-d recalls on drinks consumption: BMI and abdominal circumference	Carbonated drinks	James et al. (2004)

All studies included weight, height (measured or self-reported), *EI* daily energy intake; *ED* energy density energy/grams; *E%* percent of energy; *TEE* total energy expenditure; *DLW* doubly labeled water; *SES* socio-economic status; *y* year; *d* day

Energy and Nutrient Intake in Obese vs. Non-Obese Children

This section offers examples of research describing the association between composition of the diet and childhood obesity, based on different dietary instruments and study designs. We have identified studies reporting on energy, fat, protein and sucrose in relation to current obesity and prospective weight development in children and adolescents. Those studies also describing diet in terms of patterns will be reviewed in the section on "Food Consumption Patterns as Obesity Risk Factors".

Energy and Energy Intake

The literature on energy intake (EI) in obese vs. non-obese children includes examples of negative associations, positive associations and non-associations, using cross-sectional and prospective designs. For instance, negative associations between EI and obesity have been found in a number of cross-sectional studies (Bratteby et al. 1998; Hassapidou et al. 2006; Sjöberg et al. 2003). In one of these studies, the association was negative in girls but not in boys, a difference attributed to sex influences on underreporting (Sjöberg et al. 2003). Although it is often assumed that such associations are artifacts of obesity-related underreporting, low physical activity seems likely to be part of the explanation (Berkey et al. 2000).

In contrast, several studies have provided evidence of positive associations between energy intake and obesity. In one study using diet history, children and adolescents with obesity had significantly higher EI than non-obese children, independent of physical activity patterns and other dietary covariates (Gillis et al. 2002). In one study from UK with 7–18 year old children, a positive relation between EI based on 7-day food records, physical inactivity and BMI was found as well as a negative association between physical activity and BMI (Gibson and Neate 2007). In a French study of overweight vs. normal weight boys, the 3-day food records revealed higher EI in the overweight group (Jouret et al. 2007). In a large study ($n = 10,769$) of 9–14 year old children in the US with a 1-year follow-up, positive associations were found between EI as well as physical inactivity and weight gain (Berkey et al. 2000). Interestingly, in one longitudinal study of Hispanic children with a history of weight gain, it was observed that a further weight gain was suppressed in children who decreased their EI while also increasing their physical activity level (Butte et al. 2007).

Finally, it must be noted that a number of cross-sectional and prospective studies have not detected any relation between EI and overweight/obesity (Aeberli et al. 2007; Andersen et al. 2005; Maffeis et al. 1998; Maffeis et al. 2000; Rolland-Cachera and Bellisle 1986). One of these studies however found a positive relation only when studying EI at dinner meals (Maffeis et al. 2000).

Differences in studies can potentially be attributed to numerous methodological differences. Measurements of EI in epidemiological settings are known to be inexact (Willett 1998). One explanation for inconsistent associations with childhood obesity includes random and systematic reporting errors. These included differences in precision of different instruments and obesity-related underreporting. Another explanation is that children and adolescents with obesity have lower physical activity levels and many truly have low expenditures. Finally, if BMI reduction is being attempted during the dietary reporting period, lack of positive associations can be attributed to "reverse causation". Studies, typically small ones, using doubly labeled water to validate energy intakes have been less ambiguous than dietary surveys in their results, indicating that underlying positive associations may be attenuated by underreporting, while also confirming that voluntary energy expenditure may also be reduced in obese children (Atkin and Davies 2000; Bandini et al. 1990; Bratteby et al. 1998; McGloin et al. 2002).

Fat and Fat Type

The literature on dietary fat intake in obese vs. non-obese children is also mixed and may further depend on whether fat is measured in the absolute or as a percent of total energy (E%). For instance, in a cross-sectional study including adolescents, there was a positive association for E% of fat but not for intake of fat in grams per day (Ortega et al. 1995); however, the opposite, significant positive associations for fat in grams but not in E% has also been reported (Gillis et al. 2002). In other cross-sectional studies positive relations have been found both for absolute and energy adjusted intakes of fat (Guillaume et al. 1998; McGloin et al. 2002). In a prospective study where children were followed from birth to 15 years, energy adjusted fat was positively associated with subscapular skinfold but not with BMI or triceps skinfold (Magarey et al. 2001). In one study a positive association for fat intake was found for boys but not for girls (Jouret et al. 2007). On the contrary, following children over a 10 year period, BMI-SDS was highest in the group of children with the lowest fat intake pattern (Alexy et al. 2004). However a number of studies have reported no associations between dietary fat and childhood obesity (Aeberli et al. 2007; Andersen et al. 2005; Atkin and Davies 2000; Berkey et al. 2000; Davies 1997; Maffeis et al. 1998; Rolland-Cachera and Bellisle 1986; Scaglioni et al. 2000).

The mechanism of dietary fat in the promotion of obesity is traditionally believed to be mediated by the high energy density and its facilitating effect on positive energy balance. It has been argued that energy density is a determinant of energy intake more important than dietary fat per se, and a number of studies, almost all in adults, have confirmed this (Newby 2007). One study in children found no relation between energy density of total diet and subsequent changes in fat mass but, when energy density excluding beverages was analyzed, there was a positive relation between dietary energy density and change in % of body fat (McCaffrey et al. 2008). Seven years earlier, in the base-line study, positive associations were found between absolute and energy adjusted fat intake and obesity, but no such information was given for the follow-up (McCaffrey et al. 2008; McGloin et al. 2002). Other studies have focused on the type of fat rather than on the amount of fat as a more relevant factor in childhood obesity. For instance, one study in obese children and adolescents observed that they consumed not only more fat but more saturated fat, independent of total energy intake and physical activity level (Gillis et al. 2002). It has also been reported that the ratio between n-6/n-3 polyunsaturated fatty acids (linoleic acid, C18:2 n-6, and alpha-linolenic acid, C18:3 n-3, and long-chain metabolites) may be a factor in early obesity (Ailhaud et al. 2006; Karlsson et al. 2006). However, very little has been published about dietary intake differences in n-6/n-3 ratio in children. One study in 4-year-old children with adequate intake of n-3 fatty acids showed lower body weight than those with lower intake of n-3 fatty acids (Garemo et al. 2007). In summary, although there is evidence that total fat and high fat foods are associated with childhood obesity, the current trend is to examine specific types or attributes of dietary fat that may promote obesity, rather than total fat per se.

Protein

Longitudinal studies of feeding during first post-natal months and early childhood have demonstrated positive relation between protein intake and body size and adiposity (Rolland-Cachera et al. 1995; Scaglioni et al. 2000). Positive associations between protein intake during weaning and transition to the family diet and various indices of obesity at age 7–8 years have also been reported (Gunther et al. 2007; Skinner et al. 2004). Rolland-Cachera et al. (1995) proposed in the mid 1990s that high protein intake in infancy and early childhood was associated with obesity and with earlier adiposity rebound. Timing of and BMI at adiposity rebound (AR) are significantly related to persistent obesity (Dietz 1994; Freedman et al. 2001; He and Karlberg 2002; Whitaker et al. 1998). Other studies have shown sex-specific associations or no associations at all between protein intake in infancy and AR. There was an association between a higher protein intake between 12 and 24 months and higher BMI at AR in girls, but not in boys, and there was no consistent relation with timing of AR (Gunther et al. 2006). In another study, no association was found between high protein intake and early AR (Dorosty et al. 2000).

In cross-sectional studies percent of EI from protein has been shown to be higher among overweight children and adolescents (Aeberli et al. 2007; Azizi et al. 2001; Ortega et al. 1995; Rolland-Cachera and Bellisle 1986) but with no significant differences for absolute protein intakes.

A possible methodological complication in studies of protein intake and obesity is that protein may be underreported less than the rest of the diet, due to social desirability factors. In fact when protein is estimated as a percent of total energy there is evidence that it is proportionally overre-ported, as a consequence of corresponding underreporting of the fat and carbohydrate fractions (Heitmann and Lissner 1995; Lissner et al. 2007). To our knowledge this has not been studied in children, but might explain in part the inconsistent findings reported in adolescents, whose dietary reporting biases are likely to be similar to those in adults.

Sucrose

In the twenty-first century, sugar has become a prime suspect in the search for an obesogenic dietary composition pattern in children. Sucrose occurs both as intrinsic and added in foods and is often used as a surrogate for added sugar. In cross-sectional studies, positive associations have been found between intake of sucrose and BMI in young children (Garemo et al. 2007). There are examples of cross-sectional and prospective studies showing no associations at all between sugar intake and body fatness (Andersen et al. 2005; Buyken et al. 2008), while negative associations were found in two studies (Overby et al. 2004; Parnell et al. 2008).

Both cross-sectional (Gibson and Neate 2007) and prospective studies (Ludwig et al. 2001) about sucrose consumption in children show that consumption of calorically sweetened beverages increases the risk for obesity (Olsen and Heitmann 2009). Proposed mechanisms are that sugar from beverages can lead to a disruption in regulation of EI and satiety (physiological satiety mechanisms are not triggered and energy compensation is not functional), and liquid carbohydrates may cause lower thermogenesis. On the other hand, in a recent meta-analysis of randomized controlled studies, no association between consumption of sugar sweetened beverages and weight gain was found (Forshee et al. 2008).

Other Aspects of Nutrient Composition

There are many other aspects of nutrient intake that will be covered in the section on diet patterns. Breastfeeding is a key factor that can potentially be studied in terms of energy/nutrient content, but which is usually studied as a qualitative or semiquantitative exposure. Similarly, investigations of nutrient intake in children after infancy may benefit from observing nutrients within the context of specific meals. Nutrient content of breakfast foods are believed to differ from that of foods consumed during the rest of the day. Such information, together with differences in breakfast consumption between obese and non-obese children (documented in next section), may clarify the protective association between breakfast consumption and obesity. In this context it should be also considered that certain combinations of nutrients may be more obesogenic than others. For instance, in one prospective study, an energy-dense, high-fat and low fiber diet was followed by higher gain of fat mass from 5/7 years to 9 years (Johnson et al. 2008). However, combinations of nutrients may be more easily studied in terms of food patterns; in the same study, consumption of fast food yielded similar predictive information (Johnson et al. 2008).

It has been suggested that diets of low nutrient density and high energy density are relatively less costly (Drewnowski and Specter 2004) and dietary factors may represent one mechanism explaining the persistent socio-economic gradient in childhood obesity. Socio-economic factors are not only important for diet composition but also for risk of being obese (Guillaume et al. 1998; Rolland-Cachera and Bellisle 1986). Morevover, it has been shown that parental BMI, which is also associated with socio-economic status, may be more important for childrens' weight status than intake of fat, carbohydrate or EI (Maffeis et al. 1998, 2000; Magarey et al. 2001). Socio-ecomomic status has many components that may contribute to childhood obesity and diet may be a key component but available dietary methodology and ways of defining socio-economic status make it difficult to quantify a specific contribution of diet.

Summary Regarding Nutrient Composition and Childhood Obesity

The literature does not allow us to draw firm conclusions regarding nutrient composition and childhood obesity (Newby 2007; Rodríguez and Moreno 2006). Therefore, we turn to the evidence for food patterns which may be more promising, possibly because of better potential for accurate reporting of qualitative aspects of diet (e.g. breakfast, fast food).

Food Consumption Patterns as Obesity Risk Factors

Eating patterns are strongly associated with socio-cultural and economic characteristics of the population, and influenced by a large number of factors affecting personal and family environments. Various factors interact with each other contributing to the establishment of an obesogenic environment which increase the probability of being obese in predisposed subjects: favorable economic conditions, constant food availability, fashionable eating habits, poor family supervision, influence of TV advertisements on food selection, low price but non healthy food industry offers, poor family-social cultural level and parents knowledge about healthy habits. In spite of this hypothetic list of contemporary social factors influencing prevalence of overweight in the population, the real contribution of each one and the main exogenous cause (eating vs. physical activity patterns) remains unknown. The aim of this part of the chapter is to review food consumption patterns in relation with obesity development.

Meal Frequency and Daily Distribution of Meal

At similar energy intakes, a low meal frequency has been classically associated with overweight. In adults, four or more eating episodes per day was related to a lower risk of obesity in comparison with subjects who reported three or fewer eating episodes per day (Ma et al. 2003); and, in children, to eat few meals a day (three or fewer) may also facilitate weight gain compared with four, five or more daily meals (Toschke et al. 2005).

With respect to daily distribution of meals, obese children seem to eat less energy at breakfast, skip breakfast more frequently and consume a higher percentage of energy at dinner (Bandini et al. 1990; Livingstone and Robson 2000; Moreno et al. 2005; Serra et al. 2003). A prospective study of 9,919 adolescents and adults (age range 11–27 years) has recently shown that decreases in breakfast consumption and skipping breakfast predicted increased BMI and weight gain during this period of life (Niemeier et al. 2006). Moreover, healthy habits as a family breakfast have been associated with regular and courteous intakes in the morning (Serra et al. 2003), and the frequency of family dinner has been inversely related to fried foods and soda drinks consumption (Gillman et al. 2000).

Food Portion Size

Intake of large portion sizes of some food items (snacks, soft drinks, french fries, hamburgers, etc.) is frequently observed. Children's energy intake increases when larger portions are offered because satiety signals fail to reduce intake in response to this increment in food consumption (Colapinto et al. 2007; Fisher et al. 2007; Rolls et al. 2000; Sen 2006). Children have reported preference for larger portions of high-energy foods and smaller portions of vegetables; and, as consequence, this behavior can promote high energy intake and lower diet quality (Colapinto et al. 2007; Fisher and Kral 2008; Fisher et al. 2007). Despite increases in food portion sizes, children fail to reduce consumption by satiety signals that compensate for the feeling of "fullness" (Ello-Martin et al. 2005; Rolls et al. 2000). Growing children are not able to self-regulate their intakes in a correct way; however, in infants and small children, portion size does not affect daily energy intake (Bowman et al. 2004). Associations between portion size and overweight status in children have been described, but usually in cross-sectional studies (Fisher and Kral 2008; Lioret et al. 2009); nevertheless, this fact has not been observed in longitudinal studies looking for the risk of overweight development in children eating big portion sizes.

Family Control of Children's Eating

To eat alone without family supervision is by itself a potential risk factor for overweight development. A "family breakfast" has been associated with a regular intake in the morning (Serra et al. 2003) (while a "family dinner" has been related both to a decrease of fried foods and soda drinks consumption (Gillman et al. 2000) and reduced odds of becoming overweight after 3 years of follow-up (Sen 2006)). To eat while watching TV is very common when children are alone and it also increases the risk of overweight in children (Veugelers and Fitzgerald 2005). Results from a cross-sectional study of 4,298 students, aged 10–11 years, from Nova Scotia (Canada), showed that children were at increased risk of overweight depending on whether they bought lunch at school (odds ratio (OR) = 1.39), ate supper while watching television more than 5 times per week (OR = 1.44) or their parents were separated or divorced (OR = 1.21). The children were less likely to be overweight if they ate supper together with the family more than 3 times per week (OR = 0.68) or if their parents completed university education (OR = 0.67) (Veugelers and Fitzgerald 2005). However, no data from longitudinal studies are available describing the independent effect of eating alone or eating while watching TV on children's obesity development.

Fast Food Restaurant Consumption

When eating in fast food restaurants, children tend to consume a large amount of food and to choose high-energy foods (Colapinto et al. 2007). Both the frequency of fast food consumption and the amount of energy intake from fast foods are increasing due to a variety of factors: big portion sizes, palatable and cheap foods, the attractiveness of fast food and easy access to restaurants attractive for children and adolescents. In these fun and attractive restaurants with a wide supply of big portion sizes, children's taste perception is also influenced by branding of foods and beverages (Robinson et al. 2007). Consumption of fast food seems to have an adverse effect on dietary quality (Bowman et al. 2004; Schmidt et al. 2005). Children and adolescents who eat fast food will consume more total energy, total fat, saturated fat, carbohydrates, sodium, added sugars, and sugar-sweetened beverages; and less fiber or milk and fewer fruits and non-starchy vegetables (French et al. 2001). Therefore, excessive fast food intake may displace the consumption of other more nutritious foods.

Despite these findings, longitudinal studies have not found associations between food portion size or fast food intake and the risk of overweight development in children. In a recent study, neither the density of fast food outlets in the local neighborhood (number of outlets within a 2-km buffer around participants' homes) nor the proximity to a fast food restaurant (distance to the nearest outlet) increased the risk of obesity (Crawford et al. 2008)

Snack Consumption

"Snacks" are defined as other eating episodes out of meals, generally smaller and less structured (Gatenby 1997). The percentage of children and adolescents consuming snacks in industrialized countries and the contribution of snacking to total daily energy and fat intake have increased during the last decades (Francis et al. 2003). So, we could think that this behavior could be related to the higher prevalence of obesity due to its low nutritional value and high energy density, but research findings are not conclusive (Moreno and Rodríguez 2007; Rodríguez and Moreno 2006; Rodríguez et al. 2004). However, when snacking is associated with sedentary activities, it has been associated with unhealthy body composition changes in girls (Francis et al. 2003). Nevertheless, in large and well designed longitudinal studies based on initially non-obese children, snack consumption is not a clear predictor of weight gain among children and adolescents (Field et al. 2004; Phillips et al. 2004). In a longitudinal study performed in a cohort of 196 initially non-obese premenarcheal girls, the consumption of energy dense snacks did not seem to influence weight status or fatness change over the adolescent period (Phillips et al. 2004). Results from another prospective trial in 8,203 girls and 6,774 boys, 9–14 years of age, suggested that although snack foods may have low nutritional value, they were not an important independent determinant of weight gain among children and adolescents (Field et al. 2004).

Beverage Consumption

Beverage intake among children has also increased in the recent decades, increasing sugar caloric contribution (O'Connor et al. 2006; Wang et al. 2008).Theoretically, children's metabolism fails to reduce food consumption to compensate for the caloric contribution of sweetened drinks and, on the other hand, sweeteners such as high-fructose corn syrup contribute to an increased weight gain due to their influence on lipogenesis, insulin secretion or leptin production (Bray et al. 2004). This is one of the contemporary food consumption patterns that showed by itself a predictive influence on overweight prevalence in few longitudinal studies (Berkey et al. 2004; James et al. 2004; Ludwig et al. 2001; Welsh et al. 2005). Results from prospective cohort studies performed in children and adolescents showed that there was a positive relationship between the consumption of sugar-sweetened beverages and overweight/obesity development (Berkey et al. 2004; James et al. 2004; Ludwig et al. 2001; Welsh et al. 2005); however, a recent meta-analysis and other simultaneous longitudinal studies have found that the association between sugar-sweetened beverage consumption and BMI or weight gain is not fully convincing, based on the current body of scientific evidence (Forshee et al. 2008; Kral et al. 2008; O'Connor et al. 2006; Parnell et al. 2008).

To Eat High-Quality Foods and Food Variety

Palatability of high energy density food promotes more energy intake and compensatory eating responses may not be sufficient to suppress hunger or to delay eating in children predisposed to develop obesity (Bowman et al. 2004; French et al. 2001; Rolls et al. 2000; Schmidt et al. 2005). However, eating low-energy-dense foods (such as fruits, vegetables, and soups) maintains satiety while reducing energy intake (Bowman et al. 2004; Rolls et al. 2000). Social and taste acceptance, eating behaviors and the satiety value of several types of food tend to promote or suppress energy intake.

Individuals who consume the greatest variety of foods from all food groups have the most adequate nutrient intake (Krebs-Smith et al. 1987). It has been described both in adults and in children that dietary variety obtained from vegetables was inversely associated with body fatness; while conversely, dietary variety obtained from sweets, snacks, condiments and carbohydrates was directly associated with body fatness (McCrory et al. 1999; Miller et al. 2008; Receveur et al. 2008). Other studies have shown an association between TV/video viewing and adverse dietary practices and low diet quality (Miller et al. 2008). In our environment, less than 20% of children consumed the recommended number of portions of vegetables and fruits (Serra et al. 2003).

Summary Regarding Food Patterns and Childhood Obesity

For eating patterns, controversial results have been reported from longitudinal studies with no conclusive evidence of an association between diet habits and obesity development later in life (Moreno and Rodríguez 2007; Reilly et al. 2005; Rodríguez and Moreno 2006, 2008; Veugelers and Fitzgerald 2005). Prospective cohort studies have only found associations between obesity development and specific behaviors such as sugar-sweetened beverage consumption or skipping breakfast (James et al. 2004; Ludwig et al. 2001; Niemeier et al. 2006). Snacking, fast food and big food portion size consumption have not been consistently related to obesity development in longitudinal studies despite these dietary habits are associated with an excessive intake of energy, total fat, saturated fat, carbohydrates, added sugars, and sugar-sweetened beverages (Moreno and Rodríguez 2007; Reilly et al. 2005; Rodríguez and Moreno 2006, 2008; Veugelers and Fitzgerald 2005).

Available evidence is in general supportive of current diet recommendations, i.e. lower fat and sugar, higher fruit and vegetable consumption (Ells et al. 2008). However, better methods are needed to study diet–disease relationships, particularly in children.

Conclusions

Measuring diet is problematic in obese populations of any age and there is a clear need to develop and improve dietary instruments. The situation in children is further complicated by many factors, e.g. growth. However, with available methodologies, it has been possible to identify certain "obesogenic" dietary characteristics in children. Prospective longitudinal designs provide stronger evidence for causal associations than cross-sectional designs but unfortunately there are not many studies using this approach.

The evidence regarding obesogenic macronutrients is weak and conflicting. Considering the reviewed dietary patterns those showing more evidence on the relationship with childhood obesity development are consumption of sugar sweetened beverages and skipping breakfast. Potentially, a cluster of these and other dietary patterns could be involved in the development of obesity in children.

Acknowledgement Supported in part by the Swedish Council on Working Life and Social Research (EpiLife) and the Swedish Research Council. The authors thank Nancy Potischman for her comments.

References

Aeberli, I., Kaspar, M., & Zimmermann, M.B. (2007). Dietary intake and physical activity of normal weight and overweight 6 to 14 year old Swiss children. *Swiss Medical Weekly, 137*, 424–430.

Ailhaud, G., Massiera, F., Weill, P., Legrand, P., Alessandri, J.M., & Guesnet, P. (2006). Temporal changes in dietary fats: role of n-6 polyunsaturated fatty acids in excessive adipose tissue development and relationship to obesity. *Progress in Lipid Research, 45*, 203–236.

Alexy, U., Sichert-Hellert, W., Kersting, M., & Schultze-Pawlitschko, V. (2004) Pattern of long-term fat intake and BMI during childhood and adolescence – results of the DONALD Study. *International Journal of Obesity and Related Metabolic Disorders, 28*, 1203–1209.

Andersen, L.F., Lillegaard, I.T., Øverby, N., Lytle, L., Klepp, K.I., & Johansson, L. (2005). Overweight and obesity among Norwegian schoolchildren: changes from 1993 to 2000. *Scandinavian Journal of Public Health, 33*, 99–106.

Atkin, L.M., & Davies, B.S.W. (2000). Diet composition and body composition in preschool children. *American Journal of Clinical Nutrition, 72*, 15–21.

Azizi, F., Allahverdian, S., Mirmiran, P., Rahmani, M., & Mohammadi, F. (2001). Dietary factors and body mass index in a group of Iranian adolescents: Tehran lipid and glucose study-2. *International Journal for Vitamin and Nutrition Research, 71*, 123–127.

Bandini, L.G., Schoeller, D.A., Cyr, H.N., & Dietz, W.H. (1990). Validity of reported energy intake in obese and nonobese adolescents. *American Journal of Clinical Nutrition, 52*, 421–425.

Berkey, C.S., Rockett, H.R., Field, A.E., Gillman, M.W., Frazier, A.L., Camargo, C.A. Jr., & Colditz, G.A. (2000). Activity, dietary intake, and weight changes in a longitudinal study of preadolescent and adolescent boys and girls. *Pediatrics, 105*, E56.

Berkey, C.S., Rockett, H.R., Field, A.E., Gillman, M.W., & Colditz, G.A. (2004). Sugar-added beverages and adolescent weight change. *Obesity Research, 12*, 778–788.

Bogaert, N., Steinbeck, K.S., Baur, L.A., Brock, K., & Bermingham, M.A. (2003). Food, activity and family – environmental vs biochemical predictors of weight gain in children. *European Journal of Clinical Nutrition, 57*, 1242–1249.

Bowman, S.A., Gortmaker, S.L., Ebbeling, C.B., Pereira, M.A., & Ludwig, D.S. (2004). Effects of fast-food consumption on energy intake and diet quality among children in a national household survey. *Pediatrics, 113*, 112–118.

Bratteby, L.E., Sandhagen, B., Fan, H., Enghardt, H., & Samuelson, G. (1998). Total energy expenditure and physical activity as assessed by the doubly labeled water method in Swedish adolescents in whom energy intake was underestimated by 7-d diet records. *American Journal of Clinical Nutrition, 67*, 905–911.

Bray, G.A., Nielsen, S.J., & Popkin, B.M. (2004). Consumption of high-fructose corn syrup in beverages may play a role in the epidemic of obesity. *American Journal of Clinical Nutrition, 79*, 537–543.

Butte, N.F., Christiansen, E., & Sørensen, T.I. (2007). Energy imbalance underlying the development of childhood obesity. *Obesity (Silver Spring), 15*, 3056–3066.

Buyken, A.E., Cheng, G., Gunther, A.L., Liese, A.D., Remer, T., & Karaolis-Danckert, N. (2008). Relation of dietary glycemic index, glycemic load, added sugar intake, or fiber intake to the development of body composition between ages 2 and 7 y. *American Journal of Clinical Nutrition, 88*, 755–762.

Colapinto, C.K., Fitzgerald, A., Taper, J., & Veugelers, P.J. (2007). Children's preference for large portions: Prevalence, determinants, and consequences. *Journal of the American Dietetic Association, 107*, 1183–1190.

Coufopoulos, A.M., Maggs, C., & Hackett, A. (2001). Doing dietary research with adolescents: the problems of data collection in the school setting. *International Journal of Health Promotion* and *Education, 39*, 100–105.

Crawford, D.A., Timperio, A.F., Salmon, J.A., Baur, L., Giles-Corti, B., Roberts, R.J., Jackson, M.L., Andrianopoulus, N., & Ball, K. (2008). Neighbourhood fast food outlets and obesity in children and adults: the CLAN Study. *International Journal of Pediatric Obesity, 3*, 249–256.

Davies, P.S. (1997). Diet composition and body mass index in pre-school children. *European Journal of Clinical Nutrition, 51*, 443–448.

Dietz, W.H. (1994) Critical periods in childhood for the development of obesity. *American Journal of Clinical Nutrition, 59*, 955–959.

Dorosty, A.R., Emmett, P.M., Cowin, S., & Reilly, J.J. (2000). Factors associated with early adiposity rebound. ALSPAC Study Team. *Pediatrics, 105*, 1115–1118.

Drewnowski, A., & Specter, S.E. (2004). Poverty and obesity: the role of energy density and energy costs. *American Journal of Clinical Nutrition, 79*, 6–16.

Ello-Martin, J.A., Ledikwe, J.H., & Rolls, B.J. (2005). The influence of food portion size and energy density on energy intake: implications for weight management. *American Journal of Clinical Nutrition, 82 (1 Suppl)*, 236S–241S.

Ells, L.J., Hillier, F.C., Shucksmith, J., Crawley, H., Harbige, L., Shield, J., Wiggins, A., & Summerbell, C.D. (2008). A systematic review of the effect of dietary exposure that could have achieved through normal dietary intake on learning and performance of school-aged children of relevance to UK schools. *British Journal of Nutrition, 100*, 927–936.

Field, A.E., Austin, S.B., Gillman, M.W., Rosner, B., Rockett, H.R., & Colditz, G.A. (2004). Snack food intake does not predict weight change among children and adolescents. *International Journal of Obesity, 28*, 1210–1216.

Fisher, J.O., & Kral, T.V. (2008). Super-size me: Portion size effects on young children's eating. *Physiology & Behavior, 94*, 39–47.

Fisher, J.O., Liu, Y., Birch, L.L., & Rolls, B.J. (2007). Effects of portion size and energy density on young children's intake at a meal. *American Journal of Clinical Nutrition, 86*, 174–179.

Forshee, R.A., Anderson, P.A., & Storey, M.L. (2008). Sugar-sweetened beverages and body mass index in children and adolescents: a meta-analysis. *American Journal of Clinical Nutrition, 87*, 1662–1671.

Francis, L.A., Lee, Y., & Birch, L.L. (2003). Parental weight status and girls' television viewing, snaking, and body mass indexes. *Obesity Research, 11*, 143–151.

Frank, G.C. (1994). Environmental influences on methods used to collect dietary data from children. *American Journal of Clinical Nutrition, 59*, 207S–211S.

Freedman, D.S., Kettel Khan, L., Serdula, M.K., Srinivasan, S.R., & Berenson, G.S. (2001). BMI rebound, childhood height and obesity among adults: the Bogalusa Heart Study. *International Journal of Obesity and Related Metabolic Disorders, 25*, 543–549.

French, S.A., Story, M., Neumark-Sztainer, D., Fulkerson, J.A., & Hannan, P. (2001). Fast food restaurant use among adolescents: associations with nutrient intake, food choices and behavioral and psychosocial variables. *International Journal of Obesity and Related Metabolic Disorders, 25*, 1823–1833.

Garemo, M., Lenner, R.A., & Strandvik, B. (2007). Swedish pre-school children eat too much junk food and sucrose. *Acta Paediatrica, 96*, 266–272.

Gatenby, S.J. (1997). Eating frequency: methodological and dietary aspects. *British Journal of Nutrition, 77 (Suppl 1)*, S7–S20.

Gazanniga, J.M., & Burns, T.L. (1993). Relationship between diet composition and body fatness, with adjustment for resting energy expenditure and physical activity, in preadolescent children. *American Journal of Clinical Nutrition, 58*, 21–28.

Gibson, S., & Neate, D. (2007). Sugar intake, soft drink consumption and body weight among British children: further analysis of National Diet and Nutrition Survey data with adjustment for underreporting and physical activity. *International Journal of Food Sciences and Nutrition, 58*, 445–460.

Gillis, L.J., Kennedy, L.C., Gillis, A.M., & Bar-Or, O. (2002). Relationship between juvenile obesity, dietary energy and fat intake and physical activity. *International Journal of Obesity, 26*, 458–463.

Gillman, M.W., Rifas-Shiman, S.L., Frazier, A.L., Rockett, H.R., Camargo, C.A. Jr., Field, A.E., Berkey, C.S., & Colditz, G.A. (2000). Family dinner and diet quality among older children and adolescents. *Archives of Family Medicine, 9*, 235–240.

Guillaume, M., Lapidus, L., & Lambert, A. (1998). Obesity and nutrition in children. The Belgian Luxembourg child study IV. *European Journal of Clinical Nutrition, 52*, 323–328.

Gunther, A.L., Buyken, A.E., & Kroke, A. (2006). The influence of habitual protein intake in early childhood on BMI and age at adiposity rebound: results from the DONALD Study. *International Journal of Obesity (Lond), 30*, 1072–1079.

Gunther, A.L., Buyken, A.E., & Kroke, A. (2007). Protein intake during the period of complementary feeding and early childhood and the association with body mass index and percentage body fat at 7 y of age. *American Journal of Clinical Nutrition, 85*, 1626–1633.

Hassapidou, M., Fotiadou, E., Maglara, E., & Papadopoulou, S.K. (2006). Energy intake, diet composition, energy expenditure, and body fatness of adolescents in northern Greece. *Obesity, 14*, 855–862.

He, Q., & Karlberg, J. (2002). Probability of adult overweight and risk change during the BMI rebound period. *Obesity Research, 10*, 135–140.

Heitmann, B.L., & Lissner, L. (1995). Dietary underreporting by obese individuals–is it specific or non-specific? *British Medical Journal, 311*, 986–989.

James, J., Thomas, P., Cavan, D., & Kerr, D. (2004). Preventing childhood obesity by reducing consumption of carbonated drinks: cluster randomised controlled trial. *British Medical Journal, 328*, 1237.

Johnson, L., Mander, A.P., Jones, L.R., Emmett, P.M., & Jebb, S.A. (2008). Energy-dense, low-fiber, high-fat dietary pattern is associated with increased fatness in childhood. *American Journal of Clinical Nutrition, 87*, 846–854.

Jouret, B., Ahluwalia, N., Cristini, C., Dupuy, M., Negre-Pages, L., Grandjean, H., & Tauber, M. (2007). Factors associated with overweight in preschool-age children in southwestern France. *American Journal of Clinical Nutrition, 85*, 1643–1649.

Karlsson, M., Mårild, S., Brandberg, J., Lonn, L., Friberg, P., & Strandvik, B. (2006). Serum phospholipid fatty acids, adipose tissue, and metabolic markers in obese adolescents. *Obesity (Silver Spring), 14*, 1931–1939.

Kral, T.V., Stunkard, A.J., Berkowitz, R.I., Stallings, V.A., Brown, D.D., & Faith, M.S. (2007). Daily food intake in relation to dietary energy density in the free-living environment: a prospective analysis of children born at different risk of obesity. *American Journal of Clinical Nutrition, 86*, 41–47.

Kral, T.V., Stunkard, A.J., Berkowitz, R.I., Stalling, V.A., Moore, R.H., & Faith, M.S. (2008). Beverage consumption patterns of children born at different risk of obesity. *Obesity (Silver Spring), 16*, 1802–1808.

Krebs-Smith, S.M., Smiciklas-Wright, H., Guthrie, H.A., & Krebs-Smith, J. (1987). The effects of variety in food choices on dietary quality. *Journal of the American Dietetic Association, 87*, 897–903.

Lindroos, A.K., Lissner, L., & Sjöström, L. (1999). Does degree of obesity influence the validity of reported energy and protein intake? Results from the SOS Dietary Questionnaire. Swedish Obese Subjects. *European Journal of Clinical Nutrition, 53*, 375–378.

Lioret, S., Volatier, J.L., Lafay, L., Touvier, M., & Maire, B. (2009). Is food portion size a risk factor of childhood overweight? *European Journal of Clinical Nutrition, 63*, 382–391.

Lissner, L., Troiano, R.P., Midthune, D., Heitmann, B.L., Kipnis, V., Subar, A.F., & Potischman, N. (2007). OPEN about obesity: recovery biomarkers, dietary reporting errors and BMI. *International Journal of Obesity (Lond), 31*, 956–961.

Livingstone, M.B., & Robson, P.J. (2000). Measurement of dietary intake in children. *Proceedings of the Nutrition Society, 59*, 279–293.

Ludwig, D.S., Peterson, K.E., & Gortmaker, S.L. (2001). Relation between consumption of sugar-sweetened drinks and childhood obesity: a prospective, observational analysis. *Lancet, 357*, 505–508.

Ma, Y., Bertone, E.R., Stanek, E.J. III, Reed, G.W., Hebert, J.R., Cohen, N.L., Merriam, P.A., & Ockene, I.S. (2003). Association between eating patterns and obesity in a free-living US adult population. *American Journal of Epidemiology, 158*, 85–92.

Maffeis, C., Talamini, G., & Tato, L. (1998). Influence of diet, physical activity and parents' obesity on children's adiposity: a four-year longitudinal study. *International Journal of Obesity and Related Metabolic Disorders, 22*, 758–764.

Maffeis, C., Provera, S., Filippi, L., Sidoti, G., Schena, S., Pinelli, L., & Tatò, L. (2000). Distribution of food intake as a risk factor for childhood obesity. *International Journal of Obesity and Related Metabolic Disorders, 24*, 75–80.

Magarey, A.M., Daniels, L.A., Boulton, T.J., & Cockington, R.A. (2001). Does fat intake predict adiposity in healthy children and adolescents aged 2–15 y? A longitudinal analysis. *European Journal of Clinical Nutrition, 55*, 471–481.

McCaffrey, T.A., Rennie, K.L., Kerr, M.A., Wallace, J.M., Hannon-Fletcher, M.P., Coward, W.A., Jebb, S.A., & Livingstone, M.B. (2008). Energy density of the diet and change in body fatness from childhood to adolescence; is there a relation? *American Journal of Clinical Nutrition, 87*, 1230–1237.

McCrory, M.A., Fuss, P.J., McCallum, J.E., Yao, M., Vinken, A.G., Hays, N.P., & Roberts, S.B. (1999). Dietary variety within food groups: association with energy intake and body fatness in men and women. *American Journal of Clinical Nutrition, 69*, 440–447.

McGloin, A.F., Livingstone, M.B., Greene, L.C., Webb, S.E., Gibson, J.M., Jebb, S.A., Cole, T.J., Coward, W.A., Wright, A., & Prentice, A.M. (2002). Energy and fat intake in obese and lean children at varying risk of obesity. *International Journal of Obesity, 26*, 200–207.

Miller, S.A., Taveras, E.M., Rifas-Shiman, S.L., & Gillman, N.W. (2008). Association between television viewing and poor diet quality in young children. *International Journal of Pediatric Obesity, 4*, 1–9.

Moreno, L.A., & Rodríguez, G. (2007). Dietary risk factors for development of childhood obesity. *Current Opinion in Clinical Nutrition and Metabolic Care, 10*, 336–341.

Moreno, L.A., Kersting, M., de Henauw S, Gonzáles-Gross, M., Sichert-Hellert, W., Matthys, C., Mesana, M.I., & Ross, N. (2005). How to measure dietary intake and food habits in adolescence? – The European perspective. *International Journal of Obesity, 29 (Suppl 2)*, S66–S77.

Newby, P.K. (2007). Are dietary intakes and eating behaviors related to childhood obesity? A comprehensive review of the evidence. *Journal of Law, Medicine and Ethics, 35*, 35–60.

Niemeier, H.M., Raynor, H.A., Lloyd-Richardson, E.E., Rogers, M.L., & Wing, R.R. (2006). Fast food consumption and breakfast skipping: predictors of weight gain from adolescence to adulthood in a nationally representative simple. *Journal of Adolescent Health, 39*, 842–849.

O'Connor, T.M., Yang, S.J., & Nicklas, T.A. (2006). Beverage intake among preschool children and its effect on weight status. *Pediatrics, 118*, e1010–1018.

Olsen, N.J., & Heitmann, B.L. (2009). Intake of calorically sweetened beverages and obesity. *Obesity Reviews, 10*, 68–75.

Ong, K.K., Emmett, P.M., Noble, S., Ness, A., Dunger, D.B., & ALSPAC Study Team (2006). Dietary energy intake at the age of 4 months predicts postnatal weight gain and childhood body mass index. *Pediatrics, 117*, e503–e508.

Orlet Fisher, J.O., Rolls, B.J., & Birch, L.L. (2003). Children's bite size and intake of an entree are greater with large portions than with age-appropriate or self-selected portions. *American Journal of Clinical Nutrition, 77*, 1164–1170.

Ortega, R.M., Requejo, A.M., Andres, P., Lopez-Sobaler, A.M., Redondo, R., & Gonzalez-Fernandez, M. (1995). Relationship between diet composition and body mass index in a group of Spanish adolescents. *British Journal of Nutrition, 74*, 765–773.

Overby, N.C., Lillegaard, I.T., Johansson, L., & Andersen, L.F. (2004). High intake of added sugar among Norwegian children and adolescents. *Public Health Nutrition, 7*, 285–293.

Parizkova, J., & Rolland-Cachera, M.F. (1997). High proteins early in life as a predisposition for later obesity and further health risks. *Nutrition, 13*, 818–819.

Parnell, W., Wilson, N., Alexander, D., Wohlers, M., Williden, M., Mann, J., & Gray, A. (2008). Exploring the relationship between sugars and obesity. *Public Health Nutrition, 11*, 860–866.

Phillips, S.M., Bandini, L.G., Naumova, E.N., Cyr, H., Colclough, S., Dietz, W.H., & Must, A. (2004). Energy-dense snack food intake in adolescence: longitudinal relationship to weight and fatness. *Obesity Research, 12*, 461–472.

Receveur, O., Morou, K., Gray-Donald, K., & Macaulay, A.C. (2008). Consumption of key food items is associated with excess weight among elementary-school-aged children in a Canadian first nations community. *Journal of the American Dietetic Association, 108*, 362–366.

Reilly, J.J., Armstrong, J., Dorosty, A.R., Emmett, P.M., Ness, A., Rogers, I., Steer, C., Sherriff, A., & Avon Longitudinal Study of Parents and Children Study Team (2005). Early life risk factors for obesity in childhood: cohort study. *British Medical Journal, 330*, 1357.

Robinson, T.N., Borzekowski, D.L., Matheson, D.M., & Kraemer, H.C. (2007). Effects of fast food branding on young children's taste preferences. *Archives of Pediatrics & Adolescent Medicine, 161*, 792–797.

Rockett, H.R., Breitenbach, M., Frazier, A.L., Witschi, J., Wolf, A.M., Field, A.E., & Colditz, G.A. (1997). Validation of a youth/adolescent food frequency questionnaire. *Preventive Medicine, 26*, 808–816.

Rodríguez, G., & Moreno, L.A. (2006). Is dietary intake able to explain differences in body fatness in children and adolescents? *Nutrition, Metabolism, and Cardiovascular Diseases, 16*, 294–301.

Rodríguez, G., & Moreno, L.A. (2008). Is diet the fuel for obesity in children and adolescents? *Obesity and Metabolism, 4*, 183–188.

Rodríguez, G., Moreno, L.A., Blay, M.G., Blay, V.A., Garagorri, J.M., Sarría, A., & Bueno, M. (2004). Body composition in adolescents: measurements and metabolic aspects. *International Journal of Obesity, 28 (Suppl 3)*, S54–58.

Rolland-Cachera, M.F., & Bellisle, F. (1986). No correlation between adiposity and food intake: why are working class children fatter? *American Journal of Clinical Nutrition, 44*, 779–787.

Rolland-Cachera, M.F., Deheeger, M., Akrout, M., & Bellisle, F. (1995). Influence of macronutrients on adiposity development: a follow up study of nutrition and growth from 10 months to 8 years of age. *International Journal of Obesity and Related Metabolic Disorders, 19*, 573–578.

Rolls, B.J., Engell, D., & Birch, L.L. (2000). Serving portion size influences 5-year-old but not 3-year old children's food intakes. *Journal of the American Dietetic Association, 100*, 232–234.

Scaglioni, S., Agostoni, C., Notaris, R.D., Radaelli, G., Radice, N., Valenti, M., Giovannini, M., & Riva, E. (2000). Early macronutrient intake and overweight at five years of age. *International Journal of Obesity, 24*, 777–781.

Schmidt, M., Affenito, S.G., Striegel-Moore, R., Khoury, P.R., Barton, B., Crawford, P., Kronsberg, S., Schreiber, G., Obarzanek, E., & Daniels, S. (2005). Fast-food intake and diet quality in black and white girls: the National Heart, Lung, and Blood Institute Growth and Health Study. *Archives of Pediatrics & Adolescent Medicine, 159*, 626–631.

Sen, B. (2006). Frequency of family dinner and adolescent body weight status: evidence from the national longitudinal survey of youth, 1997. *Obesity, 14*, 2266–2276.

Serra, M.L., Ribas, B.L., Aranceta, B.J., Pérez, R.C, Saavedra, S.P., & Peña, Q.L. (2003). Childhood and adolescent obesity in Spain. Results of the enKid study (1998-2000). *Medicina Clinica (Barc), 121*, 725–732.

Sjöberg, A., Slinde, F., Arvidsson, D., Ellegård, L., Gramatkovski, E., Hallberg, L., & Hulthén, L. (2003). Energy intake in Swedish adolescents: validation of diet history with doubly labelled water. *European Journal of Clinical Nutrition, 57*, 1643–1652.

Skinner, J.D., Bounds, W., Carruth, B.R., Morris, M., & Ziegler, P. (2004). Predictors of children's body mass index: a longitudinal study of diet and growth in children aged 2-8 y. *International Journal of Obesity and Related Metabolic Disorders, 28*, 476–482.

Toschke, A.M., Küchenhoff, H., Koletzko, B., & von Kries, R. (2005). Meal frequency and childhood obesity. *Obesity Research, 13*, 1932–1938.

USDA ORC/Macro (2005). Food Assistance and Nutrition Research Program. Developing effective wording and format options for a children's nutrition behavior questionnaire for mothers of children in kindergarten. USDA contractor and cooperator report no. 10, August 2005. www.ers.usda.

Vereecken, C.A., Covents, M., Matthys, C., & Maes, L. (2005). Young adolescents' nutrition assessment on computer (YANA-C). *European Journal of Clinical Nutrition, 59*, 658–667.

Veugelers, P.J., & Fitzgerald, A.L. (2005). Prevalence of and risk factors for childhood overweight and obesity. *Canadian Medical Association Journal, 173*, 607–613.

Wang, Y.C., Bleich, S.N., & Gortmaker, S.L. (2008). Increasing caloric contribution from sugar-sweetened beverage and 100% fruit juices among US children and adolescents, 1988-2004. *Pediatrics, 121*, e1604–e1614.

Welsh, J.A., Cogswell, M.E., Rogers, S., Rockett, H., Mei, Z., & Grummer-Strawn, L.M. (2005). Overweight among low-income preschool children associated with the consumption of sweet drinks: Missouri, 1999–2002. *Pediatrics, 115*, e223–e229.

Whitaker, R.C., Pepe, M.S., Wright, J.A., Seidel, K.D., & Dietz, W.H. (1998). Early adiposity rebound and the risk of adult obesity. *Pediatrics, 101*, E5.

Willett, W. (1998). *Nutritional epidemiology*, Second edn, vol. 30. New York: Oxford University Press.

Chapter 19
Physical Activity, Fitness and Fatness in Children and Adolescents

David Jiménez-Pavón, Jonatan R. Ruiz, Francisco B. Ortega, Enrique G. Artero, Vanesa España-Romero, José Castro-Piñero, Ángel Gutiérrez, and Manuel J. Castillo

Introduction

Childhood and adolescence are crucial periods of life since dynamic changes in various metabolic systems, including hormonal regulation, changes in body fat content and body fat distribution, as well as transient changes in insulin sensitivity are known to occur during growth and puberty (Cruz et al. 2005). Dramatic psychological changes also occur during this period. Likewise, lifestyle and healthy/unhealthy behaviors are established during these years, which may influence adult behavior and health status.

A sedentary lifestyle together with a poor diet are the leading causes together with tobacco for the development of cardiovascular disease (CVD) and death (Mokdad et al. 2004). Obesity is also a major health problem that affects not only adults but also children and adolescents. Increased energy intake together with reduced energy expenditure results in body fat accumulation. The consequences on health of excess of body fat are well known. Adults who were overweight in childhood have higher levels of blood lipids and lipoproteins, blood pressure, and fasting insulin levels, and thus are at increased risk for CVD compared with adults who were thin as children (Freedman et al. 2001; Steinberger et al. 2001; Thompson et al. 2007). Moreover, over the long term, childhood overweight is strongly associated with adult obesity. Childhood overweight confers a fivefold or greater increase in risk for being overweight in early adulthood relative to children who were not overweight at the same age (Guo et al. 2002; Steinberger et al. 2001; Thompson et al. 2007).

The protective effect of intentional physical activity on the above mentioned CVD risk factors has been reported in people of all ages (Pedersen and Saltin 2006; Strong et al. 2005). However, these findings are often confined to questionnaire-based assessment of physical activity, which often lack the necessary accuracy, especially in young people (Kohl et al. 2000).

One factor related with physical activity is physical fitness. Physical activity and physical fitness are closely related in that fitness is partially determined by physical activity patterns over recent weeks or months. Cardiorespiratory fitness has received special attention during the last decades. There is increasing evidence that high levels of cardiorespiratory fitness provides strong and independent prognostic information about the overall risk of illness and death, especially that from cardiovascular causes (Castillo-Garzon et al. 2007; LaMonte and Blair 2006).

In the present chapter, we summarize the latest developments in regard to physical activity, fitness, obesity and obesity-related CVD risk factors in children and adolescents.

D. Jiménez-Pavón, J.R. Ruiz (✉), F.B. Ortega, E.G. Artero, V. España-Romero, J. Castro-Piñero,
Á. Gutiérrez, and M.J. Castillo
Department of Medical Physiology, School of Medicine, University of Granada, 18071, Granada, Spain
e-mail: ruizj@ugr.es

L.A. Moreno et al. (eds.), *Epidemiology of Obesity in Children and Adolescents*,
Springer Series on Epidemiology and Public Health 2, DOI 10.1007/978-1-4419-6039-9_19,
© Springer Science+Business Media, LLC 2011

Physical Activity and Body Fat in Children and Adolescents: Does the Intensity Matter?

Physical Activity and Total Body Fat

The prevalence of childhood and adolescence obesity is increasing at alarming rate worldwide. A sedentary lifestyle (i.e., watching television or/and playing computer/video games) as well as reduction of physical activity level seem to be the major determinants implicated in this trend. However, studies performed in children and adolescents show contradictory results, probably due to the inherent difficulties on measuring physical activity, as well as to the different technologies used to assess it. Physical activity has been commonly assessed by using questionnaires. Questionnaires have highly limited accuracy in the measurement of daily physical activity, especially in children and adolescents. More objective methods such as accelerometry, have been shown to provide adequate measures for physical activity in children and adolescents. Precise methods of measuring physical activity utilizing objective measurement such as accelerometry are needed to accurately establish the dose-response relationships between physical activity with cardiovascular health outcomes in children and adolescents (Dencker and Andersen 2008; Steele et al. 2008). In the present review, we will mostly refer to studies that used accelerometry to assess physical activity, otherwise, it will be indicated.

Cross-sectional studies examining the relationship between various measures of body fat and objectively assessed physical activity have usually indicated a negative relationship. A multicenter study conducted on 1,292 European children aged 9–10 years analyzed the associations of objectively measured physical activity with indicators of total body fat (i.e., sum of 5 skinfold thicknesses and body mass index) (Ekelund et al. 2004). The results suggested that accumulated amount of time spent at moderate and vigorous physical activity is inversely related, yet weakly, to total body fat. Wittmeier et al. (2007) investigated 251 Canadian children aged 8–11 years, and found that time spent in moderate to vigorous physical activity was inversely correlated with body mass index and skinfold-derived estimate of body fat. However, several studies suggested that vigorous physical activity may be more important than lower intensities in the prevention of obesity in children and adolescents (Abbott and Davies 2004; Ara et al. 2004; Butte et al. 2007; Dencker et al. 2008; Gutin et al. 2005; Rowlands et al. 1999; Ruiz et al. 2006d; Stallmann-Jorgensen et al. 2007). Gutin et al. (2005) reported that only vigorous physical activity was associated with lower fatness in 421 North-American adolescents aged 16 years. A report of a small study, conducted on 47 children aged 5–10, showed similar finding (Abbott and Davies 2004). Dencker et al. (2008) reported a strong inverse relationship between vigorous physical activity and body fat in 225 Swedish children aged 8–11 years. Likewise, Butte et al. (2007) observed a strong and negative association between vigorous physical activity and percent body fat in 897 children aged 4–19 years. Furthermore, Ruiz et al. (2006d) suggested that physical activity of vigorous intensity may have a greater effect on preventing obesity in children than does physical activity of lower intensity in Estonian and Swedish children participating in the European Youth Heart Study (EYHS) (Fig. 19.1). Finally, a study recently reported that lower levels of body fat were related to greater amount (≥ 1 h) of vigorous physical activity, but not with moderate physical activity or total energy intake in 661 adolescents aged 8–14 years (Stallmann-Jorgensen et al. 2007).

Longitudinal studies also support the idea that youth who participate in relatively high levels of physical activity have less body fat later in life compare to their less active peers (Berkey et al. 2000; Ekelund et al. 2002; Janz et al. 2005; Metcalf et al. 2008; Moore et al. 2003; Stevens et al. 2004). Experimental studies have been developed to obtain specific information about the influence of regular physical activity on body fat in normal-weight and/or overweight and obese children and adolescents.

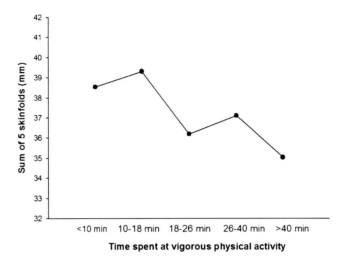

Fig. 19.1 Body fat (mean sum of five skinfolds) stratified (in fifths) by time spent at vigorous physical activity in children (*n* = 780). Modified from Ruiz et al. (2006d)

In overweight and obese children, beneficial effects in body fat control maybe attained with 30–60 min of moderate physical activity, 3–7 days/week (Barbeau et al. 1999; Gutin et al. 2002; Klijn et al. 2007; LeMura and Maziekas 2002; Owens et al. 1999). However, obese adolescents who spent more time engaged in vigorous physical activity tended to be those who decreased body fat the most (Barbeau et al. 1999; Gutin et al. 2002). For several reasons, it is reasonable to recommend moderate physical activity for obese children and adolescents until higher intensities can be attained. Moderate physical activity is better tolerated than vigorous physical activity (Barbeau et al. 1999), and tiring physical activity may lead to less physical activity on the following day (Kriemler et al. 1999), although it likely depends on the type of exercise performed (Owens et al. 1999). Therefore, for obese children and those who have been physically inactive, an incremental approach to the 45 to 60 min/day goal of moderate physical activity 5 or more days per week is recommended (Strong et al. 2005). However, these programs do not influence body fatness in normal-weight children and adolescents (Eliakim et al. 2001; Owens et al. 1999; Rowland et al. 1996; Tolfrey et al. 1998, 2004). Limited evidences suggest that more intensive and longer sessions (≥80 min/day) are needed to reduce percentage body fat in normal-weight youth (Barbeau et al. 2007; Eliakim et al. 2000; Yin et al. 2005). Finally, Gutin et al. (2008) have recently reported the effect of a 3-year after-school physical activity intervention on aerobic fitness and percent body fat. The intervention included 40 min of academic enrichment activities, during which healthy snacks were provided, and 80 min of moderate-to-vigorous physical activity. They showed a favorable effects on cardiorespiratory fitness and fatness during the school years when the children were exposed to the intervention. However, during the summers following the first and second years of intervention, the favorable effects on cardiorespiratory fitness and percentage body fat were lost, which shows the importance of maintaining exposure to vigorous physical activity.

The current literature above mentioned agrees in a fairly consistent manner that association between physical activity and obesity is stronger for vigorous physical activity than for moderate physical activity. However, when the adolescent is exercising at a higher intensity, the total energy expenditure associated with that activity is higher than for a similar time effort at moderate intensity. So the question is whether it is really the intensity what matters or is the total amount of energy expenditure the responsible for many of the outcomes reported remains to be answered. In other words, whether 30 min of moderate-intensity physical activity and 10 min of vigorous-intensity physical activity (assuming that both would have the same energy cost) have different effects on body composition indexes remains to be elucidated. Strictly, only a well-design control-randomized trial could accurately answer to this question, though some attempts can also be done using observational data.

Future research should pay effort on solving this dilemma by making equivalent the energy expenditure-linked to vigorous physical activity and moderate physical activity, so only the intensity and not the total number of calories spent will differ between these two sub-components of physical activity. The outcomes of such study designs will help to better understand how and to what extent the intensity of physical activity matters regarding obesity management and prevention.

Physical Activity and Central Body Fat

Central body fat has shown to be associated with a range of risk factors for cardiovascular disease already in young people (Gutin et al. 2007) and is becoming of increasing importance in pediatrics. Although there are accurate and sophisticated methods to evaluate central body fat, waist circumference is an accurate surrogate for central body fat (Brambilla et al. 2006) and a powerful marker associated with a number of cardiovascular risk factors and metabolic syndrome, both in non-overweight and overweight individuals (Janssen et al. 2005).

We (Ortega et al. 2007b) did not observe any association between abdominal fat and physical activity assessed by questionnaire in 2,859 Spanish adolescents who took part in the AVENA (Alimentación y Valoración del Estado Nutricional en Adolescentes) study. However, another study with 2,714 French children aged 12 years, reported a negative relationship between waist circumference and physical activity, which was also assessed by questionnaire (Klein-Platat et al. 2005).

More recent findings performed in children and adolescents have shown a negative association between central body fat and physical activity assessed by accelerometers, especially with vigorous physical activity (Dencker et al. 2008; Hussey et al. 2007; Ortega et al. 2007a; Saelens et al. 2007; Sardinha et al. 2008) (Fig. 19.2). Moreover, some of them suggest that time spent in sedentary activities, such us viewing television or/and playing computer/video games is strongly related with the increasing of central body fat (Dencker et al. 2008; Hussey et al. 2007; Ortega et al. 2007a).

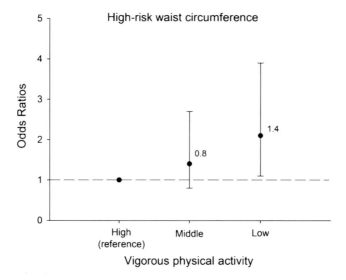

Fig. 19.2 High-risk waist circumference according to thirds of vigorous physical activity in children and adolescents ($n = 1,074$). Adapted from Ortega et al. (2007a)

Whether cardiorespiratory fitness modifies the association between physical activity and abdominal fat is another matter of interest. We (Ortega et al. 2010) have addressed the first study examining how cardiorespiratory fitness can influence the associations between objectively measured physical activity and abdominal fat in 1,075 Swedish children and adolescents from the EYHS. We showed that the associations between physical activity and abdominal fat differ by fitness levels. In low fit children and adolescents, time spent in vigorous physical activity seems to be the key component linked to abdominal body fat. Unexpectedly, we also observed that in high fit children and adolescents, physical activity was positively associated with waist circumference. Further research examining genetic and dietary factors, in addition to objectively measured physical activity and cardiorespiratory fitness are still needed for a better understanding of the associations between physical activity and central body fat in young people.

Finally, evidence from intervention studies support that physical activity in children and adolescents reduces central body fat, as well as we have mentioned for total body fat (Barbeau et al. 2007; Eliakim et al. 2000; Gutin et al. 2002; Klijn et al. 2007; Owens et al. 1999). It seems that 30 to 60 min of moderate physical activity for 3 to 7 day/week may have beneficial effects to control and reduce central body fat in obese children (Gutin et al. 2002; Klijn et al. 2007; Owens et al. 1999). However, in normal-weight children, sessions of at least 80 min/day of vigorous physical activity might be needed in order to reduce it (Barbeau et al. 2007; Eliakim et al. 2000).

Physical Activity and Obesity-Related Cardiovascular Disease Risk Factors

There is extensive evidence on the relationship between physical activity and obesity-related CVD risk factors. In adults, it has been shown an association of physical activity with slower progression towards the metabolic syndrome independently of body fatness (Ekelund et al. 2007b). However, population studies focusing on these relationships in children and adolescents are limited.

Recently, habitual physical activity levels have been associated with many obesity-related CVD risk factors such as blood pressure, total cholesterol (TC), low density lipoprotein cholesterol (LDLc), triglycerides and insulin resistance (Andersen et al. 2006; Brage et al. 2004; Ekelund et al. 2007a; Hurtig-Wennlof et al. 2007; Rizzo et al. 2008). This negative association was stronger for moderate and vigorous physical activity levels (Andersen et al. 2006; Hurtig-Wennlof et al. 2007; Rizzo et al. 2008; Sardinha et al. 2008) than for light or sedentary activity levels (Sardinha et al. 2008). In this sense, we showed that total, moderate, and vigorous physical activity were inversely correlated with insulin resistance in Swedish adolescents from the EYHS (Rizzo et al. 2008) (Fig. 19.3). In a study conducted in 2,201 children from three different countries, found that a graded decrease in metabolic risk across five levels of physical activity (Andersen et al. 2006). Children that were in the lowest activity level had an odds ratio of clustered risk around three compared with the most active children. The authors concluded that to prevent clustering of cardiovascular disease risk factors, the total accumulate physical activity level should be 90 min of daily activity. This would also prevent insulin resistance, which seems to be the central feature for clustering of cardiovascular disease risk factors.

Whether the association between physical activity and markers of cardiovascular health is mediated or confounded by body fat is controversial. The degree to which adjustment for body fat attenuates or modifies the association between physical activity and metabolic risk varies across studies. In some studies, when level of body fat is excluded from the risk score and adjusted for as a covariate, the magnitude of the association between physical activity and the non-obesity CVD risk tends remain unchanged (Brage et al. 2004; Ekelund et al. 2007a), whereas in others studies this association is attenuated (Rizzo et al. 2007). Sardinha et al. (2008) found that physical activity was associated with insulin resistance independent of total and central body fat in children.

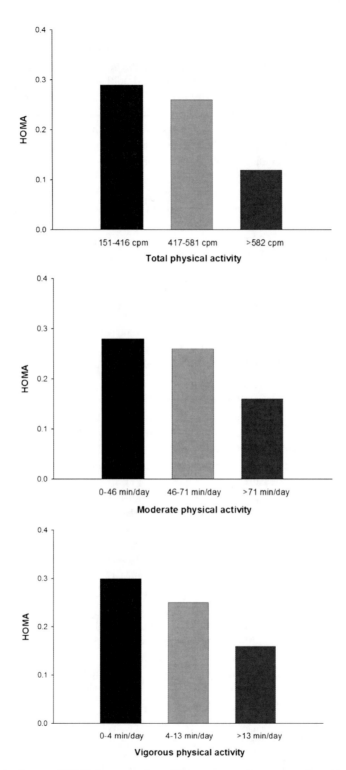

Fig. 19.3 Association between HOMA (homeostasis model assessment, a surrogate marker of insulin resistance) and thirds of total, moderate and vigorous physical activity in adolescents ($n=613$). Modified from Rizzo et al. (2008)

Attenuation may suggest a mediating effect of body fat, because this factor may lie on the causal pathway between physical activity and metabolic health. For example, physical activity may detectably impact on variables such as fasting glucose and blood lipids, whereas no effect would be observed for body fat, which is likely to be the result of long-term balance or imbalance between energy expenditure and intake. However, long-term effects of physical activity on other risk factors could plausibly exist. Different degrees of measurement precision in the assessment of body fat and physical activity may also explain attenuation of results and variation between studies.

Physical Fitness and Body Fat in Children and Adolescents

Childhood obesity is associated with a variety of adverse consequences both at early age and later in life, therefore, it is of relevance to thoroughly study the association between fatness and modifiable lifestyle-inherent factors potentially related with body fat, such as physical fitness. Not only the total fat amount may influence the youths' health status, but also how that fat is distributed in the body. In this section both total and central body fat and their relationships with physical fitness in children and adolescents are discussed.

Physical Fitness and Total Body Fat

Nowadays, children spent less time practicing sports or physical activities (Oehlschlaeger et al. 2004), and more time watching television and/or playing video games (Andersen et al. 1998). These behavioral changes may lead to decreases in daily energy expenditure, what in turns could explain, at least partially, the increasing trends in childhood obesity (Rey-Lopez et al. 2007). Despite its well known limitation to discriminate between fat and lean tissue, body mass index is internationally used to define overweight and obese in children and adolescents (Cole et al. 2000), though other anthropometrics such as skinfold thicknesses are often used in the literature as surrogates of total body fat. Several studies have been conducted to study the associations between physical fitness and fatness measures in young people.

Data from the Swedish part of the EYHS, a school based, cross-sectional study of risk factors for future CVD in a sample of children (9–10 years old) and adolescents (15–16 years old) (Poortvliet et al. 2003), indicate that those individuals having a high cardiorespiratory fitness level also have significantly lower total body fat, as measured by skinfold thicknesses (Ortega et al. 2006). When total fatness was assessed by a reference method, such as Dual Energy X-ray Absorptiometry in Spanish (Ara et al. 2004) and North American (Lee and Arslanian 2007) children, similar inverse associations were found. Cardiorespiratory fitness has shown a stronger association with total body fat, as measured by skinfold thicknesses, than other physical fitness components such as muscular fitness, speed/agility, flexibility or motor coordination (Ara et al. 2007). Even in overweight or obese children, those children who had a higher cardiorespiratory fitness have shown a lower overall body fat (Nassis et al. 2005). Longitudinal data have shown a significant relationship between adolescent cardiorespiratory fitness and later body fatness, so that the higher the cardiorespiratory fitness levels the lower the body fat levels (Ara et al. 2006; Eisenmann et al. 2005a).

Physical Fitness and Central Body Fat

The study of fat distribution among children and adolescents is complex because there are marked changes in circumferences and skinfold thickness during growth and development (Ruiz et al. 2006c).

Waist circumference has shown to be an accurate marker of abdominal fat accumulation (Taylor et al. 2000) and visceral fat (Brambilla et al. 2006) in young people. In addition, waist circumference seems to explain the variance in a range of CVD risk factors to a similar extent as measures derived from high-technology techniques, including DXA and Magnetic Resonance Imaging (Ara et al. 2007). Therefore, the use of waist circumference as a surrogate of abdominal fat, and as a powerful index associated with metabolic risk in young people, seems to be appropriate for epidemiological studies.

Data from the AVENA study showed that both moderate to high levels of cardiorespiratory fitness are associated with lower abdominal fat, as measured by waist circumference (Ortega et al. 2007b). These results are in accordance with those found in 224 Irish children aged 7–10 years (Hussey et al. 2007). Similar associations have also been reported when physical fitness was measured as lower limb explosive strength, abdominal endurance strength or speed/agility instead of cardiorespiratory fitness in 1,140 Canadian children (591 boys and 549 girls) aged 7–10 years (Brunet et al. 2007). In those studies the abdominal fat was also measured by waist circumference. The same inverse association with cardiorespiratory fitness was observed when visceral and abdominal subcutaneous adipose tissue were measured using computed tomography or magnetic imaging resonance instead of waist circumference (Lee and Arslanian 2007; Winsley et al. 2006).

Several studies showed that cardiorespiratory fitness at childhood and adolescence is a predictor of excess of overall and central body fat later in life (Andersen et al. 2004b; Boreham et al. 2002; Byrd-Williams et al. 2008; Hasselstrom et al. 2002; Janz et al. 2002; Johnson et al. 2000; Koutedakis and Bouziotas 2003; Psarra et al. 2006; Twisk et al. 2000, 2002b). In contrast, there is one study showing that cardiorespiratory fitness at the age of 16 is not associated with markers of overall and central body fat at the age of 34 (Barnekow-Bergkvist et al. 2001).

Physical Fitness and Obesity-Related Cardiovascular Disease Risk Factors

There is compelling evidence that the precursors of cardiovascular disease (CVD) have their origin in childhood and adolescence (Berenson et al. 1998). CVD risk factors such as TC, LDLc, high density lipoprotein cholesterol (HDLc), triglycerides, insulin resistance, inflammatory proteins, blood pressure and total and central body fat in childhood have been shown to track into adulthood (Andersen et al. 2004a; Raitakari et al. 2003).

Cardiorespiratory Fitness and Obesity-Related Cardiovascular Disease Risk Factors

Higher levels of cardiorespiratory fitness have been associated with a healthier cardiovascular profile in children and adolescents (Garcia-Artero et al. 2007; Hurtig-Wennlof et al. 2007; Lobelo and Ruiz 2007; Mesa et al. 2006a, b, c; Ortega et al. 2007b; Rizzo et al. 2007; Ruiz et al. 2006a, b, d, 2007b, c, d, e, f, g, 2009). This association seems to be independent of sex, age, ethnicity, and grade of obesity. Results from the AVENA study indicate that high levels of cardiorespiratory fitness are associated with a more favorable metabolic profile (computed from age and sex specific standardized values of triglycerides, LDLc, HDLc and fasting glycemia) in both overweight and non-overweight Spanish adolescents (Mesa et al. 2006c). The same association was also found between cardiorespiratory fitness and a clustering of CVD risk factors, as well as with individual CVD risk factors in Swedish and Estonian children and adolescents participating in the EYHS (Hurtig-Wennlof et al. 2007; Rizzo et al. 2007; Ruiz et al. 2007d). Data from the 1999–2002 round of the National Health and Nutrition Examination Survey (NHANES), a nationally representative sample of the non-institutionalized

U.S. adolescents (Centers for Disease Control and Prevention 2004a, b), also revealed that higher levels of cardiorespiratory fitness were associated with a more favorable cardiovascular profile (Lobelo et al. 2009).

Given the importance of cardiorespiratory fitness as a powerful marker of health in childhood and adolescence, sex-specific cut-offs for a healthy cardiorespiratory fitness level in childhood and adolescence have been proposed by several institutions and worldwide recognized organizations such as the Cooper Institute or the European Group of Pediatric Work Physiology (Table 1) (Bell et al. 1986; Cureton and Warren 1990; Ruiz et al. 2007d; The Cooper Institute for Aerobics Research 2004). The health-related cardiorespiratory fitness thresholds suggested by the FITNESSGRAM (Cureton and Warren 1990; The Cooper Institute for Aerobics Research 2004) are similar to those proposed by the European Group of Pediatric Work Physiology (Bell et al. 1986) and also to those associated with an increased risk for metabolic disease, calculated by others (Lobelo et al. 2009; Ruiz et al. 2007d) (Table 19.1). It is noteworthy that the approaches used to calculate these cardiorespiratory fitness health-related thresholds were different in these studies, as were age, race, nationality, environmental and cultural and social factors of the participants studied. However, the consistency in the findings support the existence of a hypothetical cardiorespiratory fitness value linked to a more favorable cardiovascular profile, which seems to range between 40 and 42 ml/min/kg in boys and between 35 and 38 ml/min/kg in girls.

Cardiorespiratory fitness has also been inversely associated with relatively other obesity-related CVD risk factors such as low grade inflammatory markers and homocysteine in young people (Ruiz et al. 2007e, g; Wärnberg et al. 2006b). Low-grade inflammation seems to play a role in the development of cardiovascular disease from an early age (Hansson 2005; Jarvisalo et al. 2002). It has been observed an increased low-grade inflammation in overweight adolescents compared with their non-overweight counterparts (Wärnberg et al. 2006a). We (Ruiz et al. 2007e) showed that the levels of C-reactive protein and C3 were inversely associated with cardiorespiratory fitness in prepubertal Swedish children from the EYHS, which is consistent with other studies of young people (Cooper et al. 2004; Halle et al. 1998; Isasi et al. 2003). Similarly, data from the AVENA study showed that overweight and unfit adolescents are more likely to have high levels of C-reactive protein, C3 and C4 compared to non overweight and fit peers (Wärnberg et al. 2006b). It has been shown (Halle et al. 2004) that low grade inflammation was negatively associated with cardiorespiratory fitness in normal weight and overweight children aged 12 years. They reported that IL-6 levels were as low for obese and fit as for lean and unfit children, while the higher IL-6 levels were found in the obese and unfit group. In contrast, they also showed that TNF-α seemed to be primarily dependent on

Table 19.1 Health criterion-referenced standards for cardiorespiratory fitness in children and youth

Study/institution	Methodology	Sex	Age (years)	CRF values (ml/kg/min)
FITNESSGRAM (Cureton and Warren 1990; The Cooper Institute for Aerobics Research 2004, pp. 38–39)	Linked to adult mortality/chronic disease risk	Males	12–19	42
		Females	12	37
			13	36
			≥14	35
European Group of Pediatric Work (Bell et al. 1986, pp. 39–42)	Expert judgment	Males	Adolescents	40
		Females	Adolescents	35
European Youth Heart Study (Ruiz et al. 2007d)	ROC curve	Males	9–10	42
		Females	9–10	37
NHANES 1999–2002 (Lobelo et al. 2009)	ROC curve	Males	12–15	44
			16–19	40
		Females	12–15	36
			16–19	36

ROC receiver operating characteristic; *CRF* cardiorespiratory fitness

cardiorespiratory fitness but not obesity as similar levels were found for non obese as well as obese children with a low cardiorespiratory fitness.

Epidemiologic and clinical evidence show that hyperhomocysteinemia is an independent, modifiable risk factor for atherosclerosis and CVD (Castro et al. 2006; McCully 2005). The amount of body fat has been associated with homocysteine levels in obese children and adolescents (Gallistl et al. 2000). Insulin resistance has been implicated in the relationship, since insulin levels are strongly correlated with body fat (Gallistl et al. 2000). In contrast, we did not find an association between body fatness (as expressed as skinfold thickness or as body mass) and homocysteine levels, even when the analyses were performed separately for normal-weight or overweight-obese categories (Ruiz et al. 2007a). Studies examining the association between cardiorespiratory fitness and homocysteine levels in young people are scarce, and the results published so far are contradictory. We have found conflicting results in Spanish adolescents (Ruiz et al. 2007g) and Swedish children and adolescents (Ruiz et al. 2007a) after controlling for different potential confounders including age, puberty, birth weight, smoking, socioeconomic status, skinfold thickness and methylenetetrahydro-folate reductase 677C>T genotype. Cardiorespiratory fitness was inversely and significantly associated in female Spanish adolescents (Ruiz et al. 2007g), which concur with the results reported by others (Kuo et al. 2005) in adult women. In contrast, we did not observed an association between cardiorespiratory fitness and homocysteine levels in Swedish children and adolescents (Ruiz et al. 2007a). These results should encourage discussion on whether the metabolism of homocysteine could be one way in which the benefits of high cardiorespiratory fitness are exerted.

Cardiorespiratory Fitness and Later Obesity-Related Cardiovascular Disease Risk Factors

The relationships between health-related physical fitness in youths and obesity-related CVD risk factors later in life have been examined. Several studies have showed that cardiorespiratory fitness at childhood and adolescence is a predictor of obesity-related CVD risk factors, such as abnormal blood lipids (Andersen et al. 2004b; Boreham et al. 2002; Carnethon et al. 2003; Ferreira et al. 2003, 2005; Hasselstrom et al. 2002; Janz et al. 2002; Johnson et al. 2000; Twisk et al. 2000, 2002b), high blood pressure (Andersen et al. 2004b; Carnethon et al. 2003; Hasselstrom et al. 2002; Twisk et al. 2002a), excess of overall and central body fat (Andersen et al. 2004b; Boreham et al. 2002; Byrd-Williams et al. 2008; Hasselstrom et al. 2002; Janz et al. 2002; Johnson et al. 2000; Koutedakis and Bouziotas 2003; Psarra et al. 2006; Twisk et al. 2000, 2002b), metabolic syndrome (Carnethon et al. 2003; Ferreira et al. 2005) and arterial stiffness (Boreham et al. 2004; Ferreira et al. 2003) later in life.

Musculoskeletal Fitness and Obesity-Related Cardiovascular Disease Risk Factors

In addition to cardiorespiratory fitness, the role of muscular fitness in the performance of exercise and activities of daily living, as well as in preventing disease has become increasingly recognized (Jurca et al. 2005; Wolfe 2006). Data from the AVENA study showed an inverse association between muscular fitness, as defined by an index computed from the standardized scores of maximal handgrip strength, explosive strength and endurance strength, and a CVD risk score (an average value from the standardized triglycerides, LDLc, HDLc, and glucose) in female adolescents (Garcia-Artero et al. 2007). In addition, it was reported that for a given cardiorespiratory fitness level, an increased level of muscular fitness was associated with a lower CVD risk score (Fig. 19.4).

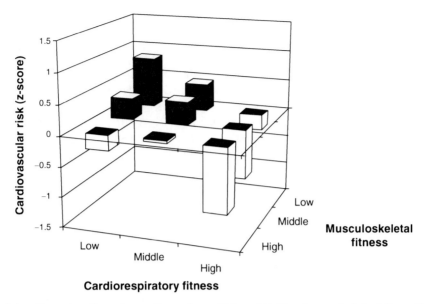

Fig. 19.4 Joint effects of cardiorespiratory fitness (low, middle and high) and musculoskeletal fitness (low, middle and high) on cardiovascular risk score (an average value from the standardized triglycerides, LDLc, HDLc and glucose) in adolescents ($n = 460$). Adapted from Garcia-Artero et al. (2007)

Findings from the same cohort indicate that muscular fitness is inversely associated with C-reactive protein, C3 and ceruloplasmin (Ruiz et al. 2008).

Results from cross-sectional studies in children and adolescents have reported a negative relationship between muscular strength and obesity-related CVD risks factors such as triglycerides, total cholesterol, high density lipoprotein cholesterol, LDLc, glucose (Garcia-Artero et al. 2007), C-reactive protein (Ruiz et al. 2008) and insulin resistance (Benson et al. 2006). Upper body muscular strength showed to be an independent predictor of insulin resistance in 126 boys and girls aged 10–15 years (Benson et al. 2006). In addition, those children in the highest third of absolute upper body muscular strength were 98% less likely to have high insulin resistance than those with the lowest strength, after adjusting for maturation, waist circumference, body mass and cardiorespiratory fitness (Benson et al. 2006). The same authors designed a study which can be considered the first randomized controlled trial of resistance training (i.e., any exercise training that uses a resistance to the force of muscular contraction, also called strength training) in children and adolescents, and reported that isolated high-intensity progressive resistance training significantly improves central and total body fat in association with muscle strength in normal-weight and overweight children and adolescents (Benson et al. 2008).

Musculoskeletal Fitness and Later Obesity-Related Cardiovascular Disease Risk Factors

There is strong evidence suggesting that increases in muscular strength in childhood and adolescence are associated with decreases in overall body fat later in life, and vice versa (decreases in muscular strength are associated with increases in overall body fat) (Janz et al. 2002; Twisk et al. 2000). This association is less evident for markers of central body fat (Hasselstrom et al. 2002; Janz et al. 2002). In contrast, there is inconclusive evidence that muscular strength changes (increases or decreases) in childhood and adolescence are associated with changes (decreases or increases) in CVD risk factors later in life (Hasselstrom et al. 2002; Janz et al. 2002).

Cardiovascular Consequences of Being Fat but Fit

There are reasons to believe that there might be potential interactions between fitness and fatness in relation to CVD risk. Regarding cardiorespiratory fitness and traits of pediatric type-II diabetes, data from the Swedish and Estonian part of the EYHS indicate that cardiorespiratory fitness explains a significant proportion of the HOMA (homeostasis model assessment, a surrogate marker of insulin resistance) and fasting insulin variance in those children with relatively high levels (i.e., the highest third) of body fat and waist circumference (Ruiz et al. 2007f). Likewise, cardiorespiratory fitness was inversely associated with C-reactive protein in those children with high levels of body fat, therefore, attenuating the negative effect of body fat on C-reactive protein (Fig. 19.5). Data from the same cohort also revealed that in girls with low levels of cardiorespiratory fitness, a higher total and central body fat were significantly associated with higher systolic blood pressure (Ruiz et al. 2007b). In contrast, none of the markers of total and central body fat were significantly associated with blood pressure in girls with high levels of cardiorespiratory fitness (Ruiz et al. 2007b). Results from the AVENA study indicate that high levels of cardiorespiratory fitness are associated with a more favorable metabolic profile in non-overweight but also in overweight Spanish adolescents (Mesa et al. 2006c) (Fig. 19.6).

It has been suggested that children and adolescents with high percent body fat and high cardiorespiratory fitness have better metabolic risk profiles than those classified as high fat but low cardiorespiratory fitness (Eisenmann et al. 2007b). It has been reported a significant difference in metabolic risk scores across four fitness-fatness groups in male adolescents and a trend for significance in females (Eisenmann et al. 2007a). High cardiorespiratory fitness did not completely remove the risk associated with high body mass index (BMI) on clustered metabolic risk, yet the study showed an attenuation of the association between BMI and clustered risk after adjustment for cardiorespiratory fitness. These result concur with others showing that clustered metabolic risk varied across fitness-fatness groups, where high cardiorespiratory fitness appeared to attenuate the metabolic risk score within BMI categories (DuBose et al. 2007). Likewise, Halle et al. (1998) reported that interleukin-6 levels were as low for obese and fit as for lean and unfit children, while the highest serum interleukin-6 concentrations were found in the obese and unfit group. Regarding muscular fitness, data from the

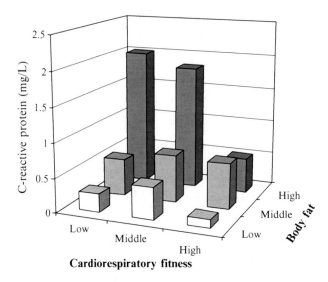

Fig. 19.5 Joint associations between cardiorespiratory fitness (low, middle and high) and body fat mass (low, middle and high of sum of 5 skinfold thickness) in children aged 9–10 years (*n*=142). Adapted from Ruiz et al. (2007e)

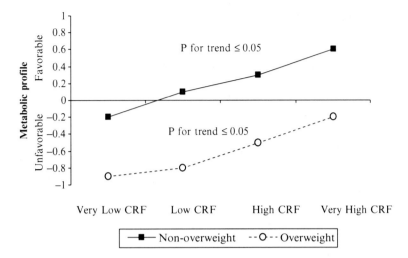

Fig. 19.6 Associations between cardiorespiratory fitness (CRF) and metabolic profile (computed with age-sex-specific standardized values of triglycerides, low density lipoprotein cholesterol, high density lipoprotein cholesterol and fasting glycemia) in non-overweight and overweight young healthy adolescents. Modified from Castillo-Garzon et al. (2007)

AVENA study revealed that C-reactive protein and transthyretin are inversely associated with muscular fitness in overweight adolescents after controlling for different confounders, including cardiorespiratory fitness (Ruiz et al. 2008).

Collectively, these findings suggest that having moderate to high levels of physical fitness may attenuate the deleterious consequences ascribed to high levels of total and central body fat in children and adolescents.

Conclusions

The available literature suggests that:

- Cross-sectional studies using objective measures of physical activity support that a high level of physical activity, particularly vigorous physical activity, is associated with a lower total and central body fat in children and adolescents. The same associations have been suggested between activity levels during childhood/adolescence and overall or central body fat later in life. However, the role of the intensity in these longitudinal associations has not been examined.
- Experimental studies suggest that 45 to 50 min of moderate-vigorous physical activity 5 or more days a week lead to significant body fat reduction in overweight or obese youths. Studies conducted in normal-weight individuals suggest that higher doses (e.g. ≥80 min moderate-vigorous physical activity) are required to decrease total body fat. The same doses of physical activity have been found useful for decreasing central body fat.
- Moderate and vigorous physical activity rather than light activity or inactivity seems to be independently associated with clustered CVD risk in normal weight children and adolescents.
- Regarding physical fitness, both cross-sectional and longitudinal studies have found an inverse association of physical fitness in childhood and adolescence and total and abdominal body fat at these ages and later in life.
- A high physical fitness level, especially cardiorespiratory and muscular fitness, is associated with more favorable levels of traditional and novel CVD risk factors in children and adolescents.

The current evidence suggests that both cardiorespiratory and muscular fitness may have a combined and accumulative effect on the cardiovascular system from an early age (i.e., childhood and adolescence).

- There is evidence of the existence of a hypothetical cardiorespiratory fitness threshold associated with a more favorable cardiovascular profile, which seems to range between 40 and 42 ml/min/kg in boys and between 35 and 38 ml/min/kg in girls.
- The deleterious consequences ascribed to high fatness could be counteracted by having high levels of cardiorespiratory fitness and/or muscular fitness. This implies that interventions to prevent states of unfavorable cardiovascular profiles should focus not only on weight reduction but also on enhancing cardiorespiratory and muscular fitness.
- Finally, the need of future research perspectives has been identified. (a) The effects of the intensity itself and the effects of energy expenditure should be separately examined or controlled in relation to body fat and obesity-related CVD risk at childhood/adolescence and later in life. (b) Whether physical fitness can modify the associations between physical activity and body fat or CVD risk, remains to be elucidated. (c) The associations between physical fitness and fatness or CVD risk are fairly consistent in the literature, but the effect of changes in fitness levels during childhood/adolescence on body fat or CVD risk need to be studied.

Acknowledgements The present work was supported by the Spanish Ministry of Education (EX-2007-1124, AP-2004-2745, AP-2005-3827 and AP2005-4358 INCLUDE: EX-2009-0899), the Swedish Council for Working Life and Social Research, and the ALPHA study, an European Union-funded study, in the framework of the Public Health Program (Ref: 2006120).

References

Abbott, R.A., & Davies, P.S. (2004). Habitual physical activity and physical activity intensity: their relation to body composition in 5.0–10.5-y-old children. *European Journal of Clinical Nutrition, 58*, 285–291.

Andersen, R.E., Crespo, C.J., Bartlet, S.J., Cheskin, L.J., & Pratt, M. (1998). Relationship of physical activity and television watching with body weight and level of fatness among children: results from the Third National Health and Nutrition Examination Survey. *Journal of the American Medical Association, 279*, 938–942.

Andersen, L., Hasselstrøm, H., Gronfeldt, V., Hansen, S., & Froberg, K. (2004a). The relationship between physical fitness and clustered risk, and tracking of clustered risk from adolescence to young adulthood: eight years follow-up in the Danish Youth and Sport Study. *The International Journal of Behavioral Nutrition and Physical Activity, 1*, 6.

Andersen, L.B., Hasselstrøm, H., Gronfeldt, V., Hansen, S.E., & Karsten, F. (2004b). The relationship between physical fitness and clustered risk, and tracking of clustered risk from adolescence to young adulthood: eight years follow-up in the Danish Youth and Sport Study. *The International Journal of Behavioral Nutrition and Physical Activity, 1*, 6.

Andersen, L.B., Harro, M., Sardinha, L.B., Froberg, K., Ekelund, U., Brage, S., & Anderssen, S.A. (2006). Physical activity and clustered cardiovascular risk in children: a cross-sectional study (The European Youth Heart Study). *Lancet, 368*, 299–304.

Ara, I., Vicente-Rodriguez, G., Jimenez-Ramirez, J., Dorado, C., Serrano-Sanchez, J.A., & Calbet, J.A. (2004). Regular participation in sports is associated with enhanced physical fitness and lower fat mass in prepubertal boys. *International Journal of Obesity and Related Metabolic Disorders, 28*, 1585–1593.

Ara, I., Vicente-Rodriguez, G., Perez-Gomez, J., Jimenez-Ramirez, J., Serrano-Sanchez, J.A., Dorado, C., & Calbet, J.A. (2006). Influence of extracurricular sport activities on body composition and physical fitness in boys: a 3-year longitudinal study. *International Journal of Obesity (Lond), 30*, 1062–1071.

Ara, I., Moreno, L.A., Leiva, M.T., Gutin, B., & Casajus, J.A. (2007). Adiposity, physical activity, and physical fitness among children from Aragon, Spain. *Obesity (Silver Spring), 15*, 1918–1924.

Barbeau, P., Gutin, B., Litaker, M., Owens, S., Riggs, S., & Okuyama, T. (1999). Correlates of individual differences in body-composition changes resulting from physical training in obese children. *American Journal of Clinical Nutrition, 69*, 705–711.

Barbeau, P., Johnson, M.H., Howe, C.A., Allison, J., Davis, C.L., Gutin, B., & Lemmon, C.R. (2007). Ten months of exercise improves general and visceral adiposity, bone, and fitness in black girls. *Obesity (Silver Spring), 15*, 2077–2085.

Barnekow-Bergkvist, M., Hedberg, G., Janlert, U., & Jansson, E. (2001). Adolescent determinants of cardiovascular risk factors in adult men and women. *Scandinavian Journal of Public Health, 29*, 208–217.

Bell, R.D., Macek, M., Rutenfranz, J., & Saris, W. (1986). Health indicators and risk factors of cardiovascular diseases during childhood and adolescence. In J. Rutenfranz, R. Mocelin, F. Klimt (Eds.), *Children and exercise XII* (pp. 39–42). Champaign: Human Kinetics Publisher.

Benson, A.C., Torode, M.E., & Singh, M.A. (2006). Muscular strength and cardiorespiratory fitness is associated with higher insulin sensitivity in children and adolescents. *International Journal of Pediatric Obesity, 1*, 222–231.

Benson, A.C., Torode, M.E., & Fiatarone Singh, M.A. (2008). The effect of high-intensity progressive resistance training on adiposity in children: a randomized controlled trial. *International Journal of Obesity (Lond), 32*, 1016–1027.

Berenson, G.S., Srinivasan, S.R., Bao, W., Newman, W.P., III, Tracy, R.E., & Wattigney, W.A. (1998). Association between multiple cardiovascular risk factors and atherosclerosis in children and young adults. The Bogalusa Heart Study. *New England Journal of Medicine, 338*, 1650–1656.

Berkey, C.S., Rockett, H.R., Field, A.E., Gillman, M.W., Frazier, A.L., Camargo, C.A., Jr., & Colditz, G.A. (2000). Activity, dietary intake, and weight changes in a longitudinal study of preadolescent and adolescent boys and girls. *Pediatrics, 105*, E56.

Boreham, C., Twisk, J., Neville, C., Savage, M., Murray, L., & Gallagher, A. (2002). Associations between physical fitness and activity patterns during adolescence and cardiovascular risk factors in young adulthood: the Northern Ireland Young Hearts Project. *International Journal of Sports Medicine 23, Suppl 1*, 22–26.

Boreham, C.A., Ferreira, I., Twisk, J.W., Gallagher, A.M., Savage, M.J., & Murray, L.J. (2004). Cardiorespiratory fitness, physical activity, and arterial stiffness: the Northern Ireland Young Hearts Project. *Hypertension, 44*, 721–726.

Brage, S., Wedderkopp, N., Ekelund, U., Franks, P.W., Wareham, N.J., Andersen, L.B., & Froberg, K. (2004). Features of the metabolic syndrome are associated with objectively measured physical activity and fitness in Danish children: the European Youth Heart Study (EYHS). *Diabetes Care, 27*, 2141–2148.

Brambilla, P., Bedogni, G., Moreno, L.A., Goran, M.I., Gutin, B., Fox, K.R., Peters D.M., Barbeau, P., De Simone, M., & Pietrobelli, A. (2006). Crossvalidation of anthropometry against magnetic resonance imaging for the assessment of visceral and subcutaneous adipose tissue in children. *International Journal of Obesity (Lond), 30*, 23–30.

Brunet, M., Chaput, J.P., & Tremblay, A. (2007). The association between low physical fitness and high body mass index or waist circumference is increasing with age in children: the "Quebec en Forme" Project. *International Journal of Obesity (Lond), 31*, 637–643.

Butte, N.F., Puyau, M.R., Adolph, A.L., Vohra, F.A., & Zakeri, I. (2007). Physical activity in nonoverweight and overweight Hispanic children and adolescents. *Medicine and Science in Sports and Exercise, 39*, 1257–1266.

Byrd-Williams, C.E., Shaibi, G.Q., Sun, P., Lane, C.J., Ventura, E.E., Davis, J.N., Kelly, L.A., & Goran, M.I. (2008). Cardiorespiratory fitness predicts changes in adiposity in overweight Hispanic boys. *Obesity (Silver Spring), 16*, 1072–1077.

Carnethon, M.R., Gidding, S.S., Nehgme, R., Sidney, S., Jacobs, D.R., Jr., & Liu, K. (2003). Cardiorespiratory fitness in young adulthood and the development of cardiovascular disease risk factors. *Journal of the American Medical Association, 290*, 3092–3100.

Castillo-Garzon, M., Ruiz, J.R., Ortega, F.B., & Gutierrez-Sainz, A. (2007). A Mediterranean diet is not enough for health: physical fitness is an important additional contributor to health for the adults of tomorrow. *World Review of Nutrition and Dietetics, 97*, 114–138.

Castro, R., Rivera, I., Blom, H.J., Jakobs, C., & Tavares de Almeida, I. (2006). Homocysteine metabolism, hyperhomocysteinaemia and vascular disease: an overview. *Journal of Inherited Metabolic Disorders, 29*, 3–20.

Centers for Disease Control and Prevention National Center for Health Statistics (2004a). *National health and nutrition examination survey 1999–2000 data.* Hyattsville: US Department of Health and Human Services, Centers for Disease Control and Prevention (September 21, 2007); http://www.cdc.gov/nchs/about/major/nhanes/nhanes99_00.htm

Centers for Disease Control and Prevention National Center for Health Statistics (2004b). *National health and nutrition examination survey 2001–2002 data.* Hyattsville: US Department of Health and Human Services, Centers for Disease Control and Prevention (September 21, 2007); http://www.cdc.gov/nchs/about/major/nhanes/nhanes01-02.htm

Cole, T.J., Bellizzi, M.C., Flegal, K.M., & Dietz, W.H. (2000). Establishing a standard definition for child overweight and obesity worldwide: international survey. *British Medical Journal, 320*, 1240–1243.

Cooper, D.M., Nemet, D., & Galassetti, P. (2004). Exercise, stress, and inflammation in the growing child: from the bench to the playground. *Current Opinion in Pediatrics, 16*, 286–292.

Cruz, M.L., Shaibi, G.Q., Weigensberg, M.J., Spruijt-Metz, D., Ball, G.D., & Goran, M.I. (2005). Pediatric obesity and insulin resistance: chronic disease risk and implications for treatment and prevention beyond body weight modification. *Annual Review of Nutrition, 25*, 435–468.

Cureton, K.J., & Warren, G.L. (1990). Criterion-referenced standards for youth health-related fitness tests: a tutorial. *Research Quarterly for Exercise and Sport, 61*, 7–19.

Dencker, M., & Andersen, L.B. (2008). Health-related aspects of objectively measured daily physical activity in children. *Clinical Physiology and Functional Imaging, 28*, 133–144.

Dencker, M., Thorsson, O., Karlsson, M.K., Linden, C., Wollmer, P., & Andersen, L.B. (2008). Daily physical activity related to aerobic fitness and body fat in an urban sample of children. *Scandinavian Journal of Medicine & Science in Sports, 18*, 728–735.

DuBose, K.D., Eisenmann, J.C., & Donnelly, J.E. (2007). Aerobic fitness attenuates the metabolic syndrome score in normal-weight, at-risk-for-overweight, and overweight children. *Pediatrics, 120*, 1262–1268.

Eisenmann, J.C., Wickel, E.E., Welk, G.J., & Blair, S.N. (2005). Relationship between adolescent fitness and fatness and cardiovascular disease risk factors in adulthood: the Aerobics Center Longitudinal Study (ACLS). *American Heart Journal, 149*, 46–53.

Eisenmann, J.C., Welk, G.J., Wickel, E.E., & Blair, S.N. (2007a). Combined influence of cardiorespiratory fitness and body mass index on cardiovascular disease risk factors among 8–18 year old youth: The Aerobics Center Longitudinal Study. *International Journal of Pediatric Obesity, 2*, 66–72.

Eisenmann, J.C., Welk, G.J., Ihmels, M., & Dollman, J. (2007b). Fatness, fitness, and cardiovascular disease risk factors in children and adolescents. *Medicine and Science in Sports and Exercise, 39*, 1251–1256.

Ekelund, U., Aman, J., Yngve, A., Renman, C., Westerterp, K., & Sjöström, M. (2002). Physical activity but not energy expenditure is reduced in obese adolescents: a case-control study. *American Journal of Clinical Nutrition, 76*, 935–941.

Ekelund, U., Sardinha, L.B., Anderssen, S.A., Harro, M., Franks, P.W., Brage, S., Cooper, A.R., Andersen, L.B., Riddoch, C., & Froberg, K. (2004). Associations between objectively assessed physical activity and indicators of body fatness in 9- to 10-y-old European children: a population-based study from 4 distinct regions in Europe (the European Youth Heart Study). *American Journal of Clinical Nutrition, 80*, 584–590.

Ekelund, U., Anderssen, S.A., Froberg, K., Sardinha, L.B., Andersen, L.B., & Brage, S. (2007a). Independent associations of physical activity and cardiorespiratory fitness with metabolic risk factors in children: The European Youth Heart Study. *Diabetologia, 50*, 1832–1840.

Ekelund, U., Franks, P.W., Sharp, S., Brage, S., & Wareham, N.J. (2007b). Increase in physical activity energy expenditure is associated with reduced metabolic risk independent of change in fatness and fitness. *Diabetes Care, 30*, 2101–2106.

Eliakim, A., Makowski, G.S., Brasel, J.A., & Cooper, D.M. (2000). Adiposity, lipid levels, and brief endurance training in nonobese adolescent males. *International Journal of Sports Medicine, 21*, 332–337.

Eliakim, A., Scheett, T., Allmendinger, N., Brasel, J.A., & Cooper, D.M. (2001). Training, muscle volume, and energy expenditure in nonobese American girls. *Journal of Applied Physiology, 90*, 35–44.

Ferreira, I., Twisk, J.W., Stehouwer, C.D., van Mechelen, W., & Kemper, H.C. (2003). Longitudinal changes in VO2max: associations with carotid IMT and arterial stiffness. *Medicine and Science in Sports and Exercise, 35*, 1670–1678.

Ferreira, I., Henry, R.M., Twisk, J.W., van Mechelen, W., Kemper, H.C., & Stehouwer, C.D. (2005). The metabolic syndrome, cardiopulmonary fitness, and subcutaneous trunk fat as independent determinants of arterial stiffness: the Amsterdam Growth and Health Longitudinal Study. *Archives of Internal Medicine, 165*, 875–882.

Freedman, D.S., Khan, L.K., Dietz, W.H., Srinivasan, S.R., & Berenson, G.S. (2001). Relationship of childhood obesity to coronary heart disease risk factors in adulthood: the Bogalusa Heart Study. *Pediatrics, 108*, 712–718.

Gallistl, S., Sudi, K., Mangge, H., Erwa, W., & Borkenstein, M. (2000). Insulin is an independent correlate of plasma homocysteine levels in obese children and adolescents. *Diabetes Care, 23*, 1348–1352.

Garcia-Artero, E., Ortega, F.B., Ruiz, J.R., Mesa, J.L., Delgado, M., Gonzalez-Gross, M., Garcia-Fuentes, M., Vicente-Rodriguez, G., Gutierrez, A., & Castillo, M.J. (2007). Lipid and metabolic profiles in adolescents are affected more by physical fitness than physical activity (AVENA study). *Revista Española de Cardiología, 60*, 581–588.

Guo, S.S., Wu, W., Chumlea, W.C., & Roche, A.F. (2002). Predicting overweight and obesity in adulthood from body mass index values in childhood and adolescence. *American Journal of Clinical Nutrition, 76*, 653–658.

Gutin, B., Barbeau, P., Owens, S., Lemmon, C.R., Bauman, M., Allison, J., Kang, H.S., & Litaker, M.S. (2002). Effects of exercise intensity on cardiovascular fitness, total body composition, and visceral adiposity of obese adolescents. *American Journal of Clinical Nutrition, 75*, 818–826.

Gutin, B., Yin, Z., Humphries, M.C., & Barbeau, P. (2005). Relations of moderate and vigorous physical activity to fitness and fatness in adolescents. *American Journal of Clinical Nutrition, 81*, 746–750.

Gutin, B., Johnson, M.H., Humphries, M.C., Hatfield-Laube, J.L., Kapuku, G.K., Allison, J.D., Gower, B.A., Daniels, S.R., & Barbeau, P. (2007). Relationship of visceral adiposity to cardiovascular disease risk factors in black and white teens. *Obesity (Silver Spring), 15*, 1029–1035.

Gutin, B., Yin, Z., Johnson, M., & Barbeau, P. (2008). Preliminary findings of the effect of a 3-year after-school physical activity intervention on fitness and body fat: the Medical College of Georgia Fitkid Project. *International Journal of Pediatric Obesity, 3 (Suppl 1)*, 3–9.

Halle, M., Berg, A., Northoff, H., & Keul, J. (1998). Importance of TNF-alpha and leptin in obesity and insulin resistance: a hypothesis on the impact of physical exercise. *Exercise Immunology Review, 4*, 77–94.

Halle, M., Korsten-Reck, U., Wolfarth, B., & Berg, A. (2004). Low-grade systemic inflammation in overweight children: impact of physical fitness. *Exercise Immunology Review, 10*, 66–74.

Hansson, G.K. (2005). Inflammation, atherosclerosis, and coronary artery disease. *New England Journal of Medicine, 352*, 1685–1695.

Hasselstrom, H., Hansen, S.E., Froberg, K., & Andersen, L.B. (2002). Physical fitness and physical activity during adolescence as predictors of cardiovascular disease risk in young adulthood. Danish Youth and Sports Study. An eight-year follow-up study. *International Journal of Sports Medicine, 23 (Suppl 1)*, 27–31.

Hurtig-Wennlof, A., Ruiz, J.R., Harro, M., & Sjöström, M. (2007). Cardiorespiratory fitness relates more strongly than physical activity to cardiovascular disease risk factors in healthy children and adolescents: the European Youth Heart Study. *European Journal of Cardiovascular Prevention and Rehabilitation, 14*, 575–581.

Hussey, J., Bell, C., Bennett, K., O'Dwyer, J., & Gormley, J. (2007). Relationship between the intensity of physical activity, inactivity, cardiorespiratory fitness and body composition in 7–10-year-old Dublin children. *British Journal of Sports Medicine, 41*, 311–316.

Isasi, C.R., Deckelbaum, R.J., Tracy, R.P., Starc, T.J., Berglund, L., & Shea, S. (2003). Physical fitness and C-reactive protein level in children and young adults: the Columbia University BioMarkers Study. *Pediatrics, 111*, 332–338.

Janssen, I., Katzmarzyk, P.T., Srinivasan, S.R., Chen, W., Malina, R.M., Bouchard, C., & Berenson, G.S. (2005). Combined influence of body mass index and waist circumference on coronary artery disease risk factors among children and adolescents. *Pediatrics, 115*, 1623–1630.

Janz, K.F., Dawson, J.D., & Mahoney, L.T. (2002a). Increases in physical fitness during childhood improve cardiovascular health during adolescence: the Muscatine Study. *International Journal of Sports Medicine, 23 (Suppl 1)*, 15–21.

Janz, K.F., Burns, T.L., & Levy, S.M. (2005). Tracking of activity and sedentary behaviors in childhood: the Iowa Bone Development Study. *American Journal of Preventive Medicine, 29*, 171–178.

Jarvisalo, M.J., Harmoinen, A., Hakanen, M., Paakkunainen, U., Viikari, J., Hartiala, J., Lehtimaki, T., Simell, O., & Raitakari, O.T. (2002). Elevated serum C-reactive protein levels and early arterial changes in healthy children. *Arteriosclerosis, Thrombosis, and Vascular Biology, 22*, 1323–1328.

Johnson, M.S., Figueroa-Colon, R., Herd, S.L., Fields, D.A., Sun, M., Hunter, G.R., & Goran, M.I. (2000). Aerobic fitness, not energy expenditure, influences subsequent increase in adiposity in black and white children. *Pediatrics, 106*, E50.

Jurca, R., Lamonte, M.J., Barlow, C.E., Kampert, J.B., Church, T.S., & Blair, S.N. (2005). Association of muscular strength with incidence of metabolic syndrome in men. *Medicine and Science in Sports and Exercise, 37*, 1849–1855.

Klein-Platat, C., Oujaa, M., Wagner, A., Haan, M.C., Arveiler, D., Schlienger, J.L., & Simon, C. (2005). Physical activity is inversely related to waist circumference in 12-y-old French adolescents. *International Journal of Obesity (Lond), 29*, 9–14.

Klijn, P.H., van der Baan-Slootweg, O.H., & van Stel, H.F. (2007). Aerobic exercise in adolescents with obesity: preliminary evaluation of a modular training program and the modified shuttle test. *BMC Pediatrics, 7*, 19.

Kohl, H.W., Fulton, J.E., & Caspersen, C.J. (2000). Assessment of physical activity among children and adolescents: a review and synthesis. *Preventive Medicine, 31*, 54–76.

Koutedakis, Y., & Bouziotas, C. (2003). National physical education curriculum: motor and cardiovascular health related fitness in Greek adolescents. *British Journal of Sports Medicine, 37*, 311–314.

Kriemler, S., Hebestreit, H., Mikami, S., Bar-Or, T., Ayub, B.V., & Bar-Or, O. (1999). Impact of a single exercise bout on energy expenditure and spontaneous physical activity of obese boys. *Pediatric Research, 46*, 40–44.

Kuo, H.K., Yen, C.J., & Bean, J.F. (2005). Levels of homocysteine are inversely associated with cardiovascular fitness in women, but not in men: data from the National Health and Nutrition Examination Survey 1999–2002. *Journal of Internal Medicine, 258*, 328–335.

LaMonte, M.J., & Blair, S.N. (2006). Physical activity, cardiorespiratory fitness, and adiposity: contributions to disease risk. *Current Opinion in Clinical Nutrition and Metabolic Care, 9*, 540–546.

Lee, S.J., & Arslanian, S.A. (2007). Cardiorespiratory fitness and abdominal adiposity in youth. *European Journal of Clinical Nutrition, 61*, 561–565.

LeMura, L.M., & Maziekas, M.T. (2002). Factors that alter body fat, body mass, and fat-free mass in pediatric obesity. *Medicine and Science in Sports and Exercise, 34*, 487–496.

Lobelo, F., & Ruiz, J.R. (2007). Cardiorespiratory fitness as criterion validity for health-based metabolic syndrome definition in adolescents. *Journal of the American College of Cardiology, 50*, 471.

Lobelo, F., Pate, R.R., Dowda, M., Liese, A.D., & Ruiz, J.R. (2009). Validity of cardiorespiratory fitness criterion-referenced standards for adolescents. *Medicine and Science in Sports and Exercise, 41*, 1222–1229.

McCully, K.S. (2005). Hyperhomocysteinemia and arteriosclerosis: historical perspectives. *Clinical Chemistry and Laboratory Medicine, 43*, 980–986.

Mesa, J.L., Ortega, F.B., Ruiz, J.R., Castillo, M.J., Hurtig-Wennlöf, A., Sjöström, M., & Gutierrez, A. (2006a). The importance of cardiorespiratory fitness for healthy metabolic traits in children and adolescents: the AVENA study. *Journal of Public Health, 14*, 178–180.

Mesa, J.L., Ortega, F.B., Ruiz, J.R., Castillo, M.J., Tresaco, B., Carreno, F., Moreno, L.A., Gutierrez, A., & Bueno, M. (2006b). Anthropometric determinants of a clustering of lipid-related metabolic risk factors in overweight and non-overweight adolescents – influence of cardiorespiratory fitness. The AVENA Study. *Annals of Nutrition & Metabolism, 50*, 519–527.

Mesa, J.L., Ruiz, J.R., Ortega, F.B., Warnberg, J., Gonzalez-Lamuno, D., Moreno, L.A., Gutierrez, A., & Castillo, M.J. (2006c). Aerobic physical fitness in relation to blood lipids and fasting glycaemia in adolescents: influence of weight status. *Nutrition, Metabolism, and Cardiovascular Disease, 16*, 285–293.

Metcalf, B.S., Voss, L.D., Hosking, J., Jeffery, A.N., & Wilkin, T.J. (2008). Physical activity at the government-recommended level and obesity-related health outcomes: a longitudinal study (EarlyBird 37). *Archives of Disease in Childhood, 93*, 772–777.

Mokdad, A.H., Marks, J.S., Stroup, D.F., & Gerberding, J.L. (2004). Actual causes of death in the United States, 2000. *Journal of the American Medical Association, 291*, 1238–1245.

Moore, L.L., Gao, D., Bradlee, M.L., Cupples, L.A., Sundarajan-Ramamurti, A., Proctor, M.H., Hood, M.Y., Singer, M.R., & Ellison, R.C. (2003). Does early physical activity predict body fat change throughout childhood? *Preventive Medicine, 37*, 10–17.

Nassis, G.P., Psarra, G., & Sidossis, L.S. (2005). Central and total adiposity are lower in overweight and obese children with high cardiorespiratory fitness. *European Journal of Clinical Nutrition, 59*, 137–141.

Oehlschlaeger, M.H., Pinheiro, R.T., Horta, B., Gelatti, C., & San'Tana, P. (2004). Prevalence of sedentarism and its associated factors among urban adolescents. *Revista de Saúde Pública, 38*, 157–163.

Ortega, F.B., Ruiz, J.R., Castillo, M.J., Moreno, L.A., Warnberg, J., Tresaco, B., Gonzalez-Gross, M., Perez, F., Garcia-Fuentes, M., & Gutierrez, A. (2006). Cardiorespiratory fitness is associated with a favorable lipid profile independent of abdominal fat in male adolescents: *Medicine and Science in Sports and Exercise, 38*, 7–8.

Ortega, F.B., Ruiz, J.R., & Sjöström, M. (2007a). Physical activity, overweight and central adiposity in Swedish children and adolescents: the European Youth Heart Study. *The International Journal of Behavioral Nutrition and Physical Activity, 4*, 61.

Ortega, F.B., Tresaco, B., Ruiz, J.R., Moreno, L.A., Martin-Matillas, M., Mesa, J.L., Warnberg, J., Bueno, M., Tercedor, P., Gutierrez, A., & Castillo, M.J. (2007b). Cardiorespiratory fitness and sedentary activities are associated with adiposity in adolescents. *Obesity (Silver Spring), 15*, 1589–1599.

Ortega, F.B., Ruiz, J.R., Hurtig-Wennlof, A., Vicente-Rodriguez, G., Rizzo, N.S., Castillo, M.J., & Sjöström, M. (2010). Cardiovascular fitness modifies the associations between physical activity and abdominal adiposity in children and adolescents. The European Youth Heart Study. *British Journal of Sports Medicine, 44*, 256–262.

Owens, S., Gutin, B., Allison, J., Riggs, S., Ferguson, M., Litaker, M., & Thompson, W. (1999). Effect of physical training on total and visceral fat in obese children. *Medicine and Science in Sports and Exercise, 31*, 143–148.

Pedersen, B.K., & Saltin, B. (2006). Evidence for prescribing exercise as therapy in chronic disease. *Scandinavian Journal of Medicine and Science in Sports, 16 (Suppl 1)*, 3–63.

Poortvliet, E., Yngve, A., Ekelund, U., Hurtig-Wennlof, A., Nilsson, A., Hagstromer, M., & Sjöström, M. (2003). The European Youth Heart Survey (EYHS): an international study that addresses the multi-dimensional issues of CVD risk factors. *Forum of Nutrition, 56*, 254–256.

Psarra, G., Nassis, G.P., & Sidossis, L.S. (2006). Short-term predictors of abdominal obesity in children. *European Journal of Public Health, 16*, 520–525.

Raitakari, O.T., Juonala, M., Kahonen, M., Taittonen, L., Laitinen, T., Maki-Torkko, N., Jarvisalo, M.J., Uhari, M., Jokinen, E., Ronnemaa, T., Akerblom, H.K., & Viikari, J.S. (2003). Cardiovascular risk factors in childhood and carotid artery intima-media thickness in adulthood: the Cardiovascular Risk in Young Finns Study. *Journal of the American Medical Association, 290*, 2277–2283.

Rey-Lopez, J.P., Vicente-Rodriguez, G., & Moreno, L.A. (2007). Sedentary behaviors and obesity development in children and adolescents. *Nutrition, Metabolism & Cardiovascular Diseases, 18*, 242–251.

Rizzo, N.S., Ruiz, J.R., Hurtig-Wennlof, A., Ortega, F.B., & Sjöström, M. (2007). Relationship of physical activity, fitness, and fatness with clustered metabolic risk in children and adolescents: the European Youth Heart Study. *The Journal of Pediatrics, 150*, 388–394.

Rizzo, N.S., Ruiz, J.R., Oja, L., Veidebaum, T., & Sjöström, M. (2008). Associations between physical activity, body fat, and insulin resistance (homeostasis model assessment) in adolescents: the European Youth Heart Study. *American Journal of Clinical Nutrition, 87*, 586–592.

Rowland, T.W., Martel, L., Vanderburgh, P., Manos, T., & Charkoudian, N. (1996). The influence of short-term aerobic training on blood lipids in healthy 10–12 year old children. *International Journal of Sports Medicine, 17*, 487–492.

Rowlands, A.V., Eston, R.G., & Ingledew, D.K. (1999). Relationship between activity levels, aerobic fitness, and body fat in 8- to 10-yr-old children. *Journal of Applied Physiology, 86*, 1428–1435.

Ruiz, J.R., Ortega, F.B., Gutierrez, A., Meusel, D., Sjöström, M., & Castillo, M.J. (2006a). Health-related fitness assessment in childhood and adolescence; A European approach based on the AVENA, EYHS and HELENA studies *Journal of Public Health, 14*, 269–277.

Ruiz, J.R., Ortega, F.B., Meusel, D., Harro, M., Oja, P., & Sjöström, M. (2006b). Cardiorespiratory fitness is associated with features of metabolic risk factors in children. Should cardiorespiratory fitness be assessed in a European health monitoring system? The European Youth Heart Study. *Journal of Public Health, 14*, 94–102.

Ruiz, J.R., Ortega, F.B., Tresaco, B., Warnberg, J., Mesa, J.L., Gonzalez-Gross, M., Moreno, L.A., Marcos, A., Gutierrez, A., & Castillo, M.J. (2006c). Serum lipids, body mass index and waist circumference during pubertal development in Spanish adolescents: the AVENA Study. *Hormone and Metabolic Research, 38*, 832–837.

Ruiz, J.R., Rizzo, N.S., Hurtig-Wennlöf, A., Ortega, F.B., Wärnberg, J., & Sjöström, M. (2006d). Relations of total physical activity and intensity to fitness and fatness in children: the European Youth Heart Study. *American Journal of Clinical Nutrition, 84*, 299–303.

Ruiz, J.R., Hurtig-Wennlöf, A., Ortega, F.B., Patersson, E., Nilsson, T.K., Castillo, M.J., & Sjöström, M. (2007a). Homocysteine levels in children and adolescents are associated with the methylenetetrahydrofolate reductase 677C > T genotype, but not with physical activity, fitness or fatness: The European Youth Heart Study. *British Journal of Nutrition, 96*, 255–262.

Ruiz, J.R., Ortega, F.B., Loit, H.M., Veidebaum, T., & Sjöström, M. (2007b). Body fat is associated with blood pressure in school-aged girls with low cardiorespiratory fitness: The European Youth Heart Study. *Journal of Hypertension, 25*, 2027–2034.

Ruiz, J.R., Ortega, F.B., Meusel, D., & Sjöström, M. (2007c). Traditional and novel cardiovascular risk factors in school-aged children: call for the further development of public health strategies with emphasis on fitness. *Journal of Public Health, 15*, 171–177.

Ruiz, J.R., Ortega, F.B., Rizzo, N.S., Villa, I., Hurtig-Wennlöf, A., Oja, L., & Sjöström, M. (2007d). High cardiovascular fitness is associated with low metabolic risk score in children: The European Youth Heart Study. *Pediatric Research, 61*, 350–355.

Ruiz, J.R., Ortega, F.B., Warnberg, J., & Sjöström, M. (2007e). Associations of low-grade inflammation with physical activity, fitness and fatness in prepubertal children; the European Youth Heart Study. *International Journal of Obesity (Lond), 31*, 1545–1551.

Ruiz, J.R., Rizzo, N.S., Ortega, F.B., Loit, H.M., Veidebaum, T., & Sjöström, M. (2007f). Markers of insulin resistance are associated with fatness and fitness in school-aged children: the European Youth Heart Study. *Diabetologia, 50*, 1401–1408.

Ruiz, J.R., Sola, R., Gonzalez-Gross, M., Ortega, F.B., Vicente-Rodriguez, G., Garcia-Fuentes, M., Gutierrez, A., Sjöström, M., Pietrzik, K., & Castillo, M.J. (2007g). Cardiovascular fitness is negatively associated with homocysteine levels in female adolescents. *Archives of Pediatrics & Adolescent Medicine, 161*, 166–171.

Ruiz, J.R., Ortega, F.B., Warnberg, J., Moreno, L.A., Carrero, J.J., Gonzalez-Gross, M., Marcos, A., Gutierrez, A., & Sjöström, M. (2008). Inflammatory proteins and muscle strength in adolescents: the AVENA study. *Archives of Pediatrics & Adolescent Medicine, 162*, 462–468.

Ruiz, J.R., Castro-Pinero, J., Artero, E.G., Ortega, F.B., Sjöström, M., Suni, J., & Castillo, M.J. (2009). Predictive validity of health-related fitness in youth: a systematic review. *British Journal of Sports Medicine, 43*, 909–923

Saelens, B.E., Seeley, R.J., van Schaick, K., Donnelly, L.F., & O'Brien, K.J. (2007). Visceral abdominal fat is correlated with whole-body fat and physical activity among 8-y-old children at risk of obesity. *American Journal of Clinical Nutrition, 85*, 46–53.

Sardinha, L.B., Andersen, L.B., Anderssen, S.A., Quiterio, A.L., Ornelas, R., Froberg, K., Riddoch, C.J., & Ekelund, U. (2008). Objectively measured time spent sedentary is associated with insulin resistance independent of overall and central body fat in 9- to 10-year-old Portuguese children. *Diabetes Care, 31*, 569–575.

Stallmann-Jorgensen, I.S., Gutin, B., Hatfield-Laube, J.L., Humphries, M.C., Johnson, M.H., & Barbeau, P. (2007). General and visceral adiposity in black and white adolescents and their relation with reported physical activity and diet. *International Journal of Obesity (Lond), 31*, 622–629.

Steele, R.M., Brage, S., Corder, K., Wareham, N.J., & Ekelund, U. (2008). Physical activity, cardiorespiratory fitness, and the metabolic syndrome in youth. *Journal of Applied Physiology, 105*, 342–351.

Steinberger, J., Moran, A., Hong, C.P., Jacobs, D.R., Jr., & Sinaiko, A.R. (2001). Adiposity in childhood predicts obesity and insulin resistance in young adulthood. *Journal of Pediatrics, 138*, 469–473.

Stevens, J., Suchindran, C., Ring, K., Baggett, C.D., Jobe, J.B., Story, M., Thompson, J., Going, S.B., & Caballero, B. (2004). Physical activity as a predictor of body composition in American Indian children. *Obesity Research, 12*, 1974–1980.

Strong, W.B., Malina, R.M., Blimkie, C.J., Daniels, S.R., Dishman, R.K., Gutin, B., Hergenroeder, A.C., Must, A., Nixon, P.A., Pivarnik, J.M., Rowland, T., Trost, S., & Trudeau, F. (2005). Evidence based physical activity for school-age youth. *The Journal of Pediatrics, 146*, 732–737.

Taylor, R.W., Jones, I.E., Williams, S.M., & Goulding, A. (2000). Evaluation of waist circumference, waist-to-hip ratio, and the conicity index as screening tools for high trunk fat mass, as measured by dual-energy X-ray absorptiometry, in children aged 3–19 y. *American Journal of Clinical Nutrition, 72*, 490–495.

The Cooper Institute for Aerobics Research (2004). *FITNESSGRAM test administration manual*, 3rd ed (pp. 38–39). Champaign: Human Kinetics.

Thompson, D.R., Obarzanek, E., Franko, D.L., Barton, B.A., Morrison, J., Biro, F.M., Daniels, S.R., & Striegel-Moore, R.H. (2007). Childhood overweight and cardiovascular disease risk factors: the National Heart, Lung, and Blood Institute Growth and Health Study. *The Journal of Pediatrics, 150*, 18–25.

Tolfrey, K., Campbell, I.G., & Batterham, A.M. (1998). Exercise training induced alterations in prepubertal children's lipid-lipoprotein profile. *Medicine and Science in Sports and Exercise, 30*, 1684–1692.

Tolfrey, K., Jones, A.M., & Campbell, I.G. (2004). Lipid-lipoproteins in children: an exercise dose-response study. *Medicine and Science in Sports and Exercise, 36*, 418–427.

Twisk, J.W., Kemper, H.C., & van Mechelen, W. (2000). Tracking of activity and fitness and the relationship with cardiovascular disease risk factors. *Medicine and Science in Sports and Exercise, 32*, 1455–1461.

Twisk, J.W., Kemper, H.C., & van Mechelen, W. (2002a). Prediction of cardiovascular disease risk factors later in life by physical activity and physical fitness in youth: general comments and conclusions. *International Journal of Sports Medicine, 23, Suppl 1*, 44–49.

Twisk, J.W., Kemper, H.C., & van Mechelen, W. (2002b). The relationship between physical fitness and physical activity during adolescence and cardiovascular disease risk factors at adult age. The Amsterdam Growth and Health Longitudinal Study. *International Journal of Sports Medicine, 23, Suppl 1*, 8–14.

Wärnberg, J., Nova, E., Moreno, L.A., Romeo, J., Mesana, M.I., Ruiz, J.R., Ortega, F.B., Sjöström, M., Bueno, M., & Marcos, A. (2006a). Inflammatory proteins are related to total and abdominal adiposity in a healthy adolescent population: the AVENA Study. *American Journal of Clinical Nutrition, 84*, 505–512.

Wärnberg, J., Ruiz, J.R., Sjöström, M., Ortega, F.B., Moreno, A., Moreno, L.A., Rizzo, N.S., & Marcos, A. (2006b). Association of fitness and fatness to low-grade systemic inflammation in adolescents. The AVENA study. *Medicine and Science in Sports and Exercise, 38*, 8.

Winsley, R.J., Armstrong, N., Middlebrooke, A.R., Ramos-Ibanez, N., & Williams, C.A. (2006). Aerobic fitness and visceral adipose tissue in children. *Acta Paediatrica, 95*, 1435–1438.

Wittmeier, K.D., Mollard, R.C., & Kriellaars, D.J. (2007). Objective assessment of childhood adherence to Canadian physical activity guidelines in relation to body composition. *Applied Physiology, Nutrition, and Metabolism, 32*, 217–224.

Wolfe, R.R. (2006). The underappreciated role of muscle in health and disease. *American Journal of Clinical Nutrition, 84*, 475–482.

Yin, Z., Gutin, B., Johnson, M.H., Hanes, J., Jr., Moore, J.B., Cavnar, M., Thornburg, J., Moore, D., & Barbeau, P. (2005). An environmental approach to obesity prevention in children: Medical College of Georgia FitKid Project year 1 results. *Obesity Research, 13*, 2153–2161.

Chapter 20
Sedentary Behaviors and Obesity in Children and Adolescents

J.P. Rey-López, G. Vicente-Rodríguez, G. Bueno, and L.A. Moreno

Introduction

From an evolutionary standpoint, human beings are hunter-gatherers (Eaton et al. 1988). Our culture has been transformed during the past 10,000 years, especially during the Industrial Revolution. Energy balance has been remarkably changed during the last few decades. The terms "obesogenic environment" and "build environment" (Papas et al. 2007) have been introduced in scientific literature. These changes include a marked change in dietary habits and physical activity (PA) patterns characterized by fast food, energy-dense diets, motorized transport, use of computers and frequent television viewing. Other factors, likely boosting this epidemic are assortative mating and epigenetic effects (Keith et al. 2006).

In spite of extensive research over the past few decades, the mechanisms by which people attain excessive body weight and adiposity are still only partially understood (Schneider et al. 2007). Debate as to the reasons for high rates of obesity among youth has centered on the two sides of the energy balance equation: energy intake and energy expenditure (Schneider et al. 2007). For some authors excessive energy intake is the primary cause (Bleich et al. 2008; Utter et al. 2003). For others, the modern inactive lifestyle is at least as important as diet and possibly represents the dominant factor (Prentice and Jebb 1995). In children and adolescents there is no evidence that excessive dietary intake explains the current increased prevalence of obesity (Rodriguez and Moreno 2006). It is likely that a combination of high dietary intake and low energy expenditure are acting together. In a systematic review of the role of sedentary behaviors in obesity development, sufficient evidence emerged to recommend a limitation of the time spent watching TV, especially in young children (Rey-López et al. 2008). TV viewing is often associated with higher caloric intake and unhealthy food (Vereecken et al. 2006). However, there are still methodological limitations in our ability to accurately measure dietary energy intake and energy expenditure in free-living populations.

J.P. Rey-López, G. Vicente-Rodríguez, G. Bueno, and L.A. Moreno
Growth, Exercise, Nutrition and Development (GENUD) Research Group, University of Zaragoza, Zaragoza, Spain

G. Vicente-Rodríguez
School of Health and Sports Sciences, Huesca, Spain

G. Bueno
Department of Pediatrics, School of Medicine, University of Zaragoza, Zaragoza, Spain

L.A. Moreno (✉)
School of Health Sciences, University of Zaragoza, Zaragoza, Spain
e-mail: lmoreno@unizar.es

L.A. Moreno et al. (eds.), *Epidemiology of Obesity in Children and Adolescents*,
Springer Series on Epidemiology and Public Health 2, DOI 10.1007/978-1-4419-6039-9_20,
© Springer Science+Business Media, LLC 2011

In this chapter, we will discuss the relationship between sedentary behaviors and obesity development. We will describe how some sedentary behaviors (mainly TV viewing, playing video games and computer use) are related to weight gain in children and adolescents. Consequently, we do not focus our review on the definition of sedentariness as the absence of moderate to vigorous physical activity.

Assessment of Sedentary Behaviors in Children and Adolescents

The study of sedentary behaviors is becoming popular. However, most studies trying to address "sedentary" behavior are in fact identifying those individuals less active than their peers or those not meeting a criterion level for physical activity (Gorely et al. 2007). It is common to find studies where nothing is said about which sedentary behaviors are taking place, for how long, or in what context. Currently, accelerometer data give objective information about the inactivity of one subject, generally in a sitting position. But the problem with the objective inactivity data is that inactivity or sitting can occur with different behaviors. We need to know how and in what context inactivity is expressed. The same lack of movement can be due to different behaviors such as TV viewing while eating snacks and drinking soft-drinks or, at the opposite end, reading in a fasting state.

Sedentary behaviors can be measured by several methods: direct observation, video recording, self-report questionnaires, diaries and parental reporting.

Direct observation means to observe the studied subject recording in a paper the type and duration of the sedentary behavior. It can be considered the reference method, but unfortunately, it is time consuming and, therefore not feasible for large epidemiological studies. In children, few tools for measuring the time watching TV have been assessed for their validity or reliability (Bryant et al. 2007). A minority of studies have employed objective techniques such as video recording or real-time capture (electronic devices that assess time when TV is on). Self-report questionnaires are quicker and easier for the researchers, but they are less accurate than direct observation. Parental reporting should be recommended in children because of their inability to report their own behavior. Diaries are used in some studies successfully but its main limitation is the low rate of fulfillment in some subjects.

Sedentary behavior is often assessed only with reference to TV viewing. Some studies provide information on TV viewing alongside other electronic-based sedentary behaviors, such as computer use and/or video games use. However, few studies have been published about other behaviors such as studying or talking. An important limitation of the use of questionnaires is that they only reflect partially inactive time. Although of the most prevalent sedentary behaviors TV viewing represents around half of the time spent (40% in a recent study of adolescents girls, Gorely et al. 2007), there is still a substantial amount of time devoted to other sedentary activities, and this may become a public health problem if the total duration of sedentariness increases, because this will produce a decrease in total energy expenditure and because total sedentary time is a metabolic risk factor, independently of amount of TV consumption.

Prevalence of Sedentary Behaviors in Children and Adolescents

Despite the importance to public health of studying inactivity among young people, to date there is no detailed review of the prevalence of diverse sedentary behaviors. The investigation of sedentary behaviors makes sense because independent of physical activity levels, inactivity has been associated with an impaired metabolic profile (insulin resistance) (Sardinha et al. 2008). Moreover, it has been suggested that the obesity epidemic is mainly due to the obesogenic environment to which children are exposed (Poston and Foreyt 1999).

In a systematic review (Marshall et al. 2006), including ninety studies published in English language journals between 1949 and 2004, it was observed that contemporary youth watch on average 1.8 to 2.8 h of TV per day, depending on age and gender. Boys and girls with access to video games spend approximately 60 and 23 min per day, respectively, using this technology. Computer use accounts for an additional 30 min per day. The authors of this review concluded that, for children with access to a television set, the number of hours spent viewing TV does not appear to have increased over the past 50 years (Marshall et al. 2006).

On the other hand, there are strong differences in TV consumption between countries. As shown in Fig. 20.1, adolescents in Nordic countries seem to watch less TV as compared with other developed countries. In contrast, the USA and Brazil present a high percentage of adolescents that are not meeting the screen time cut-off of 2 h per day. In addition, almost a third of US adolescents are considered "high TV users" (watch more than 4 h per day) (Fig. 20.2). Scottish and Welsh adolescents spend equally long hours in front of TV. Again, as is shown in Fig. 20.2, a small number of Finnish adolescents are classified as "high TV users."

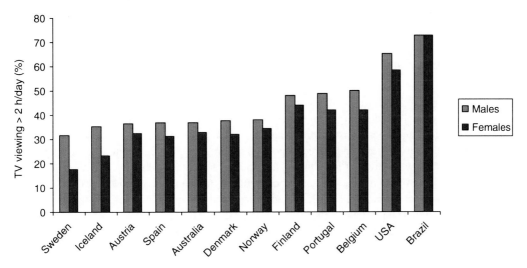

Fig. 20.1 Percentage of adolescents not meeting the TV guidelines (more than 2 h per day). Sources: Spain (te Velde et al. 2007), Finland (Tammelin et al. 2007), Austria (te Velde et al. 2007), Norway (te Velde et al. 2007), Sweden (te Velde et al. 2007), Belgium (te Velde et al. 2007), Iceland (te Velde et al. 2007), Denmark (te Velde et al. 2007), Netherlands (te Velde et al. 2007), Portugal (te Velde et al. 2007), USA (Eisenmann et al. 2008), Brazil (Wells et al. 2008), Australia (Scully et al. 2007)

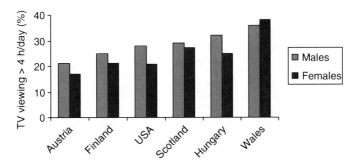

Fig. 20.2 Percentage of adolescents classified as high "TV users" (more than 4 h per day). Sources: Finland (Tammelin et al. 2007), Austria (Samdal et al. 2007), Hungary (Samdal et al. 2007), Wales (Samdal et al. 2007), Scotland (Samdal et al. 2007), USA (Dowda et al. 2001)

Strong ideological differences are found between Nordic countries and other developed countries. The television systems in the Scandinavian countries have been strictly regulated owing to political and cultural matters. Television should be used as a public service in the interest of the citizens in a democratic society. For instance, Scandinavian television stations only broadcast a few hours each day; and even in the 1970s and 1980s, the normal broadcasting time was between 5 P.M. and 11 P.M. The opposite is found in some countries like the USA, where a huge number of TV channels are provided, creating personalized TV for the consumer. It is tempting to speculate that geographic variation in the prevalence of sedentary behavior correlates with geographic variation in the prevalence of overweight in adolescents. For instance, in the Health Behavior in School-Aged Children Survey (Janssen et al. 2005), the three countries with the highest prevalence of overweight in adolescents were Malta (25.4%), the United States (25.1%), and Wales (21.2%).

However, it could happen that even if young people meet the current recommendations of screen time, the diverse sedentary behavior of young people (studying, talking with friends, passive transportation ...) could equally produce a low daily total energy expenditure and weight gain to adulthood.

Sedentary Behaviors and Obesity

Studies involving healthy children and/or adolescents aged 2–18 years and published between 1990 and April 2007 were included in a comprehensive systematic review of the relationship between sedentary behaviors and obesity in children and adolescents (Rey-López et al. 2008). Seventy-one studies met the inclusion criteria and were categorized as: cross-sectional, longitudinal or intervention studies. The studies were divided into three categories of sedentary behavior: TV viewing, use of video games (video games console) and use of computers (browsing the internet, etc). We identified 28 longitudinal studies regarding the role of sedentary behavior in the development of overweight/obesity, most of which have been carried out in the USA. For TV viewing, most of the studies reported a positive association between television viewing and adiposity, mainly in children younger than 10 at baseline, suggesting that TV viewing is a risk factor for the development of overweight/obesity in children (Rey-López et al. 2008).

Are Sedentary Behaviors Displacing Physical Activity?

Several mechanisms have been presented to explain the obesogenic effect of TV. Since TV watching does not seem to displace physical activity (Rey-López et al. 2008), one of the possibilities linking TV viewing and obesity is a higher energy intake while watching TV. In European adolescents, no associations were found between TV viewing and physical activity measured with accelerometers (Ekelund et al. 2006).

Robinson (1999) performed a randomized controlled school-based trial, including two socio-demographically and scholastically matched public elementary schools in San Jose, California. Of 198 third- and fourth-grade students, who were given parental consent to participate, 192 students (mean age, 8.9 years) completed the study. Children in one elementary school received an 18-lesson, 6-month classroom curriculum to reduce television, videotape, and video game use. The primary body composition measurement was body mass index. In this study, no changes were observed in moderate and vigorous physical activity levels, although sedentary behavior decreased.

Are All the Sedentary Behaviors Equally Obesogenic?

The use of video games (video games console) and the use of computers (playing computer games, browsing the internet, etc.) seems not to be associated with obesity risk (Rey-López et al. 2008). Regarding video games play, the majority of cross-sectional studies did not find an association between playing video games and obesity, and the same relationship was found in two longitudinal studies, although more research is needed.

O'Loughlin et al. (2000) conducted a prospective cohort study of fourth- and fifth-grade students in 16 elementary schools located in multiethnic, low-income neighborhoods in Montreal (Canada). Subjects included 2318 children aged 9–12 years with baseline and 1-year follow up data and 633 children aged 9–11 years with baseline and 2-year follow-up data. Although 1-year predictors of the highest decile of BMI increase included playing video games everyday in girls (odds ratio (OR) = 2.48, 95% confidence interval (CI) = 1.04–5.92), when 2-year predictors were examined, video games was not associated with excess weight gain in both sexes.

Gordon-Larsen et al. (2002) studied US nationally representative data from 12,759 participants in the National Longitudinal Study of Adolescent Health (1995 and 1996). Data on TV/video viewing and video game/computer use were obtained from questionnaires. Multivariate models assessed the association of overweight with initial (and 1-year change) activity and inactivity levels, controlling for age, ethnicity, socio-economic status, urban residence, cigarette smoking, and region of residence. Overweight prevalence was only positively associated with high level TV/video viewing among white boys (OR = 1.52; 95% CI = 1.08–2.14) and girls (OR = 2.45; 95% CI = 1.51–3.97). Moreover, the new generation of video games elicit a higher energy expenditure during the play than traditional ones (Graves et al. 2007). Although these active video games could prevent the weight gain, up to now, they are far of the physiological responses of exercise (Graves et al. 2007).

Finally, we did not find longitudinal studies that focused exclusively on computer use.

Television Watching and Obesity

The seminal study by Dietz and Gortmaker (1985) was the first to publish the relationship linking high TV viewing with a higher risk of overweight or obesity. Since then, the evidence has expanded to support this relationship. We have recently found in a representative sample of Spanish adolescents, that risk of overweight was increased by 15.8% per each hour of TV viewing (Vicente-Rodriguez et al. 2008). The majority of the cross-sectional studies published in the literature found significant associations with obesity in both children and adolescents. The Youth Risk Behavior Survey (YRBS) from the Centers for Disease Control and Prevention shows interesting results (Eisenmann et al. 2008). Participants were cross-tabulated into nine physical activity (PA)-TV groups using self-reported measurements to assess moderate PA (MPA) or vigorous PA (VPA) (low MPA or low VPA: doing moderate or vigorous physical activity ≤2 days per week; moderate MPA or moderate VPA: doing moderate or vigorous physical activity between 3 and 5 days per week; high MPA or high VPA: doing moderate or vigorous physical activity between 6 and 7 days per week) and TV (low: ≤1 h per day; moderate: 2 to 3 h per day; high: ≥4 h per day). In general, boys and girls watching low levels of TV did not have an increased risk of overweight regardless of PA level. Girls who watched moderate to high levels of TV had an increased risk of overweight at any level of MPA or VPA ranging from 1.27 to 3.11. In contrast, girls with high TV/low VPA had the highest risk of overweight (OR = 3.11) compared with those with a low TV/high VPA.

Although there is longitudinal evidence that TV viewing is a risk factor for the development of obesity (being more important in children than in adolescents), TV time levels seem to decrease during the transition to adulthood (Gorely et al. 2007), despite which overweight or obesity prevalences might increase. This could be explained by two factors. First, levels of physical activity decrease dramatically during adolescence; and second, adolescence is a period when new sedentary pursuits are adopted (more time studying, sitting and talking and playing with computer and video games).

TV viewing is not the opposite of physical activity. Currently, it is not well known whether sedentary time displaces time that would otherwise be used for physical activity. According to the intervention study by Robinson (1999), no changes took place in moderate and vigorous physical activity levels, although sedentary behavior decreased. A recent study in which adolescents were split into two groups according to their socioeconomic status (SES) also supports this (Mutunga et al. 2006). Adolescents in the high SES group used TVs and computers far more, despite being at lower risk of obesity. Nevertheless, this greater use of TV was compensated by higher levels of physical activity and lower energy intake. Moreover, some reviews have found that the relationship between physical activity and TV viewing is close to zero (Marshall et al. 2004; Sallis et al. 2000). TV viewing probably affects energy intake more than energy expenditure, as it is often associated with a higher intake of sweetened drinks and high energy-dense foods.

A novel risk factor for weight gain in adolescents has been introduced in relation with television viewing. The Intervention Centered on Adolescents' Physical Activity and Sedentary Behavior (ICAPS) carried out on French adolescents reported that having a TV in the bedroom was associated with higher BMI, waist circumference and body fat (in boys). However, these results were not found in girls.

Considering the relationship between TV watching and obesity, the American Academy of Pediatrics recommends that clinicians advise patients and their families to limit television and other screen time, by allowing a maximum of 2 h of screen time per day and removing televisions and other screens from children's primary sleeping area (Barlow 2007).

Finally, it must be remembered that although its obesogenic effect seems to be clear, the lack of increase in TV viewing over the last three decades means that it cannot be implicated as the main driver of the rise in obesity prevalence. Thus, there must be additional environmental factors that need to be considered to explain the obesity epidemic.

Video Games and Obesity

Up to now, research regarding the effects of video games on obesity has been rare. Four of those studies that independently analyzed the effect of playing video games found a significant obesogenic effect in both sexes, and one in only boys. The majority of longitudinal studies did not find an association between video game use and obesity risk in both sexes (Rey-López et al. 2008). For instance, overweight prevalence was not associated with video games use during 1 year of follow-up in US adolescents (OR = 1.08, 95% CI = 0.89–1.30) (Gordon-Larsen et al. 2002). When video game use was combined with computer time and TV time, the aggregated measure often resulted in a significant association with overweight and obesity, but in this case it is not possible to determine whether it was due to the total amount of sedentary behavior, or whether video games significantly accounted for this relationship. A recent study in Portuguese children (Carvalhal et al. 2007) and in Spanish adolescents (Vicente-Rodriguez et al. 2008), found that time spent playing electronic games was associated with overweight.

There are few longitudinal studies that include video game playing as sedentary behavior. Only one study revealed a significant relationship between the use of video games and excessive weight gain and that was in girls. Two other studies did not find this relationship. And no studies found the relationship in boys; all showed a lack of effect on obesity risk. The following are some factors that could explain these null effects: (a) less time devoted to playing games than watching TV; (b) the presence of a calorie intake-free behavior because the video game device is held with both hands; (c) higher energy expenditure due to this behavior. In fact, energy expenditure varies significantly depending on the video game used (Lanningham-Foster et al. 2006). In conclusion, the few published data do not suggest that video games have negative effects on body composition.

Computers and Obesity

Despite the fact that these new technologies were introduced during the last two decades, the literature regarding their effects on body composition is quite limited. As happened with video games, computer use has been scarcely investigated as a single entity isolated e.g., from TV and video games. Again, the effect on obesity observed in cross-sectional studies is not clear. Less than half of the studies showed a relationship, with the rest showing a null effect of computer use on obesity development (Rey-López et al. 2008). None of the longitudinal studies found an association between computer use and overweight and/or obesity. Nevertheless, most of the studies considered all sedentary activities together. Therefore, more studies are necessary to understand the effect of computer use on the development of obesity.

In summary, the questionnaires used to quantify computer time do not value the specific impact of computer use on body composition. However, these initial results do not suggest that computer use can cause obesity.

Food Habits Associated with Sedentary Behaviors

TV viewing has been shown to be associated with extra calorie intake during watching time (Van den Bulck and Van Mierlo 2004). Additionally, when watching TV, children are exposed to an increasing number of advertisements of foods high in fat, sugar and salt, whereas food items such as fruit and vegetables are rarely advertised.

Coon et al. (2001) showed that children from families watching TV during two or more meals a day consumed fruit and vegetables less frequently and pizza/salty snacks more frequently than did children from families where the TV was switched off at meals or switched on for just one meal. Several studies have documented the increased intake of snack foods and calories among adolescents watching more TV (Vereecken et al. 2006). The relationship with fruits and vegetables has been more recently studied. Lowry et al. (2002) found strong associations between TV viewing and eating insufficient amounts of fruits and vegetables for white students. No associations were found for black students and an inverse association was found for Hispanic male students, suggesting that the influence of TV on food habits could be gender-, race- or culture-specific (Lowry et al. 2002).

To further investigate whether the associations between TV viewing and food are country-specific or whether a general pattern exists, an international study collected data from 162,305 young people completing the 2001/2002 Health Behavior in School-Aged Children Survey, a World Health Organization cross-national study in 35 countries, on health and health behaviors among 11-, 13- and 15-year-old students (Vereecken et al. 2006). Those watching more TV were more likely to consume sweets and soft drinks on a daily basis and less likely to consume fruit and vegetables daily, although the latter associations were not so apparent among Central and Eastern European countries.

Similar results have been observed in children and young adolescents from Australia and New Zealand (Salmon et al. 2006; Utter et al. 2006). Efforts to reduce the amount of time children spend watching TV may result in better dietary habits and weight control for children and adolescents.

As much as we know, no studies have addressed the associated food pattern in some sedentary behaviors (such as internet use). The multi-center European study (HELENA Study) (Moreno et al. 2008) will soon provide comprehensive information about this issue.

Conclusions

Physical activity and sedentary behaviors are different constructs and have particular correlates. Nonetheless, despite the lack of association between TV viewing and physical activity, it is likely that promoting daily exercise in children and adolescents can reduce other unhealthy behaviors (example: long hours of TV viewing eating junk food). There is evidence that excessive TV viewing promotes obesity in children and adolescents, but this does not occur for video games and computer use. However, more healthy effects are obtained doing any kind of exercise rather than playing with active electronic games.

An expert committee, comprised of representatives from 15 US professional organizations, published a set of recommendations based on the available evidence that may help to prevent excessive weight gain (Barlow 2007). These recommendations involved eating, physical activity, and reducing time devoted to sedentary behaviors. Regarding sedentary behaviors, it was recommended that there be no television viewing before 2 years of age and thereafter no more than 2 h of television viewing per day. Moreover, TV sets and other screens should be removed from children's primary sleeping areas. Television viewing time is often associated with a higher intake of sweetened drinks and high energy-dense food (Vereecken et al. 2006), and therefore, a higher energy intake is the most likely reason of the obesogenic effect produced by television viewing.

References

Barlow, S.E. (2007). Expert committee recommendaions regarding the prevention, assessment, and treatment of child and adolescent overweight and obesity: summary report. *Pediatrics, 120*, 164–192.

Bleich, S., Cutler, D., Murray, C., & Adams, A. (2008). Why is the developed world obese? *Annual Reviews of Public Health, 29*, 273–295.

Bryant, M.J., Lucove, J.C., Evenson, K.R., & Marshall, S. (2007). Measurement of television viewing in children and adolescents: a systematic review. *Obesity Reviews, 8*, 197–209.

Carvalhal, M.M., Padez, M.C., Moreira, P.A., & Rosado, V.M. (2007). Overweight and obesity related to activities in Portuguese children, 7-9 years. *European Journal of Public Health, 17*, 42–46.

Coon, K.A., Goldberg, J., Rogers, B.L., & Tucker, K.L. (2001). Relationships between use of television during meals and children's food consumption patterns. *Pediatrics, 107*, 1–9.

Dietz, W.H., Jr., & Gortmaker, S.L. (1985). Do we fatten our children at the television set? Obesity and television viewing in children and adolescents. *Pediatrics, 75*, 807–812.

Dowda, M., Ainsworth, B.E., Addy, C.L., Saunders, R., & Riner, W. (2001). Environmental influences, physical activity, and weight status in 8- to 16-year-olds. *Archives of Pediatrics and Adolescent Medicine, 155*, 711–717.

Eaton, S.B., Konner, M., & Shostak, M. (1988). Stone agers in the fast lane: chronic degenerative diseases in evolutionary perspective. *American Journal of Medicine, 84*, 739–749.

Eisenmann, J.C., Bartee, R.T., Smith, D.T., Welk, G.J., & Fu, Q. (2008). Combined influence of physical activity and television viewing on the risk of overweight in US youth. *International Journal of Obesity, 32*, 613–618.

Ekelund, U., Brage, S., Froberg, K., Harro, M., Anderssen, S.A., Sardinha, L.B., Riddoch, C., & Andersen, L.B. (2006). TV viewing and physical activity are independently associated with metabolic risk in children: the European Youth Heart Study. *Public Library of Science Medicine, 3*, 2449–2457.

Gordon-Larsen, P., Adair, L.S., & Popkin, B.M. (2002). Ethnic differences in physical activity and inactivity patterns and overweight status. *Obesity Research, 10*, 141–149.

Gorely, T., Marshall, S.J., Biddle, S.J., & Cameron, N. (2007). The prevalence of leisure time sedentary behaviour and physical activity in adolescent girls: an ecological momentary assessment approach. *International Journal of Pediatric Obesity, 2*, 227–234.

Graves, L., Stratton, G., Ridgers, N.D., & Cable, N.T. (2007). Comparison of energy expenditure in adolescents when playing new generation and sedentary computer games: cross sectional study. *British Medical Journal, 335*, 1282–1284.

Janssen, I., Katzmarzyk, P.T., Boyce, W.F., Vereecken, C., Mulvihill, C., Roberts, C., Currie, C., & Pickett, W. (2005). Health Behaviour in School-Aged Children Obesity Working Group. Comparison of overweight and obesity prevalence in school-aged youth from 34 countries and their relationships with physical activity and dietary patterns. *Obesity Reviews, 6*, 123–132.

Keith, S.W., Redden, D.T., Katmarzyk, P.T., Boggiano, M.M., Hanlon, E.C., Benca, R.M., Ruden, D., Pietrobelli, A., Barger, J.L., Fontaine, K.R., Wang, C., Aronne, L.J., Wright, S.M., Baskin, M., Dhurandhar, N.V., Lijoi, M.C., Grilo, C.M., DeLuca, M., Westfall, A.O., & Allison, D.B. (2006). Putative contributors to the secular increase in obesity: exploring the roads less traveled. *International Journal of Obesity, 30*, 1585–1594.

Lanningham-Foster, L., Jensen, T., Foster, R., Redmond, A., Walker, B., & Heinz, D. (2006). The energetic implications of converting sedentary screen-time to active screen-time in children. *Obesity Reviews, 7*, 160.

Lowry, R., Wechsler, H., Galuska, D.A., Fulton, J.E., & Kann, L. (2002). Television viewing and its associations with overweight, sedentary lifestyle, and insufficient consumption of fruits and vegetables among US high school students: differences by race, ethnicity, and gender. *Journal of School Health, 72*, 413–421.

Marshall, S.J., Biddle, S.J., Gorely, T., Cameron, N., & Murdey, I. (2004). Relationships between media use, body fatness and physical activity in children and youth: a meta-analysis. *International Journal of Obesity, 28*, 1238–1246.

Marshall, S.J., Gorely, T., & Biddle, S.J. (2006). A descriptive epidemiology of screen-based media use in youth: a review and critique. *Journal of Adolescence, 29*, 333–349.

Moreno, L., Gonzalez-Gross, M., Kersting, M., Molnar, D., de Henauw, S., Beghin, L., Sjöström, M., Hagströmer, M., Manios, Y., Gilbert, C.C., Ortega, F.B., Dallongeville, J., Arcella, D., Wärnberg, J., Hallberg, M., Fredriksson, H., Maes, L., Widhalm, K., Kafatos, A.G., & Marcos, A. (2008). Assessing, understanding and modifying nutritional status, eating habits and physical activity in European adolescents: The HELENA (Healthy Lifestyle in Europe by Nutrition in Adolescence) Study. *Public Health Nutrition, 11*, 288–299.

Mutunga, M., Gallagher, A.M., Boreham, C., Watkins, D.C., Murray, L.J., Cran, G., & Reilly, J.J. (2006). Socioeconomic differences in risk factors for obesity in adolescents in Northern Ireland. *International Journal of Pediatric Obesity, 1*, 114–119.

O'Loughlin, J., Gray-Donald, K., Paradis, G., & Meshefedjian, G. (2000). One- and two-year predictors of excess weight gain among elementary schoolchildren in multiethnic, low-income, inner-city neighborhoods. *American Journal of Epidemiology, 15*, 739–746.

Papas, M.A., Alberg, A.J., Ewing, R., Helzlsouer, K.J., Gary, T.L., & Klassen, A.C. (2007). The built environment and obesity. *Epidemiological Reviews, 29*, 129–143.

Poston, W.S., II, & Foreyt, J.P. (1999). Obesity is an environmental issue. *Atherosclerosis, 146*, 201–209.

Prentice, A.M., & Jebb, S.A. (1995). Obesity in Britain: gluttony or sloth? *British Medical Journal, 311*, 437–439.

Rey-López, J.P., Vicente-Rodriguez, G., Biosca, M., & Moreno, L.A. (2008). Sedentary behaviour and obesity development in children and adolescents. *Nutrition, Metabolism and Cardiovascular Diseases, 18*, 242–251.

Robinson, T.N. (1999). Reducing children's television viewing to prevent obesity: a randomized controlled trial. *Journal of American Medical Association, 282*, 1561–1567.

Rodriguez, G., & Moreno, L.A. (2006). Is dietary intake able to explain differences in body fatness in children and adolescents? *Nutrition, Metabolism and Cardiovascular Diseases, 16*, 294–301.

Sallis, J.F., Prochaska, J.J., & Taylor, W.C. (2000). A review of correlates of physical activity of children and adolescents. *Medicine and Science in Sports and Exercise, 32*, 963–975.

Salmon, J., Campbell, K.J., & Crawford, D.A. (2006). Television viewing habits associated with obesity risk factors: a survey of Melbourne schoolchildren. *The Medical Journal of Australia, 184*, 64–67.

Samdal, O., Tynjala, J., Roberts, C., Sallis, J.F., Villberg, J., & Wold, B. (2007). Trends in vigorous physical activity and TV watching of adolescents from 1986 to 2002 in seven European Countries. *European Journal of Public Health, 17*, 242–248.

Sardinha, L.B., Andersen, L.B., Anderssen, S.A., Quitério, A.L., Ornelas, R., Froberg, K., Riddoch, C.J., & Ekelund, U. (2008). Objectively measured time spent sedentary is associated with insulin resistance independent of overall and central body fat in 9- to 10-year-old Portuguese children. *Diabetes Care, 31*, 569–575.

Schneider, M., Dunton, G.F., & Cooper, D.M. (2007). Media use and obesity in adolescent females. *Obesity (Silver Spring), 15*, 2328–2335.

Scully, M., Dixon, H., White, V., & Beckmann, K. (2007). Dietary, physical activity and sedentary behaviour among Australian secondary students in 2005. *Health Promotion International, 22*, 236–245.

Tammelin, T., Ekelund, U., Remes, J., & Nayha, S. (2007). Physical activity and sedentary behaviors among Finnish youth. *Medicine and Science in Sports and Exercise, 39*, 1067–1074.

te Velde, S.J., De Bourdeaudhuij, I., Thorsdottir, I., Rasmussen, M., Hagstromer, M., Klepp, K.I., & Brug, J. (2007). Patterns in sedentary and exercise behaviors and associations with overweight in 9-14-year-old boys and girls – a cross-sectional study. *BMC Public Health, 7*, 16.

Utter, J., Neumark-Sztainer, D., Jeffery, R., & Story, M. (2003). Couch potatoes or french fries: are sedentary behaviors associated with body mass index, physical activity, and dietary behaviors among adolescents? *Journal of the American Dietetic Association, 103*, 1298–1305.

Utter, J., Scragg, R., & Schaaf, D. (2006). Associations between television viewing and consumption of commonly advertised foods among New Zealand children and young adolescents. *Public Health Nutrition, 9*, 606–612.

Van den Bulck, J., & Van Mierlo, J. (2004). Energy intake associated with television viewing in adolescents: a cross sectional study. *Appetite, 43*, 181–184.

Vereecken, C.A., Todd, J., Roberts, C., Mulvihill, C., & Maes, L. (2006). Television viewing behaviour and associations with food habits in different countries. *Public Health Nutrition, 9*, 244–250.

Vicente-Rodriguez, G., Rey-López, J.P., Martin-Matillas, M., Moreno, L.A., Warnberg, J., Redondo, C., Tercedor, P., Delgado, M., Marcos, A., Castillo, M., & Bueno, M. (2008). Television watching, videogames, and excess of body fat in Spanish adolescents: the AVENA study. *Nutrition, 24*, 654–662.

Wells, J.C., Hallal, P.C., Reichert, F.F., Menezes, A.M., Araujo, C.L., & Victora, C.G. (2008). Sleep patterns and television viewing in relation to obesity and blood pressure: evidence from an adolescent Brazilian birth cohort. *International Journal of Obesity, 32*, 1042–1049.

Chapter 21
Socio-Economic Status and Obesity in Childhood

Fiona Johnson, Michelle Pratt, and Jane Wardle

Introduction

Historically, obesity was a disease of affluence; while the wealthy were able to afford ample, energy-dense food, the poor often went hungry. This pattern can still be seen in many developing countries, where lower socio-economic status (SES) is associated with food insecurity, inadequate energy intake, and malnutrition among both adults and children (UN FAO 2009). In such situations, obesity continues to be largely the preserve of those of greater affluence, although there is some evidence that this pattern is beginning to change as Western diets are increasingly adopted by middle and lower income urban populations within developing countries (Mendez et al. 2005; Wang and Lobstein 2006).

In developed countries, food scarcity rarely determines energy intake even for those at the lower end of the socio-economic spectrum, and access to high-energy palatable food is near-universal. In this context, the drivers of SES differences in rates of childhood obesity are likely to include a range of cultural, economic and educational factors. This chapter examines the evidence for an association between SES and childhood obesity across societies differing in level of economic development, and discusses the possible mechanisms underlying these differences.

Epidemiological Evidence Linking Childhood Obesity with SES

Over 100 papers have been published examining the cross-sectional association between SES and risk of childhood adiposity or obesity in different populations. In 1989, Sobal and Stunkard published a landmark review of the literature to date (together with a parallel review of adult studies) examining the association between SES and a range of continuous and categorical measures of child adiposity (Sobal and Stunkard 1989). While there were some significant associations, the relationship was not straightforward, and the 51 pediatric studies reviewed revealed a variety of positive, negative and null associations.

Results of studies from developed and developing countries were considered separately to facilitate interpretation of the findings. In developing countries, a fairly consistent association was seen,

F. Johnson and M. Pratt
Department of Epidemiology and Public Health, University College London, Gower Street, WC, 1E 6BT, UK

J. Wardle (✉)
Health Behaviour Research Centre, Department of Epidemiology and Public Health, University College London, Gower Street, WC, 1E 6BT, UK
e-mail: j.wardle@ucl.ac.uk

L.A. Moreno et al. (eds.), *Epidemiology of Obesity in Children and Adolescents*,   377
Springer Series on Epidemiology and Public Health 2, DOI 10.1007/978-1-4419-6039-9_21,
© Springer Science+Business Media, LLC 2011

with greater adiposity in children from higher SES backgrounds. Of 16 studies, 14 (88%) found that higher weight was associated with higher SES in both boys and girls, two studies (12%) found no significant relationship, and none identified an inverse relationship. The authors attributed the lower prevalence of overweight in lower SES groups to periodic or chronic food shortages together with the high energy expenditure associated with traditional, manual occupations. They also highlighted the cultural value placed on body fat in some poorer societies where adiposity is a sign of relative wealth and health (Sobal and Stunkard 1989).

Studies from developed countries produced a less conclusive picture. Of 32 studies of girls, eight (25%) reported a positive association (higher SES associated with higher rates of obesity), 11 (34%) found no relationship between SES and overweight, and 13 (41%) reported an inverse relationship. Of 34 studies of boys, nine (26%) reported a positive relationship, 14 (41%) reported no relationship, and 11 (32%) reported an inverse relationship (Sobal and Stunkard 1989). The lack of consistency in the studies from developed countries was attributed to the absence of a predominant force of the kind seen in developing countries (food shortages), and more recent work has highlighted the importance of identifying demographic and cultural moderators of the association.

In view of the rapid increases in the prevalence of childhood obesity worldwide, and the sweeping changes in food culture in both developed and developing countries in recent decades, the issue has been revisited in more recent studies. These studies have sought to establish whether the trends observed by Sobal and Stunkard (1989) have changed in the light of increasing globalization and developments in the cultural and economic environment.

Developing Countries

A small number of more recent studies from developing countries have focused specifically on children, and many have found the positive association between SES and adiposity that was observed in Sobal and Stunkard's review (Groeneveld et al. 2007; Johnson et al. 2006; Martorell et al. 2000; Wang 2001). However, there are signs that this pattern is changing, particularly in urban areas. In many developing countries urban dwellers are further removed from the traditional lifestyle of their rural compatriots, and the inhabitants of cities often adopt more westernized diets and sedentary occupations. It is among urban dwellers that the earliest signs of change to the positive association between weight and SES have become apparent (Popkin 2001; Prentice 2006). In some areas undergoing rapid economic development, the adoption of Western diets has led to a "dual-burden" situation, where both overweight and underweight are prevalent within small communities and households (Popkin 2001; Prentice 2006). However, children's nutrition and weight may respond more slowly than that of adults as countries undergo nutritional transition (Monteiro et al. 2002), and many young children remain underweight even while the prevalence of adult overweight is increasing. Studies of households and communities where underweight and overweight are both common have reported that the typical pattern is for significant levels of child underweight to be observed while the adults are becoming obese (Caballero 2005; Doak et al. 2000, 2005; Khor and Sharif 2003; Monteiro et al. 1997; Prentice 2006).

Developed Countries

The pattern is even more clearly changing in developed countries. A recent systematic review extended Sobal and Stunkard's analyses of the SES gradient in obesity in developed countries by reviewing studies of SES and adiposity in school-aged children published between 1990 and 2005

(Shrewsbury and Wardle 2008). Of a total of 45 studies that met the inclusion criteria, 19 (42%) found an inverse association, linking low SES with greater adiposity, while 12 (27%) found no association. In a further 14 studies (31%) the associations varied by subgroup (age, gender or ethnicity) with a mixture of inverse and null associations. In sharp contrast to Sobal and Stunkard's review, no studies found significant positive associations. There was evidence too that in some cases non-significant results could be attributed to lack of statistical power, since studies with sample sizes greater than 1,000 produced a higher proportion of significant inverse associations. Analyses of the magnitude of the bivariate association across the 24 studies for which this was possible, found that the odds of obesity in the lowest SES group was around twice that of the highest SES group. Since this review, further evidence supporting an inverse association has come from a very large study of data from nationally representative samples of adolescents in 35 European and North America Countries (Due et al. 2009). Here, significant negative associations between SES and overweight were seen in 21 of 24 high income countries, while associations were more mixed for the middle income countries.

Where significant SES differences in obesity have been identified, the association has often been shown to be approximately linear. Obesity is not simply restricted to the poorest group, but levels of adiposity are lower with each increment of higher SES, at least among children of white/European ethnic origin (Brophy et al. 2009; Stamatakis et al. 2010a). The association cannot, then, be attributed to the simple effects of poverty, and explanations for the effect are likely to be found in risk factors that are distributed incrementally across the SES spectrum. Explaining the link between SES and obesity in circumstances where poverty and food deprivation cannot be invoked as primary explanatory factors is complex, and the remainder of this chapter will focus on the state of understanding of the association in high income, developed countries.

Demographic Moderators of the SES-Obesity Association

A number of potential demographic moderators of the relationship between SES and childhood obesity have been proposed, although variation between studies in analytic methods and ways of reporting results has made it difficult to identify interactions between SES and other demographic factors such as age, gender or ethnicity.

Ethnicity

Many of the studies examining SES and adiposity in children have either failed to report the ethnic background of participants or have been predominantly ethnically homogenous, typically with a high proportion of children of European ancestry. Children and adults of black African or Caribbean origin have a greater risk of obesity, and this effect is independent of SES (Robert and Reither 2004; Singh et al. 2008; Wardle et al. 2006). In the few studies that have analyzed interactions between SES and ethnicity, there has been little evidence of an association between SES and adiposity in black children, while inverse relationships between SES and adiposity were seen among white children (Crawford et al. 2001; Shrewsbury and Wardle 2008). Studies of children from other ethnic groups are too few and too heterogeneous for conclusions to be drawn. This mirrors the available data for the SES-adiposity association in adults, where SES appears to play a lesser role in predicting weight and weight gain among black than white adults (Ball and Crawford 2005; Wang and Beydoun 2007; Zhang and Wang 2004).

Age

Socio-economic factors are associated with body weight from birth, although the relationship between SES and weight in very young children is not straightforward. Lower SES mothers tend to have lower birth weight babies, due to both a higher risk of premature birth (Goffinet 2005; Jansen et al. 2009; Moutquin 2003) and a higher risk of small for gestational age babies (Cammu et al. 2010; Mortensen et al. 2008; Pattenden et al. 1999). Low birth weight babies often undergo rapid "catch-up" weight gain in the first months of life and have a higher risk of later overweight regardless of SES (Ong 2006; Dubois and Girard 2006). By the pre-school years, an inverse SES gradient in child overweight is already apparent (Armstrong et al. 2003; Brophy et al. 2009; Dubois and Girard 2006; Singh et al. 2008; Wake et al. 2007).

The review by Shrewsbury and Wardle contained studies that were predominantly of children (age 5–11 years) or adolescents (aged 12–18 years), and some that included both age groups. An inverse association was found more frequently in children (10 of 18 studies) than adolescents, where only 1 of 9 studies found the association in both sexes, and a further five found it in either boys or girls. The authors note, however, that some of these studies appeared to be under-powered to detect SES differences, and another recent study using large representative adolescent samples (Due et al. 2009) found an inverse association in 21 out of 24 high income, Western countries. It seems likely that the inverse association between SES and adiposity persists throughout childhood and adolescence, but may undergo slight attenuation at adolescence.

Sex

Studies of adults have demonstrated that the association between SES and adiposity is often sex-specific. A consistent inverse association between SES and obesity has been demonstrated in women from developed countries, while the association in men is inconsistent (McLaren 2007; Sobal and Stunkard 1989). Many studies have either found no association in samples of men, or have reported a direct or curvilinear association (McLaren 2007; Sobal and Stunkard 1989). Shrewsbury and Wardle (2008) looked for sex differences across the studies included in their review to see whether there was a stronger association between SES and adiposity in girls than boys, concluding that there was little evidence for any sex differences. Where results were stratified by sex, more than half (10 of 19 studies) found consistency between the results for boys and girls. Among the remainder there was no striking trend observed for inverse associations to be more likely in one sex than the other. Although the number of studies analyzed here was too few for firm conclusions to be drawn, they provided little evidence that sex is a strong moderator of the link between adiposity and SES in either children or adolescents. It may be that sex differences in the SES-obesity association emerge only in early adulthood.

Time Trends in the Socio-Economic Gradient in Child Obesity

When results from the pre-1990 studies from developed countries reviewed by Sobal and Stunkard (1989) are compared with those from more recent work, there are striking differences. The first review reported a variety of inverse, null and positive associations in developed countries, while later studies suggest that the protective effect of lower SES seen in some pre-1990 studies has entirely disappeared.

Data from a number of Western countries suggest that the socio-economic gradient in child obesity has been increasing over time. Two UK studies have analyzed obesity prevalence trends between 1974–2003 and 1997–2007 (Stamatakis et al. 2005, 2010b) and have identified an increase in obesity disparities by SES, in both boys and girls. The most recent of these, which used data from the Health Survey for England (an annual, nationally-representative, health survey), developed an "SES position score" based on families' income position and social class in order to evaluate whether SES had a cumulative effect on obesity prevalence. The results demonstrated that while the overall prevalence of obesity in children appears to be stabilizing, this is not true for children from the lowest SES families.

Similar patterns have been seen elsewhere. An Australian study, using a school-level measure of SES that classified schools as low, medium or high SES, also found that levels of overweight and obesity in 2006 were comparable to those in 2000, except in lower SES schools where levels of obesity were continuing to increase (O'Dea and Dibley 2010). However, not all researchers have found evidence that social disparities are increasing. A study of French children reported that the socio-economic gradient in overweight remained of a similar magnitude between 1998–1999 and 2006–2007 (Lioret et al. 2009), while a US study (Wang and Beydoun 2007) concluded that the gradient weakened in the United States between 1971–1975 and 1999–2002. Nonetheless, it seems likely that, at least in some Western countries, the SES gradient is becoming greater over time due to disproportionate increases in overweight among the lowest SES groups.

Measurement of SES

A variety of different markers have been used to classify the SES of participants in studies of child overweight and obesity, and the use of different markers may partially account for differences in findings between studies. Traditional markers of SES (income, level of education and social class based on occupation) cannot be used directly with children, meaning that family, community, or school-level approaches are generally used. While these different SES markers are inter-correlated, the magnitude of these correlations (typically less than 0.50) does not justify the assumption that they are measuring a single construct (Braveman et al. 2005). This highlights the importance of selecting appropriate measures of SES for addressing a particular research question. This is particularly important in studies with an interest in causal mechanisms, since different SES markers may be associated with different risk factors (Sobal 1991). Lower family income imposes economic constraints on food purchasing, while lower levels of parental education might be linked to poor nutrition knowledge or a lower value being placed on dietary health. This is supported by an Australian study which found that nutrition knowledge partially mediated the association between low educational attainment and diet, while the association between low household income and healthy food purchasing was partially mediated by food cost concern (Turrell and Kavanagh 2006).

Area-Level Indicators

The characteristics of the neighborhood in which a child lives have often been used as a proxy for the socio-economic position of the child's family, particularly where collection of family-level data is difficult; for example in developing countries (Sobal and Stunkard 1989). It has obvious advantages in terms of the ease of data collection but there is an inevitable loss of precision when used as a proxy for family SES. Neighborhood characteristics can be seen as purely descriptive of the individuals who reside there, reflecting the social, cultural, educational, occupational or economic characteristics of the inhabitants. However area characteristics may also have a direct effect on diet and physical activity, through the availability of facilities for food purchasing, transport, leisure and through the projection of dominant social and cultural norms relating to food, eating behavior and physical activity (Black and Macinko 2008; Ford and Dzewaltowski 2008). Neighborhood indicators have been found to add explanatory value to individual level measures of disadvantage for a range of health outcomes in children (BeLue et al. 2009; Janssen et al. 2006; Sellström and Bremberg 2006), suggesting that they are not simply a less precise measure of individual SES.

Family-Level Indicators

Most measures of SES used with children are family-level markers, typically based on parental income, level of education or occupation, or a composite measure combining two or more of these. An alternative approach, which has been used in some studies with children and adolescents, is to create a "family affluence scale" that measures SES in terms of family ownership of a range of consumer and lifestyle goods and services (Currie et al. 1997, 2008; Wardle et al. 2002a). The advantage of this approach is that adolescents themselves are generally able to report accurately on consumer goods (e.g. does the family have a dishwasher), but they may not know detail of their parents education, income or occupation (Wardle et al. 2002a). Where several SES markers have been used, it has been possible to examine which of them is most closely associated with adiposity. Parental income, education and occupation have been shown to be independently associated with child overweight (Shrewsbury and Wardle 2008), and a small number of studies have used multiple markers allowing comparisons to be made. A study of child obesity trends in children of differing SES suggested that parental occupation was less strongly predictive of increases in childhood obesity over time than family income (Stamatakis et al. 2005). The majority of studies have found the strongest single SES predictor of child obesity to be parental, or particularly maternal, education (Shrewsbury and Wardle 2008). This may be partly because parental education has the benefit of being relatively stable; it does not fluctuate according to transient life events, as income or occupation can. Education also has the advantage of being a modifiable factor and it has been suggested that it provides a possible route for family intervention to reduce obesity risk (Brophy et al. 2009), although it is not clear how far education interventions directly affect lifestyle risk factors for child overweight.

Some studies have made use of composite measures of SES, composed of an aggregation of several different indicators. This approach might be thought to maximize the observed effect of risk factors associated with different aspects of SES, but composite measures that do not include an indicator for education do not always outperform education-based measures (Lioret et al. 2009). These problems have led to calls for more thoughtful attention to the choice of SES indicator in health research, linking the measurement strategy to outcomes and putative mechanisms under investigation (Braveman et al. 2005; Shavers 2007).

Putative Causal Mechanisms in the Association Between SES and Obesity

A number of possible mechanisms for the association between SES and obesity in children have been suggested. In developing countries, the single most significant factor behind the direct association between SES and adiposity is likely to be, as it was two decades ago, the effects of food shortages. Rapid changes in availability and affordability of energy dense foods and a shift from active to more sedentary lifestyles have been implicated in the increasing levels of obesity among low income families in developing countries (Popkin 2001).

A further factor that has been hypothesized to increase the vulnerability of individuals exposed to under-nutrition once food is available is the "thrifty phenotype" hypothesis (Hales and Barker 2001). According to this hypothesis, fetal exposure to inadequate nutrition can initiate metabolic and endocrine changes which are adaptive in situations where food continues to be in short supply, but predispose to weight gain if nutritional conditions subsequently improve. Both over-nutrition and under-nutrition in utero may contribute to a predisposition to adiposity in later life (Robinson and Godfrey 2008; Taylor and Poston 2007). There is some evidence that the timing of prenatal exposures may be critical (Ravelli et al. 1976), so although this hypothesis may explain some of the variance in weight gain propensity on an individual level, it seems unlikely to account for a large proportion of the SES gradient in child obesity in developed countries.

Built Environment/Neighborhood Factors

It has been suggested that characteristics of the built environment in lower SES residential areas might be less conducive to health-promoting lifestyles. Much of the evidence for reduced access to healthy foods and opportunities for physical activity in low SES neighborhoods comes from the United States, where poorer neighborhoods tend to have less access to large food stores and leisure exercise facilities, and more fast food outlets (Beaulac et al. 2009; Ford and Dzewaltowski 2008; Larson et al. 2009; Lovasi et al. 2009). A lack of studies of local environments in other Western countries means that it is unclear how far this can be extrapolated outside the United States (Papas et al. 2007). Some studies have linked features of the built environment that might encourage or discourage physical activity to child overweight, although a recent review of studies of child over-weight and physical activity-related aspects of the built environment (e.g. facilities for outside play and active modes of transportation) did not find consistent relationships, concluding that there is insufficient evidence to identify whether, and which, features of the built environment are associated with child obesity (Dunton et al. 2009). In fact it has proved difficult even to link such neighborhood characteristics to levels of physical activity in children – although associations are more likely to be found when perceived measures of neighborhood environment are used rather than objective measures (Ferreira et al. 2007; Salmon and Timperio 2007). While neighborhood is associated with obesity independently of the SES of the individual (Lovasi et al. 2009), there is little evidence for a causal relationship between the built environment of the residents and overweight.

An alternative explanation is that the prevailing social norms on a neighborhood level have an influence on the weight-related behaviors of inhabitants. Neighborhood cultural norms have been demonstrated to affect the behavior of individuals in a variety of health-related domains including smoking (Ahern et al. 2009) and alcohol consumption (Ahern et al. 2008), and the same may be true of child feeding and lifestyle practices. Therefore those whose own socio-economic circumstances are discordant with those of their neighbors may, nonetheless, adopt lifestyle behaviors characteristic of the dominant culture of their living environment.

Parental Overweight

One of the strongest risk factors for overweight in children is parental overweight (Parsons et al. 1999). The steep SES gradient in adult female adiposity means that samples of low SES families inevitably have a higher proportion of overweight mothers, and parental (or at least maternal) obesity is likely to account for at least a portion of the association between family SES and child obesity. The mode of transmission of weight phenotype from parent to child seems certain to be multifactorial. Twin studies indicate that there is a strong genetic predisposition to weight gain (Wardle and Carnell 2009), and adoption studies typically find no more than a modest effect of the shared family environment (Sørensen and Stunkard 1993). Genetic resemblance therefore probably explains a major part of the familial associations, but there are also a number of environmental exposures that could affect children of overweight mothers, regardless of SES. These include over- and under-nutrition in the fetal period (Armitage et al. 2008; Cedergren 2004; Lawlor and Chaturvedi 2006), non-adoption or early termination of breastfeeding (Amir and Donath 2007; Thulier and Mercer 2009), and lack of control over children's eating on the part of overweight mothers (Wardle et al. 2002b). Because of the strong SES gradient of weight in women, these risk factors will be more prevalent among women of low SES.

There is evidence that the link between SES and adiposity is independent of parental BMI; in five out of nine studies reviewed by Shrewsbury and Wardle (2008) that included parental BMI as a covariate, a significant inverse association persisted, demonstrating that SES is not simply a crude proxy for parental adiposity. Maternal BMI and family SES have been shown to interact in predicting childhood overweight, such that the risk associated with parental overweight is greater in low SES families (Semmler et al. 2009). This finding is consistent with the existence of a gene-environment interaction, whereby environments associated with lower SES are more conducive to the expression of genes conferring a predisposition for weight gain.

Lifestyle Factors: Eating Behavior, and Physical Activity

Differences in diet, exercise and sedentary behavior have been shown to be associated with SES in adults (Jeffery et al. 1991; Margetts et al. 1998), adolescents (Craig and Mindell 2008; Hanson and Chen 2007; van der Horst et al. 2007a, b), and children (Sisson et al. 2009). Young people from lower SES backgrounds spend more of their leisure time in sedentary pursuits (Sisson et al. 2009), have a lower intake of fruit and vegetables, and a higher intake of dietary fat and refined sugar (Hanson and Chen 2007). Such behavioral factors, which directly affect energy balance, are inevitably proximal influences on the higher prevalence of obesity in low SES children, but a range of socio-cultural influences might be assumed to underlie these differences in behavior.

Attitudes, Beliefs and Perceptions

Environmental influences operating at the socio-cultural level, such as attitudes and beliefs related to weight, overweight and health, have consistently been shown to vary by SES. Adults of higher SES have greater health consciousness, greater belief in the potential for individual control of weight and health, and perceive lifestyle factors to be more important in determining health than those of lower SES (The King's Fund 2004; Wardle and Steptoe 2003). They also have better nutrition knowledge (Parmenter et al. 2000), and respond more positively towards public health messages (Iversen and Kraft 2006; The King's Fund 2004). Attitudes towards body weight and perceptions of what constitutes a normal weight vary by SES in both adults (Wardle and Griffith 2001) and adolescents (Wardle et al. 2004), with those of lower SES perceiving a larger body shape to be more normal than those of higher SES. Lower maternal education has been associated with poor recognition of a child's excess weight on the part of mothers in some (Baughcum et al. 2000; Genovesi et al. 2005; Manios et al. 2009) but not all studies (Adams et al. 2005; Carnell et al. 2005). Higher SES women and girls are also more likely to be concerned about their weight and attempting to lose weight (Adams et al. 2000; Wardle and Griffith 2001; Wardle and Marsland 1990; Wardle et al. 2004). These differences in weight attitudes appear to emerge by late childhood, with children's weight attitudes mirroring those of their parents.

Parental Feeding and the Home Food Environment

Laissez-faire or fatalistic attitudes towards health and weight can influence the way in which parents feed their young children. Several qualitative studies of low income mothers in the US have identified attitudes and feeding practices which may contribute to a failure to promote a healthy weight in their children (Baughcum et al. 1998; Jain et al. 2001; Kaiser et al. 1999). The lower income mothers interviewed for these studies expressed a preference for a larger baby, and many worried that their child might not be getting enough to eat. Mothers of older children described using food as a parenting tool (as a reward or a bribe) and were unwilling to set limits for their children's eating. They were unable to judge whether their own children were overweight, lacked knowledge about healthy eating, and were mistrustful of the health promotion messages of health professionals; preferring to rely on the advice of their own mothers.

Because few qualitative studies have been carried out in families from higher SES backgrounds it is not possible to make direct comparisons, but quantitative studies support the proposition that maternal feeding practices vary by SES. Parental feeding styles are reliably associated with child weight (Ventura and Birch 2008) and feeding style has been shown to differ by SES from birth. Mothers from lower SES backgrounds are less likely to initiate breastfeeding and if they do, they breastfeed for a shorter duration and introduce solids at an earlier age (James et al. 1997; Robinson et al. 2007; Thulier and Mercer 2009; Wijndaele et al. 2009); both of which have been associated with higher adiposity in childhood. There is some evidence that lower SES is associated with less maternal control over the child's eating and more feeding in response to a child's emotional distress (Saxton et al. 2009). A number of other aspects of the food environment have been associated with both SES and diet quality, including the availability and accessibility of healthy and unhealthy food in the home, the social and physical characteristics of mealtimes (Patrick and Nicklas 2005), and television watching during meals (Horodynski et al. 2010).

Conclusions

The prevailing picture is that as countries move away from food poverty, obesity in children starts to become more prevalent overall and the traditional positive association between SES and obesity begins to disappear, ultimately reversing as obesity rates rise faster in lower SES groups. In most developed countries, obesity rates show a graded negative association with SES, with the effect being equally strong in boys and girls, and emerging in early childhood. This association seems to be becoming more pronounced over time, and the mixture of positive, negative and null associations seen in Sobal and Stunkard's 1989 review has resolved into a more consistent picture of greater adiposity among lower SES children (Due et al. 2009; Shrewsbury and Wardle 2008).

The causal mechanisms underlying the positive association between SES and obesity in low-income countries seem fairly straightforward; in these contexts, lower SES means greater exposure to food insecurity and chronic food scarcity. In developed countries the explanation is more complex. The fact that the SES-obesity association is graded rather than there being any particular income/education threshold, points to explanatory risk factors that are likewise incrementally distributed across levels of SES. Sobal and Stunkard's conclusions from their review of SES-obesity associations in children and adults proposed deliberate healthy lifestyle choices as protective against obesity in higher SES women; implicating personal agency in the mechanism. More recent work tends to highlight environmental factors, either physical (such as food availability or the built environment) or psychosocial (such as norms for food consumption). In practice both are likely to be important; higher SES individuals have better knowledge of nutrition, more positive attitudes towards healthy lifestyles, and are more likely to live in environments in which healthy choices are easier.

SES has been measured in a wide variety of ways, but parental education has shown the strongest and most consistent association with child overweight. This suggests that economic factors are not the primary drivers of the SES-obesity association in Western children. It is unclear however, how far the link between parental education and obesity is causal, and thus whether increasing nutrition education and improving diet and lifestyle knowledge for parents with a poor educational history might alleviate the additional obesity risk burden for low SES children.

Parenting, and particularly child feeding styles, are reliably associated with children's eating and weight gain (Ventura and Birch 2008), although this may not entirely represent a causal process from parent to child. Parental responsiveness to characteristics of the child which are themselves indicative of a higher propensity for weight gain, such as higher food responsiveness (Webber et al. 2010) are also likely to play an important role. Similarly, while differences in the home food environment are strongly implicated in the association between SES and child obesity, there is little direct evidence in the literature to date to confirm whether these are direct mediators of the association, and appropriate targets for focused intervention. These uncertainties point to the need for a major emphasis in research and policy to reduce inequalities in childhood nutritional status.

References

Adams, K., Sargent, R.G., Thompson, S.H., Richter, D., Corwin, S.J., & Rogan, T.J. (2000). A study of body weight concerns and weight control practices of 4th and 7th grade adolescents. *Ethnicity & Health, 5,* 79–94.

Adams, A.K., Quinn, R.A., & Prince, R.J. (2005). Low recognition of childhood overweight and disease risk among native-American caregivers. *Obesity Research, 13,* 146–152.

Ahern, J., Galea, S., Hubbard, A., Midanik, L., & Syme, S.L. (2008). "Culture of drinking" and individual problems with alcohol use. *American Journal of Epidemiology, 167,* 1041–1049.

Ahern, J., Galea, S., Hubbard, A., & Syme, S.L. (2009). Neighborhood smoking norms modify the relation between collective efficacy and smoking behavior. *Drug and Alcohol Dependence, 100,* 138–145.

Amir, L.H., & Donath, S. (2007). A systematic review of maternal obesity and breastfeeding intention, initiation and duration. *BMC Pregnancy and Childbirth, 7,* 9.

Armitage, J.A., Poston, L., & Taylor, P.D. (2008). Developmental origins of obesity and the metabolic syndrome: the role of maternal obesity. *Frontiers of Hormone Research, 36,* 73–84.

Armstrong, J., Dorosty, A.R., Reilly, J.J., & Emmett, P.M. (2003). Coexistence of social inequalities in undernutrition and obesity in preschool children: population based cross sectional study. *Archives of Disease in Childhood, 88,* 671–675.

Ball, K., & Crawford, D. (2005). Socioeconomic status and weight change in adults: a review. *Social Science & Medicine, 60,* 1987–2010.

Baughcum, A.E., Burklow, K.A., Deeks, C.M., Powers, S.W., & Whitaker, R.C. (1998). Maternal feeding practices and childhood obesity: a focus group study of low-income mothers. *Archives of Pediatrics & Adolescent Medicine, 152,* 1010–1014.

Baughcum, A.E., Chamberlin, L.A., Deeks, C.M., Powers, S.W., & Whitaker, R.C. (2000). Maternal perceptions of overweight preschool children. *Pediatrics, 106,* 1380–1386.

Beaulac, J., Kristjansson, E., & Cummins, S. (2009). A systematic review of food deserts, 1966–2007. *Preventing Chronic Disease, 6,* A105.

BeLue, R., Francis, L. A., Rollins, B., & Colaco, B. (2009). One size does not fit all: identifying risk profiles for overweight in adolescent population subsets. *The Journal of Adolescent Health, 45,* 517–524.

Black, J.L., & Macinko, J. (2008). Neighborhoods and obesity. *Nutrition Reviews, 66,* 2–20.

Braveman, P.A., Cubbin, C., Egerter, S., Chideya, S., Marchi, K.S., Metzler, M., & Posner, S. (2005). Socioeconomic status in health research: one size does not fit all. *The Journal of the American Medical Association, 294,* 2879–2888.

Brophy, S., Cooksey, R., Gravenor, M.B., Mistry, R., Thomas, N., Lyons, R.A., & Williams, R. (2009). Risk factors for childhood obesity at age 5: analysis of the millennium cohort study. *BMC Public Health, 9,* 467.

Caballero, B. (2005). A nutrition paradox – underweight and obesity in developing countries. *New England Journal of Medicine, 352,* 1514–1516.

Cammu, H., Martens, G., Van Maele, G., & Amy, J.J. (2010). The higher the educational level of the first-time mother, the lower the fetal and post-neonatal but not the neonatal mortality in Belgium (Flanders). *European Journal of Obstetrics, Gynecology and Reproductive Biology, 148,* 13–16.

Carnell, S., Edwards, C., Croker, H., Boniface, D., & Wardle, J. (2005). Parental perceptions of overweight in 3–5 y olds. *International Journal of Obesity (Lond), 29,* 353–355.

Cedergren, M.I. (2004). Maternal morbid obesity and the risk of adverse pregnancy outcome. *Obstetrics and Gynecology, 103,* 219–224.

Craig, R., & Mindell, J. (Eds.) (2008). *The Health Survey for England 2006: CVD and risk factors adults, obesity and risk factors children.* Leeds: Information Centre.

Crawford, P.B., Story, M., Wang, M.C., Ritchie, L.D., & Sabry, Z.I. (2001). Ethnic issues in the epidemiology of childhood obesity. *Pediatric Clinics of North America, 48,* 855–878.

Currie, C.E., Elton, R.A., Todd, J., & Platt, S. (1997). Indicators of socioeconomic status for adolescents: the WHO Health Behaviour in school-aged children survey. *Health Education Research, 12,* 385–397.

Currie, C., Molcho, M., Boyce, W., Holstein, B., Torsheim, T., & Richter, M. (2008). Researching health inequalities in adolescents: the development of the Health Behaviour in School-Aged Children (HBSC) family affluence scale. *Social Science & Medicine, 66,* 1429–1436.

Doak, C.M., Adair, L.S., Monteiro, C., & Popkin, B.M. (2000). Overweight and underweight coexist within households in Brazil, China and Russia. *The Journal of Nutrition, 130,* 2965–2971.

Doak, C.M., Adair, L.S., Bentley, M., Monteiro, C., & Popkin, B.M. (2005). The dual burden household and the nutrition transition paradox. *International Journal of Obesity (Lond), 29,* 129–136.

Dubois, L., & Girard, M. (2006). Determinants of birthweight inequalities: population-based study. *Pediatrics International, 48,* 470–478.

Due, P., Damsgaard, M.T., Rasmussen, M., Holstein, B.E., Wardle, J., Merlo, J., Currie, C., Ahluwalia, N., Sørensen, T.I., Lynch, J., HBSC Obesity Writing Group, Borraccino, A., Borup, I., Boyce, W., Elgar, F., Gabhainn, S.N., Krølner, R., Svastisalee, C., Matos, M.C., Nansel, T., Al Sabbah, H., Vereecken, C., & Valimaa, R. (2009). Socioeconomic position, macroeconomic environment and overweight among adolescents in 35 countries. *International Journal of Obesity (Lond), 33,* 1084–1093.

Dunton, G.F., Kaplan, J., Wolch, J., Jerrett, M., & Reynolds, K.D. (2009). Physical environmental correlates of childhood obesity: a systematic review. *Obesity Reviews, 10,* 393–402.

Ferreira, I., van der Horst, K., Wendel-Vos, W., Kremers, S., van Lenthe, F.J., & Brug, J. (2007). Environmental correlates of physical activity in youth – a review and update. *Obesity Reviews, 8,* 129–154.

Ford, P.B., & Dzewaltowski, D.A. (2008). Disparities in obesity prevalence due to variation in the retail food environment: three testable hypotheses. *Nutrition Reviews, 66,* 216–228.

Genovesi, S., Giussani, M., Faini, A., Vigorita, F., Pieruzzi, F., Strepparava, M.G., Stella, A., & Valsecchi, M.G. (2005). Maternal perception of excess weight in children: a survey conducted by paediatricians in the province of Milan. *Acta Paediatrica, 94,* 747–752.

Goffinet, F. (2005). Primary predictors of preterm labour *BJOG: An International Journal of Obstetrics and Gynaecology, 112 Suppl 1,* 38–47.

Groeneveld, I.F., Solomons, N.W., & Doak, C.M. (2007). Nutritional status of urban schoolchildren of high and low socioeconomic status in Quetzaltenango, Guatemala. *Revista Panamericana de Salud Pública, 22,* 169–177.

Hales, C.N., & Barker, D.J. (2001). The thrifty phenotype hypothesis. *British Medical Bulletin, 60,* 5–20.

Hanson, M.D., & Chen, E. (2007). Socioeconomic status and health behaviors in adolescence: a review of the literature. *Journal of Behavioral Medicine, 30,* 263–285.

Horodynski, M.A., Stommel, M., Brophy-Herb, H.E., & Weatherspoon, L. (2010). Mealtime television viewing and dietary quality in low-income African American and Caucasian mother-toddler dyads. *Maternal and Child Health Journal, 14,* 548–556.

Iversen, A.C., & Kraft, P. (2006). Does socio-economic status and health consciousness influence how women respond to health related messages in media? *Health Education Research, 21,* 601–610.

Jain, A., Sherman, S.N., Chamberlin, L.A., Carter, Y., Powers, S.W., & Whitaker, R.C. (2001). Why don't low-income mothers worry about their preschoolers being overweight? *Pediatrics, 107,* 1138–1146.

James, W.P., Nelson, M., Ralph, A., & Leather, S. (1997). Socioeconomic determinants of health. The contribution of nutrition to inequalities in health. *British Medical Journal, 314,* 1545–1549.

Jansen, P.W., Tiemeier, H., Jaddoe, V.W., Hofman, A., Steegers, E.A., Verhulst, F.C., Mackenbach, J.P., & Raat, H. (2009). Explaining educational inequalities in preterm birth: the generation r study. *Archives of Disease in Childhood. Fetal and Neonatal Edition, 94,* F28–F34.

Janssen, I., Boyce, W.F., Simpson, K., & Pickett, W. (2006). Influence of individual- and area-level measures of socioeconomic status on obesity, unhealthy eating, and physical inactivity in Canadian adolescents. *The American Journal of Clinical Nutrition, 83,* 139–145.

Jeffery, R.W., French, S.A., Forster, J.L., & Spry, V.M. (1991). Socioeconomic status differences in health behaviors related to obesity: the Healthy Worker Project. *International Journal of Obesity, 15,* 689–696.

Johnson, C.A., Xie, B., Liu, C., Reynolds, K.D., Chou, C.P., Koprowski, C., Gallaher, P., Spruijt-Metz, D., Guo, Q., Sun, P., Gong, J., & Palmer, P. (2006). Socio-demographic and cultural comparison of overweight and obesity risk and prevalence in adolescents in Southern California and Wuhan, China. *Journal of Adolescent Health, 39,* 925–928.

Kaiser, L.L., Martinez, N.A., Harwood, J.O., & Garcia, L.C. (1999). Child feeding strategies in low-income Latino households: focus group observations. *Journal of the American Dietetic Association, 99,* 601–603.

Khor, G.L., & Sharif, Z.M. (2003). Dual forms of malnutrition in the same households in Malaysia – a case study among Malay rural households. *Asia Pacific Journal of Clinical Nutrition, 12,* 427–437.

Larson, N.I., Story, M.T., & Nelson, M.C. (2009). Neighborhood environments: disparities in access to healthy foods in the U.S. *American Journal of Preventive Medicine, 36,* 74–81.

Lawlor, D.A., & Chaturvedi, N. (2006). Treatment and prevention of obesity – are there critical periods for intervention? *International Journal of Epidemiology, 35,* 3–9.

Lioret, S., Touvier, M., Dubuisson, C., Dufour, A., Calamassi-Tran, G., Lafay, L., Volatier, J.L., & Maire, B. (2009). Trends in child overweight rates and energy intake in France from 1999 to 2007: relationships with socioeconomic status. *Obesity (Silver Spring), 17,* 1092–1100.

Lovasi, G.S., Hutson, M.A., Guerra, M., & Neckerman, K.M. (2009). Built environments and obesity in disadvantaged populations. *Epidemiologic Reviews, 31,* 7–20.

Manios, Y., Kondaki, K., Kourlaba, G., Vasilopoulou, E., & Grammatikaki, E. (2009). Maternal perceptions of their child's weight status: the GENESIS study. *Public Health Nutrition, 12,* 1099–1105.

Margetts, B.M., Thompson, R.L., Speller, V., & McVey, D. (1998). Factors which influence "healthy" eating patterns: results from the 1993 Health Education Authority health and lifestyle survey in England. *Public Health Nutrition, 1,* 193–198.

Martorell, R., Kettel Khan, L., Hughes, M.L., & Grummer-Strawn, L.M. (2000). Overweight and obesity in preschool children from developing countries. *International Journal of Obesity and Related Metabolic Disorders, 24,* 959–967.

McLaren, L. (2007). Socioeconomic status and obesity. *Epidemiologic Reviews, 29,* 29–48.

Mendez, M.A., Monteiro, C.A., & Popkin, B.M. (2005). Overweight exceeds underweight among women in most developing countries. *The American Journal of Clinical Nutrition, 81,* 714–721.

Monteiro, C.A., Mondini, L., Torres, A.M., & dos Reis, I.M. (1997). Patterns of intra-familiar distribution of undernutrition: methods and applications for developing societies. *European Journal of Clinical Nutrition, 51,* 800–803.

Monteiro, C.A., Conde, W.L., & Popkin, B.M. (2002). Is obesity replacing or adding to undernutrition? Evidence from different social classes in Brazil. *Public Health Nutrition, 5,* 105–112.

Mortensen, L.H., Diderichsen, F., Arntzen, A., Gissler, M., Cnattingius, S., Schnor, O., Davey-Smith, G., & Nybo Andersen, A.M. (2008). Social inequality in fetal growth: a comparative study of Denmark, Finland, Norway and Sweden in the period 1981–2000. *Journal of Epidemiology and Community Health, 62,* 325–331.

Moutquin, J.M. (2003). Socio-economic and psychosocial factors in the management and prevention of preterm labour. *BJOG: An International Journal of Obstetrics and Gynaecology, 110 Suppl 20,* 56–60.

O'Dea, J.A., & Dibley, M.J. (2010). Obesity increase among low SES Australian schoolchildren between 2000 and 2006: time for preventive interventions to target children from low income schools? *International Journal of Public Health, 55,* 185–192.

Ong, K.K. (2006). Size at birth, postnatal growth and risk of obesity. *Hormone Research, 65 Suppl 3,* 65–69.

Papas, M.A., Alberg, A.J., Ewing, R., Helzlsouer, K.J., Gary, T.L., & Klassen, A.C. (2007). The built environment and obesity. *Epidemiologic Reviews, 29,* 129–143.

Parmenter, K., Waller, J., & Wardle, J. (2000). Demographic variation in nutrition knowledge in England. *Health Education Research, 15,* 163–174.

Parsons, T.J., Power, C., Logan, S., & Summerbell, C.D. (1999). Childhood predictors of adult obesity: a systematic review. *International Journal of Obesity and Related Metabolic Disorders, 23 (Suppl 8),* S1–S107.

Patrick, H., & Nicklas, T.A. (2005). A review of family and social determinants of children's eating patterns and diet quality. *Journal of the American College Nutrition, 24,* 83–92.

Pattenden, S., Dolk, H., & Vrijheid, M. (1999). Inequalities in low birth weight: parental social class, area deprivation, and "lone mother" status. *Journal of Epidemiology and Community Health, 53,* 355–358.

Popkin, B.M. (2001). The nutrition transition and obesity in the developing world. *The Journal of Nutrition, 131,* 871S–873S.

Prentice, A.M. (2006). The emerging epidemic of obesity in developing countries. *International Journal of Epidemiology, 35,* 93–99.

Ravelli, G.P., Stein, Z.A., & Susser, M.W. (1976). Obesity in young men after famine exposure in utero and early infancy. *New England Journal of Medicine, 295,* 349–353.

Robert, S.A., & Reither, E.N. (2004). A multilevel analysis of race, community disadvantage, and body mass index among adults in the US. *Social Science & Medicine, 59,* 2421–2434.

Robinson, S.M., & Godfrey, K.M. (2008). Feeding practices in pregnancy and infancy: relationship with the development of overweight and obesity in childhood. *International Journal of Obesity (Lond), 32 (Suppl 6),* S4–S10.

Robinson, S., Marriott, L., Poole, J., Crozier, S., Borland, S., Lawrence, W., Law, C., Godfrey, K., Cooper, C., & Inskip, H., & Southampton Women's Survey Study Group. (2007). Dietary patterns in infancy: the importance of maternal and family influences on feeding practice. *The British Journal of Nutrition, 98,* 1029–1037.

Salmon, J., & Timperio, A. (2007). Prevalence, trends and environmental influences on child and youth physical activity. *Medicine and Sport Science, 50,* 183–199.

Saxton, J., Carnell, S., van Jaarsveld, C.H., & Wardle, J. (2009). Maternal education is associated with feeding style. *Journal of the American Dietetic Association, 109,* 894–898.

Sellström, E., & Bremberg, S. (2006). The significance of neighbourhood context to child and adolescent health and well-being: a systematic review of multilevel studies. *Scandinavian Journal of Public Health, 34,* 544–554.

Semmler, C., Ashcroft, J., van Jaarsveld, C.H., Carnell, S., & Wardle, J. (2009). Development of overweight in children in relation to parental weight and socioeconomic status. *Obesity (Silver Spring), 17,* 814–820.

Shavers, V.L. (2007). Measurement of socioeconomic status in health disparities research. *Journal of the National Medical Association, 99,* 1013–1023.

Shrewsbury, V., & Wardle, J. (2008). Socioeconomic status and adiposity in childhood: a systematic review of cross-sectional studies 1990–2005. *Obesity (Silver Spring), 16,* 275–284.

Singh, G.K., Kogan, M.D., Van Dyck, P.C., & Siahpush, M. (2008). Racial/ethnic, socioeconomic, and behavioral determinants of childhood and adolescent obesity in the United States: analyzing independent and joint associations. *Annals of Epidemiology, 18,* 682–695.

Sisson, S.B., Church, T.S., Martin, C.K., Tudor-Locke, C., Smith, S.R., Bouchard, C., Earnest, C.P., Rankinen, T., Newton, R.L., & Katzmarzyk, P.T. (2009). Profiles of sedentary behavior in children and adolescents: the US National Health and Nutrition Examination Survey, 2001–2006. *International Journal of Pediatric Obesity, 4,* 353–359.

Sobal, J. (1991). Obesity and socioeconomic status: a framework for examining relationships between physical and social variables. *Medical Anthropology, 13,* 231–247.

Sobal, J., & Stunkard, A.J. (1989). Socioeconomic status and obesity: a review of the literature. *Psychological Bulletin, 105,* 260–275.

Sørensen, T.I., & Stunkard, A.J. (1993). Does obesity run in families because of genes? An adoption study using silhouettes as a measure of obesity. *Acta Psychiatrica Scandinavica, 370, Suppl,* 67–72.

Stamatakis, E., Primatesta, P., Chinn, S., Rona, R., & Falascheti, E. (2005). Overweight and obesity trends from 1974 to 2003 in English children: what is the role of socioeconomic factors? *Archives of Disease in Childhood, 90,* 999–1004.

Stamatakis, E., Wardle, J., & Cole, T.J. (2010a). Childhood obesity and overweight prevalence trends in England: evidence for growing socioeconomic disparities. *International Journal of Obesity (Lond), 34,* 41–47.

Stamatakis, E., Zaninotto, P., Falaschetti, E., Mindell, J., & Head, J. (2010b). Time trends in childhood and adolescent obesity in England from 1995 to 2007 and projections of prevalence to 2015. *Journal of Epidemiology and Community Health, 64,* 167–174.

Taylor, P.D., & Poston, L. (2007). Developmental programming of obesity in mammals. *Experimental Physiology, 92,* 287–298.

The King's Fund (2004). *Public attitudes to public health policy.* London: The King's Fund.

Thulier, D., & Mercer, J. (2009). Variables associated with breastfeeding duration. *Journal of Obstetric, Gynecologic, and Neonatal Nursing, 38,* 259–268.

Turrell, G., & Kavanagh, A.M. (2006). Socio-economic pathways to diet: modelling the association between socio-economic position and food purchasing behaviour. *Public Health Nutrition, 9,* 375–383.

United Nations Food and Agriculture Organization (2009). *The state of food insecurity in the world.* Retrieved from: www.fao.org/docrep/012/i0876e/i0876e00.htm (accessed 23rd March 2010).

van der Horst, K., Oenema, A., Ferreira, I., Wendel-Vos, W., Giskes, K., van Lenthe, F., & Brug, J. (2007a). A systematic review of environmental correlates of obesity-related dietary behaviors in youth. *Health Education Research, 22,* 203–226.

van der Horst, K., Paw, M. J., Twisk, J.W., & Van Mechelen, W. (2007b). A brief review on correlates of physical activity and sedentariness in youth. *Medicine and Science in Sports and Exercise, 39,* 1241–1250.

Ventura, A.K., & Birch, L.L. (2008). Does parenting affect children's eating and weight status? *The International Journal of Behavioral Nutrition and Physical Activity, 5,* 15.

Wake, M., Hardy, P., Canterford, L., Sawyer, M., & Carlin, J.B. (2007). Overweight, obesity and girth of Australian preschoolers: prevalence and socio-economic correlates. *International Journal of Obesity (Lond), 31,* 1044–1051.

Wang, Y. (2001). Cross-national comparison of childhood obesity: the epidemic and the relationship between obesity and socioeconomic status. *International Journal of Epidemiology, 30,* 1129–1136.

Wang, Y., & Beydoun, M.A. (2007). The obesity epidemic in the United States – gender, age, socioeconomic, racial/ethnic, and geographic characteristics: a systematic review and meta-regression analysis. *Epidemiologic Reviews, 29,* 6–28.

Wang, Y., & Lobstein, T. (2006). Worldwide trends in childhood overweight and obesity. *International Journal of Pediatric Obesity, 1,* 11–25.

Wardle, J., & Carnell, S. (2009). Appetite is a heritable phenotype associated with adiposity. *Annals of Behavioral Medicine, 38 (Suppl 8),* 25–30.

Wardle, J., & Griffith, J. (2001). Socioeconomic status and weight control practices in British adults. *Journal of Epidemiology and Community Health, 55,* 185–190.

Wardle, J., & Marsland, L. (1990). Adolescent concerns about weight and eating; a social-development perspective. *Journal of Psychosomatic Research, 34,* 377–391.

Wardle, J., & Steptoe, A. (2003). Socioeconomic differences in attitudes and beliefs about healthy lifestyles. *Journal of Epidemiology and Community Health, 57,* 440–443.

Wardle, J., Robb, K., & Johnson, F. (2002a). Assessing socioeconomic status in adolescents: the validity of a home affluence scale. *Journal of Epidemiology and Community Health, 56,* 595–599.

Wardle, J., Sanderson, S., Guthrie, C.A., Rapoport, L., & Plomin, R. (2002b). Parental feeding style and the intergenerational transmission of obesity risk. *Obesity Research, 10,* 453–462.

Wardle, J., Robb, K.A., Johnson, F., Griffith, J., Brunner, E., Power, C., & Tovee, M. (2004). Socioeconomic variation in attitudes to eating and weight in female adolescents. *Health Psychology, 23,* 275–282.

Wardle, J., Brodersen, N.H., Cole, T.J., Jarvis, M.J., & Boniface, D.R. (2006). Development of adiposity in adolescence: five year longitudinal study of an ethnically and socioeconomically diverse sample of young people in Britain. *British Medical Journal, 332,* 1130–1135.

Webber, L., Cooke, L., Hill, C., & Wardle, J. (2010). Associations between children's appetitive traits and maternal feeding practices. *Journal of the American Dietetic Association, 110,* 1718–1722.

Wijndaele, K., Lakshman, R., Landsbaugh, J.R., Ong, K.K., & Ogilvie, D. (2009). Determinants of early weaning and use of unmodified cow's milk in infants: a systematic review. *Journal of the American Dietetic Association, 109,* 2017–2028.

Zhang, Q., & Wang, Y. (2004). Socioeconomic inequality of obesity in the United States: do gender, age, and ethnicity matter? *Social Science & Medicine, 58,* 1171–1180.

Chapter 22
Environmental Factors: Opportunities and Barriers for Physical Activity, and Healthy Eating

Inge Huybrechts, Ilse De Bourdeaudhuij, and Stefaan De Henauw

Introduction

While genetic factors play a role in the development of obesity, the dramatic increase of its prevalence in the past 20 years strongly suggests that environmental factors are largely responsible. The history of human race during the past 20 years has seen a drastic and extremely rapid evolution of the environment (British Medical Association (BMA) 2005). While more than 100 years ago, "saving steps" documents were published (Fig. 22.1) (Van Rensselaer 1901), nowadays we are recommended to strive for 10,000 steps per day (Lindberg 2000; Mummery et al. 2006; US Department of Health and Human Services 1996).

It is clear that our global obesity epidemic is being driven by a mismatch between our environment and our metabolism. Human physiology developed to function within an environment where high levels of physical activity were needed in daily life and where food was inconsistently available (Peters et al. 2002). Control of body weight was largely accomplished through innate physiological processes and required little conscious efforts. Because of the importance of ensuring sufficient energy intake for survival and reproduction, multiple redundant physiological systems evolved to encourage eating behavior and our physiology developed the capacity to reduce metabolic rate in response to negative energy balance due to food shortage (Peters et al. 2002).

However, the current environment is characterized by a situation in which minimal physical activity is required for daily life and food is inexpensive, high in energy density and widely available. Unfortunately, there seems no strong drive to increase physical activity in response to excess energy intake and there appears to be only a weak adaptive increase in resting energy expenditure in response to excess energy intake. In our modern environment, people who are not devoting substantial conscious efforts to manage their body weight are likely to gain weight. The globally rising obesity prevalence suggests that the environment has changed in such a way that fewer and fewer people manage to maintain a healthy body weight by relying on their own biology and "instinctual" mechanisms to protect them (Peters et al. 2002).

I. Huybrechts (✉)
Department of Public Health, Ghent University, Ghent, Belgium
e-mail: inge.huybrechts@ugent.be

I. De Bourdeaudhuij
Department of Movement and Sports Sciences, Ghent University, Ghent, Belgium

S. De Henauw
Department of Public Health, Ghent University, Ghent, Belgium

L.A. Moreno et al. (eds.), *Epidemiology of Obesity in Children and Adolescents*,
Springer Series on Epidemiology and Public Health 2, DOI 10.1007/978-1-4419-6039-9_22,
© Springer Science+Business Media, LLC 2011

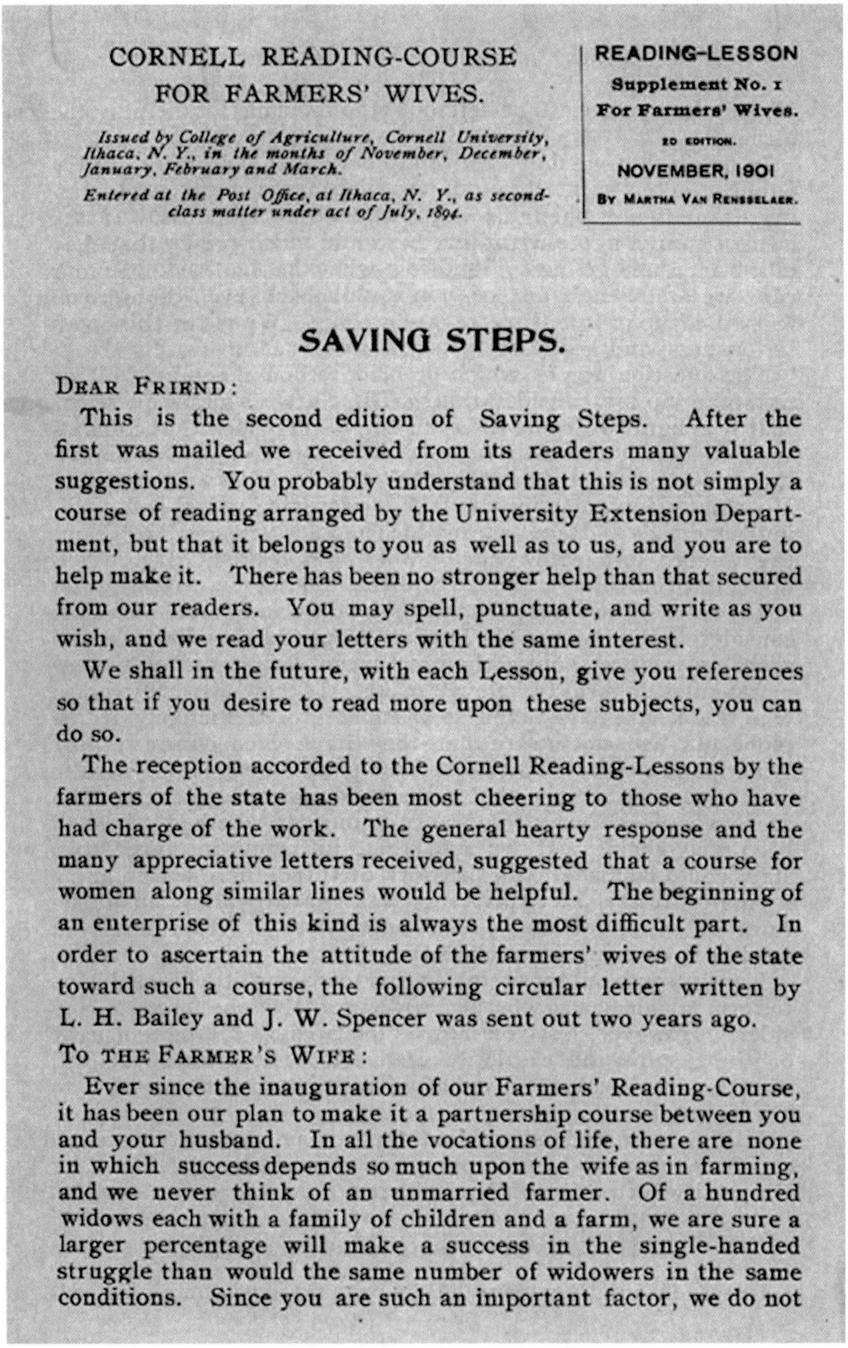

CORNELL READING-COURSE FOR FARMERS' WIVES.

Issued by College of Agriculture, Cornell University, Ithaca, N. Y., in the months of November, December, January, February and March.

Entered at the Post Office, at Ithaca, N. Y., as second-class matter under act of July, 1894.

READING-LESSON

Supplement No. 1

For Farmers' Wives.

2D EDITION.

NOVEMBER, 1901

BY MARTHA VAN RENSSELAER.

SAVING STEPS.

DEAR FRIEND:

This is the second edition of Saving Steps. After the first was mailed we received from its readers many valuable suggestions. You probably understand that this is not simply a course of reading arranged by the University Extension Department, but that it belongs to you as well as to us, and you are to help make it. There has been no stronger help than that secured from our readers. You may spell, punctuate, and write as you wish, and we read your letters with the same interest.

We shall in the future, with each Lesson, give you references so that if you desire to read more upon these subjects, you can do so.

The reception accorded to the Cornell Reading-Lessons by the farmers of the state has been most cheering to those who have had charge of the work. The general hearty response and the many appreciative letters received, suggested that a course for women along similar lines would be helpful. The beginning of an enterprise of this kind is always the most difficult part. In order to ascertain the attitude of the farmers' wives of the state toward such a course, the following circular letter written by L. H. Bailey and J. W. Spencer was sent out two years ago.

TO THE FARMER'S WIFE:

Ever since the inauguration of our Farmers' Reading-Course, it has been our plan to make it a partnership course between you and your husband. In all the vocations of life, there are none in which success depends so much upon the wife as in farming, and we never think of an unmarried farmer. Of a hundred widows each with a family of children and a farm, we are sure a larger percentage will make a success in the single-handed struggle than would the same number of widowers in the same conditions. Since you are such an important factor, we do not

Fig. 22.1 "Saving steps: cornell reading course for farmers' wives" (Van Rensselaer 1901)

In today's environment, the physiological systems that worked so well in the past are now contributing to our global obesity epidemic. Important environmental changes that contribute to the obesity epidemic are for instance an ever-increasing number of energy-dense foods, packaged in large portions, conveniently available at low cost (Berg et al. 2009; Drewnowski 2004; Ledikwe et al. 2005). Energy-dense foods contain large numbers of calories in very small portions, what promotes the over-consumption of calories. Furthermore, modern technologies allow people to be less active in their daily labor. All modern conveniences we now have access to have eliminated the need for individuals to perform much of the physical activity that was once required for daily tasks at work and at home. For example, years ago people walked to most places, while today people have access to cars and public transportation to take them to these places, thus limiting the need for physical activity. Computers, cable and satellite televisions, movies on demand, and high-tech toys like video game systems have led to a decrease in physical activity or a sedentary lifestyle in people of all ages (Wells et al. 2007).

In addition to those modern conveniences, also safety issues in the environment might stimulate those unhealthy lifestyle habits and decisions. For example, a person may not only choose not to walk to the store or to work because of laziness or convenience, but just because of a lack of alternatives (e.g., no sidewalks) and safety reasons. Communities, homes, schools and workplaces can all influence people's health decisions (Coleman et al. 2008; Dwyer et al. 2008b). Because of this influence, it is important to create environments that make it easier to engage in physical activity and to adopt a healthy diet.

Many of the physical attributes and the social and psychological structures for life and learning are acquired during the first years of life (British Medical Association (BMA) 2005) and may continue as unhealthy lifestyle patterns into adulthood (Boulton et al. 1995). Therefore, healthy lifestyle habits should be stimulated as early in life as possible (Peters et al. 2002). In addition, no strong biological mechanism seems to oppose obesity once it is established. Therefore, improving children's lifestyle by promoting healthy dietary habits and physical activity should be a priority and should be seen as an integral part of our environmental development. Failing to ensure that young children develop healthy and optimal lifestyle habits is counterproductive in the long run, since failing to invest in the young will be more costly to the whole society. By placing emphasis on the first years of life and developing healthy childhood environments and comprehensive nutrition policies, countries should be able to avert the obesity epidemic in order to avoid many preventable deaths, prevent irreversible mental damage and preserve a child's priceless endowment of emotional, intellectual and moral qualities (Michaelsen et al. 2003).

Although it is clear that the environment plays a key role in obesity prevention among children and adolescents (Government Office for Science 2007; Tauber and Jouret 2004; Woodman et al. 2008), a better understanding on how the environment impacts nutritional intake and physical activity and consequently obesity is essential to develop strategies for prevention. The purpose of this chapter is to present disparities in access to nutritious foods and in possibilities for a physically active lifestyle. Environmental barriers to obtain a healthy lifestyle will be discussed and strategies for environmental improvements that stimulate a healthy lifestyle will be proposed.

This chapter brings together wide-ranging research from health, transport, urban planning, physical activity and food policy and is of use to decision makers and researchers from all these areas.

Environmental Factors Related to Obesity

What Is Meant with "The Environment"?

Prior to discussing the environmental factors related to obesity, it is important to define the term "environment" used throughout this chapter. In its simplest meaning, the environment can be described as "the surroundings in which a person, animal, or plant lives" (Collins 2006). However, different definitions have been used to describe the term "environment," depending on the context in which the term is being used. The Analysis Grid for Environments Linked to Obesity (ANGELO) was developed for the investigation of obesogenic environments (Swinburn et al. 1999). The categories and definitions that were used in this ANGELO project to define different types of environments are now broadly used in environmental research. The ANGELO grid contains two axes.

1. One axis distinguishes between two *"sizes"* of environments (micro and macro):
   Micro-environments are defined as environmental settings where groups of people meet and get together. They are geographically distinct, with room for direct mutual influence between individuals and the environment (e.g., homes, schools, workplaces, supermarkets, recreational facilities, and neighborhoods).
   Macro-environments include the broader more anonymous infrastructures that may support or hinder health behaviors (e.g., the town planning, transport infrastructure and how produce is marketed and distributed).
2. The second axis distinguishes between four *"types"* of environments (physical, economic, political and socio-cultural).
   The physical environment refers to opportunities for healthy and unhealthy choices, such as points to purchase fruits and vegetables, soft-drink vending machines, and exercise facilities.
   The economic environment refers to the costs related to healthy and unhealthy behaviors, such as the costs of soft drinks, fruits and vegetables, and entrance fees to exercise facilities.
   The political environment refers to the rules and regulations that may influence eating and exercise behaviors, such as bans on vending machines in schools.
   The socio-cultural environment refers to the subjective and descriptive norms and other social influences such as social support for the adoption of health behavior and social pressure to engage in unhealthy habits.

The environmental factors that will be discussed in this chapter refer to the micro- or macro-environment and can belong to the different types of environments described in the ANGELO grid.

Which Environmental Factors Will Be Discussed in this Chapter?

The variety of environmental factors involved in obesity, and their mechanisms are extremely complex. In this chapter, we will discuss the most important environmental factors that might influence childhood and adolescent obesity, namely factors influencing physical activity, sedentarism (screen time), eating habits, dietary preferences and food supplies (Tauber and Jouret 2004).

Environmental Factors Influencing Physical Activity and Sedentarism

Different environmental changes during the past decades have influenced the possibilities and necessities for a physically active lifestyle. The most important environmental factors that influence physical activity and sedentary lifestyle in children and adolescents are listed below:

- *Technological advances*: technological tools like computers, remote controllers, escalators, mobile phones, and dishwashers all reduce the need for physical activity (Hill and Peters 1998; Wells et al. 2007).
- *Schools*: most children are being raised in classrooms with a main focus on intellectual education and sometimes insufficient physical education lessons (Peters et al. 2002). Even the facilities in kindergartens are often stimulating sedentary behavior rather than physical activity (e.g., due to insufficient provision of play space).
- *Sedentary pastimes*: video games, TV, internet and movies are today's pastimes of choice. Television, computers, and other modern technologies that were seen as luxury products have

become basic family products that make being sedentary much easier than ever before (Hardus et al. 2003; Hill and Peters 1998; Stettler et al. 2004).

- *Safety*: these days it is much less safe in most communities not only due to crime rates, but also due to excessive traffic. Therefore many parents are not letting their children play outside (Dwyer et al. 2008b). Sidewalks or cycling paths may not be lit up at night or there may not be any sidewalks at all (Saelens et al. 2003a, b). In some places, "parks and green spaces" are available, but they are not safe due to crime, youth gangs, unsafe equipment, etc.
- *Walkability*: high walkable neighborhoods, as defined for adults, are characterized by high population density, high land use mix and high street connectivity. Adults living in high walkable neighborhoods are more active in transport and leisure than those living in low walkable neighborhoods (De Bourdeaudhuij et al. 2003, 2005; Van Dyck et al. 2009b, 2010). However, for children and adolescents, living in lower walkable neighborhoods might stimulate playing outdoors in the streets or cycling longer distances to school or friends (Van Dyck et al. 2009a).
- *Modern transportation*: people are walking and biking less because driving is often the easiest option. Some communities are built in ways that require people to use cars to get around, instead of creating ways that make it easy and safe to walk or bike (Bellisari 2008; Hill and Peters 1998).
- *Access to sport activities*: the availability but also the quality of sport facilities is related to use. For children and adolescents, also the availability of a variety of sport clubs in their neighborhood invites them more to become member of a sport club. An important factor is also the access to sport activities at school. Schools that organize physical activity before school, during breaks or after school have pupils that are more active (Cardon et al. 2004a; Haerens et al. 2006).

Environmental Factors Influencing Eating Habits, Dietary Preferences and Food Supplies

Changes in food supply, portion sizes, food pricing, energy-density, etc. during the past decades might all contribute to unhealthy dietary habits and excessive energy intakes, which increases the risk for childhood obesity (Popkin 2001). The most important environmental factors that might influence eating habits, dietary preferences and food supplies among children and adolescents are listed below and will be further discussed in the section on "Evidences for Environmental Changes Influencing the Obesity Epidemic" of this chapter:

- *Fast food meals*: people are eating out at fast food restaurants more often because of time constraints, so they have less control over how much fat and sugar is in their food. Very often fast food restaurants also encourage *super-sizing* of meals and adding unnecessary calories (Young and Nestle 2002). However the same trend appears in other restaurants promoting "all you can eat" and even the packaging of foods in markets has increased. In 1950s, a standard size coke was 200 ml, while now it is 500 ml in the US (Young and Nestle 2002). Those growing portion sizes seem to be related to our growing obesity epidemic (Berg et al. 2009).
- *Unhealthy school environments*: school lunch programs often do not have a wide selection of healthy eating options and in many schools vending machines, school shops and canteens are still offering unhealthy snacks and beverages (Johnston et al. 2007; Kubik et al. 2003; Story et al. 1996).
- *Advertisements and strategic selling points in supermarkets*: unhealthy foods and drinks are aggressively advertised and sold to adults and children. Fast food and junk food advertisers purposely target children whom they know to have increasing purchasing power. In addition, candies, soft drinks and other tasty unhealthy foods in many supermarkets are very often exposed nearby the cash points where people have to wait to pay.
- *Access to healthy foods and food pricing*: many low-income communities do not have access to healthy food options. Even if there are options, healthy foods are usually more expensive than their processed competitors and their storage lifetime (like for fruits and vegetables) is often much less than for processed foods.

- *Night shops & food deserts (e.g., petrol stations)*: in many places, foods and beverages can be bought over 24 h during weekdays and during weekends. While night shops were still very scarce in many countries some decades ago, these days, the number of night shops has increased substantially all over the Western world. Also food deserts (districts with little or no access to foods needed to maintain a healthy diet but often served by plenty of fast food restaurants) like petrol stations and railway stations can be barriers for healthy dietary habits.
- *Foods taste better*: because of the advanced food technologies, the taste of foods has improved and many people are eating rather because of tastiness than because of hungriness. Also the smell and display of foods can make it difficult to resist.

Methods Used to Determine Environmental Factors Influencing Childhood Obesity

Different methods and designs have been used to assess the environmental factors described in the previous part of this chapter. Levels of assessment vary from entire counties down to the individual level. Methods for assessing environmental factors related to obesity include direct assessments (like in-person audits by trained observers), intermediate measures (like use of telephone book yellow pages or marketing databases to identify institutions), and indirect measures (like aggregation of census data to approximate neighborhood SES). The figure below illustrates the continuum of methods used to assess environmental factors in the current research (Booth et al. 2005) (Fig. 22.2).

Most of the studies investigating associations between environmental factors and obesity have used indirect or intermediate methods (Booth et al. 2005).

Census data (Frank et al. 2004; Kinra et al. 2000; Morland et al. 2002), GIS data (e.g., road network distance, steep hill barrier, grid of city blocks) (Frank et al. 2004; Giles-Corti and Donovan 2003), and street network data (Frank et al. 2004) were typical *indirect measures* to assess environmental factors. Other studies using indirect methods have created indexes such as material deprivation, neighborhood deprivation, and neighborhood safety (Kinra et al. 2000; van Lenthe and Mackenbach 2002) to distinguish between neighborhood SES levels.

Intermediate measures of the built environment included self-reported perceptions by neighborhood residents (Feldman and Steptoe 2004; Giles-Corti and Donovan 2003; Saelens et al. 2003a; van Lenthe and Mackenbach 2002). Other intermediate measurements of the built environment that have been used are regional land-use data from tax assessors and aerial photography (Frank et al. 2004).

Direct measurement through environmental audits has only been used in few studies with obesity as the primary outcome (Giles-Corti and Donovan 2003). Giles-Corti et al. included the type of street and the presence of sidewalks for each study participant as measurements for environmental factors.

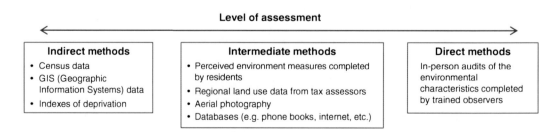

Fig. 22.2 Adapted version of the continuum of methods for measuring the environment (Booth et al. 2005)

In addition to the level of assessment the study design can differ. Therefore, different types of study designs used to investigate environmental factors related to obesity are discussed below.

Study Designs Used to Investigate Environmental Factors Related to Obesity

Observational and intervention studies can both be applied to get insight into the environmental correlates of obesogenic behaviors. In 2005, Brug et al. conducted six systematic reviews of observational studies investigating environmental correlates and environmental interventions for weight-related eating behaviors and physical activity for children (Brug et al. 2006). Although very little evidence for an association between environmental factors and weight-related behaviors was found, these reviews indicated much stronger evidences from intervention studies than from observational studies for associations between environmental factors and obesity.

The evidence that will be described in more depth in the next sections of this chapter can be derived from different study designs and types. Both, observational and intervention studies are included, using direct, intermediate and/or indirect measurement methods.

Modern Technologies Used to Investigate Environmental Factors Related to Childhood Obesity

Although technology is often blamed for childhood obesity as it disengages young people with physical activity, our modern technologies are useful for studying environmental influences of childhood obesity and also for the behavior itself. Different modern technologies like Geographical Information Systems (GIS), Global Positioning Systems (GPS), and Personal Digital Assistants (PDA's) are promising methods to support objective assessments of environmental factors.

PDA's have already been used in dietary surveys to assess dietary intakes among children (Beasley et al. 2005, 2008), while accelerometers and pedometers are widely used to assess physical activity levels in different types of surveys (Westerterp 2009). Nike and Apple recently developed a device that feeds physical activity data to an iPod. An accelerometer placed in a shoe wirelessly transmits information on distance, place and calories burned to a receiver attached to an iPod (a portable media player) contained in a pocket in the sleeve or an armband (Wells et al. 2007).

The Global Position System (GPS) is being used for both, navigational and mapping purposes in environmental research (Suminski et al. 2008). Furthermore, satellite and aerial imaging, global navigation and Web-Geographical Information System (GIS) mapping, along with advanced computing for handling and processing geo-spatial information, are new technologies broadly used in environmental studies. A geographic information system (GIS) captures, stores, analyzes, manages, and presents data that refers to or is linked to location. The GIS system has already been used in the study and prevention of childhood obesity and could be a promising method for objective environmental measurements. Person, place, and time are the three basic investigative categories needed to develop strategies for managing the obesity outbreak. The majority of epidemiologic efforts have been focusing on person and time. However, there is an urgent need to investigate how "place" (i.e., physical and social environment) contributes to the etiology of obesity. Advancement in geographic information systems over the past 20 years now provides a powerful way to conduct multivariate spatial statistical modeling of obesity in terms of its changing prevalence and environmental risk factors (Kandris and Liu 2003).

Evidences for Environmental Changes Influencing the Obesity Epidemic

The currently observed gradual weight gain all over the world is a relatively new phenomenon and likely attributable to a changing environment that provides a constant supply and has reduced the need for physical activity to survive. It is extremely difficult for most people to consistently restrict energy intake given the constant availability of good-tasting, low cost food and a physiology that promotes eating when food is available. Our physiological control system is not sufficiently strong to oppose constant unidirectional distortions in energy balance. Therefore, in today's environment, cognitive management is required to maintain a healthy body weight (Hill and Peters 1998).

Wells et al. investigated how environmental characteristics either hinder or promote healthy habits. They conceptualized a framework integrating the three themes: a broad definition of the environment, energy balance, and environmental barriers and environmental supports (Fig. 22.3). As this figure shows, physical environment characteristics that present barriers to healthy eating and physical activity are associated with increased energy intake and decreased energy output, respectively, yielding an imbalance in favor of energy input. Conversely, environmental factors that support physical activity and foster healthy eating are likely to be associated with lower caloric intakes and greater energy expenditures (Wells et al. 2007).

In the following paragraphs, we will discuss the evidences currently available for: (1) environmental barriers and opportunities for a physically active lifestyle; and (2) environmental barriers and opportunities for healthy dietary habits.

Environmental Barriers for a Physically Active Lifestyle

The link between the built environment and human physical activity behavior has recently been of interest to the field of urban planning. Different environmental factors, including walkability, public transport, safety, etc. have been studied in relation to human energy expenditure and the prevalence

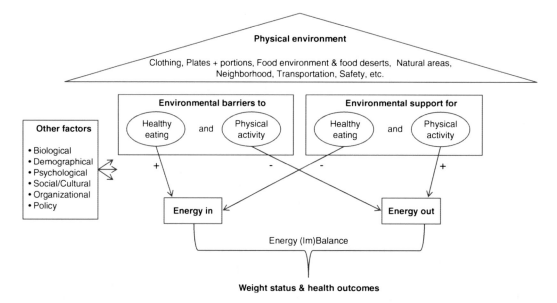

Fig. 22.3 Conceptual framework linking the environment with weight and health outcomes (Wells et al. 2007)

of overweight and obesity. The most important evidence concerning environmental barriers for energy expenditure is given below.

Technological developments during the past 100 years have played a tremendous role in reducing the physical demand of a wide range of tasks from the home environment to the workplace. Innovations have been aimed at making life easier by reducing our energy expenditure. We have strategically engineered physical activity out of our lives. For example, early research by Martha Van Rensselaer, founder of the College of Home Economics (now The College of Human Ecology) at Cornell University, was aimed at enabling housewives to "save steps" while completing daily chores (Van Rensselaer 1901; Wells et al. 2007). Today, energy-saving technologies reduce the caloric expenditure necessary to prepare meals, do laundry, wash dishes, bake bread, mow the lawn, change the television channel, and plant crops (Wells et al. 2007). In modern buildings and even in some schools, stairways are typically unattractive and inaccessible, whereas elevators and escalators are saliently located and inviting. Seldom do we find a contemporary building with a wide, stately, inviting stairway gracefully winding from one floor to another. The placement of stairs in obscure locations surely reduces their use. Another important technological development that importantly reduces physical activity in youth is the electronic access to all kinds of information like books and many more via the internet. Nowadays, almost all purchase can be done via the internet and can be delivered at home. Children and adolescents prefer chatting with each other via the internet or via text messages using their mobile instead of walking to each other's place.

These technological advances did not only reduce the need for physical activity in our home and work environment, but also in schools. Most children used to have compulsory *physical education at school* that provided substantial physical activity, while only few schools still require this physical education today (Wells et al. 2007). In addition, previous studies showed that children and adolescents are only active for less than half of the lesson time in physical education (Cardon et al. 2004b; Cardon and De Bourdeaudhuij 2008)

Moreover those technological advances importantly stimulate *sedentary pastimes* in children and adolescents. Video games, TV and movies are today's pastimes of choice. Television, computers, and other modern technologies that ever were seen as luxury products have become basic family products that make being sedentary much easier than ever before. Television watching has been the sedentary behavior measure that was most frequently measured and was directly related to weight gain in most studies (Dwyer et al. 2008a). A more in depth discussion of the relationship between sedentary lifestyle and overweight and obesity in children and adolescents can be found in Chapter 20.

Lack of *safety* in certain neighborhoods might also be a barrier to maintain a physically active lifestyle and could therefore stimulate the obesity epidemic in unsafe areas (Dwyer et al. 2008a). In a national sample of women with young children, Burdette et al. (2006) found that obesity was more prevalent among mothers who perceived their neighborhoods to be unsafe. Also Saelens et al. found that safer neighborhoods, which include a mixture of houses, commercial, retail, and recreation destinations, often result in more physical activity and social capital and less overweight and obesity (Saelens et al. 2003a, b). However, when looking at the young children themselves, Burdette found that within a population of urban low-income preschoolers, overweight was not associated with the level of neighborhood crime (Burdette and Whitaker 2004). Therefore, more research is needed to investigate the real impact of the safety in neighborhoods/environments on the physical activity level of children and adolescents.

Since recently, researchers are trying to assess the *walkability* of neighborhoods and environments in order to investigate barriers to walkability and to examine whether walkability of areas has an influence on the overweight and obesity prevalence of that area (Saelens and Handy 2008). Measurement tools that are being developed and refined to assess some built environment constructs include land use mix, street connectivity, and residential density, and other factors thought to contribute to walkability (Johnson-Taylor and Everhart 2006; Saelens and Handy 2008). Saelens et al.

identified residents of high-walkable and low-walkable neighborhoods with comparable SES using census data (Saelens et al. 2003b). Their results indicated that residents of high-walkability neighborhoods lived in neighborhoods more conducive to physical activity (i.e., higher residential density and street connectivity, more diverse and accessible land use, better aesthetics, and pedestrian safety) than did residents of low-walkability neighborhoods. Accordingly, residents of low-walkability neighborhoods tended to report higher mean BMIs (body mass index) and hence higher rates of overweight and obesity than high-walkability neighborhood residents (Saelens et al. 2003b). Other studies investigating the impact of community design or land use mix on physical activity and obesity confirmed those findings (Ewing et al. 2003; Frank et al. 2004; Wells et al. 2007). An important finding by Ewing et al. was the relation between sprawl areas (i.e., low housing density, low land-use mix, no strong centers of activity, and poor connectivity) and physical activity levels and the prevalence of obesity. County-level analyses controlling for minutes walked indicated that sprawl seemed to have a linear relationship to BMI and obesity, i.e., more sprawl resulted in higher BMIs and obesity rates (Ewing et al. 2003; Wells et al. 2007). These results were also confirmed in Europe, studying adults in low and high walkable neighborhoods in Belgium (Van Dyck et al. 2010). Living in a high-walkable neighborhood was associated with more moderate-to-vigorous physical activity as assessed by accelerometers, transportational walking and cycling, recreational walking, and less motorized transport. In addition, activity assessed by accelerometry and self-reported cycling for transport appeared to be mediators of the association between walkability and both BMI and weight-to-height ratio (Van Dyck et al. 2010).

When looking at children, it should be noted that with the exception of walking to school, children make considerably fewer utilitarian trips than adults, and even walking to school has decreased in frequency over time (Johnson-Taylor and Everhart 2006). So far, it is not known whether the characteristics that increase adult walkability actually encourage or even limit children's physical activity. For example, parents could feel that a more walkable neighborhood is less safe for their children and might therefore forbid their children to walk or play in such areas (Johnson-Taylor and Everhart 2006). A Belgian study in adolescents showed that in contrast with the expectations, adolescents living in the less walkable suburb reported 220 min/week more cycling for transport than those living in the high walkable town center. A trend was found for mean step counts/day with 1,371 more steps/day for suburban adolescents (Van Dyck et al. 2010). In contrast with previous results in adults, lower walkability and larger distance to school was associated with more physical activity in Belgian adolescents. Therefore, physical environmental interventions designed for adults, focusing on increases in connectivity, residential density and land use mix, might not be effective for adolescents.

The notion that *natural areas and green spaces* encourage physical activity is supported by evidence that people with easy access to natural areas are more likely to use the spaces (Wells et al. 2007). As natural and green spaces are becoming scarce in many industrialized countries, this lack of green spaces could be a barrier to maintain a physically active lifestyle. In a study of nearly 7,000 adults living in European cities, residents of areas with the highest levels of greenery were 3 times as likely to be physically active and 40% less likely to be overweight or obese, than those living in the least green setting (Ellaway et al. 2005; Wells et al. 2007). Similarly Giles-Corti et al. (2005) found that people who use public open spaces are 3 times more likely to achieve recommended levels of physical activity than those who do not use the spaces. Gaining a clearer understanding of the role of parks, greenways, and open spaces in physical activity levels and obesity rates among children and adolescents is particularly critical to address these issues.

Also *transportation* planners have begun to investigate factors of urban form and transportation services that influence the choice to walk. In line with the modern technologies that were discussed above, our transportation means for daily life activities have also undergone an important change over the past decades. Cars and motorbikes are very often the pre-eminently transportation means. Only few transportation studies focused on the generation of "the utilitarian walk trip" as the key variable. Edwards (2008) assessed the potential benefits of increased walking and reduced obesity associated with taking public transit in terms of dollars of medical costs saved and disability avoided. This study revealed that taking public transit is associated with walking 8.3 more minutes per day on average, or an additional 25.7 to 39.0 kcal. Edwards (2008) expects that additional walking associated with public transit could save an important amount of obesity-related medical costs. Therefore, further transportation research should examine the effects of improved mobility services in addition to alterations of the built environment and their effect on overweight and obesity. Integration of epidemiologic and transportation behavioral research could enhance our understanding of the role of urban and transportation factors on physical activity (Coogan and Coogan 2004). It is important that studies focus on the net impact of transit usage on all behaviors, including caloric intake and other types of exercise, and on whether policies can promote usage of transport at acceptable cost (Edwards 2008).

The influence of *access to physical activity facilities* on childhood obesity is one of the most common measures of the built and economic environment that has been studied in relation to the obesity epidemic (Papas et al. 2007). Two studies investigated the distance from the child's residence to the nearest playground, but both studies found no association with overweight or obesity in those children (Burdette and Whitaker 2004; Liu et al. 2002). However, Gordon-Larsen et al. (2006) investigated this issue in adolescents, and found inverse associations between the number of recreational facilities and the likelihood of being overweight. When using a measure of density (number of fitness facilities per 1,000 residents, within ZIP codes), Mobley et al. (2006) found a statistically significant negative association with BMI. In addition to the distance to physical activity facilities, also the fees for physical activity programs in such facilities might be a barrier to engage in physical activity for some children and their parents.

Environmental Opportunities to Increase Our Physical Activity Level

As Schmid et al. (1995) said "It is unreasonable to expect people to change their behaviors when the environment discourages such changes." Therefore, it is important to search for environmental opportunities that can counteract the barriers in our modern environment. In this section we will consider the evidence of strategies to change the environment in order to create opportunities for physical activity.

Increasing levels of physical activity is a real challenge within our modern environment, not just for those directly involved in public health but for groups and individuals in many sectors of the society. Adults, young people and children should try to achieve the national recommended levels by including activities such as walking, cycling or climbing stairs as part of their everyday life, when living in an environment that promotes a physically active lifestyle.

When thinking of environmental opportunities that promote physical activity, it is important to prioritize the need for people (including those whose mobility is impaired) to be physically active as a routine part of their daily life. Therefore, one should ensure that local facilities and services are easily accessible by foot, by bicycle and by other modes of transport involving physical activity and they should ensure that children can participate in physically active play (National Institute for Health and Clinical Excellence (NICE) 2008; World Health Organization (WHO) 2009).

Furthermore, it is important to ensure that pedestrians, cyclists and users of other modes of transport that involve physical activity are given the highest priority when developing or maintaining streets and roads. Possible ways to ensure this priority are by (National Institute for Health and Clinical Excellence (NICE) 2008; World Health Organization (WHO) 2009):

- Re-allocating road space to support physically active modes of transport (as an example, this could be achieved by widening pavements and introducing cycle lanes).
- Restricting motor vehicle access (for example, by closing or narrowing roads to reduce capacity).
- Introducing road-user charging schemes.

- Introducing traffic-calming schemes to restrict vehicle speeds (using signage and changes to highway design).
- Creating safe routes to schools (for example, by using traffic-calming measures near schools and by creating or improving walking and cycle routes to schools).

Planning and transport agencies should plan and provide a comprehensive network of routes for walking, cycling and using other modes of transport involving physical activity. These routes should offer convenient, safe and attractive access to workplaces, homes, schools and other public facilities (including shops, play and green areas and social destinations) (National Institute for Health and Clinical Excellence (NICE) 2008; World Health Organization (WHO) 2009).

Designers and managers of public open spaces, paths and rights of way should ensure that public open spaces and public paths can be reached by foot, by bicycle and by using other modes of transport involving physical activity and they should also be accessible by public transport. Furthermore, they should ensure that public open spaces and public paths are maintained to a high standard and that they are safe, attractive and welcoming to everyone (National Institute for Health and Clinical Excellence (NICE) 2008). Designers and managers of public open spaces, paths and rights of way could also think of outdoor and indoor physical fitness facilities that allow people to be physically active while waiting for their public transport or for an appointment (Fig. 22.4).

Furthermore, bike hiring systems could create opportunities to stimulate physical activity. In Lyon (France) for instance the city provides solid, comfortable bikes, available for anyone to use, 24 h a day, 7 days a week. You can find them at strategic locations all over Lyon and Villeurbanne, thanks to a dense network of stations located at intervals of 300 m on average. Because of this dense network and the rather cheap rent costs (first 30 min: free; 30 to 90 min: €1.00; each hour thereafter: €2.00 (cost prices in 2009)), this biking system became very popular in Lyon for young and old generations (Fig. 22.5).

Also stretching exercises (Fig. 22.6) replacing the current candy and soft drink advertisements in bus stop places could help people improving their physical fitness while waiting for the bus.

Architects, designers, developers, employers and planners involved with campus sites, including hospitals and universities, should ensure that different parts of the site are linked by appropriate walking and cycling routes. Furthermore, they should ensure that new workplaces are linked to

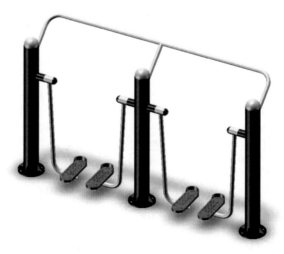

Fig. 22.4 Outdoor gym that could be part of a public waiting place like bus stop or metro station

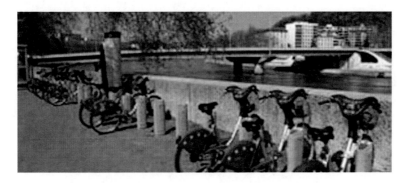

Fig. 22.5 Bike station in Lyon (vélo'v 2009 (http://www.velov.grandlyon.com/?L=1))

walking and cycling networks (National Institute for Health and Clinical Excellence (NICE) 2008).

Because it has been estimated that an additional 2 min of stair climbing per day would translate to a weight reduction of more than 0.5 kg/year (Wells et al. 2007), architects, designers and facility managers who are responsible for public buildings (including workplaces and schools) should ensure during building design or refurbishment, that staircases are designed and positioned to encourage people to use them. For example, they should be well-lit and well-decorated.

Children's services, school sport partnerships, school governing bodies and head teachers should ensure that school playgrounds are designed to encourage varied physically active play. Primary schools should create areas (for instance, by using different colors) to promote individual and group physical activities such as hopscotch (hopscotch is a hopping game that can be played on a bare patch of ground or on a floor indoors) and other games (Cardon et al. 2008; National Institute for Health and Clinical Excellence (NICE) 2008; World Health Organization (WHO) 2009).

Some areas have good conditions for walking and biking, but parents do not feel safe letting their children – especially young ones – travel alone. For many of these schools, walking school buses are the answer. They are groups of children who walk designated routes to school under adult supervision, picking up kids along the way just like a bus. For some neighborhoods it is a casual group walk, while others set up a formal plan with adults scheduled to walk on certain days. Parents are provided with maps of safe routes to school and a bus has to be launched that is suitable for a given community (Fig. 22.7).

Other opportunities to stimulate a physically active lifestyle are by offering incentives to people who cycle into work or school or who walk or cycle for shopping. In Belgium for instance many employers are offering incentives (about 0.15 €/km) for employees cycling to work (incentive based upon data available in 2009) (Departement mobiliteit en openbare werken 2010).

Tax incentives could be used to stimulate businesses within communities to meet the community standards. If it is for instance desirable that communities have sidewalks and crosswalks to promote safe walking, mechanisms should be institutionalized to ensure that these amenities are included in any new construction or renovation (Peters et al. 2002).

As changing environments takes time, in the short term, the focus could be on affecting physical activity behavior in structured environments, such as schools, workplaces and community facilities, where an infrastructure already exists that could be used to build knowledge and skills. The advantage here is that many programs to promote physical activity already exist for those venues and could quickly be disseminated. In communities, public spaces such as parks, school grounds and public buildings, should encourage physical activity by placing signage encouraging active behaviors such as taking the stairs and walking the trails. Places of commerce can play a major role here by providing both the opportunity for physical activity (e.g., walking in the shopping streets or mall)

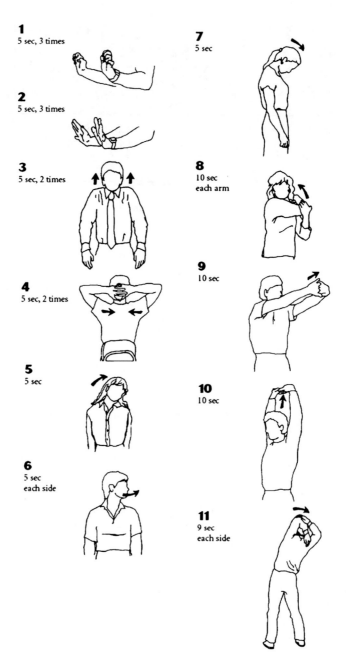

Fig. 22.6 Stretching exercise: a possible opportunity to stimulate traveler's physical fitness while waiting for the bus or train

and by giving incentives to become active (e.g., offering a bonus after a number of shopping visits by bike). This encourages more patronage at the shopping mall, so that both the walking consumer and the business gain (Peters et al. 2002).

As the recommended daily level of physical activity is rather to be achieved through lifestyle physical activity than through structured exercise, one problem is the difficulty for most people in knowing their success in achieving their physical activity target. However, the widely available step counters provide an inexpensive and easy way to monitor lifestyle physical activity (i.e., walking).

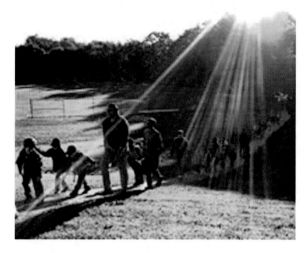

Fig. 22.7 Walking school bus

Having step counters allows people to set and monitor individual physical activity goals (De Cocker et al. 2007, 2008; Peters et al. 2002).

Environmental Barriers for Healthy Dietary Habits

Much attention has been paid on how our modern environment increases human's energy intake. Many environmental factors have been suggested to affect total energy intake and the evidence for those factors is being discussed below.

These days, people are eating out at *fast food* restaurants more often among others because of time constraints. Many fast food restaurants encourage super-sizing of meals, while other restaurants are promoting "all you can eat." However, not only *portion sizes* served in restaurants and fast food restaurants increased substantially (Diliberti et al. 2004), but also the size of soft drinks and many kinds of snack foods increased significantly (Rolls et al. 2004; Young and Nestle 2002). Different studies investigated the impact of fast food restaurants and portion sizes on adolescent's weight and/or health (see Chapter 18).

Unhealthy school environments might also contribute to the rising obesity prevalence in children and adolescents (Johnson-Taylor and Everhart 2006). Kubik et al. (2003) investigated the association between young adolescents' dietary behaviors and school vending machines, à la carte programs, and fried potatoes' being served at school lunch. Based upon their finding, they concluded that à la carte availability was inversely associated with fruit and fruit/vegetable consumption and positively associated with total and saturated fat intake. Furthermore, snack vending machines were negatively correlated with fruit consumption. Neumark-Sztainer et al. (2005) examined associations between high school students' lunch patterns and vending machine purchases and the school food environment and policies. They concluded that student snack food purchases at school were significantly associated with the number of snack machines at school. Furthermore they found that students in schools in which soft drink machines were turned off during lunch time purchased less soft drinks from vending machines on a weekly basis compared to students in schools in which soft drink machines were turned on during lunch (Neumark-Sztainer et al. 2005). These findings from cross-sectional data suggest that unhealthy school environments markedly contribute to an unhealthy lifestyle and probably to obesity in young adults. However, results from a more recent cross-sectional study provided only little evidence for associations of environmental factors in the school environment with soft drink and snack consumption among adolescents and suggest that longitudinal research is needed to confirm these findings (van der Horst et al. 2008).

Unhealthy foods and drinks are aggressively advertised via the media. However, evidence of the pervasive exposure of media on childhood overweight is still very scarce. Some studies have shown that children's request and parent purchases of advertised foods on TV are related to the hours of TV viewing (Coon and Tucker 2002; Taras et al. 1989). More recently, Dixon et al. examined (a) associations between children's regular TV viewing habits and their food-related attitudes and behavior; and (b) an experiment assessing the impact of varying combinations of TV advertisements for unhealthy and healthy foods on children's dietary knowledge, attitudes and intentions. Based upon their results, they concluded that longer TV use and more frequent commercial TV viewing were independently associated with more positive attitudes toward junk food. Furthermore, longer TV use was also independently associated with higher reported junk food consumption (Dixon et al. 2007). A more in depth discussion on the influence of the media on dietary habits in children and adolescents can be found in Chapter 20 of this book.

Availability and access to healthy foods are important for nutrition behaviors in youth and adulthood (Brug et al. 2006). The availability of supermarkets that are defined as having the most healthful food options was related to the wealth of neighborhoods. Morland et al. (2002) found 3 times as many supermarkets in the wealthier neighborhoods, while more convenience stores, small grocery stores, and specialty food stores were found in the lower-income neighborhoods. Furthermore, fast-food restaurants were more prevalent in the lower- and medium-income neighborhoods than in the higher-income neighborhoods (Morland et al. 2002). Unfortunately, those surveys did not collect data on obesity risk, so they were unable to demonstrate a relationship between the differences in the socio-economic distribution of food sources and obesity risk.

Only few studies have examined the relationship between the local food environment and dietary intake, particularly among populations at risk for obesity. Edmonds et al. found that greater availability of juice and vegetables in local restaurants was associated with higher reported juice and vegetable consumption among African American boys (Edmonds et al. 2001). Among Black Americans, the presence of a supermarket in the census tract was associated with a 30% increase in the likelihood of consuming the recommended amount of saturated fat (Morland et al. 2002). Other researchers have documented that easy access to supermarket shopping might be associated with higher household fruit consumptions (Rose and Richards 2004).

Given the important increase in *food availability 24 h a day* because of an essential rise in night shops and supermarkets that are open 24 h (e.g., some supermarkets in the UK), it would be interesting to investigate the impact of these night shops on dietary habits and obesity risks in neighborhoods where night shops are available. However, until now, no studies were found that investigated the impact of food availability 24 h a day on dietary intake and obesity risk.

Manufacturers compete for the improvement of the *taste and palatability* of their food products. Therefore, people very often eat because of tastiness rather than because of hungriness. Rolls (2007) investigated how those tasty and palatable foods might influence dietary intakes and obesity risks. Rolls showed how the physiological concepts are fundamental to understand the rise in obesity. During the last 30 years, sensory stimulation produced by the taste, smell, texture and appearance of food, as well as its availability, has increased dramatically. However, the satiety signals produced by stomach distension, satiety hormones, etc. have remained basically unchanged. Therefore, the effect on the brain's control system for appetite leads to a net average increase in the reward value and palatability of food, which overrides the satiety signals and contributes to the tendency to be over-stimulated by food and to overeat (Rolls 2007). More evidences about the relationship between sensory factors and childhood obesity can be read in Chapter 25 of this book.

Environmental Opportunities to Stimulate Healthy Dietary Habits

Although it might seem easier and less expensive to change our food environment instead of changing our physical activity environment, the fact that the scientific and medical communities (except on fruit and vegetables) rarely agree on the specifics of what a healthy diet should contain makes it a difficult task (Peters et al. 2002).

When thinking of environmental opportunities to promote healthy dietary habits, a first step could be by informing people even better about the food they consume by broadening nutrition labeling, to include calorie and nutrient information on restaurant foods and foods served in school canteens. This is especially important as more and more of today's food is consumed in restaurants, and as typical portion sizes have grown dramatically in the past decade. Most people have no idea how much they are eating and as mentioned before, there are only very weak biological mechanisms to protect against "overeating." To tackle the problem of overeating further, we could create public demand for smaller portion sizes, in order to protect against our biological and social propensity to "clean our plate" (Peters et al. 2002).

Dixon et al. (2007) found in their experiment that advertisements for nutritious foods promote selected positive attitudes and beliefs concerning these foods. Therefore changing the food advertising environment on children's TV to one where nutritious foods are promoted and junk foods are relatively unrepresented would help to normalize and reinforce healthy eating. So, governmental influences that could contribute to healthier dietary habits among children and adolescents are for instance the implementation of nutrition policies that limit advertising of unhealthy foods between television programs for children. Other examples could be the provision of tax incentives for grocery stores to open in inner cities and/or applying a "fat tax" to fast food purchases and using the money generated to create public education campaigns about obesity.

School food policies that decrease access to foods high in fats and sugars are associated with less frequent purchase of these items at school among high school students. Lowering the price of fruits and vegetables and low-fat snacks in schools and vending machines promoted purchases of those foods within schools and influenced eating behaviors (French et al. 1997, 2001; Johnson-Taylor and Everhart 2006). Therefore, schools should examine their food-related policies and decrease access to foods that are low in nutrients and high in fats and sugars (Neumark-Sztainer et al. 2005). In addition, they should foresee the provision of healthier school meals, banning of soda & snack vending machines, and the provision of fruits and vegetables at school at lower prices. Furthermore, the provision of a water fountain in schools and public places could help in the battle against soft drink consumption.

Individual dietary choices are primarily influenced by such considerations as taste, cost, convenience and nutritional value of foods. Fat and sugar provide dietary energy at very low cost. Food pricing and marketing practices are therefore an essential component of the eating environment. Recent studies have applied economic theories to changing dietary behavior. Price reduction strategies promote the choice of targeted foods by lowering their cost relative to alternative food choices. French (2003) demonstrated that price reductions are an effective strategy to increase the purchase of more healthful foods in community-based settings such as work sites and schools. As their results were generalizable across various food types and populations, reducing prices of healthful foods could be a public health strategy that should be implemented through policy initiatives and industry collaborations.

Institutionalization of Systems Required

To sustain environmental and social changes in the long-term, some level of institutionalization of systems that support the desired changes is required. If it is for instance desirable that communities have sidewalks and crosswalks to promote safe walking, they should institutionalize mechanisms that ensure that these amenities are included in any new construction or renovation. This could for instance be achievable by providing tax breaks for businesses that meet such community standards and by integrating these systems that support the desired changes in urban planning (Peters et al. 2002).

Such efforts can be sustained only through continuous funding and sustainable political will. Because of the scale of the problem that we are facing, funding will need to come from nearly every sector of society, public and private. A better understanding of the economics of physical activity and eating behaviors is urgently required to look for incentives that can support change throughout the value chain (Peters et al. 2002).

Conceptual and Methodological Considerations

Methodological Considerations with Regard to the Studies Reported in this Chapter

It is important to note that the relatively weak evidence found thus far for the association between environmental factors and obesity may not be interpreted as absence of a relationship between "the environment" and obesity-related behaviors. There is still a lack of high-quality studies and of study replications. Most of the available research was focused on only a part of the environment, especially micro-level factors in the socio-cultural and physical environment. Studies on macro-sized environmental factors are largely lacking. Furthermore, many potentially relevant environmental factors have not been studied at all (Brug et al. 2006). Many studies applied rather weak study designs and measurement instruments. For example, most of the available observational studies used cross-sectional designs, thus allowing only conjectures about associations. Only few studies used multivariate analyses, adjusting for other potential individual or environmental correlates of nutrition or physical activity behaviors and many intervention studies did not include a control group.

Other important methodological considerations should be reported for the measurement of the built environment:

Most of the studies investigating the built environment and its relationship with obesity did not directly measure the environment (Johnson-Taylor and Everhart 2006). Instead, indirect measures of the environment were used to represent it. The indirect measure most frequently used were for instance census data and GIS data (e.g., road network distance, steep hill barrier, grid of city blocks). Although these methods can approximate conditions of the built environment, they may not be as accurate as direct measurements because database information often is outdated and might not correctly reflect conditions at the time of the study (Boone et al. 2008).

Intermediate measures of the built environment have included self-reported perceptions of neighborhood residents. However, as Kirtland et al. already pointed out, only moderate to low agreement has been demonstrated between self-reports of neighborhood and community environments and objective environmental audits (Kirtland et al. 2003). Other intermediate measurements of the built environment that have been used are regional land-use data from tax assessors and aerial photography. Although these measurements can approximate the built environment, tax data are self-reported by individuals and aerial photography cannot show actual uses of buildings. Various databases (e.g., departments of environmental health, state departments of agriculture, telephone book, yellow pages online, police web sites, school district lists) also have been used to track specific entities (e.g., places where people can buy food, public playgrounds, fast-food restaurants) that are available within certain areas. The limitation of these studies, however, is that they did not audit the actual site of the entities reported within the built environment; therefore, they made assumptions about availability within the environment without actually verifying the accuracy of these data sources.

Direct measurement through environmental audits has only been used in a few studies with obesity as the primary outcome (Giles-Corti and Donovan 2003). Measurements included the type of street and the presence of sidewalks for each study participant. Although these measures specifically verified what was in the physical environment, they were not sophisticated enough to adequately capture enough characteristics of the built environment to account for all environmental factors that have influenced obesity, such as the types and frequency of different institutions available in the areas.

A last conceptual consideration is the reliance on the environment only. In the 80s psychosocial models of behavior and behavior change dominated the field, explaining health behavior by attitudes, social influences, self-efficacy, etc. People were considered conscious decision-makers deciding for healthy or unhealthy behavior in a rational way. During the last 10 years, research turned towards the environment, sometimes completely ignoring the fact that psychosocial factors are still important in explaining behavior. The importance of the environment has rather to be seen in the context of the "Ecological Model," in which the interaction of psychosocial and environmental factors is crucial in explaining and changing health behavior. It is clear that changing the environment to make it "health enhancing" in the context of obesity will be necessary but insufficient to curb the epidemic. It needs to be supplemented by strategies focusing on the personal and social determinants of nutrition and physical activity (De Bourdeaudhuij et al. 2005, 2006, 2008).

Recommendations for Future Study Designs and Analytical Strategies for Environmental Research on Obesity, Physical Activity and Diet

Several authoritative reports identified environmental and policy interventions as the most promising strategies for creating population-wide improvements in dietary habits and physical activity, in the hope to tackle the increasing obesity epidemic. However, many methodological challenges for conducting environmental and policy research still have to be overcome in order to create advances in the study area. Therefore, a meeting entitled "Study Designs and Analytic Strategies for Environmental and Policy Research on Obesity, Physical Activity, and Diet" was held 8 Apr 2008 (Sallis et al. 2009). Participants from diverse backgrounds attended this meeting and assisted in the identification of gaps in our current knowledge. In addition, they generated recommendations for promising methods to enhance environmental and policy research related to obesity. The final recommendations were based on a post-meeting participant survey, in which all meeting participants were asked to complete an online survey to rank their highest priorities in five topic areas (Sallis et al. 2009). In summary, these five resulting high priority topic areas included:

- Research status and gaps related to environment, policy, and physical activity.
- Research status and gaps related to environment, policy, and diet.
- Promising study designs for environmental and policy research and evaluation.
- Developing measures of policy for obesity, diet, and physical activity.
- Statistical approaches for environmental and policy research.

As demonstrated in the Annex, existing methods that could be applied to advance the field were identified. Those methods included for instance prospective studies, evaluations of natural experiments, and economic studies. Furthermore, training for investigators in the use of appropriate statistical methods for complex designs and interdisciplinary collaborations were highly recommended. Methodological research priorities included the development of measures of policy, health impact assessments, and the investigation of policy adoption and implementation. The results of this conference can be used to improve the quality and quantity of environmental and policy research as well as the translation to action to control obesity (Sallis et al. 2009).

One of the most important top priorities set by this study (see Annex), for research investigating associations between obesity and the environment is the need to establish causality (Sallis et al. 2009). Establishing causal relationships is an important goal because it provides a foundation for more confident policy and practice recommendations. Although ultimately longitudinal studies are necessary to establish causality, as already mentioned before, the majority of studies are cross-sectional in nature. Several authors already recognized that longitudinal or pretest-posttest intervention studies (particularly with respect to the built environment and physical activity) are still lacking and call for further research in this direction (Handy et al. 2002; Wells et al. 2007).

One opportunity for longitudinal investigations are the "natural experiments" whereby some environmental or policy changes (not intentionally induced as an experiment) allow for data collection prior to and following the environmental change. Examples of natural experiment research related to physical activity and diet include data collections prior to and following the construction of a grocery store, the opening of a vegetable stand or farmers' market, a new policy making the high school gym available to community members in the evening, etc. Although such longitudinal studies are time intensive and demanding, the clarity they can provide regarding causality makes them a worthy goal (Wells et al. 2007).

Mediators and Moderators to Explain Causality

Causality can be explained by providing insight regarding the pathway or mechanism underlying relations among variables. From a theoretical standpoint, it is crucial to understand how or why variables are related, as this allows for a clearer conceptualization of the behavior or factor being studied. A *mediator* explains "how" or "why" an independent variable affects a dependent variable as shown in Fig. 22.8. For example, physical characteristics of a neighborhood may lead to neighborhood perceptions such as sense of community, which in turn influence physical activity participation like walking or cycling. Similarly, food environment characteristics may influence food-purchasing attitudes and behaviors that in turn affect diet. Hence, mediators can operate as dependent variables (e.g., affected by neighborhood design) and independent variables (e.g., influencing physical activity) (Wells et al. 2007).

Another important direction for environmental research related to obesity is the full examination of circumstances under which relationships exist between the environment and physical activity or dietary habits. *Moderators* (or effect modifiers) affect the relationship between an independent variable like proximity to a farmers market and a dependent variable like vegetable consumption. Moderators address questions such as "for whom," "when," or "under what circumstances" (as illustrated in Fig. 22.8) and they are involved when the nature or the direction of the relation between an independent variable and a dependent variable depends on a third variable (the moderator).

With respect to environment-physical activity and environment-diet research, there is a need to know what kinds of design or environmental intervention strategies are effective for whom, under what conditions. For instance, one can question whether proximity to a park or natural area only encourages physical activity among people of a certain age, ethnicity, or gender (Wells et al. 2007).

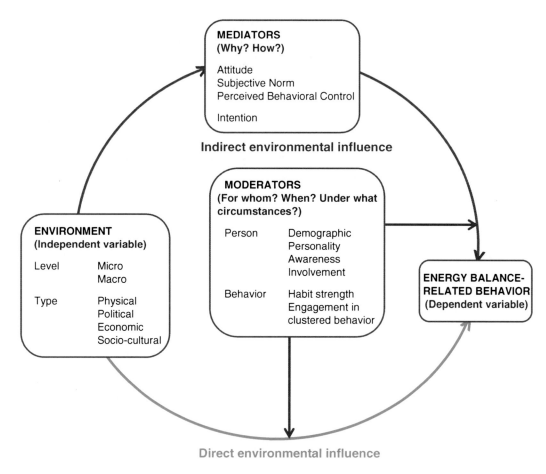

Fig. 22.8 Adapted version of the environmental research framework for weight gain prevention (EnRG) presenting the role of mediators and moderators in the environment-behavior relationship when focusing on energy–balance behavior (Kremers et al. 2006)

Kremers et al. recently provided a more detailed framework for the study of both personal and environmental determinants for nutrition and physical activity behaviors (see Fig. 22.8). They presented a dual-process view on the environment-behavior relationship. This dual-process model can be used to gain insight into the most important determinants of "energy balance-related behaviors" (EBRBs) as well as into the causal mechanisms that underlie these behaviors. In their Environmental Research framework for weight Gain prevention (EnRG), environmental influences are hypothesized to influence behavior both indirectly and directly (see Fig. 22.8). The indirect causal mechanism reflects the *mediating role* of personal behavior-specific cognitions, and the direct influence reflects the automatic, unconscious influence of the environment on behavior. In this model, six specific factors (demographic, personality, awareness, involvement, habit strength, and behavioral engagement) are postulated to *moderate* the causal path (i.e., inducing either the automatic (lower path on "Direct environmental influence" in Fig. 22.8) or the cognitive mediated environment-behavior relationship (remaining path on "Indirect environmental influence" in Fig. 22.8)) (Kremers et al. 2006). For what concerns the demographic moderators for instance, does an increasing body of evidence show a differential impact of the environment on energy balance-related behaviors with respect to age (Chinn et al. 1999), gender (Foster et al. 2004; Suminski et al. 2005), socio-economic status (Chinn et al. 1999; Giles-Corti and Donovan 2002) and ethnicity (Eyler et al. 2003; King et al. 2000).

Conclusions

Our global obesity epidemic is driven in large part by a mismatch between our environment and our metabolism. Our human physiology developed to function within an environment where high levels of physical activity were needed in daily life and food was inconsistently available. However, our current environment is characterized by a situation where minimal physical activity is required for daily life and food is abundant, inexpensive, high in energy density and widely available. Therefore, our current environment encourages overeating while discouraging physical activity, creating a consistent bias toward positive energy balance. This means that our modern environment requires substantial cognitive efforts for body weight control. As people who are not devoting substantial conscious efforts to manage their body weight are likely to gain weight, we desperately need to modify the environment to one that is less conducive to weight gain.

Because an integral part of the environment is socio-cultural, we will have to approach environmental changes in a way that ultimately will be accepted and supported by the population. It is not likely that we will easily give up our convenient modern lifestyle we have created for ourselves. Therefore, the challenge in changing the environment is not to "go back in time," but to engineer physical activity and healthy eating back into our lives in a way that is compatible with the modern world and our socio-cultural values (Peters et al. 2002). It is clear that some level of institutionalization of systems that support the desired changes is required to sustain environmental and social changes in the long-term.

Although evidence clearly shows that the environment has an impact on obesity related lifestyle factors, evidence for effective strategies combating this obesogenic environment is very scarce. Interventions that aim to change environmental factors in order to reduce obesity may include taxes or subsidies to encourage healthy eating or physical activity, extra provision of sporting facilities, efforts to improve safety and accessibility of walking and cycling or play areas or attempting to influence the social meanings and values attached to weight, food or physical activity.

Finally, it is important to note that better-designed and -conducted research on the true importance of the interaction between environmental factors and psychosocial factors, including the micro and the macro level, for obesogenic behavioral change is needed to reassure the success of large-scale environmental change interventions.

Research priorities identified include improving the design of effectiveness evaluations and, particularly, using designs which include a control group for evaluating policy; including cost-effectiveness analysis and improving measures for other outcomes; measuring impact for population subgroups; investigating impact on health inequalities; conducting and integrating qualitative research, and developing a common framework.

Finally, features of the built and social environments should be combined with psychosocial variables to propose mediational models that can be tested to develop theories of how environment influences behavior and obesity.

Annex

Top-scoring recommendations for improving the methodology of environment and policy research related to obesity, diet, and physical activity.[1] A meeting titled "Study Designs and Analytic Strategies for Environmental and Policy Research on Obesity, Physical Activity, and Diet" was held 8 Apr 2008. Meeting participants were asked to complete an online survey to rank their highest priorities from each of nine lists in five topic areas. The top-ranked two to five recommendations for each list are provided in the table below. Surveys were completed by 41 of 53 conference

[1] Based on rankings of conference participants ($n=41$).

participants, for a 77% response rate. The full report of the conference, including slide presentations, is available on websites (Active Living Research 2009 (www.activelivingresearch.org); Healthy Eating Research 2009 (www.healthyeatingresearch.org)) (Sallis et al. 2009).

	Rating average (1 = lowest; 5 = highest)
TOPIC 1: Research status and gaps related to environment, policy, and physical activity	
Top five promising methods that can be used in research now	
Natural experiments with good measures that are practical and cost effective	3.97
Surveillance systems with good measures of environmental variables	3.44
Define individual and environmental factors using mixed methods and other new models to study both simultaneously	3.08
Evaluation of policy process	2.93
Opportunity to study synergies of environmental factors with health outcomes and ecologic sustainability (e.g., carbon reduction and walking/bicycling)	2.78
Top five research priorities	
Prospective studies and evaluations of natural experiments to improve evidence of causality	4.14
Test multiple levels of social–ecologic model and evaluate interaction of variables across levels (e.g., environmental and social)	3.54
Develop appropriate measurement tools for target populations, particularly those at high risk for obesity (physical activity and correlates)	3.35
Understand how local communities can be mobilized to initiate policy change	3.25
Understand how local (and other) policies are implemented (e.g., how implementation varies across different locales or populations and what factors affect implementation)	3.05
Top two priorities for funding and communicating research	
Dedicated funding and study sections for multilevel, environmental, and policy studies	2.64
Speed up dissemination of results so that they can be translated more quickly to policy and practice changes (alternatives to journals, including blogs, working papers, websites)	2.57
TOPIC 2: Research status and gaps related to environment, policy, and diet	
Top five promising methods that can be used in research now	
Policy change evaluations that assess (1) implementation, (2) enforcement, (3) community acceptance, and (4) impact over time on rates of obesity or obesogenic nutrition behaviors	3.78
Surveillance research to track changes in food-industry activities with the potential to influence nutrition behaviors (e.g., packaged portion sizes, reduced-calorie options) would allow researchers to (1) identify opportunities for natural experiments, (2) examine the influence of industry activities on nutrition behaviors and obesity, and (3) determine how industry activities shift in response to policy changes	3.08
Observational multilevel studies, including research designed to examine interactions between individuals and food environments (e.g., what individual factors increase susceptibility to obesogenic food environments)	2.89
Studies designed to examine (or quantify) the influence of multiple environmental domains and their interactions on rates of obesity (or obesogenic nutrition behaviors)	2.79
Cross-disciplinary and transdisciplinary collaborations that incorporate complementary methodologies (e.g., qualitative and quantitative approaches)	2.76
Top five research priorities	
Conduct research in minority and low-income populations, such as the evaluation of policies to reduce/eliminate disparities in access to food (e.g., tax incentives for stores in low-income neighborhoods)	3.86

(continued)

(continued)

Develop standardized measures of food environment and nutrition policies (for various types of environments and contexts) to improve the comparability of findings across studies)	3.67
Examine motivations for food choices, including tensions between internal and external (environmental) factors on behavior	2.94
Conduct research relating to home and family food environments	2.76
Conduct research guided by systems theory	2.6
Top two priorities for funding and communicating research	
Create special funding mechanisms for conducting time-sensitive natural experiments and collaborative research	1.73
Encourage cross-disciplinary collaborations and mentoring of junior scientists by those experienced in this area	1.57
TOPIC 3: Promising study designs for environmental and policy research and evaluation	
Top five promising study designs	
Promote rapid evaluation of natural experiments	4.17
Develop policy surveillance measures and data-collection systems	3.84
Promote health impact assessment techniques	3.38
Support international research and comparisons to expand range of environments and policies assessed	2.95
Exploit and promote analysis of cohort/panel data	2.85
TOPIC 4: Developing measures of policy for obesity, diet, and physical activity	
Top five priorities for developing measures of policy	
Measures to support surveillance of food- and activity-related policies	3.54
Measures of strength of policy, policy enforcement, policy implementation that can be compared across policy domains	3.5
Improved measures of valuation: what do different communities value? Valuation models in the health field	3.07
Develop HIA methods and funding mechanisms	3
Develop measures of community support for policy changes	3
TOPIC 5: Statistical approaches for environmental and policy research	
Top five priorities for statistical approaches	
Develop an accessible compendium of metrics or indicators derived from available environmental measures	3.43
Conduct training workshops in designing and analyzing multilevel studies	3.14
Use both quantitative and qualitative methods, including case studies	3.13
Training in analytic techniques tailored for small samples	2.95
Consider variability of environmental and policy factors in designing studies: how much variability is necessary?	2.89

HIA = health impact assessment

References

Active Living Research (2009). *Building the evidence to prevent childhood obesity and support active communities.* Robert Wood Johnson Foundation, San Diego (February 8, 2010); http://www.activelivingresearch.org.

Beasley, J.M., Riley, W.T., & Jean-Mary, J. (2005). Accuracy of a PDA-based dietary assessment program. *Nutrition, 21,* 672–677.

Beasley, J.M., Riley, W.T., Davis, A., & Singh, J. (2008). Evaluation of a PDA-based dietary assessment and intervention program: a randomized controlled trial. *Journal of American College of Nutrition, 27,* 280–286.

Bellisari, A. (2008). Evolutionary origins of obesity. *Obesity Reviews, 9,* 165–180.

Berg, C., Lappas, G., Wolk, A., Strandhagen, E., Toren, K., Rosengren, A., Thelle, D., & Lissner, L. (2009). Eating patterns and portion size associated with obesity in a Swedish population. *Appetite, 52,* 21–26.

Boone, J.E., Gordon-Larsen, P., Stewart, J.D., & Popkin, B.M. (2008). Validation of a GIS facilities database: quantification and implications of error. *Annals of Epidemiology, 18,* 371–377.

Booth, K.M., Pinkston, M.M., & Poston, W.S. (2005). Obesity and the built environment. *Journal of the American Dietetic Association, 105,* S110–S117.

Boulton, T.J., Magarey, A.M., & Cockington, R.A. (1995). Tracking of serum lipids and dietary energy, fat and calcium intake from 1 to 15 years. *Acta Paediatrica, 84,* 1050–1055.

British Medical Association (BMA) (2005). *Preventing childhood obesity.* London: BMA publications unit.

Brug, J., van Lenthe, F.J., & Kremers, S.P. (2006). Revisiting Kurt Lewin: how to gain insight into environmental correlates of obesogenic behaviors. *American Journal of Preventive Medicine, 31,* 525–529.

Burdette, H.L., & Whitaker, R.C. (2004). Neighborhood playgrounds, fast food restaurants, and crime: relationships to overweight in low-income preschool children. *Preventive Medicine, 38,* 57–63.

Burdette, H.L., Wadden, T.A., & Whitaker, R.C. (2006). Neighborhood safety, collective efficacy, and obesity in women with young children. *Obesity (Silver Spring), 14,* 518–525.

Cardon, G.M., & De Bourdeaudhuij, I.M. (2008). Are preschool children active enough? Objectively measured physical activity levels. *Research Quarterly for Exercise and Sport, 79,* 326–332.

Cardon, G., De Clercq, D., De Bourdeaudhuij, I., & Breithecker, D. (2004a). Sitting habits in elementary schoolchildren: a traditional versus a "moving school". *Patient Education and Counselling, 54,* 133–142.

Cardon, G., Verstraete, S., De Bourdeaudhuij, I.M., & De Clercq, D.L. (2004b). Physical activity levels in elementary-school physical education: a comparison of swimming and non-swimming classes. *Journal of Teaching in Physical Education, 23,* 252–263.

Cardon, G., Van Cauwenberghe, E., Labarque, V., Haerens, L., & De Bourdeaudhuij, I. (2008). The contribution of preschool playground factors in explaining children's physical activity during recess. *International Journal of Behavioral Nutrition and Physical Activity, 5,* 11.

Chinn, D.J., White, M., Harland, J., Drinkwater, C., & Raybould, S. (1999). Barriers to physical activity and socioeconomic position: implications for health promotion. *Journal of Epidemiology and Community Health, 53,* 191–192.

Coleman, K.J., Geller, K.S., Rosenkranz, R.R., & Dzewaltowski, D.A. (2008). Physical activity and healthy eating in the after-school environment. *Journal of School Health, 78,* 633–640.

Collins (2006). *Collins essential English dictionary.* New York: HarperCollins Publishers.

Coogan, P.F., & Coogan, M.A. (2004). When worlds collide: observations on the integration of epidemiology and transportation behavioral analysis in the study of walking. *American Journal of Health Promotion, 19,* 39–44.

Coon, K.A., & Tucker, K.L. (2002). Television and children's consumption patterns. A review of the literature. *Minerva Pediatrica, 54,* 423–436.

De Bourdeaudhuij, I., Sallis, J.F., & Saelens, B.E. (2003). Environmental correlates of physical activity in a sample of Belgian adults. *American Journal of Health Promotion, 18,* 83–92.

De Bourdeaudhuij, I., Teixeira, P.J., Cardon, G., & Deforche, B. (2005). Environmental and psychosocial correlates of physical activity in Portuguese and Belgian adults. *Public Health Nutrition, 8,* 886–895.

De Bourdeaudhuij, I., Yngve, A., te Velde, S.J., Klepp, K.I., Rasmussen, M., Thorsdottir, I., Wolf, A., & Brug, J. (2006). Personal, social and environmental correlates of vegetable intake in normal weight and overweight 9 to 13-year old boys. *International Journal of Behavioral Nutrition and Physical Activity, 3,* 37.

De Bourdeaudhuij, I., te Velde, S., Brug, J., Due, P., Wind, M., Sandvik, C., Maes, L., Wolf, A., Perez Rodrigo, C., Yngve, A., Thorsdottir, I., Rasmussen, M., Elmadfa, I., Franchini, B., & Klepp, K.I. (2008). Personal, social and environmental predictors of daily fruit and vegetable intake in 11-year-old children in nine European countries. *European Journal of Clinical Nutrition, 62,* 834–841.

De Cocker, K.A., De Bourdeaudhuij, I.M., Brown, W.J., & Cardon, G.M. (2007). Effects of "10,000 steps Ghent": a whole-community intervention. *American Journal of Preventive Medicine, 33,* 455–463.

De Cocker, K.A., De Bourdeaudhuij, I.M., Brown, W.J., Cardon, G.M. (2008). The effect of a pedometer-based physical activity intervention on sitting time. *Preventive Medicine, 47,* 179–181.

Departement mobiliteit en openbare werken (2010). *Mobiel Vlaanderen, voor uw vragen over mobiliteit en openbare werken: Fietsvergoeding woon-werk verkeer.* Brussel (February 8, 2010); http://www.mobielvlaanderen.be/wegverkeer/fietsen-013.php.

Diliberti, N., Bordi, P.L., Conklin, M.T., Roe, L.S., & Rolls, B.J. (2004). Increased portion size leads to increased energy intake in a restaurant meal. *Obesity Reserach, 12,* 562–568.

Dixon, H.G., Scully, M.L., Wakefield, M.A., White, V.M., & Crawford, D.A. (2007). The effects of television advertisements for junk food versus nutritious food on children's food attitudes and preferences. *Social Science & Medicine, 65,* 1311–1323.

Drewnowski, A. (2004). Obesity and the food environment: dietary energy density and diet costs. *American Journal of Preventive Medicine, 27,* 154–162.

Dwyer, G.M., Higgs, J., Hardy, L.L., & Baur, L.A. (2008a). What do parents and preschool staff tell us about young children's physical activity: a qualitative study. *International Journal of Behavioral Nutrition and Physical Activity, 5,* 66.

Dwyer, J., Needham, L., Simpson, J.R., & Heeney, E.S. (2008b). Parents report intrapersonal, interpersonal, and environmental barriers to supporting healthy eating and physical activity among their preschoolers. *Applied Physiology, Nutrition, and Metabolism, 33,* 338–346.

Edmonds, J., Baranowski, T, Baranowski, J., Cullen, K.W., & Myres, D. (2001). Ecological and socioeconomic correlates of fruit, juice, and vegetable consumption among African-American boys. *Preventive Medicine, 32,* 476–481.

Edwards, R.D. (2008). Public transit, obesity, and medical costs: assessing the magnitudes. *Preventive Medicine, 46,* 14–21.

Ellaway, A., Macintyre, S., & Bonnefoy, X. (2005). Graffiti, greenery, and obesity in adults: secondary analysis of European cross sectional survey. *British Medical Journal, 331,* 611–612.

Ewing, R., Schmid, T., Killingsworth, R., Zlot, A., & Raudenbush, S. (2003). Relationship between urban sprawl and physical activity, obesity, and morbidity. *American Journal of Health Promotion, 18,* 47–57.

Eyler, A.A., Matson-Koffman, D., Young, D.R., Wilcox, S., Wilbur, J., Thompson, J.L., Sanderson, B., & Evenson, K.R. (2003). Quantitative study of correlates of physical activity in women from diverse racial/ethnic groups: The Women's Cardiovascular Health Network Project – summary and conclusions. *American Journal of Preventive Medicine, 25,* 93–103.

Feldman, P.J., & Steptoe, A. (2004). How neighborhoods and physical functioning are related: the roles of neighborhood socioeconomic status, perceived neighborhood strain, and individual health risk factors. *Annals of Behavioral Medicine, 27,* 91–99.

Foster, C., Hillsdon, M., & Thorogood, M. (2004). Environmental perceptions and walking in English adults. *Journal of Epidemiology and Community Health, 58,* 924–928.

Frank, L.D., Andresen, M.A., & Schmid, T.L. (2004). Obesity relationships with community design, physical activity, and time spent in cars. *American Journal of Preventive Medicine, 27,* 87–96.

French, S.A. (2003). Pricing effects on food choices. *Journal of Nutrition, 133,* 841S–843S.

French, S.A., Jeffery, R.W., Story, M., Hannan, P., & Snyder, M.P. (1997). A pricing strategy to promote low-fat snack choices through vending machines. *American Journal of Public Health, 87,* 849–851.

French, S.A., Jeffery, R.W., Story, M., Breitlow, K.K., Baxter, J.S., Hannan, P., & Snyder, M.P. (2001). Pricing and promotion effects on low-fat vending snack purchases: the CHIPS Study. *American Journal of Public Health, 91,* 112–117.

Giles-Corti, B., & Donovan, R.J. (2002). Socioeconomic status differences in recreational physical activity levels and real and perceived access to a supportive physical environment. *Preventive Medicine, 35,* 601–611.

Giles-Corti, B., & Donovan, R.J. (2003). Relative influences of individual, social environmental, and physical environmental correlates of walking. *American Journal of Public Health, 93,* 1583–1589.

Giles-Corti, B., Broomhall, M.H., Knuiman, M., Collins, C., Douglas, K., Ng, K., Lange, A., & Donovan, R.J. (2005). Increasing walking: how important is distance to, attractiveness, and size of public open space? *American Journal of Preventive Medicine, 28,* 169–176.

Gordon-Larsen, P., Nelson, M.C., Page, P., & Popkin, B.M. (2006). Inequality in the built environment underlies key health disparities in physical activity and obesity. *Pediatrics, 117,* 417–424.

Government Office for Science (2007). *Foresight "Tackling obesities: future choices – project report", 2nd edition.* London: Department for Business Innovation and Skills (BIS), URN: 07/1184X.

Haerens, L., Deforche, B., Maes, L., Cardon, G., Stevens, V., & De Bourdeaudhuij, I. (2006). Evaluation of a 2-year physical activity and healthy eating intervention in middle school children. *Health Education Research, 21,* 911–921.

Handy, S.L., Boarnet, M.G., Ewing, R., & Killingsworth, R.E. (2002). How the built environment affects physical activity: views from urban planning. *American Journal of Preventive Medicine, 23,* 64–73.

Hardus, P.M., van Vuuren, C.L., Crawford, D., & Worsley, A. (2003). Public perceptions of the causes and prevention of obesity among primary school children. *International Journal of Obesity and Related Metabolic Disorders, 27,* 1465–1471.

Healthy Eating Research (2009). *Building evidence to prevent childhood obesity.* Robert Wood Johnson Foundation, Minneapolis (February 8, 2010); http://www.healthyeatingresearch.org.

Hill, J.O., & Peters, J.C. (1998). Environmental contributions to the obesity epidemic. *Science, 280,* 1371–1374.

Johnson-Taylor, W.L., & Everhart, J.E. (2006). Modifiable environmental and behavioral determinants of overweight among children and adolescents: report of a workshop. *Obesity (Silver Spring), 14,* 929–966.

Johnston, L.D., Delva, J., & O'Malley, P.M. (2007). Soft drink availability, contracts, and revenues in American secondary schools. *American Journal of Preventive Medicine, 33,* S209–S225.

Kandris, S., & Liu, G. (2003). *Indianapolis site-specific neighborhood health analysis: environmental factors and risk of childhood obesity.* Indianapolis: The Polis Center, IUPUI.

King, A.C., Castro, C., Wilcox, S., Eyler, A.A., Sallis, J.F., & Brownson, R.C. (2000). Personal and environmental factors associated with physical inactivity among different racial-ethnic groups of U.S. middle-aged and older-aged women. *Health Psychology, 19,* 354-364.

Kinra, S., Nelder, R.P., & Lewendon, G.J. (2000). Deprivation and childhood obesity: a cross sectional study of 20 973 children in Plymouth, United Kingdom. *Journal of Epidemiology and Community Health, 54,* 456–460.

Kirtland, K.A., Porter, D.E., Addy, C.L., Neet, M.J., Williams, J.E., Sharpe, P.A., Neff, L.J., Kimsey, C.D. Jr, & Ainsworth, B.E. (2003). Environmental measures of physical activity supports: perception versus reality. *American Journal of Preventive Medicine, 24,* 323–331.

Kremers, S.P., de Bruijn, G.J., Visscher, T.L., van Mechelen, W., de Vries, N.K., & Brug, J. (2006). Environmental influences on energy balance-related behaviors: a dual-process view. *International Journal of Behavioral Nutrition and Physical Activity, 3,* 9.

Kubik, M.Y., Lytle, L.A., Hannan, P.J., Perry, C.L., & Story, M. (2003). The association of the school food environment with dietary behaviors of young adolescents. *American Journal of Public Health, 93,* 1168–1173.

Ledikwe, J.H., Ello-Martin, J.A., & Rolls, B.J. (2005). Portion sizes and the obesity epidemic. *Journal of Nutrition, 135,* 905–909.

Lindberg, R. (2000). Active living: on the road with the 10,000 Steps Program. *Journal of the American Dietetic Association, 100,* 878–879.

Liu, G.C., Cunningham, C., Downs, S.M., Marrero, D.G., & Fineberg, N. (2002). A spatial analysis of obesogenic environments for children. *Proceedings of the AMIA Symposium,* Indianapolis, 459–463.

Michaelsen, K.F., Weaver, L., Branca, F., & Robertson, A. (2003). *Feeding and nutrition of infants and young children: Guidelines for the WHO European Region, with emphasis on the former Soviet countries.* Copenhagen, Denmark, World Health Organization, Regional Office for Europe: WHO Regional Publications, European Series, No. 87.

Mobley, L.R., Root, E.D., Finkelstein, E.A., Khavjou, O., Farris, R.P., & Will, J.C. (2006). Environment, obesity, and cardiovascular disease risk in low-income women. *American Journal of Preventive Medicine, 30,* 327–332.

Morland, K., Wing, S., Roux, A.D., & Poole, C. (2002). Neighborhood characteristics associated with the location of food stores and food service places. *American Journal of Preventive Medicine, 22,* 23–29.

Mummery, W.K., Schofield, G., Hinchliffe, A., Joyner, K., & Brown, W. (2006). Dissemination of a community-based physical activity project: the case of 10,000 steps. *Journal of Science and Medicine in Sport, 9,* 424–430.

National Institute for Health and Clinical Excellence (NICE) (2008). *Physical activity and the environment: Guidance on the promotion and creation of physical environments that support increased levels of physical activity.* London (April 13, 2009); http://www.nice.org.uk/Guidance/PH8.

Neumark-Sztainer, D., French, S., Hannan, P., Story, M., & Fulkerson, J. (2005). School lunch and snacking patterns among high school students: associations with school food environment and policies. *International Journal of Behavioral Nutrition and Physical Activity, 2,* 14.

Papas, M.A., Alberg, A.J., Ewing, R., Helzlsouer, K.J., Gary, T.L., & Klassen, A.C. (2007). The built environment and obesity. *Epidemiologic Reviews, 29,* 129–143.

Peters, J.C., Wyatt, H.R., Donahoo, W.T., & Hill, J.O. (2002). From instinct to intellect: the challenge of maintaining healthy weight in the modern world. *Obesity Reviews, 3,* 69–74.

Popkin, B.M. (2001). Nutrition in transition: the changing global nutrition challenge. *Asia Paific Journal of Clinical Nutrition, 10 Suppl,* S13–S18.

Rolls, E.T. (2007). Understanding the mechanisms of food intake and obesity. *Obesity Reviews, 8,* 67–72.

Rolls, B.J., Roe, L.S., Kral, T.V., Meengs, J.S., & Wall, D.E. (2004). Increasing the portion size of a packaged snack increases energy intake in men and women. *Appetite, 42,* 63–69.

Rose, D., & Richards, R. (2004). Food store access and household fruit and vegetable use among participants in the US Food Stamp Program. *Public Health Nutrition, 7,* 1081–1088.

Saelens, B.E., & Handy, S.L. (2008). Built environment correlates of walking: a review. *Medicine and Science in Sports and Exercise, 40,* S550–S566.

Saelens, B.E., Sallis, J.F., Black, J.B., & Chen, D. (2003a). Neighborhood-based differences in physical activity: an environment scale evaluation. *American Journal of Public Health, 93,* 1552–1558.

Saelens, B.E., Sallis, J.F., & Frank, L.D. (2003b). Environmental correlates of walking and cycling: findings from the transportation, urban design, and planning literatures. *Annals of Behavioral Medicine, 25,* 80–91.

Sallis, J.F., Story, M., & Lou, D. (2009). Study designs and analytic strategies for environmental and policy research on obesity, physical activity, and diet: recommendations from a meeting of experts. *American Journal of Preventive Medicine, 36,* S72–S77.

Schmid, T.L., Pratt, M., & Howze, E. (1995). Policy as intervention: environmental and policy approaches to the prevention of cardiovascular disease. *American Journal of Public Health, 85,* 1207–1211.

Stettler, N., Signer, T.M., & Suter, P.M. (2004). Electronic games and environmental factors associated with childhood obesity in Switzerland. *Obesity Research, 12,* 896–903.

Story, M., Hayes, M., & Kalina, B. (1996). Availability of foods in high schools: is there cause for concern? *Journal of the American Dietetic Association, 96,* 123–126.

Suminski, R.R., Poston, W.S., Petosa, R.L., Stevens, E., & Katzenmoyer, L.M. (2005). Features of the neighborhood environment and walking by U.S. adults. *American Journal of Preventive Medicine, 28,* 149–155.

Suminski, R.R., Fritzsinger, J., Leck, T., & Hyder, M.M. (2008). Observing physical activity in suburbs. *Health & Place, 14,* 894–899.

Swinburn, B., Egger, G., & Raza, F. (1999). Dissecting obesogenic environments: the development and application of a framework for identifying and prioritizing environmental interventions for obesity. *Preventive Medicine, 29,* 563–570.

Taras, H.L., Sallis, J.F., Patterson, T.L., Nader, P.R., & Nelson, J.A. (1989). Television's influence on children's diet and physical activity. *Journal of Developmental & Behavioral Pediatrics, 10,* 176–180.

Tauber, M., & Jouret, B. (2004). Role of environmental factors in childhood obesity. In W. Kiess, C. Marcus, & M. Wabitsch (Eds.), *Obesity in childhood and adolescence* (pp. 91–102). Basel: Karger.

US Department of Health and Human Services (1996). *Physical activity and health: a report of the surgeon general.* Atlanta: US Department of Health and Human Services, Centers for Disease Control and Prevention, National Center for Chronic Disease Prevention and Health Promotion.

van der Horst, K., Timperio, A., Crawford, D., Roberts, R., Brug, J., & Oenema A. (2008). The school food environment associations with adolescent soft drink and snack consumption. *American Journal of Preventive Medicine, 35,* 217–223.

Van Dyck, D., Cardon, G., Deforche, B., & De Bourdeaudhuij, I. (2009a). Lower neighbourhood walkability and longer distance to school are related to physical activity in Belgian adolescents. *Preventive Medicine, 48,* 516–518.

Van Dyck, D., Deforche, B., Cardon, G., & De Bourdeaudhuij, I. (2009b). Neighbourhood walkability and its particular importance for adults with a preference for passive transport. *Health & Place, 15,* 496–504.

Van Dyck, D., Cardon, G., Deforche, B., Sallis, J.F., Owen, N., & De Bourdeaudhuij, I. (2010). Neighborhood SES and walkability are related to physical activity behavior in Belgian adults. *Preventive Medicine, 50,* 74–79.

Van Dyck, D., Cerin, E., Cardon, G., Deforche, B., Sallis, J.F., Owen, N., & De Bourdeaudhuij, I. (2010). Physical activity as a mediator of the associations between neighborhood walkability and adiposity in Belgian adults. *Health Place. 16,* 952–960.

van Lenthe, F.J., & Mackenbach, J.P. (2002). Neighbourhood deprivation and overweight: the GLOBE study. *International Journal of Obesity, 26,* 234–240.

Van Rensselaer, M. (1901). Saving steps. *Suppl. 1.* Ithaca: Cornell University; College of Agriculture. Cornell Reading Course for Farmers' Wives.

vélo'v (2009). Lyon (February 8, 2010); http://www.velov.grandlyon.com/?L=1.

Wells, N.M., Ashdown, S.P., Davies, E.H.S., & Cowett, F.D. (2007). Environment, design, and obesity, opportunities for interdisciplinary collaborative research. *Environment and Behavior, 39,* 6–33.

Westerterp, K.R. (2009). Assessment of physical activity: a critical appraisal. *European Journal of Applied Physiology, 105,* 823–828.

Woodman, J., Lorenc, T., Harden, A., & Oakley, A. (2008). Social and environmental interventions to reduce childhood obesity: a systematic map of reviews. London: Social Science Research Unit. EPPI-Centre report.

World Health Organization (WHO) (2009). *Diet and physical activity: a public health priority.* Geneva (April 13, 2009); http://www.who.int/dietphysicalactivity/en.

Young, L.R., & Nestle, M. (2002). The contribution of expanding portion sizes to the US obesity epidemic. *American Journal of Public Health, 92,* 246–249.

Chapter 23
Psychosocial Aspects of Childhood Obesity

Amy E. Sgrenci and Myles S. Faith

Introduction

The obesity epidemic is increasing in youths at a startling rate. By 2010, it is projected that approximately 50% of North American children and 30% of children from the European Union will be overweight (Wang and Lobstein 2006). In the United States, obesity in children and adolescents is defined as a body mass index (BMI; weight in kilograms divided by the height squared in meters) at or above the 95th percentile for individuals of the same age and sex as established by the Centers for Disease Control (Dietz 2004). In European countries, cut-offs created by the International Obesity Task Force are used typically to establish overweight and obesity (Cole et al. 2000). There are many medical disorders associated with childhood obesity, including Type 2 diabetes and hypertension (Stunkard and Wadden 1993), however the psychological consequences can be equally devastating (Puhl and Latner 2007). This is especially concerning when severe pediatric obesity continues into adulthood (Dietz 2004). Thus, it is important to become aware of the psychosocial risk factors for excess weight gain in childhood, as well as the psychological consequences of pediatric obesity.

This chapter first explores psychosocial risk factors for the development of pediatric obesity, including depression and abuse/neglect, during childhood. The next section discusses the potential psychological sequelae of childhood obesity, including poorer self-esteem, suicidal behaviors, reduced quality of life and interpersonal relationships, and disordered eating patterns. We conclude that there is a need for new interventions to help obese children better cope with the psychosocial problems that can occur in order to enhance their quality of life and, potentially improve their weight control.

Psychosocial Risk Factors for the Development of Obesity

Childhood depression and chronic stress are associated with increased BMI and the onset of obesity in childhood. We review these studies below.

A.E. Sgrenci
Department of Psychology, La Salle University, 1900 West Olney Avenue, Philadelphia, PA, 19141, USA

M.S. Faith (✉)
Center for Weight and Eating Disorders, University of Pennsylvania School of Medicine, 3535 Market Street – 3rd Floor, Philadelphia, PA, 19104, USA
e-mail: mfaith@mail.med.upenn.edu

L.A. Moreno et al. (eds.), *Epidemiology of Obesity in Children and Adolescents*,
Springer Series on Epidemiology and Public Health 2, DOI 10.1007/978-1-4419-6039-9_23,
© Springer Science+Business Media, LLC 2011

Childhood Depression

Depression in childhood has been linked to adulthood BMI. Pine et al. (2001) conducted a prospective study investigating the relationship between the presence or absence of major depression during childhood and future adulthood BMI. The sample included 199 six-to-seventeen-year-old children and adolescents who presented with a clinical diagnosis of major depression and an age matched control group of 176 children who had no lifetime psychiatric history. Follow-up assessment was conducted 10–15 years after the initial assessment, at which time BMI data was collected from 90 probands and 87 controls. Results indicated that adult BMI was significantly greater among participants who had a diagnosis of childhood depression compared to controls. Participants who had a history of childhood depression reported lower levels of physical activity, lower income, and greater cigarette, medication, and alcohol use as adults compared to the control group. Thus, these behaviors may partially mediate the association between childhood depression and adulthood obesity. Interestingly, other studies have reported that adults with current depression or a lifetime diagnosis of depression were more likely to smoke, be obese, be physically inactive, and drink heavily (Strine et al. 2008).

Other investigators have reported that adolescents with major depression are at increased risk to become overweight or obese in adulthood, especially females (Pine et al 2001; Richardson et al. 2003). Goodman and Whitaker (2002) explored the prospective relationships between depression and weight gain to determine which factor preceded the other. Participants were 9,374 adolescents in 7th–12th grade who were enrolled in the National Longitudinal Study of Adolescent Health. Baseline data were collected in 1995 and then 1 year later for follow-up assessment. Obesity was defined as a BMI equal to or greater than the 95th percentile, and overweight status was greater or equal to the 85th percentile and less than the 95th percentile. Depression was assessed by the Center for Epidemiologic Studies Depression Scale. Results indicated that depression at baseline was not significantly correlated with baseline BMI. After controlling for baseline BMI, age, race, gender, parental obesity, family socioeconomic status, number of parents in the home, and other behavioral covariates, baseline depression predicted the onset of obesity at follow-up among those not obese at baseline. However, obesity at baseline did not predict the onset of depression at follow-up (Goodman and Whitaker 2002).

Summary

In sum, there is evidence to support a "causal" association between depression during childhood/adolescence and excess weight gain or the onset of obesity. This association may be mediated by a number of behavioral factors that are being investigated. Evidence to support the hypothesis that pediatric obesity "causes" depression is lacking (Herva et al. 2006; Pine et al. 2001; Richardson et al. 2003; Roberts et al. 2003).

Chronic Stress (Sexual Abuse, Neglect)

Chronic stress and abuse in childhood has been found to be associated with increased childhood and adulthood BMI. Lissau and Sorensen (1994) investigated school teachers' and nurses' impressions of students' parental support, family structure, and general hygiene in relationship to their BMI at a 10-year follow-up. Results indicated that children previously described as "dirty and neglected" were 10 times more likely to become obese in adulthood compared to those described as having "average" hygiene.

Williamson et al. (2002) explored the relationship between childhood abuse and its risk in the development of adult obesity. Data were collected through the Adverse Childhood Experiences (ACE) Study which was designed to evaluate the influence of childhood experiences on health behaviors and outcomes in adults. The ACE study's sample included 13,777 adults, whose mean age was 55.7 years, enrolled in the Kaiser Permanente Health Maintenance Organization (HMO) in southern California. Participants' heights and weights were evaluated at the organization's health appraisal clinic, and then a questionnaire was mailed a week later inquiring about their childhood experiences and current health behaviors. The study compared incidences of 4 types of abuse (sexual, verbal, fear of physical abuse, and physical abuse) in the participants' first 18 years of life with their current BMI. Results indicated that two-thirds of participants reported at least one type of abuse as a child. The most prevalent type was verbal abuse (47.3%), followed by physical abuse (44.5%), fear of physical abuse (42.7%), and sexual abuse (21.7%). All forms of abuse were positively correlated with increased weight in adulthood, with individuals who reported childhood abuse being about 0.6 to 4.0 kg heavier than adults who did not report childhood abuse. The population attributable fraction (PAF) was 8% for participants with a BMI ≥ 30, meaning that 8% of the cases of obesity in the population would be prevented if any type of abuse had not occurred. The PAF was 17% for participants with a BMI ≥ 40.

Gustafson and Sarwer (2004) conducted a literature review to investigate the existing research on the relationship between childhood sexual abuse and adult obesity. One study reviewed the charts of 131 patients who were enrolled in a weight loss program. Results revealed that 60% of patients who reported rape or sexual molestation in their history were at least 50 lbs overweight compared to 28% of individuals (matched with sex and age) who did not report sexual abuse history. Additionally, victims of childhood sexual abuse were more likely to suffer from extreme obesity. Twenty-five percent of victims were found to be at least 100 lbs overweight compared to 6% of the control group (Felitti 1991).

Springs and Friedrich (1992) found that individuals who reported a history of childhood sexual abuse had a higher rate of being overweight compared to individuals who did not report abuse. Their study investigated 511 females who were surveyed in a family practice in a Midwestern rural community. Overweight was measured as at least 40% above their ideal body weight (Springs and Friedrich 1992).

Adverse childhood experiences have been found to be associated with adult obesity. Felitti (1993) discovered that overweight individuals (measured by 65 or more pounds over ideal body weight) were more likely than average weight individuals to have a history of childhood sexual abuse (25 vs. 6%), any type of childhood abuse (29 vs. 14%), lose a parent under the age of 18 (48 to 23%), and parental alcoholism (40 vs. 17%).

A possible explanation for the link between childhood abuse and the development of adult obesity is the mediating role of binge eating (Gustafson and Sarwer 2004). Binge eating has been observed as a common coping mechanism for those who have been sexually abused. Research has suggested that a history of sexual abuse is more common in individuals who are diagnosed with binge eating disorder (BED) compared to normal controls (Grilo and Masheb 2001; Striegel-Moore et al. 2002). Grilo and Masheb (2001) discovered that 30.3% of 145 individuals with BED reported a history of childhood sexual abuse compared to only 18.4% of healthy controls. Likewise, 35.5% of 162 women in a community sample reported childhood sexual abuse compared to 12.2% of normal controls (Striegel-Moore et al. 2002).

Generally, chronic stress has been considered to be associated with the onset of obesity. Clinical experience with youth lends some support to this. However, empirical data on this relationship have been lacking (Greeno and Wing 1994). Mellin et al. (2002) found that overweight adolescents reported higher levels of emotional distress than their normal weight peers. Study participants included 9,118 7th, 9th, and 11th graders from a 1996 statewide school-based survey.

Stress has been measured by the increased activity of the hypothalamic-pituitary-adrenal (HPA) axis, and has been linked to health problems in adults, such as visceral obesity (Chrousos 2000).

Additionally, it has been found that psychological stress related to early serious life events activates the HPA axis in children (Turner-Cobb 2005). One study (Koch et al. 2008) found a significant relationship between psychological stress in the family and childhood obesity. Participants were a part of the All Babies in Southeast Sweden-project (ABIS), which followed a population cohort from birth to adolescence. A total of 5,221 families provided data at all age points for this study (birth, age 1, age 2, and age 5). Weight and height was collected, and psychological stress was assessed at each age. Psychological stress was assessed by the parents with four domains: serious life events (i.e.: divorce, death of a relative, unemployment, exposure to violence), parenting stress, lack of social support, and parental worries related to the child's health. Exposure to family stress is thought to likely impact the child, although it is understood all individuals respond to events differently. Study findings suggested serious life events were related significantly to childhood obesity, even when controlling for background factors. Parental worries were significantly related as well to childhood obesity. Parenting stress and lack of social support were not found to be significantly related to childhood obesity in this study. The overall findings suggested that long-term chronic stress in families is related to childhood obesity. The percentage of children with obesity increases with the number of psychological stressors being experienced (Koch et al. 2008).

Summary

In sum, research suggests an association between childhood adverse events and excess weight gain or the development of obesity. Also, obesity appears to develop more often in adulthood for these individuals, but little research has been done to display whether weight gain may develop earlier, such as in childhood or adolescence. Furthermore, additional research looking at the association of chronic stress and the development of obesity is needed. The direction of this relationship is unclear, as stress likely may develop as a result of factors that are associated with obesity.

Childhood Behavioral Problems

Childhood behavioral problems have also been found to be associated with the development of obesity in childhood and adulthood. Mamun et al. (2009) investigated whether behavioral problems in childhood compared to adolescence have a greater influence on young adult's BMI and obesity. Behavioral problems were assessed through maternal reports of the Achenbach's Child Behavior Checklist (CBCL; Achenbach 1991). Children who scored above the 90th percentile were classified as having significant behavior problems. Participants included 2,278 21 year olds from Australia who were part of the Mater-University of Queensland Study of Pregnancy and Its Outcomes (1981), a longitudinal study beginning from birth. Of the 2,278 young adults, 20.85% were considered overweight and 12.77% were obese at 21 years of age. Those young adults who were documented to have had behavioral problems at the age of 5 or 14 on average were found to have a greater BMI and more likely to be obese than young adults without behavioral problems at those ages. Specifically, these individuals had on average 3.44 kg/m² greater BMI scores than young adults without behavioral problems. Even after controlling for child dietary patterns, family communication, family meals, time spent watching television, and involvement in physical activity, this significant association between childhood behavioral problems and obesity at the age of 21 still existed. Additionally, those with childhood behavioral problems were 2.08 times (and 3.86 times for persistent childhood behavioral problems) more likely to be obese by 21 years of age than children without behavioral problems (Mamun et al. 2009).

Lumeng et al. (2003) found that behavioral problems in children between the ages of 8 and 11 were associated with a greater risk of concurrent overweight status and becoming overweight in normal weight children. Participants were from the National Longitudinal Survey of Youth (NLSY), and included 755 mother-child pairs. Data was collected at two separate times, 1996 and 1998, for 700 of these participants. The findings suggested that six percent of normal weight children in 1996 became overweight in 1998 (Lumeng et al. 2003).

Research suggests childhood behavioral disorders are associated with childhood and adult obesity. Mustillo et al. (2003) found a significant association between children diagnosed with oppositional defiant disorder (ODD) and chronic obesity. Chronically obese children were found to have higher rates of ODD. Additionally, another study found a link between conduct disorder in adolescence and obesity in young adulthood (Pine et al. 1997). The sample consisted of 776 adolescents who were assessed in 1983 and later as adults in 1992. At the second assessment, adult weight (BMI) was significantly related to adolescent conduct disorder (Pine et al. 1997).

Summary

In sum, research suggests behavioral problems in childhood and adolescence predict overweight and obese status concurrently and in young adulthood. It appears obesity develops more often in young adulthood for those with behavioral problems, however, the link between concurrent obesity and behavioral problems question which factor precedes the other. Thus, it is possible excess weight may predict behavioral problems as well.

Psychosocial Sequelae of Childhood Obesity

Childhood obesity may lead to the following outcomes: stigmatization, low self-esteem, suicidal behaviors and thoughts, poor quality of life, poor peer relationships, and body dissatisfaction. We review studies devoted to these problems below.

Stigmatization

There is increasing evidence indicating that obese children and adolescents are significantly affected by stigmatization, as they are judged by others to be "unattractive, ugly, lazy, and dumb" (Allon 1981). These views have not changed over the past several decades (Latner et al. 2005) and were found to be equally endorsed by obese and non-obese youth (Goodman and Whitaker 2002; Latner et al. 2005; Puhl and Brownell 2003; Quinn and Crocker 1999). Obesity stigma may vary among races and social economic strata, however it generally permeates in the American culture and is reinforced by the media (Adams et al. 2000; Crandall 1994; Harrison 2001; Puhl and Brownell 2003). As part of stigmatization, obese youth are more likely to be bullied, isolated, and ostracized than normal weight peers (Halpern et al. 2005; Janssen et al. 2004; Strauss and Pollack 2003).

Research shows that obese children are exposed to negative biases and stereotypes from peers, educators, and parents. As childhood and adolescence is a developmental period when social relationships are vital in shaping self-identity, these findings are concerning. Weight stigmatization can impede youths' social, emotional, and academic achievement. For example, Crosnoe (2007) investigated the association between obesity status and college attendance among adolescents in a study of 10,829 7th–12th graders in the Longitudinal Study of Adolescent Health. Results indicated that obese girls in 1995 were 50% less likely to attend college in 2002 than non-obese girls. Interestingly, this finding only occurred among girls who attended a high school where obesity was rare but not among girls who attended a high school where obesity was common. For boys, there was no link between obesity and college attendance (Crosnoe 2007).

Other research has shown that the probability of women being overweight doubles if they have less than a high school degree compared to if they have a graduate degree (Kenkel et al. 2006). Adolescent and adulthood obesity is more prevalent in individuals with lower compared to higher education (Himes and Reynolds 2005), which ultimately affects income and work experience later in life. The average obese woman is 10% more likely to live in poverty than the average non-obese woman (Wadden and Stunkard 1985).

Self-Esteem

Research has revealed mixed findings on the cross-sectional relationship between obesity and self-esteem. Wardle and Cooke (2005) concluded in their comprehensive review that obese youth were not more vulnerable to a lower self-esteem than non-obese youth in community and clinical samples. However, clinical samples of obese youth reported lower levels of self-esteem than community control youth who were obese and average weight. In another review article, French et al. (1995) concluded that thirteen out of twenty-five cross-sectional studies displayed lower self-esteem in obese children and adolescents compared to normal weight individuals.

Davison and Birch (2001) found that weight teasing by peers and weight criticism by parents mediated the relationship between poor self-esteem and obesity in adolescents. Eisenberg et al. (2003) found that weight teasing was correlated with poorer self-esteem in female and male adolescents. Moreover, overweight adolescents whose self-esteem declined over a 4-year period were more likely to engage in unhealthy behaviors, including smoking and alcohol use, compared to children whose self-esteem did not decrease (Strauss 2000).

Among a clinical sample of obese youth, those that believed they were responsible for their excess weight had a poorer self-esteem. Children who attributed their weight to external factors exhibited a more positive self-esteem (Pierce and Wardle 1997). In a different clinical sample of obese youth, self-esteem was poorer when treatment included messages of personal responsibility for obesity or blame for not being able to lose weight (Wardle and Cooke 2005).

Suicidal Behavior

One of the most disconcerting consequences of childhood obesity is an increased risk of suicidal behaviors. Obese adolescents are more likely to endorse suicidal thoughts and to attempt suicide than normal weight peers (Ackard et al. 2003; Eaton et al. 2005; Falkner et al. 2001). One study found that obese girls were 1.7 times more likely to report a suicide attempt in the past year compared to thinner peers (Falkner et al. 2001). Additionally, among Caucasian, Hispanic, and Black students, a higher BMI and greater self-perceptions of being overweight were found to be positively correlated with suicidal ideation. More specifically, perceiving oneself to be very overweight was associated with greater suicide attempts among Caucasian students (Eaton et al. 2005). Eisenberg et al. (2003) found that teasing was associated with greater suicidal ideation and attempts in both sexes, and adolescents who were teased were 2–3 times more likely to report suicidal ideation than those who were not teased.

Neumark-Sztainer et al. (2002) found that 51% of girls who reported being teased by peers and teachers about their weight reported having suicidal ideation compared to 25% of girls who did not report being teased. Among boys who reported weight-based teasing by family members, 13% reported attempting suicide compared to only 4% who were not teased. It has been suggestive that females are affected significantly more by the obesity stigma than boys (Crosnoe 2007).

Quality of Life

Obesity impacts detrimentally on children's health related quality of life. Schwimmer et al. (2003) compared health related quality of life scores on the Pediatric Quality of Life Inventory, 4.0 (Varni et al. 2001) among 106 obese children attending a gastroenterology/nutrition clinic, 401 healthy controls, and 106 children and adolescents diagnosed with cancer and receiving chemotherapy. Cancer patients were included as a comparison group because this population has been shown to have the lowest health related quality of life. The investigators found that obese children reported lower health-related quality of life (physical health, psychosocial health, emotional and social well-being, and school functioning) than non-obese children, and that their scores were comparable to children with cancer.

Landgraf (2001) found that overweight children in a population-based sample had poorer psychosocial health outcomes (e.g.: reduced self-esteem, emotional well-being, physical functioning, and overall general health) compared to normal weight children. Overweight children were 2–4 times more likely than healthy weight controls to have low scores on psychosocial health, self-esteem, and physical functioning (Friedlander et al. 2003).

Among 642 overweight youth who were 11–19 years old from community and clinical settings, self-reported quality of life was inversely related to BMI. In addition, when comparing the clinical population of obese adolescents with community population of obese adolescents, those who sought weight management treatment (clinical population) reported poorer weight related quality of life scores than those who did not seek treatment (Kolotkin et al. 2006).

Peer Relationships

Strauss and Pollack (2003) investigated 90,118 adolescents (13–18 years of age) who were enrolled in the National Longitudinal Study of Adolescent Health. They found that overweight adolescents were more likely to be socially isolated compared to normal weight adolescents. For peer nominations, overweight adolescents received significantly fewer friendship nominations from other peers than normal weight adolescents received. Furthermore, overweight adolescents were more likely to have no friendship nominations compared to normal weight adolescents (12 vs. 7%). Increased friendship nominations were associated with decreased television viewing, increased levels of sports participation, and increased participation in school clubs.

Overweight children (10–14 years old) recruited from a fitness camp were found to have higher preferences for sedentary/isolative activities compared to non-overweight children in the general population and reduced preference for social activities (Hayden-Wade et al. 2005). Faith et al. (2002) found that weight teasing during sports was associated with reduced preference for physical activity.

Overweight children seem to be aware about weight biases, and its effect on social rejection. Pierce and Wardle (1997) found that overweight children in a clinical sample believed that their excess weight hindered their interactions with peers. Additionally, 69% of the sample believed that if they lost weight they would have more friends (Pierce and Wardle 1997). Some research suggests that weight bias may be spreading to individuals who have relationships with obese individuals (Hebl and Mannix 2003).

Disordered Eating Behaviors

Weight stigma and teasing are associated with disordered eating patterns, drug use, and alcohol use. Hayden-Wade et al. (2005) investigated 70 overweight and 85 non-overweight children ages 10–14 years old. They found that appearance related teasing was more prevalent among overweight children, and that weight related teasing was positively correlated with bulimic behaviors. Other research has shown that weight teasing and parental weight criticism are linked with dieting, restrictive eating, poor body image, binge eating, and bulimic behaviors. Thompson et al. (1995) found that teasing history mediated the relationship between obesity and poor body image. Moreover, teasing and body image were linked with increased restrictive eating patterns.

Neumark-Sztainer et al. (2007) investigated 2,516 adolescents in a longitudinal population-based study examining the prevalence and co-occurrence of overweight, binge eating, and extreme weight control behaviors. They found that 40% of overweight females and 20% of overweight males engaged in binge eating, restricted eating, or both. Among the overweight females, 10% reported binge eating and extreme weight control behaviors, 6.4% reported only binge eating, and 23.5% reported only extreme weight control behaviors. Among overweight boys, adverse weight-related behaviors were less common. Specifically, 1.9% reported both binge eating and extreme weight-control behavior, 3.7% reported binge eating behaviors only, and 12.3% reported extreme weight-control behaviors. Boutelle et al. (2002) found that overweight female adolescents are more than twice as likely to report extreme weight-control behaviors such as vomiting, and unhealthy uses of laxatives and diet pills.

Conclusions

There are psychosocial risk factors for the development of pediatric obesity, as well as psychological sequelae. Factors such as childhood depression and early adverse experiences have been found as possible precursors to excess weight gain later in life. Identifying these factors and understanding their related roles will help psychologists improve their interventions at an early age for certain populations before obesity develops. Target populations should include children with depression and those who may be exposed to adverse events at a young age, especially sexual and physical abuse.

For those children who already suffer from obesity, it is important to recognize common psychological problems that they confront. The stigmatization of obesity continues, which puts certain obese children at greater risk for low self-esteem, suicidal thoughts and/or behavior, poor quality of life, poor peer relationships, and disordered eating behaviors. Understanding the relationships between these factors and childhood obesity will help childcare providers become more aware of psychological problems these children may be facing. Obesity is a subject many individuals do not like to discuss, and often ignore without existing medical complications. However, it may be important to discuss with obese children their emotions and experiences to prevent psychological distress.

References

Achenbach, T.M. (1991). *Integrative guide for the 1991 CBCL/4-18, YSR, and TRF profiles.* Burlington, VT: University of Vermont Department of Psychiatry.

Ackard, D.M., Neumark-Sztainer, D., Story, M., & Perry, C. (2003). Overeating among adolescents: prevalence and associations with weight-related characteristics and psychological health. *Pediatrics, 111(1),* 67–74.

Adams, K., Sargent, R.G., Thompson, S.H., Richter, D., Corwin, S.J., & Rogan, T. (2000). A study of body weight concerns and weight control practices of 4th and 7th grade adolescents. *Ethnicity and Health, 5,* 79–94.

Allon, N. (1981). The stigma of overweight in everyday life. In B.J. Wolman (Ed.), *Psychological aspects of obesity: A handbook*. New York: Van Nostrand.

Boutelle, K., Neumark-Sztainer, D., Story, M., & Resnick, M. (2002). Weight control behaviors among obese, overweight, and nonoverweight adolescents. *Journal of Pediatric Psychology, 27(6)*, 531–540.

Chrousos, G.P. (2000). The role of stress and the hypothalamic-pituitary-adrenal axis in the pathogenesis of the metabolic syndrome: neuro-endocrine and target tissue-related causes. *International Journal of Obesity Related Metabolic Disorders, 24*, 50–55.

Cole, T.J., Bellizzi, M.C., Flegal, K.M., & Dietz, W.H. (2000). Establishing a standard definition for child overweight and obesity worldwide: International study. *British Medical Journal, 320*, 1240–1243.

Crandall, C. (1994). Prejudice against fat people: Ideology and self-interest. *Journal of Personality and Social Psychology, 66*, 882–894.

Crosnoe, R. (2007). Gender, obesity, and education. *Sociology of Education, 80*, 241–260.

Davison, K.K. & Birch, L.L. (2001). Childhood overweight: A contextual model and recommendations for future research. *Obesity Reviews, 2*, 159–171.

Dietz, W.H. (2004). Overweight in childhood and adolescence. *New England Journal of Medicine, 350(9)*, 855–857.

Eaton, D., Lowry, R., Brener, N., Galuska, D., & Crosby, A. (2005). Associations of body mass index and perceived weight with suicide ideation and suicide attempts among US high school students. *Archives of Pediatric and Adolescent Medicine, 159*, 513–519.

Eisenberg, M.E., Neumark-Sztainer, D. & Story, M. (2003). Associations of weight-based teasing and emotional well-being among adolescents. *Archives of Pediatrics & Adolescent Medicine, 157(8)*, 733–738.

Faith, M.S., Leone, M.A., Ayers, T.S., Heo, M., & Pietrobelli, A. (2002). Weight criticism during physical activity, coping skills, and reported physical activity in children. *Pediatrics, 110*, e23.

Falkner, N., Neumark-Sztainer, D., Story, M., Jeffrey, R., Beuhring, T., & Resnick, M. (2001). Social, educational, psychological correlates of weight status in adolescents. *Obesity Research, 9*, 32–42.

Felitti, V.J. (1991). Long-term medical consequences of incest, rape, and molestation. *Southern Medicine Journal, 84*, 328–331.

Felitti, V.J. (1993). Childhood sexual abuse, depression, and family dysfunction in adult obese patients: a case control study. *Southern Medicine Journal, 86*, 732–736.

French, S.A., Story, M., & Perry, C.L. (1995). Self-esteem and obesity in children and adolescents: a literature review. *Obesity Research, 3(5)*, 479–490.

Friedlander, S.L., Larkin, E.K., Rosen, C.L., Palmero, T.M., & Redline, S. (2003). Decreased quality of life associated with obesity in school-aged children. *Archives of Pediatric and Adolescent Medicine, 157*, 1206–1211.

Goodman, E., & Whitaker, R.C. (2002). A prospective study of the role of depression in the development and persistence of adolescent obesity. *Pediatrics, 109*, 497–504.

Greeno, C.G., & Wing, R.R. (1994). Stress-induced eating. *Psychological Bulletin, 115(3)*, 444–464.

Grilo, C.M., & Masheb, R.M. (2001). Childhood psychological, physical, and sexual maltreatment in outpatients with binge eating disorder: frequency and associations with gender, obesity, and eating-related psychopathology. *Obesity Research, 9*, 320–325.

Gustafson, T.B., & Sarwer, D.B. (2004). Childhood sexual abuse and obesity. *Obesity Reviews, 5*, 129–135.

Halpern, C. T., King, R.B., Oslak, S.G., & Udry, J.R. (2005). Body mass index, dieting, romance, and sexual activity in adolescent girls: Relationships over time. *Journal of Research on Adolescence, 15*, 535–559.

Harrison, K. (2001). Ourselves, our bodies: Thin-ideal, media, self-discrepancies, and eating disorder symptomatology in adolescents. *Journal of Social and Clinical Psychology, 20*, 289–323.

Hayden-Wade, H.A., Stein, R.I., Ghaderi, A., Saelens, B.E., Zabinski, M.F., & Willfley, D.E. (2005). Prevalence, characteristics, and correlates of teasing experiences among overweight children vs. non-overweight peers. *Obesity Research, 13*, 1381–1392.

Hebl, M.R., & Mannix, L.M. (2003). The weight of obesity in evaluating others: A mere proximity effect. *Personality and Social Psychology Bulletin, 29*, 28–38.

Herva, A., Laitinen, J., Miettunen, J., Veijola, J., Karvonen, J.T., Läksy, K., & Joukamaa, M. (2006). Obesity and depression: Results from the longitudinal Northern Finland 1966 Birth Cohort Study. *International Journal of Obesity, 30*, 520–527.

Himes, C. L., & Reynolds, S. L. (2005). The changing relationship between obesity and educational status. *Gender Issues, 22(2)*, 45–57.

Janssen, I., Craig, W.M., Boyce, W.F., & Pickett, W. (2004). Associations between overweight and obesity with bullying behaviors in school-age children. *Pediatrics, 113*, 1187–1194.

Kenkel, D., Lillard, D., & Mathios, A. (2006). The roles of high school completion and GED receipt in smoking and obesity. *Journal of Labor Economics, 24(3)*, 635–660.

Koch, F.-S., Sepa, A., & Ludvigsson, J. (2008). Psychological stress and obesity. *The Journal of Pediatrics, 153*, 839–844.

Kolotkin, R.L., Zeller, M., Modi, A.C., Samsa, G.P., Quinlan, N.P., Yanovski, J.A., Bell, S.K., Maahs, D.M., de Serna, D.G., & Roehrig, H.R. (2006). Assessing weight related quality of life in adolescents. *Obesity, 14 (3)*, 448–457.

Landgraf, J.M. (2001). Measuring and monitoring quality of life in children and youth: A brief commentary. *Sozial-und Präventivmedizin, 46*, 281–282.

Latner, J.D., Stunkard, A.J., & Wilson, G.T. (2005). Stigmatizated students: Age, sex, and ethnicity effects in the stigmatization of obesity. *Obesity Research, 13*, 1226–1231.

Lissau, I., & Sorensen, T.I.A. (1994). Parental neglect during childhood and increased risk of obesity in young adulthood. *Lancet, 343*, 324–327.

Lumeng, J.C., Gannon, K., Cabral, H.J., Frank, D.A., & Zuckerman, B. (2003). Association between clinically meaningful behavior problems and overweight in children. *Pediatrics, 112*, 1138–1145.

Mamun, A.A., O'Callaghan, M.J., Cramb, S.M., Najman, J.M., Williams, G.M., & Bor, W. (2009). Childhood behavioral problems predict young adults' BMI and obesity: Evidence from a birth cohort study. *Obesity, 17*, 761–766.

Mellin, A.E., Neumark-Sztainer, D., Story, M., Ireland, M., & Resnick, M.D. (2002). Unhealthy behaviors and psychosocial difficulties among overweight adolescents: the potential impact of familial factors. *Journal of Adolescent Health, 31*, 145–153.

Mustillo, S., Worthman, C., Erkanli, A., Keeler, G., Angold, A., & Costello, E.J. (2003). Obesity and psychiatric disorder: Developmental trajectories. *Pediatrics, 111*, 851–859.

Neumark-Sztainer, D., Falkner, N., Story, M., Perry, C., Hannan, P.J., & Mulert, S. (2002). Weight-teasing among adolescents: correlations with weight status and disordered eating behaviors. *International Journal of Obesity Related Metabolic Disorders, 26*, 123–131.

Neumark-Sztainer, D., Wall, M., Haines, J., Story, M., Sherwood, N., & Van Den Berg, P. (2007). Shared risk and protective factors for overweight and disordered eating adolescents. *American Journal of Preventive Medicine, 33*, 359–369.

Pierce, J.W., & Wardle, J. (1997). Cause and effect beliefs and self-esteem of overweight children. *Journal of Child Psychology and Psychiatry and Allied Disciplines, 38(6)*, 645–650.

Pine, D.S., Cohen, P., Brook, J., & Coplan, J.D. (1997). Psychiatric symptoms in adolescence as predictors of obesity in early adulthood: A longitudinal study. *American Journal of Public Health, 87*, 1303–1310.

Pine, D.S., Goldstein, R.B., Wolk, S., & Weissman, M.M. (2001). The association between childhood depression and adulthood body mass index. *Pediatrics, 107(5)*, 1049–1056.

Puhl, R.M., & Brownell, K.D. (2003). Psychological origins of obesity stigma: Toward changing a powerful and pervasive bias. *Obesity Reviews, 4*, 213–227.

Puhl, R.M., & Latner, J.D. (2007). Stigma, obesity, and the health of the nation's children. *Psychological Bulletin, 133 (4)*, 557–580.

Quinn, D.M., & Crocker, J. (1999). When ideology hurts: Effects of belief in the Protestant ethic and feeling overweight on the psychological well-being of women. *Journal of Personality and Social Psychology, 77*, 402–414.

Richardson, L.P., Davis, R., Poulton, R., McCauley, E., Moffitt, T.E., Caspi, A., & Connell, F. (2003). A longitudinal evaluation of adolescent depression and adult obesity. *Archival Pediatric Adolescent Medicine, 157*, 739–745.

Roberts, R.E., Deleger, S., Strawbridge, W.J., & Kaplan, G.A. (2003). Prospective association between obesity and depression: Evidence from the Alameda Count Study. *International Obesity Related Metabolism Disorders, 27*, 514–521.

Schwimmer, J.B., Burwinkle, T.M., & Varni, J.W. (2003). Health-related quality of life of severely obese children and adolescents. *Journal of the American Medical Association, 289 (14)*, 1813–1819.

Springs, F.E., & Friedrich, W.N. (1992). Health risk behaviors and medical sequelaw of childhood sexual abuse. *Mayo Clinic Proceedings, 67*, 527–532.

Strauss, R.S. (2000). Childhood obesity and self-esteem. *Pediatrics, 105(1)*, e15.

Strauss, R.S., & Pollack, H.A. (2003). Social marginalization of overweight children. *Archives of Pediatric & Adolescent Medicine, 157*, 746–752.

Striegel-Moore, R.H., Dohm, F., Pike, K.M., Wilfley, D.E., & Fairburn, C.G. (2002). Abuse, bullying, and discrimination as risk factors for binge eating disorder. *American Journal of Psychiatry, 159*, 1902–1907.

Strine, T.W., Mokdad, A.H., Dube, S.R., Balluz, L.S., Gonzalez, O., Berry, J.T., Manderscheid, R., & Kroenke, K. (2008). The association of depression and anxiety with obesity and unhealthy behaviors among community-dwelling US adults. *General Hospital Psychiatry, 30*, 127–137.

Stunkard, A.J., & Wadden, T. (Eds.) (1993). *Obesity: Theory and therapy (2nd ed.).* New York: Raven Press.

Thompson, J.K., Coovert, M., Richards, K., Johnson, S., & Cattarin, J. (1995). Development of body image, eating disturbance, and general psychological functioning in female adolescents: Covariance structure modeling and longitudinal investigations. *International Journal of Eating Disorders, 18*, 221–236.

Turner-Cobb, J.M. (2005). Psychological stress hormone correlates in early life: A key to HPA-axis dysregulation and normalization. *Stress, 8*, 47–57.

Varni, J.W., Seid, M., & Kurtin, P.S. (2001). PedsQL4.0: Reliability and validity of the Pediatric Quality of Life Inventory Version 4.0 Generic Core Scales in healthy and patient populations. *Medical Care, 39*, 800–812.

Wadden, T.A., & Stunkard, A.J. (1985). Social and psychological consequences of obesity. *Annals of Internal Medicine, 103*, 1062–1067.

Wang, Y., & Lobstein, T. (2006). Worldwide trends in childhood overweight and obesity. *International Journal of Obesity, 19,* 562–569.

Wardle, J., & Cooke, L. (2005). The impact of obesity on psychological well-being. *Best Practice & Research Clinical Endocrinology & Metabolism, 19,* 421–440.

Williamson, D.F., Thompson, T.J., Anda, R.F., Dietz, W.H., & Felitti, V. (2002). Body weight and obesity in adults and self-reported abuse in childhood. *International Journal of Obesity, 26,* 1075–1082.

Chapter 24
Consumer Behavior in Childhood Obesity Research and Policy

Lucia A. Reisch, Wencke Gwozdz, and Suzanne Beckmann

The Background

Within the last 30 years, a remarkable weight gain could be observed in nearly all developed countries independent of sex, age, and social class. Thus, this epidemic affects not only one single social stratum or one specific group of consumers, but rather whole populations. Nowadays, more than 30% of all European children are overweight or obese – with an increasing tendency (European Commission 2007). Overweight and obesity become even more important when taking into account their strong relationship with the increase in cardio-vascular diseases or type-two-diabetes. These consequences result in high costs for individuals and societies. Despite a plethora of activities and initiatives to reverse this development, there is no identifiable downward trend in sight. Rather, future economic and social consequences seem to be unpredictable and unmanageable.

While the severity of obesity's consequences for the individual is known, its societal implications reveal themselves in diverse areas bit by bit. Economic consequences occur in national health systems – chronically under funded anyway – as well as in the labor markets. With regard to the latter, obese individuals have lower employment rates, which are often ascribed to the assumption that obese people are less productive, have more sick days and are likely to die prematurely (McCormick and Stone 2007). Indeed, obesity and its co-morbidities are the second most frequent cause – after tobacco consumption – of premature death (HM Government 2008). The mix of poorer employment opportunities, deteriorating health, premature death, reduced mobility, lower self-esteem, and higher living expenses (Government Office for Science 2007; Harper 2000; Morris 2006) clearly impacts on quality of life.

However, causalities between these factors are far from being understood. A pretty robust result is that the prevalence of overweight and obesity is higher in low socio-economic status (SES) families than in any other social group (McLaren 2007). The explanation given for this phenomenon is the poorer access to and the higher prices of healthy food as well as fewer opportunities for physical activities for low SES families (Robertson et al. 2007). Scientific evidence discloses a vicious circle: belonging to a lower socio-economic status family increases the probability of becoming overweight or obese while being obese decreases chances to generate well-being. The described consequences

L.A. Reisch (✉) and W. Gwozdz
Department of Intercultural Communication and Management, Copenhagen Business School, Porcelænshaven 18B, 2000 Frederiksberg, Denmark
e-mail: lr.ikl@cbs.dk

S. Beckmann
Department of Marketing, Copenhagen Business School, Copenhagen, Denmark

L.A. Moreno et al. (eds.), *Epidemiology of Obesity in Children and Adolescents*,
Springer Series on Epidemiology and Public Health 2, DOI 10.1007/978-1-4419-6039-9_24,
© Springer Science+Business Media, LLC 2011

not only undermine social cohesion, but also derogate from social equity and fairness. Thus, it is high time to implement effective strategies to fight the obesity epidemic.

In the long run, children play a decisive role in the fight against obesity since obese children are more likely to become obese adults (Procter 2007). Scientific evidence points out that learned behavior in childhood affects not only the current health status but also lifestyles and weight-related health problems in adulthood (Lobstein et al. 2004). Thus, preventing and reducing overweight and obesity already in childhood should be a major objective and the concerted responsibility of politics, consumer organizations, industry, advertisers, preschool and school authorities, caretakers and teachers, as well as parents. Recently, there has been a tremendous increase in obesity-prevention activities and programs, which complement and reinforce one another. On the policy level, food based dietary guidelines have been compiled and authorized by the responsible health authorities in practically all European countries and beyond. Some countries also have issued evidence-based recommendations for children's level of physical activity (e.g., Belgium (Nutrition Information Center 2006), Canada (Health Canada 2005), Denmark (Nordic Council of Ministers 2005), UK (National Heart Forum 2007), and the US (U.S. Department of Health and Human Services and U.S. Department of Agriculture 2005)). Moreover, in most European countries and also in other countries worldwide – e.g., in the US (US Department of Health and Human Services 2001), in Canada (Heart Stroke Foundation Canada 2006 and Social Development Canada 2002), in Australia (National Obesity Task Force 2004) – health and consumer authorities have developed national action plans that aim at preventing and reducing childhood obesity (Hawkes 2004). These action plans and guidelines target increased awareness of the obesity problem in families, schools, communities, and in the food industry, and they promote behavior change towards a more health supporting diet and physical activity (overview in Acs and Lyles 2007).

Prevention and intervention are the only practicable and cost-efficient solutions. Nevertheless, strategies to overcome the obesity epidemic and its consequences are still rather unexplored. Research has shown that the earlier in the lifespan target-orientated preventive actions are taken, the better the chances of successful intervention (Procter 2007). This holds especially true for the very young age group from 2 to 12 years on – the age group on which the IDEFICS study is focusing.

The main purpose of this chapter is to review the factors that influence health-relevant behavioral patterns of children and then deduce effective and efficient options the various actors have. The focus is on children aged between 2 and 12 years. We attempt to explain why many children do not follow a healthy diet, do not exercise enough, and hence end up with problems of overweight and obesity. After presenting a multilevel approach that relates the various factors on a theoretical basis to one another (section on "Overview of Factors of Consumer Behavior Influencing Childhood Obesity"), we elaborate on children's impact as consumers in the market place. In order to understand children's consumption behavior, we show the relevance of existing concepts of children's socialization as consumers and the impact of so called social agents such as parents, caretakers, and the media. Empirical evidence on the key factors – media use, advertisements, "pester power," the food industry, and social class – is provided (section on "Influence of Socialization Agents as Regards Food and Physical activity"). Finally, the roles and scope of action of the various stakeholders in preventing and reducing childhood obesity are discussed (section on "Empirical Evidence of Influencing Factors").

Overview of Factors of Consumer Behavior Influencing Childhood Obesity

It has long been an established truth that the mental and physical environment – i.e., the family, neighborhood, childcare institutions and schools, community, and society – affects not only children's dietary behavior and their physical activity, but also their preferences, beliefs, and knowledge as regards diet and exercise. Socialization theory in general and social learning theory in particular tell us that young children learn mainly via imitating dietary habits, food preferences, eating patterns, as well as exercise habits from their immediate environment (Dennison et al. 1996; Sellers et al. 2005). Understanding the underlying mechanisms, i.e., the internal and external factors determining childhood obesity is one of the most prominent aims of current research (Baranowski 1997). These days, research tends to focus on the complexity between factors influencing children's dietary and physical activity behavior rather than on simple bivariate relationships. Most of the offered models are based on either Bandura's social learning theory (Bandura 1977) and/or on Bronfenbrenner's (1989) ecological systems theory. The former approach is useful for an understanding of children's health behavior by looking at the interactions between personal factors, environmental influences, and behavior. The latter integrates the various environments ("ecological systems") to which children are directly or indirectly exposed. Some researchers have combined these two approaches into one comprehensive concept (Story et al. 2002). Following the comprehensive framework proposed by Story et al. (2002), we use a multilevel approach that distinguishes four different dimensions of factors influencing health behavior among children: intrapersonal, interpersonal, community, and societal level. Figure 24.1 depicts the model and provides some examples of factors at each level.

In the following, the levels of the conceptual framework are briefly described:

1. Intrapersonal level: The intrapersonal level represents *individual factors*, incorporating psychological factors (e.g., stress, mood, or attitudes) and lifestyle aspects such as meal and activity patterns. It is well known that irregular meal patterns, heavy television viewing, and low levels of physical activity increase the risk of being obese. These factors do not only influence food choices but also short and long term responses to preventions and interventions (EUFIC 2005). Additionally, the role of biological factors such as genetics (Allison et al. 2001), hunger (EUFIC 2005),

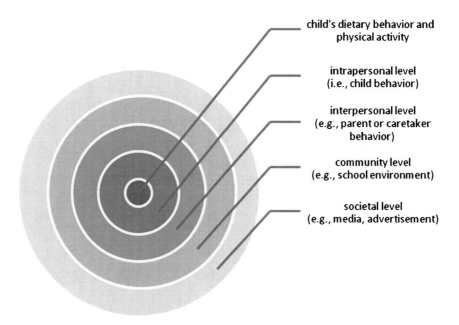

Fig. 24.1 Conceptual model of factors influencing childhood obesity, based on Davison and Birch (2001) and Story et al. (2002)

or sensory properties (Wild-Stiftung 2008) should be considered as an individual's basic endowment. Nevertheless, the rapid rise of obesity in a comparatively short biological time suggests that other than genetic endowments are decisive (Smith and Cummins 2009).

2. Interpersonal level: Of particular interest are the effects of social agents such as family members, peers, and caretakers. Socialization theory in general and social learning theory in particular assume that young children learn mainly by imitating dietary habits, food preferences, eating habits, and physical activities from their immediate environment (Sellers et al. 2005). For instance, parents' attitudes towards the use of food as reward/punishment are important parameters. Via the learning mechanism of operant conditioning, children learn to reward/punish themselves with food and to use food for mood management (Taper et al. 1991).

3. Community level: Focusing only on the intrapersonal and interpersonal levels, one might overlook the important effects and interactions going on between food choice and the physical environment. The physical environment can be more or less "obesogenic," i.e. providing more or fewer stimuli to become obese (Lobstein et al. 2004). Here, the emphasis is on the availability and accessibility of healthy food and physical activities. There is some empirical evidence that low cost and/or easy access to healthy foods and beverages can increase their intake (Hearn et al. 1998). This has also been shown in studies that investigate the role of the school and preschool environment on food preferences, food choices, and physical activities of children (Goldberg and Gunasti 2007; Leviton 2008). The community level comprises the immediate pre-school/school environment as well as restaurants, supermarkets, playgrounds, and so forth, within the reach of children.

4. Societal level: Information on children's buying power and "pester power" as well as on media exposure and media literacy enters the model on the societal level (Livingstone and Helsper 2004). Children today have a lot of "pester power" as well as direct buying power, which makes them an attractive target group for commercial communication. Basically, pester power describes the influence children have on their parents' buying behavior (sometimes called "the nagging factor"), while buying power is the money that is directly available for children. Moreover, prior research has provided empirical evidence that advertising does influence health behavior (Lobstein and Baur 2005; Procter 2007); hence, the scope and scale of advertisements are relevant factors in this model.

A better knowledge about internal and external factors should provide policy makers with the empirical evidence needed to develop effective prevention and intervention strategies. An ecological system model such as the one used in the present study, helps to identify and categorize factors that influence children's food choice and physical activities. However, the empirical research evidence relating to obesity at each level is still scant and not always clear-cut, while the relative importance of each factor in the highly complex interplay of factors and levels is not yet very well discovered (Livingstone et al. 2005).

Children's Impact as Consumers

Children as consumers represent three markets in one: the classical children's market where they spend their own money; the second market where children influence the purchases of their parents; and the third market, i.e., the future market where children become potential adult customers (McNeal 1992).

First, children today experience an increased purchasing power and spending autonomy. Witkowski (2007) pointed out that increased purchasing power led to increased dietary intake, also in the case of children. Children's purchasing power makes them very attractive customers for the food and beverage industry, leading to newly developed, specifically targeted products that are systematically advertised.

The direct children's markets comprise goods especially designed for children such as clothing, toys, personal-care products, media, and foods. These markets have grown in large numbers, outstripping the population growth of children. Within the last decades, children's spending power increased significantly. As in all developed countries, the US shows an obvious trend: While in 1968 children aged between 4 and 12 spent about $2.2 billion on these markets, in 2006 their direct buying power exceeded $51 billion (Dotson and Hyatt 2005). In Germany, children aged six to thirteen had about 6.5 billion Euros at their disposal while in 2007 the amount had risen to more than 1,100 Euros per child per year (Effertz 2008). Nowadays, within UK children markets, children themselves spend about 18.7% of total money spent, using their own money from cash gifts, pocket money, or allowances. One reason for this trend is the growing disposable income of children in recent years (Nicholls and Cullen 2004).

Second, children exert a strong influence on parental purchase decisions: In the US, children's impact on parental spending was roughly about $350 billion in 2005 (McNeal 2007). In Great Britain it was about £30 billion annually (Wilson and Wood 2004), and in Germany about €50 billion in 2003 (Effertz 2008). Moreover, children heavily influence purchases of "family" products such as computers, cars, houses, or holidays. The past decades have witnessed a shift in the perception of the roles of parents and children as consumers: While in the 1950s, parents were considered as gatekeepers to children's consumption, today, marketers address children directly (ibid.). This also leads to a higher conflict potential between children and parents in purchasing situations where children often make use of their "pester power," which is defined as a "child's attempt to exert control over a purchase situation as a simple battle of wills" (Nicholls and Cullen 2004, p. 80). Pester power is not mitigated by industry and retailers as they have long ago recognized the potential of young consumers and have consequently invested in targeted development of products and marketing. Some studies suggest that nagging is one of the most successful techniques that children can apply to influence parental consumption (Gunter and Furnham 1998).

Third, there is evidence that brand loyalty develops already during childhood. Children's brand loyalty depends on two aspects: First, on the familiarity with the brand and second on marketing and media stimuli and parents' brand preferences (Dotson and Hyatt 2005). When children have become young adults, 70% of their brand portfolio is already determined (McNeal 1992). If companies succeed in building a strong brand loyalty during childhood, this can be carried over into adulthood (Dotson and Hyatt 2005). This high potential of children as consumers leads marketers to "invest" in children in the long run, next to the short term manipulation of children's own purchasing decisions and the attempt to steer their use of pester power in the desired direction.

Roles of Socialization Agents as Regards Food and Physical Activity

Obesity evolves whenever calorie intake exceeds calorie consumption over a longer period. A long-term energy imbalance is determined by characteristics of lifestyle, food styles, and level of physical activity – all three factors being the primary responsibility of the individual. However, as behavioral economists and other behavioral scientists point out, we do not usually observe the perfectly informed, highly disciplined, utility maximizing consumer that neoclassical economics assumes. In fact, consumers are often aware of acting against their own interests but are still not able to change their behavior. This is certainly true when it comes to overweight and obesity where widespread knowledge about how – and why – to live healthily does exist, but people are unable to follow up to their best intentions such as working out regularly (Prendergrast et al. 2008). One explanation of this phenomenon is that of an inconsistency between long-term (inherent) and short-term (constructive) preferences of individuals (Scharff 2008). Behavioral economics (e.g., Thaler and Sunstein 2008) and the psychology of consumer behavior stress the power of "default options" of the consumption context for consumer decisions: Since consumers tend to minimize decision costs, they usually follow heuristics, rule of thumb, emotional stimuli, habits, and defaults which are presented by their environment. Decisions made "upstream" by others (e.g., by the government, by suppliers) are less complex and less troublesome. Hence, "making the healthier choice the simple choice" is an important drive towards promoting healthy nutrition.

This is all the more true for children's consumption decisions. Depending on their stage of development, they can only partly assume responsibility for their own food and exercise behavior. They are mainly influenced by parents and social agents with whom they interact (Roedder John 1999). As far as children are concerned, the major responsibility for obesity lies with their parents and families as well as with secondary socialization agents such as caretakers and teachers. Even if nowadays children have more of a say within the family and school environment, parents and caretakers are still acting as gatekeepers. This means that they have also, to a larger or lesser degree, the power to control the impact the media exercises on children's preferences for food and physical activities. Another relevant socialization agent is only touched upon in this chapter: peer groups. They become more important in adolescence and are less influential in the regarded age group (2–10 years).

Models of Children's Behavior and Development

According to consumer socialization theory, which explains the development of consumer knowledge, skills, and values from childhood to adolescence (Ward 1974), there are four main socialization agents: parents, caretakers, peers, and media. Socialization takes place within a socio-cultural environment by learning essential skills for functioning as consumers (Caruana and Vassallo 2003). Following developmental theories (e.g., Kohlberg and Lickona 1976; Piaget 1983 cited in Chan and McNeal 2004; Roedder John 1999), children pass through several stages of cognitive and social development from birth to adulthood. These concepts aim to explain how children are shaped into becoming a member of the consumer society and how they exert their influence within the relationship system they are embedded in. The transition from one stage to another is usually rather smooth and based on the acquisition of essential abilities. The development process is about how to perceive the social environment, and about acquiring information processing skills to organize and use knowledge about this environment. Development also means understanding social interactions and gaining competencies in decision-making as consumers. Typically, three different stages of consumer socialization are identified that can be separated by knowledge development, decision-making skills, and strategies of influencing purchases: perceptual stage, analytical stage, and reflective stage (Roedder John 1999):

1. Children pass through the *perceptual stage* at the age of 3–7 years. Here, observable, "perceivable" characteristics of consumer markets are most important for children of this age. Single dimensions or attributes observed in person, characterize consumer knowledge. Decisions are based on limited information without questioning and consumer orientation is neither more nor less than simple, expedient, and egocentric). Already at this age, children are aware of several specific products, brands, and retail stores.
2. Subsequently, children aged 7–11 years go through the *analytical stage* where some of the most relevant abilities and competencies of consumers are developed. A better understanding of the functioning of consumer markets as well as of the complex structures of advertising is gained due to the ability to recognize symbolic attributes beyond perceptual ones. At this stage, children do not rely on one single dimension, but adapt consumer decision strategies based on multiple, observable, and unobservable dimensions such as price, product category, and previous experiences. Due to increasing social abilities they reflect incrementally on concepts such as brands or advertising. They also learn how to negotiate with parents and other social agents about desired products in a more rational way.

3. The *reflective stage* begins at the age of 11 years and ends in adolescence, at the age of about 16 years. Social and cognitive abilities increase further; information processing becomes more sophisticated, leading to a higher understanding of brands, pricing, or advertising. At this stage, reflecting on and reasoning consumer decisions are new and not only perceived as isolated from other individuals. Now, the beliefs and attitudes of others become important and thus, behavior becomes more strategic.

Nowadays, it is recommended to reconsider the age groups cited above as children today are involved in consumer decisions at an earlier age and quickly become fully-fledged members of the consumer society. This can be shown by children's significantly increased media usage and ever-high exposure to all kind of commercial settings (e.g., sponsoring of mass media).

Roles of Parents and the Family

Parents are the key agents in children's early food socialization by forming their nutritional habits and preferences (Hughner and Maher 2006), starting already pre- and continuous postnatal (Procter 2007). During the first years after birth, they are the main persons responsible for the child's nutrition – not only by feeding the child but also by socially interacting with the child, exerting punishment, and reward and so forth. Once children get older, other actors enter the stage. On entering preschool and school, caretakers and teachers as individuals and as representatives of their institutions (and hence following the institutions' rules) influence children's dietary behavior and physical activity. Depending on the parental style, mass media, and the internet can also play a relevant role (Holm 2008). The increasing influence of these actors does not release parents from their responsibility for the health of their child. The opposite might be true, since parents have also a say in what type of social environment their child is exposed to (e.g., their family policy on media use).

Parents exert a powerful influence on their children via role modeling, communication models, and parental styles (Nicklas and Hayes 2008). Moreover, with their daily family lifestyle management and pocket money policy, parents can forcefully influence the food and the physical activity environment, i.e., the available choices children have (easy) access to (e.g., Hearn et al. 1998). Davison and Birch (2001) categorize families into two groups with different behavioral patterns: In the "obsogenic" family type, energy intake is rather high and at the same time energy use via physical activity is low. "Nonobesogenic" families have lower levels of energy intake and higher levels of physical activity, resulting in a lower probability of being overweight.

The younger the child, the stronger is the influence of parental food management and food styles. Even in many day-care institutions, parents have a say in when, where, and what food is consumed. One key to the development of healthy food styles is seen in making use of the impact of habits that are familiarized and sustained by parents or caretakers. Parents' fruit and vegetable intake proved to be a good indicator for children's fruit and vegetable consumption (Cooke et al. 2003; Wardle et al. 2005). Experiments have shown that the mere exposure to healthy food increases its intake (Baranowski et al. 1993; Kirby et al. 1995) and the more frequently parents and children eat together, the healthier the children's diets (Gillman et al. 2000). Research has shown, for instance, that children in families having regular breakfast and/or children with parents who put together a healthy diet – i.e., based on food recommendations – have a healthier diet compared to others (Nicklas et al. 2001). Moreover, it has been shown that children actively impersonate their parents' food styles and learn by observation, e.g., they prefer eating fruits and vegetables when their parents do (Cullen et al. 2000).

Another field of research has been to look into the influence of communication about food during meals on children's food preferences (Nicklas et al. 2001): Experiencing a meal in negative family surroundings resulted in a lesser future preference for the food which was served during this meal. Parents restricting access to or forcing children to eat specific foods evoke a reaction in an undesired direction (Birch 1999). It is important to note that the learning process is not just about skills (what is edible? how do I eat it?) but also about motivation and positive reinforcements (Bandura 1977). Research has shown that children accept unknown food more easily if parents or other role models such as siblings eat – and give positive comments on – this food in front of children (Birch 1980). Reducing sedentary behavior such as television or video viewing succeeds when parents restrict access via programming an automatically limited television usage (Gortmaker et al. 1999; Robinson 1999). This, in turn can significantly contribute to weight loss (Lobstein et al. 2004).

The child–parent communication on food is highly dependent on the general parental style that is practiced in the family (Gunter and Furnham 1998). In the pedagogic literature, three different parental styles are distinguished (Baumrind 1973): the authoritarian, the authoritative, and the permissive style. The authoritarian parenting style displays a high level of control over children's food intake by parents, including the usage of food for punishment or reward, resulting in a negative effect on children's dietary behavior and body weight. The authoritative style is characterized by negotiations and discussions, based on the expert knowledge of parents but taking into account the needs of children. It can be hypothesized that an authoritative style enables children to learn a more self-controlled diet since authoritative parents discuss consumption issues more than other parents. As opposed to permissive parents, they do monitor and restrict children's food choice and media exposure (Nicklas et al. 2001). Moreover, parents supporting physical activity have children that are more active (Lobstein et al. 2004), but empirical evidence on this parental style is scarce. On the other hand, "laissez-faire" reflects the behavioral method of the permissive parental style. This style also goes along with a larger economic independence of children's buying decisions. Children experiencing the latter style suffer more often from overweight (Nicklas et al. 2001).

In real life, a mixture of these three parenting styles will be found in families, with one style being more pronounced than the other two. Research has shown that parental styles depend on cultural and ethical backgrounds, socio-economic status (SES), age, and sex of the child (e.g., French et al. 2001; Lobstein et al. 2004): Parents' input very often relies on access to healthy foods, physical activity, and their own knowledge which is all reflected by SES (McLaren 2007). How parents deal with their children depends also very much on the age of the child (Dotson and Hyatt 2005). Concerning spending autonomy, a family's SES is U-shaped, which means that lower and higher SES parents allow their children a greater spending autonomy once they reach adolescence than parents living in medium SES families (Gunter and Furnham 1998).

In a nutshell: Parents are observed and modeled by their offspring. Communicational patterns between children and parents are important and rely very much on the parental style. Parents serve as role models for their offspring, but the socialization process is not the same in all families. There are limits to the extent of parents' capability to act as gatekeepers. This is not only due to the influence of peers and the pushing of the market, but is also due to existing social norms and installed practices – such as using candies to reward children – that are seldom challenged and difficult to circumnavigate once they are installed (Thaler and Sunstein 2008).

Roles of Caretakers

Whenever children enter childcare institutions, caretakers[1] take over a part of the responsibility for children's eating behavior and physical activity and thus serve as a role model in much the

---

[1] Here, we use the term caretaker for both kindergarten and school teacher. If we are talking only about one of these types of caretakers, we highlight this.

same way as parents do. Since children spend a good deal of their day within the childcare/ school system, and eat, on average, at least one meal and one snack based on British settings (Edmunds et al. 2001), the key role of preschool and school settings for children's body weight is not surprising. While earlier research has shown that, in the US, infants and toddlers are generally well nourished regardless of the type of child care arrangement (child care center or home care) (Goodwin et al. 1999), it is well known that eating together means much more than just intake of calories and the right amount of nutritional elements. In childcare settings, common meals as a central daily routine play an important role by structuring the day, offering breaks, forming eating habits, experimenting with new tastes, likes and dislikes, and offering the possibility of spending time together outside the play or class room. Sellers et al. (2005, p. 229) argue that "since dietary practices and activity patterns are influenced by what occurs in the childcare environment, it is reasonable to suggest that childcare providers are important mediators in the prevention of childhood overweight." A study from the 1990s (Briley et al. 1994) found that the factors that have the most direct influence on the menus at childcare centers are: food program requirements, staff perceptions of children's food preferences, history of the food program at the center, and cost. Moreover, research has shown that children's food intake and physical activity offered at school are important determinants of body weight (Edmunds et al. 2001), and that childcare providers exert a significant influence on the young children's lives.

Many studies (e.g., Black 2002; Hearn et al. 1998; Lakin and Littledyke 2008; Nicklas et al. 2001; Rossiter et al. 2007; Sellers et al. 2005) highlight the importance of these institutional settings on dietary practices and activity patterns. They conclude that schools and childcare facilities as well as teachers and caretakers can adopt a mediating role in the prevention of childhood obesity by steering food consumption patterns in a more favorable direction: by acting as positive role models themselves, by educating children on these issues as well as by controlling the availability and accessibility of foods and drinks within the institution and – in cooperation with the local community – in its neighborhood. The same holds true for the available facilities and conveyed motivation for physical activity. Moreover, Hendy and Raudenbush (2000) found that children are more likely to eat food when they observe an adult eating it. Yet, schoolteachers rarely take their meals together with the children (Nahikian-Nelms 1997), while caretakers in day care centers (e.g., kindergartens, preschools) usually do. In general, parents' and caretakers' pedagogic styles impact on communication about food (Nicklas et al. 2001).

Often parents do not recognize their child's overweight problem (Dennison and Boyer 2004) or they tend to underestimate it (Sellers et al. 2005). Caretakers have a more realistic perspective on children's overweight status (Sellers et al. 2005) and might act as facilitators or caretakers to parents. However, they often experience difficulties in communicating with parents about the child's overweight problem. Since relationships between parents and caretakers are crucial for a health-promoting environment for young children (Nicklas et al. 2001), this calls for further training and tools to communicate effectively. In order to enable the caretakers to conduct effective prevention activities, it is vital to understand the knowledge, behaviors, attitudes, and expectations of educators as regards healthy living (O'Dea and Abraham 2001; Yager and O'Dea 2005). If caretakers are themselves overweight, they might not be successful in promoting the "healthy living" message since they are not seen as credible sources of nutrition and weight control information. Sellers et al. (2005) found that educators often do realize their influence on children's food and physical activity choices, but also feel powerless in the face of competition with other influences such as peers and an obesogenic environment. Faced by limited means, they often resent being held responsible for the state of children's health by parents and the media.

Roles of Media

Children's dietary practices and physical activity patterns are affected by the physical and social contexts in which food and activities are offered. Preschoolers and elementary school pupils are particularly apt to imitate dietary habits, food preferences, eating patterns, use of food, and habits of exercise or sedentary activities such as television viewing from adults and peers (Dennison et al. 1996; Sellers et al. 2005). To date, television is still the most frequently used media for younger children; however, computers and mobile phones are catching up (Livingstone et al. 2005).

Consumption preferences and patterns cannot be disentangled from traditional and new media use. Children's socialization is taking place earlier and their media use is heavier these days compared to 20 or 30 years ago. They experience purchasing and consumption situations more frequently already at an earlier stage via the accelerated information processing and development of media technology (Eckstrøm and Tufte 2007). The newly learned consumption behavior is sometimes shared with parents who learn new consumption roles from their offspring. Here, children act as "front runners" (Tufte et al. 2005). Media's influential potential as well as children's buying power, and thus their impact on families' purchase decisions make children a very appealing target for marketers who use all kinds of media channels to transmit their messages. Hence, young children are both: Particularly susceptible to commercial influences via media and ideal targets for preventive strategies.

While very young children do not possess explicit brand awareness, they do recognize brand logos already at the age of three (Bachmann-Achenreiner and Roedder John 2003), i.e., at the perceptual stage. By the age of five, children are able to distinguish between "normal" television programs and commercials (Mallalieu et al. 2005), even if this is rather on a perceptual level – e.g., shorter length of commercial spots – than understanding the selling purpose of commercials (Roedder John 1999). The latter does not appear before children are aged 7 or 8 years. Children at the analytical stage have a broader understanding of commercials even if they do not fully question the sent messages. They know that commercials are not always telling the truth. Children aged 7–11 years become aware of the intention of advertising to sell products. Nevertheless, preferences for and familiarity with particular brands are developed exactly at this stage (Roedder John 1999). Media play a major role in transmitting commercials messages to children and are thus decisive for shaping consumption behavior.

About 20 to 25% of children's daily energy intake is consumed in front of the television (Matheson et al. 2004). The media are quite influential in forming children's food habits: They have the power for both interrupting habituation to food cues and impeding the development of eating habituations (Temple et al. 2007). A habituation to food cues is known across all species and is regulated by biological signals of the body from the sensory, the neuronal, or the digestive system (Swithers and Hall 1994). Television can distract children's attention away from eating and, in the long run, even wean them from known habits (Temple et al. 2007). Moreover, children respond to emotional stimuli: Repeated exposure to a specific positive atmosphere in combination with a product might lead to emotional conditioning (Phelps 2006). This emotional effect works in a similar way to Pavlovian "classical" conditioning: At a later stage, children do not need the stimuli anymore to experience the positive atmosphere; the mere sight of the respective product is enough to evoke positive emotions (Effertz 2008). Also, while parents – and caretakers in childcare – exert most influence in early childhood, teachers and peers enter the stage at a later point in time, while the media are steady companions of most children of the regarded age group.

Independent of timing, all social agents impact children's knowledge, skills and behavior as consumers within a society (Dotson and Hyatt 2005). The matter of childhood socialization becomes even more complex when considering that all agents interact with one another and influence children more or less simultaneously – often with conflicting messages.

Empirical Evidence of Influencing Factors

Empirical consumer behavior research has detected several factors that impact on children's overweight. The previously presented multilevel approach based on French et al. (2001) emphasizes the complexity and interdependencies of relevant dimension: intrapersonal, interpersonal, community, and societal level. While it is beyond the scope of this chapter to present a comprehensive overview (e.g., Procter 2007), the present section focuses on those key factors where substantial empirical evidence is available. These are: children's pester power, the role of social class, influences of the food industry, the impact of media use, and advertising. Pester power describes children's behavior in consumer settings and thus, stands at the intrapersonal level. The role of social class presents behavioral influences at the interpersonal level. However, both pester power and social class are embedded in the societal context and hence, societal factors such as the food industry, media, and advertisements play an important role in shaping children's health behavior.

Pester Power

Pester power, describing children's purchase request behavior, seems to be one of the most successful techniques children apply to exert influence on parents purchase decisions (Nicholls and Cullen 2004). McNeal (1999) found that on average children nag for 15 products per shopping trip and that many of these desires are aroused by advertisements. The outcomes of these "pester conflicts" strongly depend on the parent-child communication relationship, the parental style, as well as on the product category (Valkenburg and Cantor 2001). How sophisticated pestering is depends on the child's stage of consumer socialization. The strategies can vary from asking, begging, and whining to persuading and employing emotional strategies (Marshall et al. 2007). As regards product categories, food is probably the one with highest pester power potential: Food purchases are more complex than, e.g., shopping for toys or clothing, since many different tastes, family requests, and needs have to be taken into account. Moreover, while parents usually want to buy food efficiently, children often take an interest in food shopping and want to participate in the decision processes. It is hence not surprising that research has found that conflict potential is fairly high in supermarket shopping environments (Nicholls and Cullen 2004).

McDermott and colleagues reviewed some of the more influential studies on the controversially discussed relationship between children's purchase request behavior and parental purchase decisions (McDermott et al. 2006). They found "strong evidence that food promotion does encourage children to request food purchases from their parents" (p. 532). In the best case it complicates the parent-child purchasing relationship and in the worst case, parents buy unhealthy food due to the nagging against better knowledge. Parents often perceive children's pestering as a negative influence on their family relationships and thus get fed up with endless negotiations about purchases and the associated financial decisions (Middleton et al. 1994). Nutritional considerations are most important for parents while shopping; preferences of their children in deciding what food to buy come a close second (Spungin 2004). Pestering seems to be a successful strategy in that children get their way about half the time (McDermott et al. 2006). Meanwhile, parents also develop tactics for responding to pestering by their parental and communication patterns (Marshall et al. 2007). Such a strategy involves, for instance, avoiding visits to supermarkets with children as far as possible (Petterson et al. 2004).

Parents' challenges for dealing with children's pester power in purchasing situations are further complicated by the media, advertisements, and – when the children are getting older – peer pressure (BCI 2003). Analyzing almost 200 studies on the effect of food promotion on children, Stead et al. (2007) conclude that there is strong evidence that children's pester behavior is influenced by advertising.

Retailers and marketers have long identified the potential of children's power over parental purchase decisions and actively create shopping environments where such conflicts arise (Mayo 2005). A well-known example is that supermarket chains position candy and unhealthy treats at child-eye level in the checkout lines. Parents and consumer activists have long battled against these types of "tantrum tamers," but while nowadays some supermarkets offer candy-free checkout lanes, industry finds less overt ways to shape children's food preferences such as school sponsoring, guerrilla marketing, and viral marketing.

The Role of Social Class

One of the most robust results on child obesity research is the positive correlation between low socio-economic status (SES) and a higher prevalence of obesity (McLaren 2007). Compared with the rest of the population, children and women in lower social classes show higher rates of obesity with a steepening trend of the gradient (Robertson et al. 2007).

Remembering the U-shaped relationship between spending autonomy and social status, children of middle SES families have the lowest consumer experience: Children from low SES families are exposed earlier and more often to commercial settings and thus, are more experienced (Gunter and Furnham 1998). Due to different communication processes and higher consumption autonomy, children from upper class families also acquire consumer knowledge at an early life stage. They also seek more information before making a purchase decision and are said to have stronger brand loyalties than children of the other two groups (ibid.). It is questionable whether the social class is also related to diverging communication processes. Here, empirical evidence is contradictory. However, the main barrier to healthy food behavior seems not to be a lack of information, but rather the ability to transfer this knowledge into practice (Robertson et al. 2007).

McLaren (2007) provided a comprehensive review including more than 300 studies on the relationship between SES and obesity that have been conducted over the past 20 years. The majority of European, American, Canadian, and Australian studies confirm an existence of the relationship between social class and diet. However, there are conflicting results when it comes to childhood overweight and obesity with regard to social class in that there is little empirical evidence (Parsons et al. 1999). Nevertheless, children, growing up in deprived families, have a higher probability of being overweight in adulthood. This has been explained by poor access to and higher prices for healthy food as well as by fewer opportunities for physical activity (Robertson et al. 2007).

With regard to dietary behavior, higher SES families tend to have a healthier diet and to be more physically active. Nutrition in lower SES families tends to be higher in energy and lower in micronutrients, leading to a higher probability of having a positive energy balance (Robertson et al. 2007). Children tend to drink more soft drinks, eat less vegetables and fruits, are less physically active and adopt more sedentary lifestyles (McLaren 2007). Among others, there is a financial reason for this behavior: Lower social classes have to spend a larger proportion of their household income for food, even if they go for the cheaper alternatives. In general, food expenditure is the most flexible part of a household budget (Leather 1996). Thus, low SES families save on money by a different composition of the shopping basket compared to higher SES families: Fewer foods that are recommended for healthy diets and more cheap foods that satisfy hunger but simultaneously are higher in fat, salt, and sugar.

In a broader sense, SES can also be seen as an indicator for the social environmental circumstances in which children are living. Thus, it is correlated with the physical environment, i.e., the neighborhood, which has also been depicted as a factor influencing childhood obesity (Kinra et al. 2000). Moreover, lower SES limits access to reasonably priced food of good quality, to inexpensive and safe opportunities for physical activities, and to knowledge about healthy dietary and physical activity behavior. Yet, it is known that economic security, adequate housing, and food and nutrition security are social health factors that reduce the risk of disease (Robertson et al. 2007). In low SES areas, prices for fruit and vegetables are 30–40% higher and availability is lower when compared to better-off areas (Popkin et al. 2005). Moreover, the number of fast food outlets in economically deprived areas is four times as high as in less deprived areas (Cummins et al. 2005; Macdonald et al. 2007). As Procter (2007) argues, a lower public transport supply decreases the scope of action for consumer choices, e.g., fewer shopping possibilities are in reachable distance when families do not have a car. While only little research is available about the relationship between children's access to safe parks and green areas within a neighborhood and obesity (Timperio et al. 2005), some qualitative investigations of low SES families within the IDEFICS study support the assumption that it is the subjectively perceived safety of the environment that counts. After all, crime rates are higher in deprived areas than in better off ones.

Food Industry

Irrespective of social class, children's intake of energy dense food has increased drastically (Robertson et al. 2007). This is not only due to intensified media use, increased advertising pressure, and the ubiquitous availability of food; it is also due to other aspects of food marketing: The increased offer of processed food and ready-made meals which contain more energy per food or drink unit (Jeffery and Utter 2003) as well as to increasingly larger package sizes marketed over the past 20 years (Diliberti et al. 2004; Rolls et al. 2004; Young and Nestle 2003). Hence, food industry is accused of facilitating obesogenic dietary behavior in order to realize higher profits (Procter 2007). Industry and retail largely shape the context in which food choice takes place. Behavioral economics has shown that the influence of the immediate context (e.g., in-store marketing, product offers, built environment) has a decisive impact on consumers' decisions, that access and availability of healthy alternatives are crucial and that many preferences are "constructed" right at the point of sale ("constructive preferences") (Thaler and Sunstein 2008).

Indeed, the food environment has drastically changed over the last four decades. In the US, the convenience food industry experienced strong growth and the number of easy-to-access and ready-to-eat food stores doubled within this period (Jeffery and Utter 2003). Consumers tend to spend more for eating out than for eating at home (Procter 2007). Developments in Europe are similar. Characteristics of preferred food stores are: limited choice, quick service and opportunities for take away (National Restaurant Association 1998). The composition of food supply in traditional food stores also changed towards more processed food-stuff (Jeffery and Utter 2003). These developments indicate that food is easier available and more convenient, which contributes to a higher energy intake.

The food industry has increased portion sizes over the last 20 years (Diliberti et al. 2004; Young and Nestle 1995) and offers these larger servings for comparatively lower prices (Wansink 1996). The same development took place in restaurants (Diliberti et al. 2004). Large package sizes nudge consumers to over consume: Many large packages contain multiple servings, which is not always obvious to consumers. Moreover, consumers tend to eat or drink up a package once it is opened – rather unimpressed by its size. This has been shown, e.g., by Wansink and Park (2001) in varying movie-goers popcorn sizes as well as by Rolls et al. (2004) in serving different sizes of pasta in a restaurant. Similarly, consumers tend to increase their energy intake in restaurants where larger portions are offered. Diliberti et al. (2004) analyzed whether larger entrées would be finished off in the same manner as smaller portions: They were, and whether consumers would compensate for larger entrée sizes: They did not.

As regards ready-made and processed meals, it is quite difficult for consumers to assess their energy density and nutritional value – unless industry provides this information on the package.

Hence, there is a heated and ongoing debate amongst industry, regulators, and science on how to best label and present relevant nutritional information to consumers. In general, consumers are interested in nutrition information on packages, but these have to be understandable and easy to read (Grunert and Wills 2007). It has been shown that information about included fat impacts purchasing decisions in favor of buying lower fat products (Roefs and Jansen 2004). In Europe, consumers can find different competing systems on the supermarket shelves: positive vs. negative labeling, with vs. without colors, absolute vs. relative specifications, varying quite a lot in details. The Swedish "Keyhole" for instance is a positive, relative system, comparing foods within one category. The Guideline Daily Amount (GDA) provides information about absolute nutritional values based on a priori undetermined unit, which can be grams, servings, etc. The traffic light system is also an absolute scheme using colors depending on the nutritional value according to dietary recommendations. All available systems are highly controversial and either preferred by industry, or policy regulators, or consumer organizations.

While some studies have shown that the traffic light system is more useful for consumers than the GDA system (Lobstein and Davies 2009), others have found that consumers tend to misunderstand the colors and get confused (Grunert and Wills 2007). What is widely accepted, however, is the fact that consumers in general prefer simple, easily understandable information cues on the front of the packages. Experimental studies suggest that the label information provided is indeed used by consumers. However, there is still little evidence about how different systems are accepted and understood in real world shopping and how they affect dietary patterns (Cowburn and Stockley 2005; Grunert and Wills 2007). The requirements for a working food labeling scheme is the synthesis of key nutritional information such as fat, sugar, and salt content, energy density and portion size that is understandable to consumers, applicable across food categories, and manageable via transparent regulations (Lobstein and Davies 2009). For sure, it would be of tremendous importance to have one common system that consumers can recognize and learn to understand.

While it is unclear how effective food labeling is in influencing consumers' choices (so called "primary effects"), the traffic light system seems to have notable "secondary effects" on the industry: In the UK, product recipes have been changed towards less transfats and less sugar, and package sizes have been reduced (Lobstein and Davies 2009). This is good news for the age group of young children who will usually neither have the competence nor the interest to read food labels – however thoughtfully they may be designed.

Media Use

Children these days are highly exposed to mass media. Children in the US and Europe watch, on average, more than two and a half hours television daily (Diehl 2005; Holt et al. 2007). Basically, this exposure can have both negative and positive effects. Public television and radio programs, for instance, present high quality educative programs, and are sometimes media partners in public campaigns for children's diet and physical activity. Mass media have hence the potential to reach a very large target group in attractive formats to raise problem awareness and offer solutions. On the other hand, food and drink advertisements are heavily focused on less healthy product choices: Most television ads these days promote sweet, fatty, or salty snacks or drinks (Desrochers and Holt 2007; Hastings et al. 2003; Livingstone 2005) and hence tend to mould preferences for rather unhealthy food. Moreover, the use of mass media is normally a sedentary behavior and adds to children's physical inactivity (Holt et al. 2007). The negative consequences of heavy television, video and computer use for children are manifold and widely acknowledged.

While computer and video game use has dramatically increased in the past decade, for the age group of the 2–12 year olds, television is still the most frequently used mass media in today's consumer societies (Desrochers and Holt 2007). In Germany, children aged between 3 and 5 years watch on average 1 h daily; when they are 6–9 years old, this increases to one and a half hours and to more than 2 h when aged 10–13 years (Diehl 2005). Similar television viewing hours are found for British (Halford et al. 2004) and American children (Crespo et al. 2001). Children's parents and grandparents are not the best role models since their television consumption exceeds these numbers by far (Diehl 2005). In principle, when children watch television or play video games, they are physically inactive. Only few studies have investigated whether the number of television viewing hours is a representative indicator for sedentary lifestyles and the prevalence of overweight and obesity. However, results differ and show a rather weak correlation (Durant and Baranowski 1994; Robinson et al. 1993) or provide no support (Andersen et al. 1998). Nevertheless, television viewing is recognized as one important factor that correlates with poor diets, poor health and obesity (Ofcom 2004). While viewing television, energy intake increases in the form of snacking behavior, fast food and pre-prepared meals consumption (Coon and Tucker 2002; Crespo et al. 2001; Temple et al. 2007). It goes without saying that television viewing includes the exposure of children to advertisements (Ofcom 2004).

Consumer research has investigated the relationship between television viewing and children's weight. Several studies have found a strong positive relationship between the prevalence of obesity and the amount of television viewing (Andersen et al. 1998; Crespo et al. 2001; Dietz and Gortmaker 1985; Gortmaker et al. 1996; Lowry et al. 2002; Proctor et al. 2003). Yet, a few studies have found no significant relationship (Durant and Baranowski 1994; Robinson et al. 1993; Vandewater et al. 2004). The contrariness of these results is partly due to the data and methods used, but it gives sufficient cause for challenging the assumption of a causal relationship. Experiments are usually the better method for tracing causalities. Indeed, some experimental studies found a decrease in children's weight when television-viewing times were reduced in a trial (Epstein et al. 2000; Gortmaker et al. 1999; Robinson 1999). Epstein and colleagues found that viewing time reduction led to a lower energy intake but not to more physical activity (Epstein et al. 2008). Thus, reducing television (and video game, computer) hours could be one possible factor in reducing overweight and obesity.

Advertising

Food industry's commercial communication makes use of different channels to advertise their food and drinks to children and their parents. Besides the classical tool of television advertising, companies these days use more subtle forms of advertising such as product placement in TV programs, internet websites, games, and communities, toys or games created in partnerships with food companies (sometimes shown in program-length commercials), in-school marketing activities such as vending machines, sponsoring, or supply of educational material (Story and French 2004). Specific instruments are used to raise brand awareness and brand liking – such as celebrities ballyhooing their favorite foods, or funny cartoons rather than health issues (Dotson and Hyatt 2005; Stead et al. 2007). As expected, advertisements concentrate on fun and taste rather than on issues such as health and nutritional value (Hastings et al. 2003). Several experiments support the assumption that food branding changes children's preferences in favor of the branded food (Robinson et al. 2007). Advertisements are successful strategies for brand building in children's food (Dammler and Middelmann-Motz 2002) and they are intensively used, as shown in a major report on research into the effects of food promotion on children (Hastings et al. 2003). Despite the spread of the internet and other types of media, television remains the major promotional channel for food producers, retailers, and restaurants to advertise their products to children (Brown et al. 2005; IOM 2006).

Nevertheless, advertisers reject any responsibility for the obesity crisis. They claim that advertisements cannot coerce consumers into buying unhealthy foods, but that they can – at best – change preferences within a food category (Hoek and Gendall 2006). To date, there is some evidence for brand switching (Diehl 2005) and some for category switching (Hastings et al. 2003). Some authors argue that commercial communication in its many forms might not be able to induce, but just reinforce existing unhealthy behavioral patterns. Livingstone and Helsper 2004 concludes cautiously from her comprehensive literature review on the direct effect of television advertisements on children's food preferences, consumption, and health behavior that at least moderate direct effect does exist. Likewise, Hastings et al. (2003) state that there is an effect of television viewing and exposure to advertisements on children's food behavior and diet, independent of other factors. However, the size of the effect is not yet clear (Ofcom 2004).

For the age group of 2–10 year olds, television advertisements are assumed to be the most effective and most heavily used marketing instrument these days (Stead et al. 2007). Children are aware of commercial television spots and enjoy watching them while parents notice that commercials influence families' communication and shopping behavior (Hastings et al. 2003). Due to high television viewing, children aged between 2 and 11 years are increasingly exposed to advertisements – about 25,000 commercials (food and non-food) per year (Coon and Tucker 2002; Desrochers and Holt 2007). About 20% of this communication is about food products (Desrochers and Holt 2007). Most food advertisements are for rather unhealthy food products, high in sugar, transfats, and/or salt (Diehl 2005; Kelly et al. 2007; Linn 2000). Highly promoted product groups are sugared breakfast cereals, confectionary, soft drinks, savory snacks, and fast food restaurants (Hastings et al. 2003). There is empirical evidence that the unhealthy content of advertisements often leads to unhealthier food choices (Borzekowski and Robinson 2001; Lewis and Hill 1998; Taveras et al. 2006). Not only do overweight and obese children recognize advertised products significantly more often, but also they have a higher intake of advertised products (Coon and Tucker 2002; Halford et al. 2004). Moreover, a higher exposure to ads of unhealthy food leads to a lower intake of fruits and vegetables (Livingstone and Helsper 2004). On the other hand, some studies suggest a weak, but positive relationship between the exposure to healthy food commercials and the intake of fruits and vegetables (Klepp et al. 2007).

Summarizing the above, the empirical studies available on the relationship between advertisements and childhood obesity are controversial: Some find a significant positive relationship (Hastings et al. 2003; Lobstein and Dibb 2005), others have found no relationship at all (Diehl 2005). The latter position might be backed up by the observation that in countries where TV advertising targeted at children has been banned for many years – such as Sweden – obesity rates are no different from those countries with less strict regulatory regimes. The former position, however, can point to the fact that if advertising does not "work" in the intended direction (i.e., shaping preferences), why then should industry spend huge amounts of money on advertising.

Policy Implications

The factors presented above are valuable starting points for changing young consumers' behavior in a more socially and individually sustainable direction. While the goal to reduce obesity is broadly accepted, the motives, strategies, possibilities, and dependencies of the various actors in the food chain and in food and health politics differ. In the following we argue that policy actions are necessary, but that they can only be effective if all stakeholders support these policies with all the means within their reach. Given the number of stakeholders that are involved in the obesity issue and their different perspectives, fainting profiles of individual roles get redefined. Responsibilities of governments, industry, parents and caretakers, and consumer organizations are constantly discussed and negotiated anew. This is partly due to a lack of empirical evidence on the effects of regulations, interventions, preventions, and voluntary activities. Thus, there is an ongoing debate over theory, methods, and evidence parallel to a policy debate over policy tools (Livingstone 2005).

Implications for Parents and Caretakers

Parents are the first instance of children's socialization as consumers. Caretakers assume a part of this responsibility when children enter secondary socialization institutions. The European Commission (2007) notes that parents, having the main responsibility for their children, should be able to make informed choices and transfer their knowledge to their offspring. Parents and caretakers adopt several responsibilities at the same time, e.g., they are role models for their children who learn via observing and imitating. Parents also introduce their offspring into the world of consumers: They provide shopping experiences, teach market knowledge, evaluate brands and products, and regulate access to consumption and purchase situations. Via these instruments, parents and caretakers also shape children's knowledge, attitudes, and beliefs concerning nutrition. Also, parents are the main stakeholders responsible for the diet and physical activity of their children. Thus, parents (and caretakers) should have good knowledge on how to act as "sovereign" consumers themselves. They need to acquire and apply knowledge about healthy life styles; they should be able to reflect on their own consumption behavior, find appropriate communication patterns towards children, and understand market mechanisms and consumer rights; they should have a basic understanding of how to evaluate prices, read labels, and interpret advertisements. We can easily add more "shoulds" to this list. As shown above, particularly low SES parents will not be able to live up to these expectations and will need further education and support.

Implications for Consumer Organizations

Consumer organizations are the advocates of consumers and represent their interests in the political realm. By combining their power in platforms of action and via the media, consumer organizations are able to find an attentive ear, especially among food producers and retailers. They can ask governments to provide support for healthy lifestyles and industry to provide healthy products. The other role of consumer organizations is to raise awareness of the responsibilities consumers have. One way of doing this is by educating parents and children about what a healthy lifestyle means and implies, and how it can be realized. Arranging campaigns and establishing networks are other means these organizations can apply. Thus, consumer organizations act as information brokers, guiding hands, and political activists between consumers, media, industry, and policy makers.

Implications for Regulators

Taking on a macro-economic point of view, it is financially worthwhile for a government to intervene in the rising prevalence of obesity (Acs and Lyles 2007). Health system expenditure for the consequences of overweight and obesity are enormous, and if prevention and intervention are not successful, taxpayers will be burdened with the additional costs. It might be rational for single consumers to stick to an unhealthy lifestyle; but it is not rational for governments not to counteract the escalating health costs. Nevertheless, policy makers need convincing evidence before implementing new strategies to fight obesity (Lobstein and Baur 2005). One key assumption made by most policy makers is that ultimately, each individual is responsible for its own consumption decisions and thus, consumer policy should limit its role to empowering individuals to make informed choices (European Commission 2007).

Yet, with regard to the growing prevalence of childhood obesity, this view is not entirely convincing. Children are vulnerable consumers and lack cognitive skills and market place experience. While parents should not be set free from their responsibility to provide healthy nutrition and opportunities for physical activity, their influence is limited, as shown above. Consumer policy should in the first place inform, educate, empower, support, and engage consumers in general, but especially those as parents responsible for their children's health. In the case of obesity, three main strategic goals have been identified: raise awareness of the risks of obesity, reduce energy intake, and increase energy output (Witkowski 2007). To reach these goals, consumer information, education, and advice are relevant tools, but they might not be far-reaching enough, especially not if constructive preferences triumph over inherent preferences when it comes to nutritional or physical activity decision-making processes. Strengthening consumer organizations and listening to them in a constant dialog consumer interest is another relevant tool (Viswanathan and Gau 2005). In some cases, it might be most effective to actively steer consumption subtly – "to nudge" (Thaler and Sunstein 2008) – into healthier choices by shaping the consumption context, i.e., designing access and default settings. Examples in case are guidelines or regulations on vending machines in schools, smart defaults in canteens, and a ban on food advertising and sponsoring in children's programs. Access to healthy food and physical activity can be assured via the school or community environment.

Implications for Industry and Advertising

In 2004, the European Commission brought together all stakeholders of the obesity crisis to start a discussion on appropriate approaches to tackling obesity. Among them were the food industry and retailers who are, of course, primarily interested in satisfying their shareholders. Nevertheless, a voluntary contribution by the food industry could comprise a shift in focus from short-term goals to investment in long-term programs (Layton and Grossbart 2006) in order to alleviate the means whereby children as well as parents can make healthier and more sustainable choices. The national action plans as well as food based dietary guidelines – even if being constantly questioned and adapted – are a sound basis for nutritional values and activities. These can be used to inform consumers in an easy and understandable way via food labeling. There is a large potential for improving and standardizing the existing food labeling systems in order to reduce consumers' confusion (Procter 2007). In order to ease the decision process for consumers, there is a need for easy and low cost access to healthy food, such as vegetables and fruits, by improving the availability by food producers as well increasing in store promotion by retailers (Government Office for Science 2007). Moreover, recipes could be reformulated by modifying levels of fat, sugar, or salt. Another approach would be to decrease package and portion sizes (European Commission 2008). Recent trends and developments of products such as diet sodas or reduced-calorie foods illustrate the way the industry is trying to meet consumer needs, financial targets, and healthy product images.

Marketers and advertisers know that advertisements influence children's food preferences (Hastings et al. 2003) and exacerbate parents' role as gatekeepers by tailoring appealing promotion strategies towards children. Marketers are already subjected to policy regulations at national levels, but within these boundaries, they become very innovative in discovering new channels and methods. There are attempts to force the industry to act accordingly by regulations, but evidence of success is weak (Lang and Rayner 2007). Furthermore, a ban on unhealthy food advertisements would have unknown consequences, especially with regard to where the banned advertisements would end up and what the replacement would be (Desrochers and Holt 2007). Thus, policy-makers seek to establish best practices to curb food advertisements targeted at children. For instance, the European Commission implemented a round table for this purpose, where not only the policy-makers were present, but also representatives from the European Advertising Standards Alliance and interested NGOs (European Commission 2006). In the US, the Council of Better Business and the National Advertising Review Council implemented self-regulated limits for unhealthy advertisements (Desrochers and Holt 2007). In Denmark, a voluntary code of responsible food marketing communication to children has recently been implemented (Forum of Responsible Food Marketing Communication 2008). These are promising starting points.

References

Acs, Z.J., & Lyles, A. (Eds.) (2007). *Obesity, business and public policy*. Cheltenham: Edward Elgar.

Allison, D.B., Matz, P.E., Pietrobelli, A., Zannolli, R., & Faith, M.S. (2001). Genetic and environmental influences on obesity. In A. Bendich & R. J. Deckelbaum (Eds.), *Primary and secondary preventive nutrition* (pp. 147–164). Totowa: Humana Press.

Andersen, R.E., Crespo, C.J., Bartlett, S.J., Cheskin, L.J., & Pratt, M. (1998). Relationship of physical activity and television watching with body weight and level of fatness among children: results from the third national health and nutrition examination survey. *Journal of American Medical Association, 279(12)*, 938–942.

Bachmann-Achenreiner, G., & Roedder John, D. (2003). The meaning of brand names to children: a developmental investigation. *Journal of Consumer Psychology, 13(3)*, 205–219.

Bandura, A. (1977). *Social learning theory*. Englewood Cliffs: Prentice-Hall.

Baranowski, T. (1997). Families and health action. In D. Gochman (Ed.), *Handbook of behavioral medicine*, Vol. 1 (pp. 179–205). New York: Plenum Press.

Baranowski, T., Domel, S., Gould, R., Baranowski, J., Leonard, S., Treiber F., & Mulli, R. (1993). Increasing fruit and vegetable consumption among 4th and 5th grade students: results from focus groups using reciprocal determinism. *Journal of Nutrition Education, 25*, 114–120.

Baumrind, D. (1973). The development of instrumental competence through socialization. In A. D. Pick (Ed.), *Minnesota symposium on child psychology*, Vol. 7 (pp. 3–46). Minneapolis: University of Minnesota Press.

BCI (Broadcasting Commission of Ireland) (2003). What do you think? Summary of the responses received from children and young people to the phase two consultation (December 5, 2005); http://www.bci.ie/documents/phase2_childsummary.pdf

Birch, L.L. (1980). Effects of peer models' food choices and eating behaviors on preschoolers' food preferences. *Child Development, 51(2)*, 489–496.

Birch, L.L. (1999). Development of food preferences. *Annual Review of Nutrition, 19*, 41–62.

Black, M.M. (2002). Society of pediatric psychology presidential address: Opportunities for health promotion in primary care. *Journal of Pediatric Psycholology, 27(7)*, 637–6.

Borzekowski, D.L., & Robinson, T.N. (2001). The 30-second effect: an experiment revealing the impact of television commercials on food preferences of preschoolers. *Journal of American Dietetic Association, 101*, 42–46.

Briley, M.E., Buller, A.C., Roberts-Gray, C., & Simpson, D. (1994). Identifying factors that influence the menu at the child care center: a grounded theory approach. *Journal American Dietetic Association, 94*, 276–281.

Bronfenbrenner, U. (1989). Ecological systems theory. In R. Vasta (Ed.), *Annals of child development*, Vol. 6 (pp. 187–251). Greenwich: JAI.

Brown, K.R., Endicott, C., MacDonald, S., Shumann, M., Sierra, J., & Gina, E. (2005). *50th annual 100 leading national advertisers*. The ad age group (June 21, 2007); http://adage.com/images/random/lna2005.pdf

Caruana, A., & Vassallo, R. (2003). Children's perception of their influence over purchases: the role of parental communication patterns. *Journal of Consumer Marketing, 20(1)*, 55–66.

Chan, K., & McNeal, J.U. (2004). *Advertising to children in China*. Hong Kong: The Chinese University of Hong Kong.

Cooke, L.J., Wardle, J., Gibson, E.L., Saponchnik, M., Sheiham, A., & Lawson, M. (2003). Demographic, familial and trait predictors of fruit and vegetable consumption by pre-school children. *Public Health Nutrition, 7(2)*, 295–302.

Coon, K.A., & Tucker, K.L. (2002). Television and children's consumption patterns. A review of the literature. *Minerva Pediatrics, 54*, 423–436.

Cowburn, G., & Stockley, L. (2005). Consumer understanding and use of nutrition labelling: a systematic review. *Public Health Nutrition, 8(1)*, 21–28.

Crespo, C.J., Smit, E., Troiano, R.P., Bartlett, S.J., Macera, C.A., & Andersen, R.E. (2001). Television watching, energy intake, and obesity in US children: results from the third national health and nutrition examination survey, 1988–1994. *Archives of Pediatric Adolescent Medicine, 155(3)*, 360–365.

Cullen, K., Weber, K., Baranowski, T., Rittenberry, L., & Olvera, N. (2000). Social-environmental influences on children's diets: results from focus groups with African-, Euro- and Mexican-American children and their parents. *Health Education Research, 15(5)*, 581–590.

Cummins, S., McKay, L., & MacIntyre, S. (2005). McDonald's restaurants and neighborhood deprivation in Scotland and England. *American Journal of Preventive Medicine, 29(4)*, 308–310.

Dammler, A., & Middelmann-Motz, A.V. (2002). I want one with Harry Potter on it. *Young Consumers: Insight and Ideas for Responsible Marketers, 3(2)*, 3–8.

Davison, K.K., & Birch, L.L. (2001). Childhood overweight: a contextual model and recommendations for future research. *Obesity Reviews, 2(3)*, 159–171.

Dennison, B.A., & Boyer, P.S. (2004). Risk evaluation in pediatric practice: aids in prevention of childhood overweight. *Pediatric Annuals, 33(1)*, 25–30.

Dennison, B.A., Jenkins, P.L., & Chen, T. (1996). Excess TV viewing by preschoolers is associated with high fat and SFA diets. *Circulation, 94(1)*, 1–578.

Desrochers, D.M., & Holt, D.J. (2007). Children's exposure to television advertising: implications for childhood obesity. *Journal of Public Policy & Marketing, 26(2)*, 182–201.

Diehl, J.M. (2005). Macht Werbung dick? Einfluss der Lebensmittelwerbung auf Kinder und Jugendliche. *Ernährungs-Umschau, 52*, 40–46.

Dietz, W.H., & Gortmaker, S.L. (1985). Do we fatten our children at the television set? Obesity and television viewing in children and adolescents. *Pediatrics, 75(5)*, 807.

Diliberti, N., Bordi, P.L., Conklin, M.T., Roe, L.S., & Rolls, B.J. (2004). Increased portion size leads to increased energy intake in a restaurant meal. *Obesity, 12(3)*, 562–568.

Dotson, M.J., & Hyatt, E.M. (2005). Major influence factors in children's consumer socialization. *Journal of Consumer Marketing, 22(1)*, 35–42.

Durant, R.H., & Baranowski, T. (1994). The relationship among television watching, physical activity, and body composition of young. *Pediatrics, 94(4)*, 449.

Eckstrøm, K.M., & Tufte, B. (2007). Introduction. In K.M. Eckstrøm & B. Tufte (Eds.), *Children, media and consumption – on the front edge* (pp. 11–30). Gothenburg: Nordicum.

Edmunds, L., Waters, E., & Elliot, E.J. (2001). Evidence based management of childhood obesity. *British Medical Journal, 323(7318)*, 916–919.

Effertz, T. (2008). *Kindermarketing: Analyse und rechtliche Empfehlungen*. Frankfurt: Peter Lang.

Epstein, L.H., Paluch, R.A., Gordy, C.C., & Dorn, J. (2000). Decreasing sedentary behaviors in treating pediatric obesity. *Archives of Pediatric Adolescent Medicine, 154(3)*, 220–226.

Epstein, L.H., Roemmich, J.N., Robinson, J.L., Paluch, R.A., Winiewicz, D.D., Fuerch, J.H., & Robinson, T.N. (2008). A randomized trial of the effects of reducing television viewing and computer use on body mass index in young children. *Archives of Pediatric Adolescent Medicine, 162(3)*, 239–245.

EUFIC (2005). *The determinants of food choice*. EUFIC Review, European Food Information Council, No. 8/2005.

European Commission (2006). *Self-regulation in the EU advertising sector: A report of some discussion among interested parties*. Brussels: DG Sanco.

European Commission (2007). *White paper on a strategy for Europe on nutrition, overweight and obesity related health issues* [COM(2007) 279]. Brussels: DG Sanco.

European Commission (2008). *EU platform on diet, physical activity and health – 2008 annual report*. Brussels: DG Sanco.

Forum of Responsible Food Marketing Communication (eds.) (2008), *Kodeksfor fødevarereklamer til børn*, Copenhagen. [11 Februar 2009]. http://kodeksforfoedevarereklamer.di.dk/NR/rdonlyres/90789762-72B9-44AD-BDA2-83BD09EF61BA/0/guideline_EnglishJan2008.pdf

French, S.A., Jeffery, R.W., Story, M., Breitlow, K.K., Baxter, J.S., Hannan, P., & Snyder, M.P. (2001). Pricing and promotion effects on low-fat vending snack purchases: the chips study. *American Journal of Public Health, 91(1)*, 112–117.

Gillman, M.W., Rifas-Shiman, S.L., Frazier, A.L., Rockett, H.R.H., Camargo, C.A., Field, A.E., Jr., Berkey, C.S., & Colditz, G.A. (2000). Family dinner and diet quality among older children and adolescents. *Archives of Family Medicine, 9(3)*, 235–240.

Goldberg, M.E., & Gunasti, K. (2007). Creating an environment in which youths are encouraged to eat a healthier diet. *Journal of Public Policy & Marketing, 26(2)*, 162–181.

Goodwin, M.A., Flocke, S.A., Borawski, E.A., Zyzanski, S.J., & Stange, K.C. (1999). Direct observation of health-habit counseling of adolescents. *Archives of Pediatrics & Adolescent Medicine, 153(4)*, 367–373.

Gortmaker, S.L., Must, A., Sobol, A.M., Peterson, K., Colditz, G.A., & Dietz, W.H. (1996). Television viewing as a cause of increasing obesity among children in the United States, 1986–1990. *Archives of Pediatric Adolescent Medicine, 150(4)*, 356–362.

Gortmaker, S.L., Peterson, K., Wiecha, J., Sobol, A.M., Dixit, S., Fox, M.K., & Laird, N. (1999). Reducing obesity via a school-based interdisciplinary intervention among youth: planet health. *Archives of Pediatric Adolescent Medicine, 153(4)*, 409–418.

Government Office for Science, UK. (2007). Foresight Tackling obesities: Future choices project, Department for Innovation, Universities and Skills. www.bis.gov.uk/assets/bispartners/foresight/docs/obesity/03.pdf (November 21, 2010).

Grunert, K., & Wills, J. (2007). A review of European research on consumer response to nutrition information on food labels. *Journal of Public Health, 15,* 385–399.

Gunter, B., & Furnham, A. (1998), *Children as consumers – a psychological analysis of the young people's market.* New York: Routledge.

Halford, J.C.G., Gillespie, J., Brown, V., Pontin, E.E., & Dovey, T.M. (2004). Effect of television advertisements for foods on food consumption in children. *Appetite, 42(2),* 221–225.

Harper, B. (2000). Beauty, Stature and the Labour Market: A British Cohort Study. *Oxford Bulletin of Economics and Statistics, 62(S1),* 771–800.

Hastings, G., Stead, M., McDermott, L., Forsyth, A., MacKintosh, A., Rayner, M., Godfrey, C., Caraher, M., & Angus, K. (2003). *Review of the research on the effects of food promotion to children.* Glasgow: Centre for Social Marketing, University of Glasgow.

Hawkes, C. (2004). *Marketing food to children: the global regulatory environment.* Geneva: World Health Organization.

Health Canada (2005). *Canada's food guide.* Vancouver: Government of Canada.

Hearn, M.D., Baranowski, T., Baranowski, J.C., Doyle, C., Smith, M., Lin, L.S., & Resnicow, K. (1998). Environmental influences on dietary behavior among children: availability and accessibility of fruits and vegetables enable consumption. *Journal of Health Education, 29(1),* 26–32.

Heart Stroke Foundation of Canada (2006). *The heart and stroke foundation's health promotion: Action plan on obesity.* Ottawa: Heart & Stroke Foundation of Canada.

Hendy, H.M., & Raudenbush, B. (2000). Effectiveness of teacher modeling to encourage food acceptance in preschool children. *Appetite, 34(1),* 61–76.

HM Government UK (2008). *Healthy weight, healthy lives: A cross-government strategy for England.* No. 9087, London: Cross-Government Obesity Unit, Department of Health and Department of Children, School and Families.

Hoek, J., & Gendall, P. (2006). Advertising and obesity: a behavioral perspective. *Journal of Health Communication, 11(4),* 409–423.

Holm, S. (2008). Parental responsibility and obesity in children. *Public Health Ethics, 1 (1),* 21–29.

Holt, D.J., Ippolito, P.M., Desrochers, D.M., & Kelley, C.R. (2007). *Children's exposure to TV advertising in 1977 and 2004 – Information for the obesity debate.* Bureau of Economics Staff Report, Federal Trade Commission, No. 133. Washington: Federal Trade Commission.

Hughner, R.S., & Maher, J.K. (2006). Factors that influence parental food purchases for children: implications for dietary health. *Journal of Marketing Management, 22(9/10),* 929–954.

IOM (2006). *Food marketing to children and youth: threat or opportunity?* Washington: The National Academies Press.

Jeffery, R.W., & Utter, J. (2003). The changing environment and population obesity in the United States. *Obesity, 11 (10S),* 12S–22S.

Kelly, B., Smith, B., King, L., Flood, V., & Bauman, A. (2007). Television food advertising to children: the extent and nature of exposure. *Public Health Nutrition, 10(11),* 1234–1240.

Kinra, S., Nelder, R.P., & Lewendon, G.J. (2000). Deprivation and childhood obesity: a cross sectional study of 20,973 children in Plymouth, United Kingdom. *Journal of Epidemiology and Community Health, 54(6),* 456–460.

Kirby, S., Baranowski, T., Reynolds, K.D., Taylor, G., & Binkley, D. (1995). Children's fruit and vegetable intake: socioeconomic, adult-child, regional, and urban-rural influences. *Journal of Nutrition Education, 27,* 261–271.

Klepp, K.-I., Wind, M., de Bourdeaudhuij, I., Rodrigo, C., Due, P., Bjelland, M., & Brug, J. (2007). Television viewing and exposure to food-related commercials among European school children, associations with fruit and vegetable intake: a cross sectional study. *International Journal of Behavioral Nutrition and Physical Activity, 4(1),* 46.

Kohlberg, L., & Lickona, T. (Eds.) (1976). *Moral stages and moralization: the cognitive-developmental approach.* Holt: Rinehart and Winston.

Lakin, L., & Littledyke, M. (2008). Health promoting schools: integrated practices to develop critical thinking and healthy lifestyles through farming, growing and healthy eating. *International Journal of Consumer Studies, 32(3),* 253–259.

Lang, T., & Rayner, G. (2007). Overcoming policy cacophony on obesity: an ecological public health framework for policymakers. *Obesity Reviews, 8,* 165–181.

Layton, R.A., & Grossbart, S. (2006). Macromarketing: past, present, and possible future. *Journal of Macromarketing, 26(2),* 193–213.

Leather, S. (1996). *The making of modern malnutrition: An overview of food poverty in the UK.* The Caroline Walker Lecture 1996. London: The Caroline Walker Trust.

Leviton, L.C. (2008). Children's healthy weight and the school environment. *The Annals of the American Academy of Political and Social Science, 615(1),* 38–55.

Lewis, M.K., & Hill, A.J. (1998). Food advertising on British children's television: a content analysis and experimental study with nine-year olds. *International Journal of Obesity Related Metabolic Disorders, 22*, 206–214.

Linn, S. (2000). *Marketing to children harmful: experts urge candidates to lead nation in setting limits.* Washington: Center for Media Education (May 11, 2009); http://www.cme.org/press/001018pr.html

Livingstone, S. (2005). Assessing the research base for the policy debate over the effects of food advertising to children. *International Journal of Advertising, 24(3)*, 273–296.

Livingstone, S., & Helsper, E. (2004). *Advertising "unhealthy" foods to children: understanding promotion on children.* London: Ofcom.

Livingstone, S., Boper, M., & Helsper, E. (2005). *Internet literacy among children and young people. Findings from the UK Children Go Online project.* 4. OFCOM/ESRC. London: Ofcom.

Lobstein, T., & Baur, L.A. (2005). Policies to prevent childhood obesity in the European Union. *European Journal of Public Health, 15(6)*, 576–579.

Lobstein, T., Baur, L.A., & Uauy, R. (2004). Obesity in children and young people: a crisis in public health. *Obesity Reviews, 5*, 4–85.

Lobstein, T., & Davies, S. (2009). Defining and labelling "healthy" and "unhealthy" food. *Public Health Nutrition, 12*, 331–340.

Lobstein, T., & Dibb, S. (2005). Evidence of a possible link between obesogenic food advertising and child overweight. *Obesity Reviews, 6(3)*, 203–208.

Lowry, R., Wechsler, H., Galuska, D.A., Fulton, J.E., & Kann, L. (2002). Television viewing and its associations with overweight, sedentary lifestyle, and insufficient consumption of fruits and vegetables among US high school students: differences by race, ethnicity, and gender. *Journal of School Health, 72*, 413–421.

Macdonald, L., Cummins, S., & Macintyre, S. (2007). Neighbourhood fast food environment and area deprivation – substitution or concentration? *Appetite, 49(1)*, 251–254.

Mallalieu, L., Palan, K., & Laczniak, R.N. (2005). Understanding children's knowledge and beliefs about advertising: a global issue that spans generations. *Journal of Current Issues and Research in Advertising, 27,* 53–64.

Marshall, D., O'Donohoe, S., & Kline, S. (2007). Families, food, and pester power: beyond the blame game? *Journal of Consumer Behaviour, 6(4)*, 164–181.

Matheson, D.M., Killen, J.D., Wang, Y., Varady, A., & Robinson, T.N. (2004). Children's food consumption during television viewing. *American Journal of Clinical Nutrition, 79,* 1088–1094.

Mayo, E. (2005). Hopping generation. *Young Consumers: Insight and Ideas for Responsible Marketers, 6(4)*, 43–49.

McCormick, B., & Stone, I. (2007). Economic costs of obesity and the case for government intervention. *Obesity Reviews, 8(s1)*, 161–164.

McDermott, L., O'Sullivan, T., Stead, M., & Hastings, G. (2006). International food advertising, pester power and its effects. *International Journal of Advertising, 25(4)*, 513–539.

McLaren, L. (2007). Socioeconomic status and obesity. *Epidemiology Reviews, 29(1)*, 29–48.

McNeal, J.U. (1992). *Kids as customers.* New York: Lexington Books.

McNeal, J.U. (1999). *The kids market: myth and realities.* Ithaca: Paramount Market Publishing.

McNeal, J.U. (2007). *On becoming a consumer – development of consumer behavior patterns in childhood.* Oxford: Elsevier.

Middleton, S., Ashworth, K., & Walker, R. (1994). *Family fortunes.* London: Child Poverty Action Group.

Morris, S. (2006). Body mass index and occupational attainment. *Journal of Health Economics, 25(2)*, 347–64.

Nahikian-Nelms, M. (1997). Influential factors of caregiver behavior at mealtime: a study of 24 child-care programs. *Journal of the American Dietetic Association, 97(5)*, 505–509.

National Heart Forum (2007). *Lightening the load: tackling overweight and obesity.* London: National Heart Forum.

National Obesity Task Force (2004). Healthy Weight 2008 – *Australia's Future: The National Action Agenda for Children and Young People and their Families.* Canberra: The National Obesity Task force Secretariat Department of Health and Ageing

National Restaurant Association (1998). *Restaurant industry numbers: 25-year history, 1970–1995.* Washington: National Restaurant Association.

Nicholls, A.J., & Cullen, P. (2004). The child-parent purchase relationship: "Pester power," human rights and retail ethics. *Journal of Retailing and Consumer Services, 11(2)*, 75–86.

Nicklas, T.A., Baranowski, T., Baranowski, J.C., Cullen, K., Rittenberry, L.T., & Olvera, N. (2001). Family and child-care provider influences on preschool children's fruit, juice, and vegetable. *Nutrition Reviews, 59(7)*, 224–235.

Nicklas, T.A., & Hayes, D. (2008). Position of the American Dietetic Association: nutrition guidance for healthy children ages 2 to 11 years. *Journal of the American Dietetic Association, 108(6)*, 1038–1047.

Nordic Council of Ministers (2005). *Nordic nutrition recommendations 2004 – integrating nutrition and physical activity*, Vol. 4. Copenhagen: Nordic Council of Ministers.

Nutrition Information Center (2006). *De actieve voedingsdriehoek.* Brussels: Nutrition Information Center (NICE).

O'Dea, J., & Abraham, S. (2001). Knowledge, beliefs, attitudes and behaviors related to weight control, eating disorders and body image in Australian trainee home economics and physical education teachers. *Journal of Nutrition Education, 33,* 332–340.

OFCOM (2004). Childhood obesity – *Food advertising in context: Children's food choices, parents' understanding and influence, and the role of food promotion.* London: Ofcom.

Parsons, T.J., Powers, C., Logan, S., & Summerbell, C.D. (1999). Childhood predictors of adult obesity: a systematic review. *International Journal of Obesity and Related Metabolic Disorders, 23,* 1–107.

Petterson, A., Olsson, U., & Fjellström, C. (2004). Family life in grocery stores: a study of interaction between adults and children. *International Journal of Consumer Studies, 28(4),* 317–328.

Phelps, E. (2006). Emotion and cognition: insights from studies of the human amygdala. *Annual Review of Psychology, 57,* 27–53.

Piaget, J. (1983). Piaget's theory. In P. Mussen (Ed.), *Handbook of child psychology,* Vol. 1 (pp. 703–732). New York: Wiley.

Popkin, B.M., Duffey, K., & Gordon-Larsen, P. (2005). Environmental influences on food choice, physical activity and energy balance. *Physiology and Behavior, 86(5),* 603–613.

Prendergrast, J., Foley, B., Menne, V., & Isaac, A.K. (2008). *Creatures of habit? The art of behavioural change.* London: The Social Market Foundation.

Procter, K.L. (2007). The aetiology of childhood obesity: a review. *Nutrition Research Reviews, 20(1),* 29–45.

Proctor, M.H., Moore, L.L., Gao, D., Cupples, L.A., Bradlee, M.L., Hood, M.Y., & Ellison R.C. (2003). Television viewing and change in body fat from preschool to early adolescence: the Framingham children's study. *International Journal of Obesity and Related Metabolic Disorders, 27(7),* 827–833.

Robertson, A., Lobstein, T., & Knai, C. (2007). *Obesity and socio-economic groups in Europe: evidence review and implications for action.* Brussels: DG Sanco.

Robinson, T.N. (1999). Reducing children's television viewing to prevent obesity. *Journal of the American Medical Association, 282(16),* 1561–1567.

Robinson, T.N., Hammer, L.D., Killen, J.D., Kraemer, H.C., Wilson, D.M., Hayward, C., & Taylor, C.B. (1993). Does television viewing increase obesity and reduce physical activity? Cross-sectional and longitudinal analyses among adolescent girls. *Pediatrics, 91(2),* 273–280.

Robinson, T.N., Borzekowski, D.L.G., Matheson, D.M., & Kraemer, H.C. (2007). Effects of fast food branding on young children's taste preferences. *Archives of Pediatrics and Adolescent Medicine, 161(8),* 792–797.

Roedder John, D. (1999). Consumer socialization of children: a retrospective look at twenty-five years of research. *Journal of Consumer Research, 26(3),* 183–213.

Roefs, A., & Jansen, A. (2004). The effect of information about fat content on food consumption in overweight/obese and lean people. *Appetite, 43(3),* 319–322.

Rolls, B.J., Roe, L.S., Meengs, J.S., & Wall, D.E. (2004). Increasing the portion size of a sandwich increases energy intake. *Journal of the American Dietetic Association, 104(3),* 367–372.

Rossiter, M., Glanville, T., Taylor, J., & Blum, I. (2007). School food practices of prospective teachers. *Journal of School Health, 77(10),* 694–700.

Scharff, R. (2009). Obesity and hyperbolic discounting: Evidence and implications. *Journal of Consumer Policy, 32(1),* 3–21.

Sellers, K., Russo, T.J., Baker, I., & Dennison, B.A. (2005). The role of childcare providers in the prevention of childhood overweight. *Journal of Early Childhood Research, 3(3),* 227–242.

Smith, D.M., & Cummins, S. (2009). Obese cities: how our environment shapes overweight. *Geography Compass, 3(1),* 518–535.

Spungin, P. (2004). Parent power, not pester power. *Young Consumers, 5(3),* 37–40.

Stead, M., McDermott, L., & Hastings, G. (2007). Towards evidence-based marketing: the case of childhood obesity. *Marketing Theory, 7(4),* 379–406.

Story, M., & French, S. (2004). Food advertising and marketing directed at children and adolescents in the US. *International Journal of Behavioral Nutrition and Physical Activity, 1(1),* 3.

Story, M., Neumark-Sztainer, D., & French, S. (2002). Individual and environmental influences on adolescent eating behaviors. *Journal of the American Dietetic Association, 102(3),* S40–S51.

Swithers, S.E., & Hall, W.G. (1994). Does oral experience terminate ingestion? *Appetite, 29,* 213–224.

Taper, L.J., Frigge, C., & Rogers C.S. (1991). Paternal child-feeding attitudes and obesity in school-age sons. *Family and Consumer Sciences Research Journal, 19(3),* 215–223.

Taveras, E.M., Sandora, T.J., Shih, M.-C., Ross-Degnan, D., Goldmann, D.A., & Gillman M.W. (2006). The association of television and video viewing with fast food intake by preschool-age children. *Obesity, 14(11),* 2034–2041.

Temple, J.L., Giacomelli, A.M., Kent, K.M., Roemmich, J.N., & Epstein, L.H. (2007). Television watching increases motivated responding for food and energy intake in children. *American Journal of Clinical Nutrition, 85(2),* 355–361.

Thaler, R.H., & Sunstein, C.R. (2008). *Nudge – improving decisions about health, wealth, and happiness.* New Haven: Yale University Press.

Timperio, A., Salmon, J., Telford, A., & Crawford, D. (2005). Perceptions of local neighborhood environments and their relationship to childhood overweight and obesity. *International Journal of Obesity, 29(2)*, 170–175.

Tufte, B., Kampmann, J., & Christensen, L.B. (2005). *Frontrunners or copycats*. Copenhagen: Copenhagen Business School Press.

US Department of Health & Human Services & U.S. Department of Agriculture (2005). *Dietary guidelines for Americans 2005*. Washington: U.S. Department of Health and Human Services & U.S. Department of Agriculture.

US Department of Health and Human Services (2001). *The Surgeon General's call to action to prevent and decrease overweight and obesity*. Rockville, MD: U.S. Department of Health and Human Services, Public Health Service, Office of the Surgeon General.

Valkenburg, P.M., & Cantor, J. (2001). The development of a child into a consumer. *Journal of Applied Developmental Psychology, 22(1)*, 61–72.

Vandewater, E.A., Shim, M., & Caplovitz, A.G. (2004). Linking obesity and activity level with children's television and video game use. *Journal of Adolescence, 27(1)*, 71–85.

Viswanathan, M., & Gau, R. (2005). Functional illiteracy and nutritional education in the United States: a research-based approach to the development of nutritional education materials for functionally illiterate consumers. *Journal of Macromarketing, 25(2)*, 187–201.

Wansink, B. (1996). Can package size accelerate usage volume? *Journal of Marketing, 60*, 1–14.

Wansink, B., & Park, S.B. (2001). At the movies: how external cues and perceived taste impact consumption volume. *Food Quality and Preferences, 12*, 69–74.

Ward, S. (1974). Consumer socialization. *Journal of Consumer Research, 1(2)*, 1–14.

Wardle J., Carnell, S., & Cooke, L. (2005). Parental control over feeding and children's fruit and vegetable intake: how are they related? *Journal of the American Dietary Association, 105(2)*, 227–232.

Wild-Stiftung, R. (2008). Geschmäcker sind verschieden. *Fakten, Trends und Meinungen* – Gesunde Ernährung interdisziplinär aufbereitet, *3*, 1–5.

Wilson, G., & Wood, K. (2004). The influence of children on parental purchases during supermarket shopping. *International Journal of Consumer Studies, 28(4)*, 329–336.

Witkowski, T.H. (2007). Food marketing and obesity in developing countries: Analysis, ethics, and public policy. *Journal of Macromarketing, 27(2)*, 126–137.

Yager, Z., & O'Dea, J.A. (2005). The role of teachers and other educators in the prevention of eating disorders and child obesity: what are the issues? *Eating Disorders, 13*, 261–278.

Young L.R., & Nestle, M.S. (1995). Portion sizes in dietary assessment: issues and policy implication. *Nutrition Reviews, 53*, 149–158.

Young, L.R., & Nestle, M.S. (2003). Expanding portion sizes in the US marketplace: implications for nutrition coun-selling. *Journal of the American Dietetic Association, 103(2)*, 231–234.

Chapter 25
Eating Behavior and Weight in Children

Clare Llewellyn, Susan Carnell, and Jane Wardle

Introduction

The idea that eating styles might influence weight is not new. In 1968, Stanley Schachter published a seminal paper proposing the "externality theory" of obesity (Schachter 1968). It described a series of innovative experiments in which the eating behavior of a clinical sample of severely obese individuals was compared with the eating behavior of normal-weight individuals, using a variety of physiological and environmental manipulations. The conclusion was that the obese were more reactive to external cues of food (such as smell or taste) and less responsive to internal physiological sensations related to hunger and satiety, indicating a weakening of normal appetitive controls. In modern environments where highly palatable food is abundant and cheap, high external responsiveness could lead to overeating and weight gain, especially if it is not buffered by strong satiety sensitivity.

Another focus of early research was how emotions differentially influence eating behavior in the obese and the normal-weight. Focusing again on clinical populations, Kaplan and Kaplan (1957) put forward the "psychosomatic theory" of obesity, which proposed that obese individuals were unable to distinguish the physiological arousal caused by emotional states such as fear or anger from hunger, possibly as a result of learning experiences in early childhood (Bruch 1964). This led to over-eating in response to emotional arousal. Schachter et al. (1968) took a slightly different point of view, suggesting that while normal-weight individuals eat less in response to negative emotional states, the eating activity of the obese remains unaffected. But both theories proposed that differences in food intake between the obese and the normal-weight would be observed in states of emotional arousal.

The pediatric obesity literature grew out of this early work with adults, and likewise focused largely on clinical populations including children who "fail to thrive" (the underweight population). Research into "externality theory" has continued with attempts to unpick the dimensions of this trait and understand the specific conditions under which children overeat. Fisher and Birch (1999a) assessed the tendency of children to overeat when presented with palatable foods under conditions of satiety [so-called eating in the absence of hunger (EAH)], and also the role of differences in satiety sensitivity (Johnson and Birch 1994). Another important line of work examined whether

C. Llewellyn and J. Wardle (✉)
Health Behaviour Research Centre, Department of Epidemiology and Public Health,
University College London, Gower street, WC, IE 6BT, UK
e-mail: j.wardle@ucl.ac.uk

S. Carnell
The New York Obesity Research Center, St. Luke's-Roosevelt Hospital Center, Columbia University College
of Physicians and Surgeons, New York, NY, USA

L.A. Moreno et al. (eds.), *Epidemiology of Obesity in Children and Adolescents*,
Springer Series on Epidemiology and Public Health 2, DOI 10.1007/978-1-4419-6039-9_25,
© Springer Science+Business Media, LLC 2011

some children value food more highly than others, based on their choice of palatable food over access to enjoyable activities (Temple et al. 2008).

Emotional eating has also been studied in children, but research has addressed some children's tendency to eat less in response to negative emotions (which may represent a natural biological response to stress as gut activity is inhibited under heightened emotional states (Wardle and Gibson 2001)). While emotional over-eating increases risk of weight gain, emotional under-eating may be a trait that protects against overweight (Wardle et al. 2001a).

Other behaviors associated with underweight that have been of interest include fussiness or pickiness about food, which may protect against overweight by reducing the number of foods a child is willing to eat (Wright and Birks 2000). On the other hand, preferences for energy-dense foods (high in sugar and fat) may increase the risk of overweight. Evidence that a high-fat diet is involved in the development and maintenance of overweight has led to efforts to understand food choices (e.g. Hill et al. 1992). It is generally agreed that food choice is significantly influenced by taste preferences (Bere and Klepp 2004; Raynor et al. 2004), making this another area that researchers have been interested in investigating weight gain.

Methods and Measures Used in Eating Behavior Research

Behavioral Measures of Eating Behaviors in Children

Researchers who developed "externality theory" in the adult population drew heavily on experimental behavioral work, and pediatric studies have followed suit. A number of different behavioral paradigms have been developed to quantify sensitivity to satiety and responsiveness to external cues of food.

Energy Compensation

This paradigm tests the idea that an individual who is responsive to internal satiety cues will adjust their intake at a meal according to the energy content of a "preload" of food given before the meal; satiety insensitive individuals will not. Typically the preload varies along a continuum of calories and is carried out over two or more testing sessions. Each participant receives a compensation score (COMPX) indicating how much their meal intake compensated for the preload using a standardized formula $((\text{Ad-libitum intake KJ}_{\text{low energy preload}} - \text{Ad-libitum intake KJ}_{\text{high energy preload}}) / (\text{Drink preload KJ}_{\text{high}} - \text{Drink preload KJ}_{\text{low}}) \times 100\%))$ (Johnson and Birch 1994).

Microstructural Analysis of Ingestive Patterns

This method involves observing the child eating a meal and characterizing the eating behavior in detail in smaller structures such as quantity of food per unit of time, and stages. This allows for within-meal and between-participant comparisons of behaviors throughout the course of the meal (Guss and Kissileff 2000). An eating rate that slows down, as characterized by a deceleration curve, is assumed to reflect a "normal," biologically determined satiation process, while non-deceleration has been hypothesized to indicate impaired satiety responsiveness (Meyer and Pudel 1972). The average rate at which food is consumed throughout the meal is thought to indicate hunger level or motivation to eat, with a faster eating rate also compromising satiety by outpacing the physiological control mechanisms. The microstructure of infant feeding can also be assessed using sucking behavior variables such as sucking rate, sucking pressure and volume per suck (Agras et al. 1987).

Sensory Activation of Eating

This technique involves exposing children to sensory food cues (e.g. smell and taste of highly palatable foods) versus no food cues (control task), and assessing how much of that same food is consumed following exposure (Jansen et al. 2003). It is hypothesized that hyper-responsive children will consume more of the food following exposure to the sight and smell of it, than in the control condition.

Eating in the Absence of Hunger

This paradigm measures intake of highly palatable foods under conditions of satiety, and is assumed to indicate the extent to which palatable foods override internal satiety regulation. Typically, a child will be fed a meal and instructed to eat until full. Following the meal each child is tested individually and tastes and rates a variety of snack foods, after which they are left alone with free access to the snacks and toys and intake is assessed (Fisher and Birch 1999a). In order to exclude the confounding effects of hunger on intake, children are sometimes asked to rate their hunger level following the meal and those who are still hungry are excluded from the analyses, although a limitation of this method is uncertainty about the reliability of this information in children. One drawback of the EAH paradigm is that subsequent intake of palatable foods may reflect both hypersensitivity to external food cues and insensitivity to internal satiety cues.

Behavioral Economic Analysis of Food Choice

Individual differences in the level of pleasure or reward experienced when eating highly palatable foods may drive motivation to eat those foods. This can be explored by assessing the relative reinforcing value (RRV) of food, which quantifies how hard an individual is willing to "work" to gain access to food of higher versus lower palatability, or food versus non-food rewards. Concurrent schedules of reinforcement are set up such that the work requirement to obtain the desirable food becomes progressively more effortful, while the non-food schedule remains constant (Lappalainen and Epstein 1990). The point at which the child opts for the alternative reward over the palatable food reward provides an index of the reinforcing value of the desirable food. The harder an individual is prepared to work for the desirable food, the more food responsive they are deemed to be.

Food Preference Studies

Typically, behavioral assessment of food preferences involves the children taking part in some kind of "taste test" in which they sample foods from a range of food groups, and then either rank the foods in order of preference (e.g. Fisher and Birch 1995) or rate them.

Limitations of Behavioral Studies of Eating in Children

While observational studies are often seen as producing the best possible data because of their objectivity, they can be expensive to organize on the scale necessary for adequate statistical power to detect small relationships with weight. Furthermore, there is always the possibility that the process of being observed alters the children's behavior. Additionally many studies use only a single behavioral observation, limiting generalization from that instance of behavior to the underlying trait (Epstein 1983) because the outcome is vulnerable to the extrinsic factors at play on that day; that is, behavior is always a state measure, even if it is being used to impute traits.

Quantitative Psychometric Measurement of Eating Behaviors in Children

Psychometric measures (standardized quantitative questionnaires) lose the objectivity of behavioral assessment but have the advantage of reflecting behavioral characteristics over a range of situations. An additional advantage is that they are convenient to administer on a large scale, maximizing statistical power. Of course, self-report measures can be problematic at ages when children lack the comprehension skills or self-awareness to answer questions about their behavior, and parent-report questionnaires are often used for younger children. Although parent-reports of behavior are necessarily subjective and may reflect socially desirable responses (especially from parents with overweight or obese children), parents have privileged observational access to their children, arguably making them the most accurate informants of their child's behavioral traits.

A number of studies have used modified versions of adult self-report questionnaires in studies with children, usually to detect eating disorder symptomatology (e.g. Lluch et al. 2000; Snoek et al. 2007; Shunk and Birch 2004). One is the Three Factor Eating Questionnaire [TFEQ] (Stunkard and Messick 1985) which measures dietary restraint, disinhibition and hunger, and has been used sporadically with older adolescents (e.g. de Lauzon et al. 2004). The Dutch Eating Behaviour Questionnaire [DEBQ] (van Strien et al. 1986), measuring external eating (eating in response to external food-related stimuli), emotional eating (the tendency to overeat in response to negative emotional states) and restrained eating (deliberate suppression of eating), has been used far more extensively with children. Some studies have used the adult self-report version with children (e.g. Lluch et al. 2000; Snoek et al. 2007; Shunk and Birch 2004), but a parent-report version of the DEBQ also exists [DEBQ-P] (Caccialanza et al. 2004), as does a child self-report version which has been validated for use in 7–12 year olds [DEBQ-C] (Van Strien and Oosterveld 2008).

The most recent development is the Child Eating Behaviour Questionnaire [CEBQ], a parent-report measure designed to assess the main eating styles implicated in the development of both under- and overweight (Wardle et al. 2001a). Scales include behaviors that have typically been implicated in the failure to thrive literature such as "fussiness about food" and "emotional under-eating," as well as scales that assess the eating styles associated with overweight and obesity in the behavioral literature, such as satiety responsiveness (akin to sensitivity of satiety), slowness in eating (similar to eating rate), food responsiveness and enjoyment of food (both similar to the behavioral measure of responsiveness to external cues of food). Each scale correlates well with the behavioral measures on which the scales were based (Carnell and Wardle 2007) and the scores have been shown to be stable from 4 to 11 years of age (Ashcroft et al. 2008).

Assessing the Relationship Between Eating Behavior and Weight in Children

Most studies relating eating behavior to weight have utilized case-control designs, comparing normal-weight with overweight or obese participants, often from clinical populations. Two limitations of case-control designs should be considered. Firstly, eating behaviors may have been modified by the individual as a result of being classified clinically as overweight or obese, which would also affect parent-report measures. Secondly, the overweight and obese categories are essentially arbitrary cut-offs toward the upper end of an adiposity continuum, and the population as a whole is gaining weight with heavier individuals at higher risk of future health problems than leaner individuals, and it is important to be able to explain all weight variation, not just the categories of overweight and obesity.

In addition to sampling limitations, because cross-sectional designs have predominated, conclusions about causal direction have been tentative. There is a need for more studies using longitudinal designs to explore how different eating behaviors are associated with the development of adiposity over time, and better still, intervention studies, which can elucidate causal processes.

Lastly, there are other obstacles to identifying eating behaviors that are implicated in the development and maintenance of overweight. Weight gain is in many cases the result of tiny aberrations in energy balance compounded over many years. An excess of 100 kcal/day is sufficient to add over 5 kg of fat over 1 year assuming energy is stored at 50% efficiency and an excess of 3,500 kcal leads to a net gain of about 1 pound of fat (Hill et al. 2003). Identifying behaviors that explain such small differences in intake is a challenge, and measurement error may obscure such marginal effects.

Current Evidence Relating Eating Behaviors to Weight in Children

Responsiveness to Food Cues

Using a "sensory activation of eating" approach, Jansen et al. (2003) compared intake of highly palatable snack foods by obese and normal-weight children in two exposure conditions (tasting or smelling the snack foods) and a control condition (following a 10-min non-food activity). Obese children showed a stronger behavioral reaction to exposure to food cues, with a greater difference in intake between control and exposure (smelling), whereas the normal-weight children actually ate less than in the control condition. Using a similar design in infants, with parental weight status as an indicator of obesity risk, Millstein (1980) found that babies with two overweight parents sucked more avidly in response to a sweetened solution compared with plain water, compared to babies with two normal-weight parents, suggesting that responsiveness to external cues of food may be an antecedent rather than a consequence of overweight. This implicates responsiveness to food cues in the causal process.

A number of studies have provided evidence in support of the externality theory using the EAH paradigm. Intake of palatable snack foods has been found to be higher in overweight girls than normal-weight girls (Fisher and Birch 2002), and in another study in overweight children compared with normal-weight children (Fisher et al. 2007). Francis et al. (2007) showed EAH to be higher in girls at higher risk of obesity (indexed by having two overweight parents versus only one or no overweight parents), and daughters of overweight mothers had a greater increase in EAH from age 5–9 years compared with daughters of normal-weight mothers, as well as a significantly greater increase in BMI across the same time period (Francis and Birch 2005). However, although this may indicate that EAH would predict weight gain over time, Butte et al. (2007) using the same sample found that EAH did not significantly predict weight gain over a 1 year period; perhaps 1 year is not long enough to show the weight gain sequelae from this trait.

Recently we assessed the relationship between EAH and weight in community samples in two naturalistic settings – within a school and at home. In both samples EAH was positively and linearly associated with BMI for boys, but the association was weaker for girls (Hill et al. 2008). Interestingly, in the study that used school-based testing, where the task was carried out in a classroom, girls demonstrated progressively higher EAH from underweight through the top and bottom 50% of healthy weight (lower and higher healthy weight), but a sharp decline within the overweight and obese range. In the other study in which the task was completed in sibling pairs at home, girls showed a graded increase in EAH across the entire range, although it did not reach significance. Two other studies have also reported associations for boys only (Faith et al. 2006; Moens and Braet 2007).

Social desirability bias may explain some of these sex differences – the social exposure inherent in the collective testing situation in our study may have modified girls' eating behavior (Hill et al. 2008), while the children in Moens and Braet's study (2007) were on a waiting list for a weight loss intervention and the girls may have restricted their intake in an attempt to demonstrate their good intentions. Also the relationship between weight and EAH may be smaller in girls such that a larger sample size is required to find an association reliably (e.g. Fisher et al. 2007). EAH has been found to be higher in boys than in girls in some studies (e.g. Fisher et al. 2007; Hill et al. 2008) with implications of reduced power to find differences among girls due to lower variability in their data. However in contrast to these findings, Cutting et al. (1999) found an association between EAH and weight for girls but not for boys. It is clear that more research is needed to assess this eating behavior in different settings and across weight groups, to elucidate when and why this behavior is expressed in girls and boys.

An important group of studies have operationalized responsiveness to food as the reinforcing value of food. Temple et al. (2008) recently reported on two different food reinforcement studies with groups of overweight and normal-weight children. In the first study, the researchers compared the reinforcing value of pizza versus a (favorite) non-food activity such as a hand-held video game, coloring or a magazine. The task used a progressive schedule of reinforcement for food (the number of buttons required to gain each additional slice of pizza doubled) concurrent with a variable ratio schedule for non-food (an average of four presses was required throughout the session). The second study compared the reinforcing value of a selection of snack foods and a (favorite) non-food activity, using progressive schedules of reinforcement for both the food and non-food alternatives, which doubled each time in each case. In both studies, the overweight children found food more reinforcing than normal-weight children: in Study 1 the overweight children made significantly more responses for food as the reinforcement schedules progressed (characterized by an interaction between weight group and reinforcement schedule) and consumed significantly more energy than the normal-weight children; in Study 2 the overweight children found food more reinforcing than the non-food alternative whereas the normal-weight children found the alternative activity more reinforcing than food.

In a similar study, the same research group compared decline over the course of 10 2-min (fixed interval) trials during which normal-weight and overweight children "worked" for access to a cheeseburger (Temple et al. 2007). Overweight children showed a slower decline in responding for food over the whole 20-min period than their leaner peers (characterized by a higher number of responses during each 2-min trial), and the overweight group consumed more energy than their leaner peers, indicating that overweight children habituate slower to food cues than their leaner counterparts.

We recently used a longitudinal design to investigate the association between the relative reinforcing value of food and change in adiposity in children, using a simplified version of the task (Hill et al. 2009). Higher reinforcing value of food at baseline predicted change into a higher weight category over the year, and this was the case for children across all levels of the weight spectrum, suggesting that the reinforcing value of food plays a causal role in weight gain.

Psychometric measures of responsiveness to external cues of food have generally supported the hypothesis that fatter children are more food responsive than thinner children, although not all studies have demonstrated the association. One study with the DEBQ-P found that a clinical sample of obese children scored significantly higher on the External Eating subscale than normal-weight matched controls (Braet and Van Strien 1997), although similar data from an Italian community sample showed no association (Caccialanza et al. 2004). The two CEBQ subscales of Food Responsiveness and Enjoyment of Food have consistently demonstrated a positive association with adiposity across six samples of children (Carnell and Wardle 2008; Sleddens et al. 2008; Viana et al. 2008; Webber et al. 2009). Where the full weight spectrum has been assessed, results showed a linear association between these eating behaviors and adiposity (Carnell and Wardle 2008; Viana et al. 2008; Webber et al. 2009), suggesting that these traits do not simply distinguish the clinical from the non-clinical but are systematically related to adiposity across the continuum.

Sensitivity to Internal Cues of Satiety

Speed of Eating

In cross-sectional studies heavier children tend to eat faster than lighter children. Early studies assessing eating speed during a meal in naturalistic settings found differences between groups of overweight and normal-weight children (Drabman et al. 1979; Waxman and Stunkard 1980), and a later laboratory-based study replicated these findings (Barkeling et al. 1992). In a more recent laboratory-based study, Lindgren et al. (2000) found a trend for faster eating in obese children than normal-weight controls, although this did not quite reach significance and we recently demonstrated a linear association between eating speed and adiposity across the weight continuum (Llewellyn et al. 2008).

Two longitudinal studies with infants used sucking rate as a marker of speed. More rapid sucking at 2- and 4-weeks of age predicted adiposity at 2 and 3 years of age (Agras et al. 1990). Using maternal weight status (lean or obese) as an indicator of the infant's later obesity risk (maternal obesity is a strong early-childhood predictor of adult obesity – Whitaker et al. 1997), Stunkard et al. (2004) found that sucking behavior differentiated infants at higher or lower risk, and vigorous sucking behavior at 3 months of age predicted adiposity at 1 and 2 years of age, suggesting a causal role for this behavior. An early intervention study succeeded in slowing eating speed in children (by encouraging them to put their utensils down between bites of food) and this resulted in them consuming less food over a 6-month period (Epstein et al. 1976).

Other studies have used the Slowness in Eating subscale of the CEBQ and found a significant association with adiposity in the hypothesized direction (Carnell and Wardle 2008; Sleddens et al. 2008; Viana et al. 2008; Webber et al. 2009), which increases linearly with weight across the spectrum (Carnell and Wardle 2008; Viana et al. 2008; Webber et al. 2009). Collectively, these studies indicate that as eating speed increases, so does weight.

Few studies have assessed whether overweight children exhibit less deceleration in their eating rate over the course of a meal than their normal-weight counterparts. Two laboratory-based studies reported that obese children did not decelerate their eating rate towards the end of the meal to the extent demonstrated by normal-weight children (Barkeling et al. 1992; Lindgren et al. 2000), and another study (Laessle et al. 2001) found that obese children only demonstrated non-decelerated eating patterns when their mother was present. In our recent study, although we found an association between eating rate and weight, we did not find that deceleration over the course of the meal differed by weight (Llewellyn et al. 2008); however, there may be a range of environmental factors that influence this effect. Sophisticated experimental studies with adults, in which a number of different variables have been manipulated, have indicated that eating rate and deceleration over the course of a meal are influenced by food deprivation, food palatability, age, sex, and even portion size (Spiegel 2000). Further research in the microstructure of eating in children and infants is needed to shed light on when and why faster eating rates and non-decelerated eating patterns emerge.

Preload Compensation

Studies that have assessed differences in satiety sensitivity using preload paradigms have found mixed results. Johnson and Birch (1994) were the first to assess weight-related differences in compensation accuracy in children. On two separate occasions, children were given drinks matched for volume, mass and sensory properties but differing in energy content, and 20 min later their ad libitum energy intake from a standardized mixed buffet was measured. Poorer compensation after high-energy drinks was modestly associated with greater adiposity in girls but not boys. We replicated this study in a school setting, adding two conditions – a familiar low-energy drink (water) and a familiar high-energy drink (strawberry-flavored milkshake) (unpublished data by Carnell, Gibson and Wardle). The data indicated a significant positive association between adiposity and poorer compensation in both sexes. Another case control study found that obese children did not down-regulate intake of palatable snacks approximately 10 min after a preload, compared with a no pre-load condition, while the normal-weight children compensated, suggesting greater satiety sensitivity (Jansen et al. 2003).

However, two other studies failed to find an association. Faith et al. (2004) used Johnson and Birch's (1994) protocol with a 25-min interval between preloads and subsequent food, but did not find any association with adiposity, rather finding that the children as a whole demonstrated remarkable compensation accuracy and Cecil et al. (2005) compared a no-energy condition (250 ml water), and low- and high-energy condition which both used a 250 ml orange drink and a muffin matched for taste and mass but differing in energy content. Ninety minutes later intake was measured during a test meal. No association was observed between intake and weight; instead all children compensated with better compensation in the younger children. Methodological differences between these studies may go part way towards explaining the different findings. Cecil et al. (2005) had solid food as well as liquids in their different preloads and a longer interval, which may have improved compensation across the board and Faith et al. (2004) suggested their study was underpowered to detect a small effect. Larger sample sizes may be needed to reliably detect the typical association between compensation ability and weight.

Four psychometric studies have used the CEBQ to associate the Satiety Responsiveness subscale with adiposity, and all have found a negative association with adiposity (Carnell and Wardle 2008; Sleddens et al. 2008; Viana et al. 2008; Webber et al. 2009). Satiety responsiveness appeared to decrease linearly as weight increased (Carnell and Wardle 2008; Viana et al. 2008; Webber et al. 2009).

Food Preferences and Food Fussiness

Food Preferences

A number of studies have investigated the relationship between food preferences and adiposity in children, but findings are not consistent. Fisher and Birch (1995) found that fat preferences were related to triceps skinfold measurements, although not to BMI or subscapular skinfold, while Ricketts (1997) found that fat preferences were related to BMI and triceps skinfold, but not to subscapular skinfold. On the other hand, a study with adolescents found no difference in fat preferences between the obese and normal-weight (Fieldstone et al. 1997). Using parental BMI as an index of obesity risk, we found that higher-risk children had greater preference for higher fat foods (assessed behaviorally), and lower liking for various vegetables (as reported by the mother) (Wardle et al. 2001b). However, in a recent study, we found no associations between adiposity and preferences for fatty and sugary foods, or fruits and vegetables (Hill et al. 2009).

The inconsistencies in these findings may reflect the distinction between "liking" and "wanting," demonstrated in the neurobiological characteristics (Berridge 1996, 2004). While it is primarily liking (or reports of liking) that is tapped in taste tests, wanting may be the crucial drive of food choices in the real world. Wanting a food might be indexed more effectively by behavioral reinforcement paradigms in which a child is forced to choose between alternative foods. In support of this, Temple et al. (2008) found a significant correlation between the reinforcing value of food and energy intake, but no relation between food liking and intake, and the reinforcing value of food was not correlated with food liking, highlighting the importance of distinguishing between the drive to eat certain foods and the pleasure gained from eating them.

Food Fussiness

Food fussiness has primarily been assessed clinically (Harris 1993), and has been linked with lower weight, lower rates of overweight, and failure to thrive (Galloway et al. 2005; Wright and Birks 2000), although these findings have not always been replicated (Carruth et al. 1998; Jacobi et al. 2003; Rydell et al. 1995). Recently, a number of studies have examined the nature of the relationship between fussiness and weight in non-clinical samples using the CEBQ. We found a significant linear negative association between food fussiness and weight in two samples of children (Webber et al. 2009), and this was replicated by Viana et al. (2008), suggesting that fussiness could be protective against over-eating, perhaps by reducing the number of foods a child is willing to eat. The same effect was not replicated in a recent Dutch study using the same measure, although the pattern of results indicated a trend in the same direction (Sleddens et al. 2008).

However, research showing how fussiness is linked to weight in the longer-term is lacking. Data from animal studies have suggested that similar behavior, termed "finickiness," was associated with a higher risk of obesity (Schachter 1971). Finicky animals ate less when the food was bitter-tasting, but if they were offered good-tasting food, they ate more than the non-finicky animal. On this basis we might find that the association between fussiness and weight depends on the quality and palatability of the food supply. Longitudinal studies will be needed if we are to understand the longer-term outcomes associated with this eating style.

Emotional Eating

Studies relating emotional eating to weight in children have found mixed results. The Emotional Eating subscale of the DEBQ (and DEBQ-P) has shown all possible relationships with weight. Only one study found that obese children scored significantly higher than non-obese children, but this study utilized a clinical sample (Braet and Van Strien 1997). Two other studies, both using non-clinical samples, found no association between emotional eating and weight (Caccialanza et al. 2004; Wardle et al. 1992). To complicate matters further, two studies have reported a negative association between emotional eating and weight Hill et al. (1994) found underweight girls in a community sample to have the highest score on emotional eating, with the overweight girls scoring lower, while a negative association has been reported in a study using a bespoke psychometric measure of emotion-induced eating (Striegel-Moore et al. 1999).

A number of studies using the CEBQ have assessed the relationship between weight and both emotional over-eating and under-eating (EOE, EUE). While a recent study with a community sample found no association between either EOE or EUE and weight (Sleddens et al. 2008), Viana et al. (2008) found a positive graded between EOE and weight, and a weaker negative association between EUE and weight. We also found a positive association between EOE and weight, but not EUE and weight, indicating that EOE and EUE do not represent opposite ends of the same dimension (Webber et al. 2009).

Methodological heterogeneity may account for some of the different findings (different age groups, ethnicities and measures), but an alternative is that the association can vary. Stress research with animals has indicated that both over- and under-eating occurs in response to stress. A recent study with students found that change in weight (both gaining and losing it) was associated with more stress than weight stability, suggesting that individuals may vary in their response to stress, with hypophagic and hyperphagic eating behaviors being possible, depending on the nature and intensity of the stressor and subsequent stress response (Serlachius et al. 2007).

Future Research into Eating Behaviors and Child Weight

Few studies have used designs that can identify the direction of causation. Longitudinal studies are informative: if eating behavior characteristics can be shown to precede weight gain prospectively, it is less likely that the obesity caused the eating behaviors, although there could still be a third variable that causes both the eating behavior and the obesity. In addition, assessing eating behaviors longitudinally in very young infants would allow researchers to understand more fully how they develop.

Few longitudinal studies have been reported, although one of the earliest studies in the field showed that externality was related to weight gain in girls attending a summer camp (Rodin and Slochower 1976). Our research group has recently set up a new study called Gemini – Health and Development in Twins. This will assess the unfolding of eating behaviors from birth through to 5 years of age, alongside development of weight. Gemini will allow researchers to gain a better understanding of how eating behaviors develop, and how they relate to weight gain in infancy and early childhood.

Etiology of Eating Behaviors

Eating behaviors have largely been defined by the paradigms used to measure them, with broader traits such as responsiveness to food cues or food preferences being inferred from experimental findings. However, it is important to understand the neurological and physiological pathways associated with these various behavioral phenomena, and to evaluate whether they are manifestations of the same broad underlying traits, or represent many different pathways. Collaborations between researchers in endocrinology, neurology, and behavioral science have started to uncover the physiological and neurological traits tapped by these behaviors, while genetic research is making progress in determining their molecular origins.

Physiological Correlates of Eating Behaviors

While neuroimaging studies in children present a number of challenges such as the requirement for restricted motion in the scanner (Davidson et al. 2003), a group of researchers have successfully used functional MRI scanning to study children with Prader–Willi syndrome (a complex condition that includes a voracious appetite and obesity in childhood) and normal controls. Interestingly, they found that the children showed post-meal increases in areas of the brain involved in motivation and reward, including the orbitofrontal cortex, medial prefrontal cortex, insula, hippocampus and para-hippocampal gyrus, compared with decreases in these areas in normal-weight children (Holsen et al. 2006). The same research group has recently found similar hyperactivation of motivation and reward areas in children with "common" obesity (Bruce et al. 2010).

Examination of the endocrinological pathways that underlie eating behaviors is an important area of study, in that relevant biomarkers may be used to predict later obesity risk. There is evidence in the adult literature that grehlin stimulates appetite (Horvath et al. 2001), and that a number of hormones are involved in post-prandial satiety, including: peptide YY (PYY), glucagon-like peptide 1 (GLP-1), oxyntomodulin (Oxm), cholecystokinin (CCK), and pancreatic polypeptide (PP) (Chaudhri et al. 2008). In addition, the hormone leptin is produced by adipocytes in white adipose tissue in levels proportionate to fat mass and is believed to regulate appetite over the longer-term by stimulating central appetite controls when adiposity levels are low (Druce and Bloom 2006).

Research into the hormonal basis of eating behaviors in children is difficult. Ethical approval for invasive protocols, especially with infants and children, is not easily granted and only a handful of studies have examined these hormones in relation to eating behavior with children, although some investigators have used placental cordal blood as an alternative. Haqq et al. (2003) found that grehlin levels are markedly increased in children with Prader–Willi syndrome compared with controls, which implicates grehlin as one of the factors behind the insatiable appetite and consequent obesity seen in this condition. However, cross-sectional studies comparing circulating grehlin levels of normal-weight and overweight children, and in relation to weight gain in early infancy, have found an inverse relationship with weight suggesting that grehlin concentrations may change as part of an adaptive response with obese children demonstrating down-regulated levels and slower-growing infants demonstrating higher levels (Bellone et al. 2002; Savino et al. 2005), indicating the need for prospective studies very early on to inform cause and effect relationships. Using cordal blood collected at birth, James et al. (2004) found that low cord blood grehlin levels was associated prospectively with slow weight gain over the first 3 months of life, although no association was found between cordal grehlin and milk intake or feed frequency over the first 6 days of life (James et al. 2007).

Cord blood leptin levels have been found to be significantly negatively associated with all parameters of size at birth, and with weight gain from birth to 24 months, independently of birthweight (Ong et al. 1999). Furthermore, Mantzoros et al. (2009) found that lower cordal leptin predicted increased weight in the first 6 months of life, and higher BMI at 3 years, but did not relate to feeding behavior in the study by James et al. (2007).

Lastly, PYY has been related to weight in children. Roth et al. (2005) found that obese children demonstrated significantly lower levels of PYY than lean controls, and fasting PYY correlated negatively with the degree of overweight, suggesting that decreased PYY levels could predispose children to develop obesity, although decreased levels could also be secondary to obesity. Lomenick et al. (2008) also found different meal-related changes in PYY in obese children, compared with lean controls.

Genetic Influences on Eating Behaviors

Heritability of Eating Behaviors

Family studies and twin designs have long been used by behavioral researchers to establish the heritability of weight-related traits. The essence of the method is to compare the magnitude of associations between relatives on a particular trait to the values that would be expected from their genetic relatedness. If associations follow genetic relatedness, we infer genetic influence; if they do not, then environmental influences may be assumed. Twin data are particularly powerful and allow the relative contribution of genes and environment to be determined by comparing the resemblance between monozygotic (MZ) twins (who are genetically identical), with that between dizygotic twins (DZ) who share approximately 50% of their segregating genes, but are similar to MZ twins in that they are the same age and grow up at the same time, in the same family. Twin resemblance not attributable to genes is considered to reflect shared environmental influences while remaining variance is apportioned to unique, non-shared environmental effects and measurement error (Plomin et al. 2008). Family and twin studies produce heritability estimates which are an index of genetic effect size for any given trait.

The heritability of adult body weight is a long-established finding (Maes et al. 1997; Malis et al. 2005; Stunkard et al. 1990) with 55–85% of variation in adult BMI being attributed to genetic influences, with a similar value (77%) in childhood (Wardle et al. 2008a). It is important to recognize that high genetic influence on body weight does not preclude the influence of behavioral traits. Genes are known to influence a number of different behavioral traits as powerfully as physiological processes (Plomin et al. 2008), and the idea that genes could influence body weight through behavioral pathways (e.g. through effects on eating behaviors) allows for those most susceptible to the temptations of the environment to gain the most weight. There is a large body of research investigating the heritability of eating behaviors in adults and a much smaller literature in children, so both are included in the summary of evidence below.

Heritability of Psychometric Measures of Eating Behaviors. In adults, most psychometric studies of eating behavior heritability have used the TFEQ, which has been administered to large epidemiological cohorts as part of larger ongoing studies. Using a family design to estimate heritability, Provencher et al. (2005) found heritability estimates of 6% for cognitive restraint, 18% for disinhibition, and 28% for susceptibility to hunger and a similar study (Steinle et al. 2002) found slightly higher estimates (28% for restraint, 40% for disinhibition, 23% for hunger). But adult twin studies have produced mixed results. De Castro and Lilenfeld (2005) found significant heritability for cognitive restraint (44%) and hunger (24%), but not for disinhibition (0%) which was accounted for by shared environmental influences. However, another twin study found high heritability (45%) for disinhibition but low heritability for hunger and restraint (Neale et al. 2003) while a study of male twins (Tholin et al. 2005) and using a 21-item version of the TFEQ found comparatively high heritability estimates for cognitive restraint (59%) and two aspects of disinhibition (emotional eating (60%) and uncontrolled eating (45%)). Neale et al. (2003) also conducted multivariate modeling and found that disinhibition and hunger covaried significantly and that the traits represented by these two scales are influenced by the same set of genetic factors, while restraint was found to be empirically distinct.

It is not clear why findings have been so varied, but small sample sizes may be a factor as larger sample sizes are needed to give robust estimates. Sex differences are another possibility, and these have been reported previously in TFEQ scores (Neumark-Sztainer et al. 1999; Provencher et al. 2004). The TFEQ scales also contain attitudinal as well as behavioral components which may make it more difficult to pick up on simple additive genetic effects on eating behavior. This problem may be compounded in samples of adults who may have modified their eating behavior, or reports, according to socially prescribed attitudes. In addition to these limitations, studies with adult twins and families who have been living apart for a number of years may not detect *shared* environmental effects present in childhood which may have diminished by adulthood when children are living away from their siblings and parents (Koeppen-Schomerus et al. 2001). This makes it important to carry out pediatric studies.

Our group has used the CEBQ to assess the heritability of two eating behaviors fundamental to obesity research – satiety responsiveness and enjoyment of food – in twin children (Carnell et al. 2008). For satiety responsiveness, model-fitting indicated heritability to be 63%, shared environment effects to be 21%, and non-shared individual environment effects to be 16%. For enjoyment of food, heritability was estimated to be even higher at 75%, shared environment to be lower at 10% and non-shared environment to be 15%. These are the highest heritability estimates yet reported for eating behavior traits, and suggest that eating behavior in children is highly influenced by genetic factors.

The same sample was also used to assess the heritability of food neophobia (fear of unfamiliar foods) using a parent-report questionnaire, and it was found to be a highly heritable trait (78%) with the remaining variance being accounted for by non-shared environmental effects (22%), and no evidence for any shared environment effects (Cooke et al. 2007). We also estimated the heritability of food preferences using parents' reports for 77 different foods, in a sub-sample of these twin children. Heritability estimates differed for different types of foods, with estimates of 0.20 for desserts, 0.37 for vegetables, 0.51 for fruits, and 0.78 for protein foods. Shared environmental effects were higher than those of appetitive traits ("satiety responsiveness" and "enjoyment of food"), with 0.64 for desserts, 0.34 for fruits, 0.51 for vegetables, and 0.12 for proteins, indicating that shared influences such as parental feeding styles or exposure to certain types of foods may increase preference for those foods in children (Breen et al. 2006).

Heritability of Behavioral Measures of Eating Behaviors. In the adult literature, heritability studies using behavioral measures of eating behaviors have mainly relied on self-report methods including diet-diaries and food frequency questionnaires. The studies in this area are diverse and include a range of different populations and sample sizes, as well as many different types of eating behavior such as total daily energy and macronutrient intake (de Castro 1993, 1999a; Fabsitz et al. 1978; Faith et al. 1999; Heller et al. 1988; Mitchell et al. 2003; Perusse et al. 1988; Vauthier et al. 1996; Wade et al. 1981), dietary energy density (De Castro 2006), breakfast meal intake (Billon et al. 2002), patterns of food intake such as "healthy" versus "unhealthy" (Gunderson et al. 2006; van den Bree et al. 1999), the effect of pre-meal stomach contents on food intake (de Castro 1999b), pre- and post-meal hunger and palatability ratings and their relationship with food intake (de Castro 1999c, 2001a), and diurnal changes in food intake (de Castro 2001b). Not surprisingly, heritability estimates range widely, from 0% (Billon et al. 2002; Perusse et al. 1988; Vauthier et al. 1996) to 65% (de Castro 1999a) which may be the result of heterogeneity within sample characteristics, the different nature of the behaviors studied, and the unreliability of self-report measures of intake. However, one study with adults used measured observations of eating behavior in a laboratory and estimated the heritability of total caloric intake to be between 24 and 33% (Faith et al. 1999).

A handful of studies have assessed the heritability of eating behaviors using measured observations in children. Faith et al. (2004) used an energy compensation design with sibling pairs to assess familial aggregation of total energy intake following different preloads, and of the COMPX scores. They found significant familial aggregation for total energy intake ($\rho=0.39$), for percentages of fat, carbohydrate and protein intakes ($\rho=0.66$, 0.67, 0.61, respectively), but no significant familial aggregation for COMPX scores. Fisher et al. (2007) assessed ad libitum dinner intake and EAH within a laboratory setting. Significant heritability estimates were seen for energy intake during the ad libitum dinner (52%) as well as for EAH following the dinner (51%), suggesting that genes influence objective measures of appetite in children.

Twin designs have also indicated heritability for behavioral measures of food choice in children, using the child's 24 h food intake to indicate his or her food choices, measured by recall interview with parents. Faith et al. (2008) assessed genetic influences on nine composite food and beverage categories consumed over 24 h and found significant heritability estimates for seven categories of food among boys (ranging from 12 to 79%), and for three among girls (ranging from 20 to 56%), suggesting sex differences in the development of eating patterns.

Our group recently tested the heritability of eating rate using twin children (Llewellyn et al. 2008). We assessed "bites per minute" consumed during a standard lunch at home. Heritability of eating rate was strikingly high at 62%, while non-shared environmental effects explained the remaining variance (38%) with no evidence of shared environmental influence.

Lastly, Keski-Rahkonen et al. (2004) investigated breakfast eating patterns in twin adolescents using a 1-item question within a larger questionnaire. Their modeling suggested that genetic effects explained 41% of the variance of breakfast eating in girls and 66% in boys, with shared environmental effects being higher in girls (45%) than in boys (14%).

Molecular Genetic Basis of Eating Behaviors

The research base on the heritability of eating behaviors has demonstrated the importance of genes in determining appetitive traits. Genome-wide association and linkage studies can indicate regions of the human genome that relate to weight and eating behavior. The search for common genetic variants with links to obesity has been underway for some time (Rankinen et al. 2006; Saunders et al. 2007; Willer et al. 2009; Yang et al. 2007). A recent meta-analysis of 15 genome-wide association studies ($n = 32,387$) identified 8 loci associated with BMI, including FTO, MC4R, TMEM18, KCTD15, GNPDA2, SH2B1, MTCH2, and NEGR1 (Willer et al. 2009). Importantly, 7 of the 8 loci highlight genes that are highly expressed in the brain, and several in the hypothalamus, consistent with multiple roles of the central nervous system on body weight regulation, including appetite, which indicates that genes may influence weight through eating behaviors.

Genome-Wide Association and Linkage Studies and Eating Behavior. A number of linkage studies have found associations between specific eating behaviors and loci. Bouchard et al. (2004) conducted a genome-wide scan to identify quantitative trait loci associated with the three eating behaviours of the TFEQ. They found that the peak linkage was between markers surrounding the neuromedin-β gene, and homozygotes for a missense mutation located within this gene were twice as likely to exhibit high levels of disinhibition and susceptibility to hunger as were the non-mutation homozygotes. Steinle et al. (2002) also conducted a genome-wide scan to investigate the genetic underpinnings of the TFEQ, and found two chromosomal regions with linkage for cognitive restraint, two with linkage for disinhibition, and another with linkage for perceived hunger. Three other studies have used this technique to look at actual energy intake or macronutrient intake and have found a number of different linkages (Cai et al. 2004; Choquette et al. 2008; Collaku et al. 2004).

Genotype Studies and Energy Intake. The next step is to associate eating behaviors with actual genotypes (located through designs described above, or hypothesized to be functionally relevant), and some progress has been made. The genetic variant that has had most attention in relation to weight and energy intake is FTO, a gene on human chromosome 16. FTO has shown a robust association with weight in both adults and children (Cha et al. 2008; Chang et al. 2008; Dina et al. 2007; Frayling et al. 2007; Loos and Bouchard 2008), with those who carry two copies of the high risk allele being 3 kg heavier than non-carriers. They represent approximately 16% of the population, making FTO the first common obesity gene. A recent report using 7-day weighed food diaries found differences in energy intake by FTO genotype, but no differences in energy expenditure, consistent with the idea that FTO influences weight through appetite pathways (Speakman et al. 2008). In a sample of children an association was observed between FTO genotype and dietary energy intake and fat intake, using 7-day food diaries (Timpson et al. 2008), although another recent study with children failed to find an association between FTO genotype and energy intake using a 4-day food record (Hakanen et al. 2009). The authors, however, suggested that this null finding maybe the result of the unreliability of the 4-day food measure. Johnson et al. (2009) recently investigated whether there is a gene-environment interaction between FTO and energy density in the determination of weight in children, such that FTO and energy density conspire to bestow a synergistic (rather than simply an additive) effect on weight, using 7-day diet diary data, but although they replicated the association with weight, they did not indicate an interaction with dietary energy density.

A number of other genotypes have been related to energy and macronutrient intakes. The serotonin receptor gene has been associated with lower energy intake and the data indicated a linear gene dosage effect such that homozygotes for the variant consumed the least, homozygotes for the wild type consumed the most, and heterozygotes were intermediate in two samples (clinical and non-clinical) of overweight adults, using a diet history questionnaire and diet diary data (Aubert et al. 2000). This association was later investigated in a sample of children and adolescents and once again the variant was also associated with lower energy as well as fat intakes and indicated a linear gene dosage effect (Herbeth et al. 2005). A polymorphism in the apolipoprotein A-II gene promoter was associated with higher BMI, higher daily energy intake (measured by a food frequency questionnaire), and higher fat and protein intakes, suggesting a role for this gene in regulating energy intake as well as body weight (Corella et al. 2007). Interestingly, this gene is located within the region of chromosome 1 that was found to be linked with total energy and fat intake in a genome-wide linkage study (Collaku et al. 2004). Other studies have also found genotypic variants that relate to different macronutrient intakes (Eny et al. 2008; Loos et al. 2005).

Genotype Studies and Taste Perception. It has been established that bitter taste perception (recognition of phenylthiocarbamide (PTC) and propylthiouracil (PROP)) is strongly influenced by variants of the TAS2R38 gene on chromosome 7q (Drayna et al. 2003; Kim et al. 2003), with gene effects appearing to determine three broad taste perception phenotypes: those that are sensitive to PCT and PROP, those that have little or no sensitivity to them, and those with intermediate sensitivity (Mennella et al. 2005). Interestingly, Mennella et al. 2005) found that children who were carriers of the gene variant bestowing PROP-sensitivity preferred sweet flavors, but this finding was not replicated in the mothers. This could indicate that during childhood this genotype may affect food preferences, but cultural forces override the genetic effects as children mature into adulthood.

Genotype Studies and Classical Eating Behaviors. FTO is highly expressed in areas of the hypothalamus associated with feeding (Stratigopoulos et al. 2008), and expression varies with acute food deprivation (Gerken et al. 2007), indicating that one of the pathways through which it influences body weight (and energy intake, as cited above) is likely to be appetite or satiety. Using an energy compensation paradigm with children Cecil et al. (2008) found that the higher risk allele was associated with increased energy intake but did not appear to be involved in the regulation of energy expenditure. Our group investigated the relationship between eating behaviors and FTO variants in two studies with children. Using the EAH paradigm we found that carriers of the higher risk allele ate significantly more than children homozygous for the low risk allele, indicating a dominance effect, while there was no association with physical activity (Wardle et al. 2009). In another study we found that children homozygous for the higher risk FTO allele scored significantly lower on the Satiety Responsiveness Scale of the CEBQ (Wardle et al. 2008b).

Genetic effects on food reward and motivation have also been examined. Epstein et al. (2004) assessed the relation between food reinforcement (using a modified questionnaire-based version of the relative reinforcing value of food paradigm), variants of two dopamine genotypes, and food intake (measured behaviorally) in adults. Neither of the genotypes showed a straightforward association with energy or macronutrient intake but food reinforcement was associated with energy intake, and its effect was moderated by variants of the two genotypes.

Summary of Research into the Genetic Influence on Eating Behaviors

There is reasonable evidence for the heritability of several eating behaviors in adults, but less research has been carried out with children, and as yet no study has investigated feeding behaviors in infants. Heritability estimates are known to change over the lifespan therefore it is important to understand the relative influences of genes and shared and non-shared environments from very early on in the developmental trajectory. Research into the molecular genetic basis for eating traits, although in its infancy, has begun to provide some exciting insights into exactly how genes influence our eating behaviors, but further studies are needed to unveil the role of more obesity-related genes. Lastly, very little work has addressed how genes and environments interact to determine behavioral traits. Our new study, Gemini, will permit us to quantify the heritability of variation in eating behaviors (and weight), as well as the contribution of shared and non-shared environmental factors, and genotyping the children will make it possible to explore how genotypic variants influence eating behavior in this important developmental period. More details on genetic factors are to be found in Chapters 14 and 15.

Environmental Influences on Eating Behaviors

Understanding if there are modifiable influences on the development of "obesogenic" eating behaviors is important because interventions might be developed to prevent the development of excessive weight gain. A number of different environmental factors have been implicated, with some occurring very early in development during fetal and early post-natal life, and others occurring later on in infancy and childhood.

Perinatal Nutritional Influences on Eating Behaviors

Some epidemiological studies have found a U- or J-shaped relationship between birth weight and later adiposity (Curhan et al. 1996; Fall et al. 1995; Kensara et al. 2005) which has led researchers to hypothesize that very early (intra-uterine or early post-natal) under- or over-nutrition (using birth weight as an indicator for nutritional status) may influence later obesity risk (Gluckman and Hanson 2008; Grattan 2008; Taylor and Poston 2007). This finding has been further supported by some observational and clinical research. Female infants born to women who were under-nourished during the early gestational period as a result of the Dutch famine in 1944–1945 were found to have an increased risk of obesity in later life (Ravelli et al. 1999); infants born to mothers with gestational diabetes are larger and at greater risk of obesity (Catalano et al. 2007; Hillier et al. 2007; Silverman et al. 1998) with maternal hyperglycaemia hypothesized to mediate increased birth weight and later obesity risk (Eidelman and Samueloff 2002; Gluckman and Hanson 2008). However, these designs do not rule out the possibility that the observed associations are due to confounding factor(s) that covary with nutritional status (or birth weight) and later body size.

Among the strongest evidence implicating a causal role for nutrition in "programming" later obesity risk comes from experimental research with animals. A number of imaginative and highly controlled studies have provided convincing evidence for a causal relationship that may arise from developmental changes to appetite resulting from epigenetic effects in cases of both under- and over-nutrition (Gluckman and Hanson 2008). Animal studies that have restricted maternal nutrition have indicated that: (1) offspring have a tendency towards obesity (McMillen and Robinson 2005), and (2) there are developmental changes to centers that control appetite and food preferences, with nutritionally challenged offspring demonstrating hyperphagia and a preference for high fat foods (Bellinger et al. 2004; Vickers et al. 2000). It has been hypothesized that such developmental changes provide adaptive traits in anticipation of a nutritionally limited environment once the infant is born (Gluckman and Hanson 2008). Similarly, studies whereby mice have been over-fed on a diet that is high in fat while pregnant or during lactation have offspring that are fatter, hyperphagic, and have a preference for high fat foods over protein-rich foods (Bayol et al. 2007; Samuelsson et al. 2008), indicating that maternal eating habits during pregnancy and breast-feeding can set the infant's own eating behaviors. Interestingly, both over- and under-nutrition appear to result in permanent alteration to the same hypothalamic circuits controlling appetite and energy intake

(McMillen et al. 2005), indicating a common mechanism for obesity programming, with a key player hypothesized to be leptin (reduced availability in under-nourishment and hypothalamic leptin resistance in over-nourishment) (Grattan 2008).

Insights such as these from the animal literature have led some researchers to suggest that the different macronutrient composition of formula milk (up to 70% greater protein – (Heinig et al. 1993)) compared with breast milk may be one of the factors that contributes to faster growth often associated with formula feeding, and the protective effect of breast-feeding on later obesity risk sometimes observed in epidemiological studies (Gillman et al. 2001; Gluckman and Hanson 2008; Harder et al. 2005; Owen et al. 2005).

These findings indicate that there is the potential for large environmental influence on taste preferences. This is apparent with new-born breast- and bottle-fed infants who within days of birth orient towards the smell of their respective milk type (Mela 2001). It is also revealed in developmental changes in food preferences; tastes that are aversive in childhood such as black coffee and alcohol are enjoyed by many in adulthood, and likes and dislikes vary with different cultures. This is in keeping with our finding that the environmental influence on dessert foods and vegetables was high for children (80% and 63% respectively), indicating that environmental factors play the most important role in influencing taste preferences for these foods in children.

Parental Influences on Eating Behaviors During Infancy and Childhood

Psychological, social and behavioral processes may play a role in the development of eating behaviors during infancy and childhood. Five feeding styles have received particular attention in psychological theorizing about eating behavior etiology: (1) *restriction* of particular kinds of (unhealthy) foods or amounts of food; (2) *pressure or excessive encouragement* to eat particular kinds of (healthy) foods or more food, especially at a meal; (3) *instrumental feeding* – using food as a reward to manipulate behavior; (4) *emotional feeding* – using food to manage the child's negative emotional states; and (5) *exposure* – children eat what their parents give them, and may copy their parents' own eating behaviors. Research studies have measured the feeding styles with psychometric tests and assessed the association of these with child eating behavior, and have emulated the different styles in a research context and observed effects on subsequent eating behavior. It has proved difficult to tie particular eating behaviors with particular feeding styles, but key studies are summarized below.

Restriction. It has been hypothesized that overly restricting a child's access to a particular food can lead to an increased desire in the child for the restricted food. As the foods that are most often restricted are the "unhealthy" foods, on this theory, children will overeat on forbidden unhealthy foods given the opportunity. Experimental studies in which children's access to snack foods was manipulated (free access versus restricted access) have shown that children increase their desire for, and selection and intake of that food when it is available, and that this is the case for healthy (fruit) as well as unhealthy foods (Fisher and Birch 1999b; Jansen et al. 2007, 2008). Consistent with this, psychometric measures of maternal restriction have been found to predict higher intake in EAH paradigms both cross-sectionally (Fisher and Birch 1999a, 2000) and longitudinally (Fisher and Birch 2002; Birch et al. 2003). Maternal restriction has also been associated with poorer short-term energy regulation (Birch and Fisher 2000), higher daily energy intake (Montgomery et al. 2006), and higher dietary fat intake (Lee et al. 2001) suggesting that this parenting style may influence the development of preferences for restricted foods and cause over-responsiveness to forbidden foods. However, some research has indicated that restriction may influence some children more than others, with overweight girls being most likely to show the predicted effect (Birch et al. 2003), and others have failed to find an association with eating behavior (Montgomery et al. 2006), indicating that other factors such as sex and child weight status may moderate this effect.

The important issue for this area of work is whether the effects are causal. As they stand, the findings are equally consistent with the idea that poorer regulation in the child elicits more restrictive behavior from the parent in an attempt to curb the child's tendency towards over-eating.

Pressure and Encouragement. Pressuring a child to eat when the child is not hungry, or to eat particular kinds of foods, has been hypothesized to result in the child not learning to self-regulate their food intake according to their internal hunger or satiety cues, and eating in response to external cues instead (Faith et al. 2004; Savage et al. 2007). Some cross-sectional studies have supported this theory in that they have found an association between a psychometric measure of "pressure to eat" and greater energy intake (Campbell et al. 2006; Fisher and Birch 2002), but others (Montgomery et al. 2006) have failed to find an association. Observational studies have similarly produced mixed findings, with some studies finding that children who were prompted to eat more frequently by their mothers ate for longer (Klesges et al. 1983, 1986) and ate more (McKenzie et al. 1991), whereas others found that maternal prompting was negatively associated with total energy intake and total meal time, although positively associated with eating rate (Drucker et al. 1999). These inconsistent findings may result from the different measures of pressure that have been used. Measures include forceful pressuring behavior, as well as more gentle forms of encouragement, and different approaches may result in different outcomes (Faith et al. 2004). Research in which different forms of pressure or encouragement are assessed in more detail is needed to ascertain if this is the case.

Instrumental Feeding. Using palatable foods to reward consumption of healthy foods (such as vegetables during a meal) has been hypothesized to result in an increased dislike for the healthy food, and increased liking for the reward food (Faith et al. 2004). A number of studies have found that instrumental feeding decreases preference for the food that is rewarded, and increases preference for the food that is used to reward (Birch et al. 1980, 1984; Kroller and Warschburger 2008; Newman and Taylor 1992; Vereecken et al. 2004). However, some studies have found that using non-foods to reward healthy food consumption does not have this detrimental effect – e.g. stickers have successfully increased consumption of fruit and vegetables (Hendy et al. 2007; Horne et al. 1995, 2004; Lowe et al. 2004). More research is needed to clarify the role of different rewards in food consumption, particularly non-object rewards such as praise (Horne et al. 1995).

Emotional Feeding. One of the oldest psychological theories of obesity was the psychosomatic theory which posited that individuals who are repeatedly fed under conditions of negative affective states will come to crave those foods under the same psychological states through the processes of classical conditioning. This can lead to a cycle of eating in response to negative emotions, whether or not the individual is hungry (Kaplan and Kaplan 1957). Some retrospective studies have found that obese participants report more instrumental and emotional feeding as a child compared to successful dieters and normal-weight controls (Brink et al. 1999), but no study has yet explored whether emotional feeding by the parent is associated with emotional eating in the child, and longitudinal studies whereby emotional feeding precedes emotional eating, will provide more convincing evidence.

Exposure. One of the most important influences on food preferences and intake for children is familiarity (Cooke 2007). Experimental research and naturalistic interventions have demonstrated that repeated exposure to unfamiliar foods increases liking and consumption of those foods, including fruits and vegetables (Sullivan and Birch 1990, 1994; Wardle et al. 2003a, b). In addition, the amount of exposure needed to influence liking and consumption appears to increase with age indicating that it may be important to introduce healthy foods such as fruits and vegetables as early as possible during weaning (Cooke 2007). Parents' own food choices also appear to influence children's eating behavior. Cooke and colleagues found that the strongest predictor of both fruit and vegetable intake was the parents' own intake of those foods (Cooke et al. 2004), which could be a combination of availability of those foods in the home, modeling effects, exposure, and shared genetic influences.

Summary of Research into the Environmental Influences on Eating Behaviors

It is likely that nutritional factors during the perinatal period are important for obesity risk later on in childhood and adulthood. The animal literature indicates that this risk is in part mediated through epigenetic effects on pathways that influence eating behaviors and appetite. Although animal models are useful for initial models of programming effects, more substantial research with human infants is necessary to test whether the theory appears to stand true with regard to nutritional factors with human infants. Our Gemini study will allow us to investigate the effects of early nutritional factors (such as breast- or bottle-feeding and the timing of introduction of solid foods and junk foods) on the development of eating behaviors in infancy and early childhood.

Work with parental feeding styles has also been informative in that a number of associations have been found. However, the majority of work in this area has been cross-sectional and it is unclear whether the causal direction that is often assumed – parents influencing children – may in fact be reversed, with parental feeding styles being responses to their child's eating behavior. Longitudinal studies may help elucidate effects (e.g. Gemini) but it is possible that parents may adjust their feeding style as quickly as children's eating behaviors develop, making it difficult to detect cause and effect relationships within the time-intervals between data collection. Careful planning of critical periods will be important in elucidating this dynamic. More details on the influence of imprinting and breastfeeding on childhood obesity can be found in Chapter 17.

Implications for Treatment and Prevention

This chapter has presented evidence suggesting that a number of eating behaviors which can be seen early in childhood are associated with adiposity, including lower sensitivity to satiety, food-cue responsiveness, a higher "reinforcing" value of food, and preferences for energy-dense foods. All of these behaviors appear to have some genetic basis. A common misconception about genetic influences on behavioral traits is that they negate the possibility of environmental intervention. However, a number of family environmental influences have been shown to also play a role, some of which are modifiable, including early over- or under-nutrition, parental feeding style, parental behaviors, and exposure, all of which may modify the expression of genetically determined behavioral tendencies.

In the light of evidence that eating behaviors relate to weight in children, what might be the most effective way of preventing and treating overweight in children? Firstly, it may be helpful to use behavioral or psychometric measures to identify infants or children behaviorally "at risk." For example, the CEBQ has recently been modified for use with very young infants during the period when they are exclusively milk-fed, presenting a possibility for very early identification of infants demonstrating vigorous feeding behaviors. Specific eating behaviors could then be targeted with appropriate behavioral interventions. For children with low satiety sensitivity, parents may be encouraged to offer smaller portion sizes and to provide foods lower in energy-density to prevent over-eating, and children themselves may be educated about satiety as they get older. Two encouraging studies have indicated that such behavioral interventions may be effective: Johnson (2000) successfully improved preschool children's intake regulation by teaching them how to attend to their internal satiety cues using a demonstration doll, and Bergh et al. (2008) have shown promising results in an intervention study in which extremely obese girls were taught to regulate their eating rate to improve satiety signals using computerized feedback. For children high in food cue responsiveness, exposure to palatable foods could be limited by parents keeping such foods out of sight or out of the home, in line with behavioral techniques used with adults. In addition, if children demonstrate high relative reward of palatable foods, parents may endeavor to find enjoyable non-food activities that may be able to compete with those foods.

Research into taste preferences has indicated the importance of early exposure to many different kinds of foods for taste preferences later on. These findings suggest it may be helpful to limit foods high in sugar and fat during the early years, and to offer fruits and vegetables as early as possible. It may also be possible to influence early preferences for fruit and vegetables through modeling by parents and older siblings (Cooke et al. 2003, 2004).

Research into the hormonal control of hunger and satiety is making progress, and it is possible that future interventions will include physiological screening for individuals with high-risk hormonal profiles. This could be followed by targeted pharmacological intervention using drugs that manipulate appetite and satiety hormones (Druce and Bloom 2006).

At the same time, the importance of wider interventions must not be understated. As a number of studies reviewed in this chapter have demonstrated, the relationship between eating behaviors and weight is quantitative, so it is likely that large-scale changes to the environment that encourage greater energy expenditure and less energy intake may benefit everyone, and reduce the overall population weight, along with the incidence of weight-related disease.

References

Agras, W.S., Kraemer, H.C., Berkowitz, R.I., Korner, A.F., & Hammer, L.D. (1987). Does a vigorous feeding style influence early development of adiposity. *Journal of Pediatrics, 110*, 799–804.

Agras, W.S., Kraemer, H.C., Berkowitz, R.I., & Hammer, L.D. (1990). Influence of early feeding style on adiposity at 6 years of age. *Journal of Pediatrics, 116*, 805–809.

Ashcroft, J., Semmler, C., Carnell, S., Van Jaarsveld, C., & Wardle, J. (2008). Continuity and stability of eating behaviour traits in children. *European Journal of Clinical Nutrition, 62*, 985–990.

Aubert, R., Betoulle, D., Herbeth, B., Siest, G., & Fumeron, F. (2000). 5-HT2A receptor gene polymorphism is associated with food and alcohol intake in obese people. *International Journal of Obesity and Related Metabolic Disorders, 24*, 920–924.

Barkeling, B., Ekman, S., & Rossner, S. (1992). Eating behavior in obese and normal weight 11-year-old children. *International Journal of Obesity, 16*, 355–360.

Bayol, S.A., Farrington, S.J., & Stickland, N.C. (2007). A maternal 'junk food' diet in pregnancy and lactation promotes an exacerbated taste for 'junk food' and a greater propensity for obesity in rat offspring. *British Journal of Nutrition, 98*, 843–851.

Bellinger, L., Lilley, C., & Langley-Evans, S.C. (2004). Prenatal exposure to a maternal low-protein diet programmes a preference for high-fat foods in the young adult rat. *British Journal of Nutrition, 92*, 513–520.

Bellone, S., Rapa, A., Vivenza, D., Castellino, N., Petri, A., Bellone, J., Me, E., Broglio, F., Prodam, F., Ghigo, E., & Bona, G. (2002). Circulating ghrelin levels as function of gender, pubertal status and adiposity in childhood. *Journal of Endocrinological Investigation, 25*, RC13–RC15.

Bere, E., & Klepp, K.I. (2004). Correlates of fruit and vegetable intake among Norwegian schoolchildren: parental and self-reports. *Public Health Nutrition, 7*, 991–998.

Bergh, C., Sabin, M., Shield, J., Hellers, G., Zandian, M., Palmberg, K., Olofsson, B., Lindeberg, K., Björnström, M., & Södersten, P. (2008). A framework for the treatment of obesity: early support. In E.M. Blass (Ed.), *Obesity: causes, mechanisms and prevention*. Sunderland, MA: Sinauer Associates.

Berridge, K.C. (1996). Food reward: brain substrates of wanting and liking. *Neuroscience and Biobehavioral Reviews, 20*, 1–25.

Berridge, K.C. (2004). Motivation concepts in behavioral neuroscience. *Physiology and Behavior, 81*, 179–209.

Billon, S., Lluch, A., Gueguen, R., Berthier, A.M., Siest, G., & Herbeth, B. (2002). Family resemblance in breakfast energy intake: the Stanislas Family Study. *European Journal of Clinical Nutrition, 56*, 1011–1019.

Birch, L.L., & Fisher, J.O. (2000). Mothers' child-feeding practices influence daughters' eating and weight. *American Journal of Clinical Nutrition, 71*, 1054–1061.

Birch, L.L., Zimmerman, S.I., & Hind, H. (1980). The influence of social-affective context on the formation of children's food preferences. *Child Development, 51*, 856–861.

Birch, L.L., Marlin, D.W., & Rotter, J. (1984). Eating as the "means" activity in a contingency: effects on young children's food preference. *Child Development, 55*, 431–439.

Birch, L.L., Fisher, J.O., & Davison KK. (2003). Learning to overeat: maternal use of restrictive feeding practices promotes girls' eating in the absence of hunger. *American Journal of Clinical Nutrition*, *78*, 215–220.

Bouchard, L., Drapeau, V., Provencher, V., Lemieux, S., Chagnon, Y., Rice, T., Rao, D.C., Vohl, M-C., Tremblay, A., Bouchard, C., & Perusse, L. (2004). Neuromedin beta: a strong candidate gene linking eating behaviors and susceptibility to obesity. *American Journal of Clinical Nutrition*, *80*, 1478–1486.

Braet, C., & Van Strien, T. (1997). Assessment of emotional, externally induced and restrained eating behaviour in nine to twelve-year-old obese and non-obese children. *Behaviour Research and Therapy*, *35*, 863–873.

Breen, F.M., Plomin, R., & Wardle, J. (2006). Heritability of food preferences in young children. *Physiology & Behavior*, *88*, 443–447.

Brink, P.J., Ferguson, K., & Sharma, A. (1999). Childhood memories about food: the Successful Dieters Project. *Journal of Child and Adolescent Psychiatric Nursing*, *12*, 17–25.

Bruce, A.S., Holsen, L.M., Chambers, R.J., Martin, L.E., Brooks, W.M., Zarcone, J.R., Butler, M.G., & Savage, C.R. (2010). Obese children show hyperactivation to food pictures in brain networks linked to motivation, reward and cognitive control. *International Journal of Obesity*, *34*, 1494–500.

Bruch, C.H. (1964). Psychological aspects of overeating and obesity. *Psychosomatics*, *5*, 269–274.

Butte, N.F., Cai, G., Cole, S.A., Wilson, T.A., Fisher, J.O., Zakeri, I.F., Ellis, K.J., & Comuzzie, A.G. (2007). Metabolic and behavioral predictors of weight gain in Hispanic children: the Viva la Familia Study. *American Journal of Clinical Nutrition*, *85*, 1478–1485.

Caccialanza, R., Nicholls, D., Cena, H., Maccarini, L., Rezzani, C., Antonioli, L., Dieli, S., & Roggi, C. (2004). Validation of the Dutch Eating Behaviour Questionnaire parent version (DEBQ-P) in the Italian population: a screening tool to detect differences in eating behaviour among obese, overweight and normal-weight preadolescents. *European Journal of Clinical Nutrition*, *58*, 1217–1222.

Cai, G., Cole, S.A., Bastarrachea, R.A., MacCluer, J.W., Blangero, J., & Comuzzie AG. (2004). Quantitative trait locus determining dietary macronutrient intakes is located on human chromosome 2p22. *American Journal of Clinical Nutrition*, *80*, 1410–1414.

Campbell, K.J., Crawford, D.A., & Ball, K. (2006). Family food environment and dietary behaviors likely to promote fatness in 5-6 year-old children. *International Journal of Obesity*, *30*, 1272–1280.

Carnell, S., & Wardle, J. (2007). Measuring behavioural susceptibility to obesity: validation of the Child Eating Behaviour Questionnaire. *Appetite*, *48*, 104–113.

Carnell, S., & Wardle, J. (2008). Appetite and adiposity in children: evidence for a behavioral susceptibility theory of obesity. *American Journal of Clinical Nutrition*, *88*, 22–29.

Carnell, S., Haworth, C.M., Plomin, R., & Wardle, J. (2008). Genetic influence on appetite in children. *International Journal of Obesity*, *32*, 1468–1473.

Carruth, B.R., Skinner, J., Houck, K., Moran, J., Coletta, F., & Ott, D. (1998). The phenomenon of "picky eater": a behavioral marker in eating patterns of toddlers. *Journal of the American College of Nutrition*, *17*, 180–186.

Catalano, P.M., Thomas, A., Huston-Presley, L., & Amini, S.B. (2007). Phenotype of infants of mothers with gestational diabetes. *Diabetes Care*, *30*, 156–160.

Cecil, J.E., Palmer, C.N., Wrieden, W., Murrie, I., Bolton-Smith, C., Watt, P., Wallis, D.J., & Hetherington, M.M. (2005). Energy intakes of children after preloads: adjustment, not compensation. *American Journal of Clinical Nutrition*, *82*, 302–308.

Cecil, J.E., Tavendale, R., Watt, P., Hetherington, M.M., & Palmer, C. (2008). An obesity-associated *FTO* gene variant and increased energy intake in children. *New England Journal of Medicine*, *359*, 2558–2566.

Cha, S.W., Choi, S.M., Kim, K.S., Park, B.L., Kim, J.R., Kim, J.Y., & Shin, H.D. (2008). Replication of genetic effects of FTO polymorphisms on BMI in a Korean population. *Obesity*, *16*, 2187–2189.

Chang, Y.C., Liu, P.H., Lee, W.J., Chang, T-J., Jiang, Y-D., Li, H-Y., Kuo, S-S., Lee, K-C., & Chuang, L-M. (2008). Common variation in the fat mass and obesity-associated (FTO) gene confers risk of obesity and modulates BMI in the Chinese population. *Diabetes*, *57*, 2245–2252.

Chaudhri, O.B., Field, B.C., & Bloom, S.R. (2008). Gastrointestinal satiety signals. *International Journal of Obesity*, *32*, 28–31.

Choquette, A.C., Lemieux, S., Tremblay, A., Chagnon, Y.C., Bouchard, C., Vohl, M-C., & Perusse, L. (2008). Evidence of a quantitative trait locus for energy and macronutrient intakes on chromosome 3q27.3: the Quebec Family Study. *American Journal of Clinical Nutrition*, *88*, 1142–1148.

Collaku, A., Rankinen, T., Rice, T., Leon, A.S., Rao, D.C., Skinner, J.S., Wilmore, J.H., & Bouchard, C. (2004). A genome-wide linkage scan for dietary energy and nutrient intakes: the Health, Risk Factors, Exercise Training, and Genetics (HERITAGE) Family Study. *American Journal of Clinical Nutrition*, *79*, 881–886.

Cooke, L. (2007). The importance of exposure for healthy eating in childhood: a review. *Journal of Human Nutrition and Dietetics*, *20*, 294–301.

Cooke, L., Wardle, J., & Gibson, E.L. (2003). Relationship between parental report of food neophobia and everyday food consumption in 2-6-year-old children. *Appetite*, *41*, 205–206.

Cooke, L.J., Wardle, J., Gibson, E.L., Sapochnik, M., Sheiham, A., & Lawson, M. (2004). Demographic, familial and trait predictors of fruit and vegetable consumption by pre-school children. *Public Health Nutrition*, 7, 295–302.

Cooke, L.J., Haworth, C., & Wardle, J. (2007). Genetic and environmental influences on children's food neophobia. *American Journal of Clinical Nutrition*, 86, 428–433.

Corella, D., Arnett, D.K., Tsai, M.Y., Kabagambe, E.K., Peacock, J.M., Hixson, J.E., Straka, R.J., Province, M., Lai, C-Q., Parnell, L.D., Borecki, I., & Ordovas, J.M. (2007). The −256T>C polymorphism in the apolipoprotein A-II gene promoter is associated with body mass index and food intake in the genetics of lipid lowering drugs and diet network study. *Clinical Chemistry*, 53, 1144–1152.

Curhan, G.C., Chertow, G.M., Willett, W.C., Spiegelman, D., Colditz, G.A., Manson, J.E., Speizer, F.E., & Stampfer, M.J. (1996). Birth weight and adult hypertension and obesity in women. *Circulation*, 94, 1310–1315.

Cutting, T.M., Fisher, J.O., Grimm-Thomas, K., & Birch, L.L. (1999). Like mother, like daughter: familial patterns of overweight are mediated by mothers' dietary disinhibition. *American Journal of Clinical Nutrition*, 69, 608–613.

Davidson, M.C., Thomas, K.M., & Casey, B.J. (2003). Imaging the developing brain with fMRI. *Mental Retardation and Developmental Disabilities Research Reviews*, 9, 161–167.

de Castro, J.M. (1993). Independence of genetic influences on body size, daily intake, and meal patterns of humans. *Physiology and Behavior*, 54, 633–639.

de Castro, J.M. (1999a). Behavioral genetics of food intake regulation in free-living humans. *Nutrition*, 15, 550–554.

de Castro, J.M. (1999b). Inheritance of premeal stomach content influences on eating and drinking in free living humans. *Physiology and Behavior*, 66, 223.

de Castro, JM. (1999c). Heritability of hunger relationships with food intake in free-living humans. *Physiology and Behavior*, 67, 249–258.

de Castro, J.M. (2001a). Palatability and intake relationships in free-living humans: the influence of heredity. *Nutrition Research*, 21, 935–945.

de Castro, J.M. (2001b). Heritability of diurnal changes in food intake in free-living humans. *Nutrition*, 17, 713.

de Castro, J.M. (2006). Heredity influences the dietary energy density of free-living humans. *Physiology and Behavior*, 87, 192–198.

de Castro, J.M., & Lilenfeld, L. (2005). Influence of heredity on dietary restraint, disinhibition, and perceived hunger in humans. *Nutrition*, 21, 446–455.

de Lauzon, B., Romon, M., Deschamps, V., Lafay, L., Borys, J-M., Karlsson, J., Ducimetière, P., & Charles, M.A. (2004). The Three-Factor Eating Questionnaire-R18 is able to distinguish among different eating patterns in a general population 1. *Journal of Nutrition*, 134, 2372–2380.

Dina, C., Meyre, D., Gallina, S., Durand, E., Korner, A., Jacobson, P., Carlsson, L.M.S., Kiess, W., Vatin, V., Lecoeur, C., Delplanque, J., Vaillant, E., Pattou, F., Ruiz, J., Weill, J., Levy-Marchal, C., Horber, F., Potoczna, N., Hercberg, S., Le Stunff, C., Bougneres, P., Kovacs, P., Marre, M., Balkau, B., Cauchi, S., Chevre, J-C., & Froguel, P. (2007). Variation in FTO contributes to childhood obesity and severe adult obesity. *Nature Genetics*, 39, 724–726.

Drabman, R.S., Cordua, G.D., Hammer, D., Jarvie, G.J., & Horton, W. (1979). Developmental-trends in eating rates of normal and overweight preschool-children. *Child Development*, 50, 211–216.

Drayna, D., Coon, H., Kim, U.K., Elsner, T., Cromer, K., Otterud, B., Baird, L., Peiffer, A.P., & Leppert, M. (2003). Genetic analysis of a complex trait in the Utah Genetic Reference Project: a major locus for PTC taste ability on chromosome 7q and a secondary locus on chromosome 16p. *Human Genetics*, 112, 567–572.

Druce, M., & Bloom, S.R. (2006). The regulation of appetite. *Archives of Disease in Childhood*, 91, 183–187.

Drucker, R.R., Hammer, L.D., Agras, W.S., & Bryson, S. (1999). Can mothers influence their child's eating behavior? *Journal of Developmental and Behavioural Pediatrics*, 20, 88–92.

Eidelman, A.I., & Samueloff, A. (2002). The pathophysiology of the fetus of the diabetic mother. *Seminars in Perinatology*, 26, 232–236.

Eny, K.M., Wolever, T.M., Fontaine-Bisson, B., & El-Sohemy, A. (2008). Genetic variant in the glucose transporter type 2 is associated with higher intakes of sugars in two distinct populations. *Physiological Genomics*, 33, 355–360.

Epstein, S. (1983). Aggregation and beyond: some basic issues on the prediction of behavior. *Journal of Personality*, 51, 360–392.

Epstein, L.H., Parker, L., Mccoy, J.F., & Mcgee, G. (1976). Descriptive analysis of eating regulation in obese and nonobese children. *Journal of Applied Behavior Analysis*, 9, 407–415.

Epstein, L.H., Wright, S.M., Paluch, R.A., Leddy, J.J., Hawk, L.W., Jaroni, J.L., Saad, F.G., Crystal-Mansour, S., Shields, P.G., & Lerman, C. (2004). Relation between food reinforcement and dopamine genotypes and its effect on food intake in smokers. *American Journal of Clinical Nutrition*, 80, 82–88.

Fabsitz, R.R., Garrison, R.J., Feinleib, M., & Hjortland, M. (1978). A twin analysis of dietary intake: evidence for a need to control for possible environmental differences in MZ and DZ twins. *Behavior Genetics*, 8, 15–25.

Faith, M.S., Rha, S.S., Neale, M.C., & Allison, D.B. (1999). Evidence for genetic influences on human energy intake: results from a twin study using measured observations. *Behavior Genetics, 29*, 145–154.

Faith, M.S., Keller, K.L., Johnson, S.L., Pietrobelli, A., Matz, P.E., Must, S., Jorge, M.A., Cooperberg, J., Heymsfield, S.B., & Allison, D.B. (2004). Familial aggregation of energy intake in children. *American Journal of Clinical Nutrition, 79*, 844–850.

Faith, M.S., Berkowitz, R.I., Stallings, V.A., Kerns, J., Storey, M., & Stunkard, A.J. (2006). Eating in the absence of hunger: a genetic marker for childhood obesity in prepubertal boys? *Obesity, 14*, 131–138.

Faith, M.S., Rhea, S.A., Corley, R.P., & Hewitt, J.K. (2008). Genetic and shared environmental influences on children's 24-h food and beverage intake: sex differences at age 7 y. *American Journal of Clinical Nutrition, 87*, 903–911.

Fall, C.H., Osmond, C., Barker, D.J., Clark, P.M.S., Hales, C.N., Stirling, Y., & Meade, T.W. (1995). Fetal and infant growth and cardiovascular risk factors in women. *British Medical Journal, 310*, 428–432.

Fieldstone, A., Zipf, W.B., Schwartz, H.C., & Berntson, G.G. (1997). Food preferences in Prader–Willi syndrome, normal weight and obese controls. *International Journal of Obesity and Related Metabolic Disorders, 21*, 1046–1052.

Fisher, J.O., & Birch, L.L. (1995). Fat preferences and fat consumption of 3- to 5-year-old children are related to parental adiposity. *Journal of the American Dietetic Association, 95*, 759–764.

Fisher, J.O., & Birch, L.L. (1999a). Restricting access to foods and children's eating. *Appetite, 32*, 405–419.

Fisher, J.O., & Birch, L.L. (1999b). Restricting access to palatable foods affects children's behavioral response, food selection, and intake. *American Journal of Clinical Nutrition, 69*, 1264–1272.

Fisher, J.O., & Birch, L.L. (2000). Parents' restrictive feeding practices are associated with young girls' negative self-evaluation of eating. *Journal of the American Dietetic Association, 100*, 1341–1346.

Fisher, J.O., & Birch, L.L. (2002). Eating in the absence of hunger and overweight in girls from 5 to 7 y of age. *American Journal of Clinical Nutrition, 76*, 226–231.

Fisher, J.O., Cai, G.W., Jaramillo, S.J., Cole, S.A., Comuzzie, A.G., & Butte, N.F. (2007). Heritability of hyperphagic eating behavior and appetite-related hormones among Hispanic children. *Obesity, 15*, 1484–1495.

Francis, L.A., & Birch, L.L. (2005). Maternal weight status modulates the effects of restriction on daughters' eating and weight. *International Journal of Obesity and Related Metabolic Disorders, 29*, 942–949.

Francis, L.A., Ventura, A.K., Marini, M., & Birch, L.L. (2007). Parent overweight predicts daughters' increase in BMI and disinhibited overeating from 5 to 13 years. *Obesity, 15*, 1544–1553.

Frayling, T.M., Timpson, N.J., Weedon, M.N., Zeggini, E., Freathy, R.M., Lindgren, C.M., Perry, J.R.B., Elliott, K.S., Lango, H., Rayner, N.W., Shields, B., Harries, L.W., Barrett, J.C., Ellard, S., Groves, C.J., Knight, B., Patch, A-M., Ness, A.R., Ebrahim, S., Lawlor, D.A., Ring, S.M., Ben-Shlomo, Y., Jarvelin, M-R., Sovio, U., Bennett, A.J., Melzer, D., Ferrucci, L., Loos, R.J.F., Barroso, I., Wareham, N.J., Karpe, F., Owen, K.R., Cardon, L.R., Walker, M., Hitman, G.A., Palmer, C.N.A., Doney, A.S.F., Morris, A.D., Davey Smith, G., Hattersley, A.T., & McCarthy, M.I. (2007). A common variant in the FTO gene is associated with body mass index and predisposes to childhood and adult obesity. *Science, 316*, 889–894.

Galloway, A.T., Fiorito, L., Lee, Y., & Birch, L.L. (2005). Parental pressure, dietary patterns, and weight status among girls who are "picky eaters." *Journal of the American Dietetic Association, 105*, 541–548.

Gerken, T., Girard, C.A., Tung, Y., Webby, C.J., Saudek, V., Hewitson, K.S., Yeo, G.S.H., McDonaugh, M.A., Cunliffe, S., McNeill, L.A., Galvanovskis, J., Rorsman, P., Robins, P., Prieur, X., Coll, A.P., Ma, M., Jovanovic, Z., Farooqi, I.S., Sedgwick, B., Barroso, I., Lindahl, T., Ponting, C.P., Ashcroft, F.M., O'Rahilly, S., & Schofield, C.J. (2007). The obesity-associated *FTO* gene encodes a 2-oxoglutarate-dependent nucleic acid demethylase. *Science, 318*, 1469–1472.

Gillman, M.W., Rifas-Shiman, S.L., Camargo, C.A., Jr., Berkey, C.S., Frazier, A.L., Rockett, H.R.H., Field, A.E., & Colditz, G.A. (2001). Risk of overweight among adolescents who were breastfed as infants. *Journal of the American Medical Association, 285*, 2461–2467.

Gluckman, P.D., & Hanson, M.A. (2008). Developmental and epigenetic pathways to obesity: an evolutionary perspective. *International Journal of Obesity, 32*, 62–71.

Grattan, D.R. (2008). Fetal programming from maternal obesity: eating too much for two? *Endocrinology, 149*, 5345–5347.

Gunderson, E.P., Tsai, A.L., Selby, J.V., Caan, B., Mayer-Davis, E.J., & Risch, N. (2006). Twins of mistaken zygosity (TOMZ): evidence for genetic contributions to dietary patterns and physiologic traits. *Twin Research and Human Genetics, 9*, 540–549.

Guss, J.L., & Kissileff, H.R. (2000). Microstructural analyses of human ingestive patterns: from description to mechanistic hypotheses. *Neuroscience and Biobehavioral Reviews, 24*, 261–268.

Hakanen, M., Raitakari, O.T., Lehtimaki, T., Peltonen, N., Pahkala, K., Sillanmaki, L., Lagstrom, H., Viikari, J., Simell, O., & Ronnemaa, T. (2009). FTO genotype is associated with Body Mass Index after the age of 7 years but not with energy intake or leisure-time physical activity. *Journal of Clinical Endocrinology and Metabolism, 94(4)*, 1281–1287.

Haqq, A.M., Farooqi, I.S., O'Rahilly, S., Stadler, D.D., Rosenfeld, R.G., Pratt, K.L., LaFranchi, S.H., & Purnell, J.Q. (2003). Serum ghrelin levels are inversely correlated with body mass index, age, and insulin concentrations in normal children and are markedly increased in Prader–Willi syndrome. *Journal of Clinical Endocrinology and Metabolism, 88*, 174–178.

Harder, T., Bergmann, R., Kallischnigg, G., & Plagemann, A. (2005). Duration of breastfeeding and risk of overweight: a meta-analysis. *American Journal of Epidemiology, 162*, 397–403.

Harris, G. (1993). Feeding problems and their treatment. In S.T. James, I. Roberts, G. Harris & D.J. Messer (Eds.), *Infant crying, feeding and sleeping: development, problems and treatments. The developing body and mind* (pp. 118–132). London: Harvester Wheatsheaf.

Heinig, M.J., Nommsen, L.A., Peerson, J.M., Lonnerdal, B., & Dewey, K.G. (1993). Energy and protein intakes of breast-fed and formula-fed infants during the first year of life and their association with growth velocity: the DARLING Study. *American Journal of Clinical Nutrition, 58*, 152–161.

Heller, R.F., O'Connell, D.L., Roberts, D.C., Allen, J.R., Knapp, J.C., Steele, P.L., & Silove, D. (1988). Lifestyle factors in monozygotic and dizygotic twins. *Genetic Epidemiology, 5*, 311–321.

Hendy, H.M., Williams, K.E., Camise, T.S., Alderman, S., Ivy, J., & Reed, J. (2007). Overweight and average-weight children equally responsive to "Kids Choice Program" to increase fruit and vegetable consumption. *Appetite, 49*, 683–686.

Herbeth, B., Aubry, E., Fumeron, F., Aubert, R., Cailotto, F., Siest, G., & Visvikis-Siest, S. (2005). Polymorphism of the 5-HT2A receptor gene and food intakes in children and adolescents: the Stanislas Family Study. *American Journal of Clinical Nutrition, 82*, 467–470.

Hill, J.O., Lin, D., Yakubu, F., & Peters, J.C. (1992). Development of dietary obesity in rats: influence of amount and composition of dietary fat. *International Journal of Obesity and Related Metabolic Disorders, 16*, 321–333.

Hill, A.J., Draper, E., & Stack, J. (1994). A weight on children's minds: body shape dissatisfactions at 9-years old. *International Journal of Obesity and Related Metabolic Disorders, 18*, 383–389.

Hill, J.O., Wyatt, H.R., Reed, G.W., & Peters, J.C. (2003). Obesity and the environment: where do we go from here? *Science, 299*, 853–855.

Hill, C., Llewellyn, C.H., Saxton, J., Webber, L., Semmler, C., Carnell, S., van Jaarsveld, C.H.M., Boniface, D., & Wardle, J. (2008). Adiposity and 'eating in the absence of hunger' in children. *International Journal of Obesity, 32*, 1499–1505.

Hill, C., Wardle, J., & Cooke, L. (2009). Adiposity is not associated with children's reported liking for selected foods. *Appetite, 52*(3), 603–608.

Hill, C., Saxton, J., Webber, L., Blundell, J., & Wardle, J. (2009). The relative reinforcing value of food predicts weight gain in a longitudinal study of 7-10-y-old children. *American Journal of Clinical Nutrition, 90*, 276–81.

Hillier, T.A., Pedula, K.L., Schmidt, M.M., Mullen, J.A., Charles, M.A., & Pettitt, D.J. (2007). Childhood obesity and metabolic imprinting: the ongoing effects of maternal hyperglycemia. *Diabetes Care, 30*, 2287–2292.

Holsen, L.M., Zarcone, J.R., Brooks, W.M., Butler, M.G., Thompson, T.I., Ahluwalia, J.S., Nollen, N.L., & Savage, C.R. (2006). Neural mechanisms underlying hyperphagia in Prader–Willi syndrome. *Obesity, 14*, 1028–1037.

Horne, P.J., Lowe, C.F., Fleming, P.F., & Dowey, A.J. (1995). An effective procedure for changing food preferences in 5-7-year-old children. *Proceedings of the Nutrition Society, 54*, 441–452.

Horne, P.J., Tapper, K., Lowe, C.F., Hardman, C.A., Jackson, M.C., & Woolner, J. (2004). Increasing children's fruit and vegetable consumption: a peer-modelling and rewards-based intervention. *European Journal of Clinical Nutrition, 58*, 1649–1660.

Horvath, T.L., Diano, S., Sotonyi, P., Heiman, M., & Tschop, M. (2001). Minireview: ghrelin and the regulation of energy balance – a hypothalamic perspective. *Endocrinology, 142*, 4163–4169.

Jacobi, C., Agras, W.S., Bryson, S., & Hammer, L.D. (2003). Behavioral validation, precursors, and concomitants of picky eating in childhood. *Journal of the American Academy of Child & Adolescent Psychiatry, 42*, 76–84.

James, R.J., Drewett, R.F., & Cheetham, T.D. (2004). Low cord ghrelin levels in term infants are associated with slow weight gain over the first 3 months of life. *Journal of Clinical Endocrinology and Metabolism, 89*, 3847–3850.

James, R.J., James, A., Drewett, R.F., & Cheetham, T.D. (2007). Milk intake and feeding behavior in the first week of life and its relationship to cord blood ghrelin, leptin, and insulin concentrations. *Pediatric Research, 62*, 695–699.

Jansen, A., Theunissen, N., Slechten, K., Nederkoorn, C., Boon, B., Mulkens, S., & Roefs, A. (2003). Overweight children overeat after exposure to food cues. *Eating Behaviors, 4*, 197–209.

Jansen, E., Mulkens, S., & Jansen, A. (2007). Do not eat the red food!: prohibition of snacks leads to their relatively higher consumption in children. *Appetite, 49*, 572–577.

Jansen, E., Mulkens, S., Emond, Y., & Jansen, A. (2008). From the Garden of Eden to the land of plenty. Restriction of fruit and sweets intake leads to increased fruit and sweets consumption in children. *Appetite, 51*, 570–575.

Johnson, S.L. (2000). Improving preschoolers' self-regulation of energy intake. *Pediatrics, 106*, 1429–1435.

Johnson, S.L., & Birch, L.L. (1994). Parents' and children's adiposity and eating style. *Pediatrics, 94*, 653–661.

Johnson, L., Van Jaarsveld, C., Emmett, P.M., Rogers, I.S., Ness, A.R., Hattersley, A.T., Timpson, N.J., Davey Smith, G., & Jebb, S.A. (2009) Dietary energy density affects fat mass in early adolescence and is not modified by *FTO* variants. *PLoS ONE, 4*, e4594.

Kaplan, H.I., & Kaplan, H.S. (1957). The psychosomatic concept of obesity. *Journal of Psychosomatic Research, 16*, 305–308.

Kensara, O.A., Wootton, S.A., Phillips, D.I., Patel, M., Jackson, A.A., & Elia, M. (2005). Fetal programming of body composition: relation between birth weight and body composition measured with dual-energy X-ray absorptiometry and anthropometric methods in older Englishmen. *American Journal of Clinical Nutrition, 82*, 980–987.

Keski-Rahkonen, A., Viken, R.J., Kaprio, J., Rissanen, A., & Rose, R.J. (2004). Genetic and environmental factors in breakfast eating patterns. *Behavior Genetics, 34(5)*, 503–514.

Kim, U.K., Jorgenson, E., Coon, H., Leppert, M., Risch, N., & Drayna, D. (2003). Positional cloning of the human quantitative trait locus underlying taste sensitivity to phenylthiocarbamide. *Science, 299*, 1221–1225.

Klesges, R.C., Coates, T.J., Brown, G., Sturgeon-Tillisch, J., Moldenhauer-Klesges, L.M., Holzer, B., Woolfrey, J., & Vollmer, J. (1983). Parental influences on children's eating behavior and relative weight. *Journal of Applied Behavior Analysis, 16*, 371–378.

Klesges, R.C., Malott, J.M., Boschee, P.F., & Weber, J.M. (1986). The effects of parental influences on childrens food-intake, physical-activity, and relative weight. *International Journal of Eating Disorders, 5*, 335–346.

Koeppen-Schomerus, G., Wardle, J., & Plomin, R. (2001). A genetic analysis of weight and overweight in 4-year-old twin pairs. *International Journal of Obesity and Related Metabolic Disorders, 25*, 838–844.

Kroller, K., & Warschburger, P. (2008). Associations between maternal feeding style and food intake of children with a higher risk for overweight. *Appetite, 51*, 166–172.

Laessle, R.G., Uhl, H., & Lindel, B. (2001). Parental influences on eating behavior in obese and nonobese preadolescents. *International Journal of Eating Disorders, 30*, 447–453.

Lappalainen, R., & Epstein, L.H. (1990). A behavioral economics analysis of food choice in humans. *Appetite, 14*, 81–93.

Lee, Y., Mitchell, D.C., Smiciklas-Wright, H., & Birch, L.L. (2001). Diet quality, nutrient intake, weight status, and feeding environments of girls meeting or exceeding recommendations for total dietary fat of the American Academy of Pediatrics. *Pediatrics, 107*, 95–102.

Lindgren, A.C., Barkeling, B., Hagg, A., Ritzen, E.M., Marcus, C., & Rossner, S. (2000). Eating behavior in Prader–Willi syndrome, normal weight, and obese control groups. *Journal of Pediatrics, 137*, 50–55.

Llewellyn, C.H., van Jaarsveld, C.H., Boniface, D., Carnell, S., & Wardle, J. (2008). Eating rate is a heritable phenotype related to weight in children. *American Journal of Clinical Nutrition, 88*, 1560–1566.

Lluch, A., Herbeth, B., Mejean, L., & Siest, G. (2000). Dietary intakes, eating style and overweight in the Stanislas Family Study. *International Journal of Obesity and Related Metabolic Disorders, 24*, 1493–1499.

Lomenick, J.P., Clasey, J.L., & Anderson, J.W. (2008). Meal-related changes in Grehlin, Peptide YY, and appetite in normal weight and overweight children. *Obesity, 16*, 547–552.

Loos, R.J., & Bouchard, C. (2008). FTO: the first gene contributing to common forms of human obesity. *Obesity Reviews, 9*, 246–250.

Loos, R.J., Rankinen, T., Rice, T., Rao, D.C., Leon, A.S., Skinner, J.S., Bouchard, C., & Argyropoulos, G. (2005). Two ethnic-specific polymorphisms in the human Agouti-related protein gene are associated with macronutrient intake. *American Journal of Clinical Nutrition, 82*, 1097–1101.

Lowe, C.F., Horne, P.J., Tapper, K., Bowdery, M., & Egerton, C. (2004). Effects of a peer modelling and rewards-based intervention to increase fruit and vegetable consumption in children. *European Journal of Clinical Nutrition, 58*, 510–522.

Maes, H.H., Neale, M.C., & Eaves, L.J. (1997). Genetic and environmental factors in relative body weight and human adiposity. *Behavioral Genetics, 27*, 325–351.

Malis, C., Rasmussen, E.L., Poulsen, P., Petersen, I., Christensen, K., Beck-Nielsen, H., Astrup, A., & Vaag, A.A. (2005). Total and regional fat distribution is strongly influenced by genetic factors in young and elderly twins. *Obesity Research, 13*, 2139–2145.

Mantzoros, C.S., Rifas-Shiman, S.L., Williams, C.J., Fargnoli, J.L., Kelesidis, T., & Gillman, M.W. (2009). Cord blood leptin and adiponectin as predictors of adiposity in children at 3 years of age: a prospective cohort study. *Pediatrics, 123*, 682–689.

McKenzie, T.L., Sallis, J.F., Nader, P.R., Patterson, T.L., Elder, J.P., Berry, C.C., Rupp, J.W., Atkins, C.J., Buono, M.J., & Nelson, J.A. (1991). BEACHES: an observational system for assessing children's eating and physical activity behaviors and associated events. *Journal of Applied Behavior Analysis, 24*, 141–151.

McMillen, I.C., & Robinson, J.S. (2005). Developmental origins of the metabolic syndrome: prediction, plasticity, and programming. *Physiological Reviews, 85*, 571–633.

McMillen, I.C., Adam, C.L., & Muhlhausler, B.S. (2005). Early origins of obesity: programming the appetite regulatory system. *Journal of Physiology, 565*, 9–17.

Mela, D.J. (2001). Determinants of food choice: relationships with obesity and weight control. *Obesity Research*, *9*, 249–255.

Mennella, J.A., Pepino, Y., & Reed, D.R. (2005). Genetic and environmental determinants of bitter perception and sweet preferences. *Pediatrics*, *115*, 216–222.

Meyer, J.E., & Pudel, V. (1972). Experimental studies on food-intake in obese and normal weight subjects. *Journal of Psychosomatic Research*, *16*, 305–308.

Millstein, R.M. (1980). Responsiveness of newborn infants of overweight and normal weight parents. *Appetite*, *1*, 65–74.

Mitchell, B.D., Rainwater, D.L., Hsueh, W.C., Kennedy, A.J., Stern, M.P., & MacCluer, J.W. (2003). Familial aggregation of nutrient intake and physical activity: results from the San Antonio Family Heart Study. *Annals of Epidemiology*, *13*, 128–135.

Moens, E., & Braet, C. (2007). Predictors of disinhibited eating in children with and without overweight. *Behaviour Research and Therapy*, *45*, 1357–1368.

Montgomery, C., Jackson, D.M., Kelly, L.A., & Reilly, J.J. (2006). Parental feeding style, energy intake and weight status in young Scottish children. *British Journal of Nutrition*, *96*, 1149–1153.

Neale, B.M., Mazzeo, S.E., & Bulik, C.M. (2003). A twin study of dietary restraint, disinhibition and hunger: an examination of the eating inventory (three factor eating questionnaire). *Twin Research*, *6*, 471–478.

Neumark-Sztainer, D., Sherwood, N.E., French, S.A., & Jeffery, R.W. (1999). Weight control behaviors among adult men and women: cause for concern? *Obesity Research*, *7*, 179–188.

Newman, J., & Taylor, A. (1992). Effect of a means-end contingency on young children's food preferences. *Journal of Experimental Child Psychology*, *53*, 200–216.

Ong, K.K., Ahmed, M.L., Sherriff, A., Woods, K.A., Watts, A., Golding, J., & Dunger, D.B. (1999). Cord blood leptin is associated with size at birth and predicts infancy weight gain in humans. ALSPAC Study Team. Avon Longitudinal Study of Pregnancy and Childhood. *Journal of Clinical Endocrinology and Metabolism*, *84*, 1145–1148.

Owen, C.G., Martin, R.M., Whincup, P.H., Smith, G.D., & Cook, D.G. (2005). Effect of infant feeding on the risk of obesity across the life course: a quantitative review of published evidence. *Pediatrics*, *115*, 1367–1377.

Perusse, L., Tremblay, A., Leblanc, C., Cloninger, C.R., Reich, T., Rice, J., & Bouchard, C. (1988). Familial resemblance in energy intake: contribution of genetic and environmental factors. *American Journal of Clinical Nutrition*, *47*, 629–635.

Plomin, R., DeFries, J.C., McClearn, G.E., & McGuffin, P. (2008). *Behavioral genetics*. New York: Worth Publishers.

Provencher, V., Drapeau, V., Tremblay, A., Despres, J.P., Bouchard, C., & Lemieux, S. (2004). Eating behaviours, dietary profile and body composition according to dieting history in men and women of the Quebec Family Study. *British Journal of Nutrition*, *91*, 997–1004.

Provencher, V., Perusse, L., Bouchard, L., Drapeau, V., Bouchard, C., Rice, T., Rao, D.C., Tremblay, A., Despres, J-P., & Lemieux, S. (2005). Familial resemblance in eating behaviors in men and women from the Quebec Family Study. *Obesity Research*, *13*, 1624–1629.

Rankinen, T., Zuberi, A., Chagnon, Y.C., Weisnagel, S.J., Argyropoulos, G., Walts, B., Perusse, L., & Bouchard, C. (2006). The human obesity gene map: the 2005 update. *Obesity*, *14*, 529–644.

Ravelli, A.C., Van der Meulen, J.H., Osmond, C., Barker, D.J., & Bleker, O.P. (1999). Obesity at the age of 50 y in men and women exposed to famine prenatally. *American Journal of Clinical Nutrition*, *70*, 811–816.

Raynor, H.A., Polley, B.A., Wing, R.R., & Jeffery, R.R. (2004). Is dietary fat intake related to liking or household availability of high-and low-fat foods? *Obesity Research*, *12*, 816–823.

Ricketts, C.D. (1997). Fat preferences, dietary fat intake and body composition in children. *European Journal of Clinical Nutrition*, *51*, 778–781.

Rodin, J., & Slochower, J. (1976). Externality in the nonobese: effects of environmental responsiveness on weight. *Journal of Personality and Social Psychology*, *33*, 338–344.

Roth, C.L., Enriori, P.J., Harz, K., Woelfle, J., Cowley, M.A., & Reinehr, T. (2005). Peptide YY is a regulator of energy homeostasis in obese children before and after weight loss. *Journal of Clinical Endocrinology and Metabolism*, *90*, 6386–6391.

Rydell, A.M., Dahl, M., & Sundelin, C. (1995). Characteristics of school children who are choosy eaters. *Journal of Genetic Psychology*, *156*, 217–229.

Samuelsson, A.M., Matthews, P.A., Argenton, M., Christie, M.R., McConnell, J.M., Jansen, E.H.J.M., Piersma, A.H., Ozanne, S.E., Fernandez Twinn, D., Remacle, C., Rowlerson, A., Poston, L., & Taylor, P.D. (2008). Diet-induced obesity in female mice leads to offspring hyperphagia, adiposity, hypertension, and insulin resistance: a novel murine model of developmental programming. *Hypertension*, *51*, 383–392.

Saunders, C.L., Chiodini, B.D., Sham, P., Lewis, C.M., Abkevich, V., Adeyemo, A.A., de Andrade, M., Arya, R., Berenson, G.S., Blangero, J., Boehnke, M., Borecki, I.B., Chagnon, Y.C., Chen, W., Comuzzie, A.G., Deng, H-W., Duggirala, R., Feitosa, M.F., Froguel, P., Hanson, R.L., Hebebrand, J., Huezo-Dias, P., Kissebah, A.H., Li,

W., Luke, A., Martin, L.J., Nash, M., Ohman, M., Palmer, L.J., Peltonen, L., Perola, M., Price, R.A., Redline, S., Srinivasan, S.R., Stern, M.P., Stone, S., Stringham, H., Turner, S., Wijmenga, C., & Collier, D.A. (2007). Meta-analysis of genome-wide linkage studies in BMI and obesity. *Obesity*, *15*, 2263–2275.

Savage, J.S., Fisher, J.O., & Birch, L.L. (2007). Parental influence on eating behavior: conception to adolescence. *Journal of Law, Medicine and Ethics*, *35*, 22–34.

Savino, F., Liguori, S.A., Fissore, M.F., Oggero, R., Silvestro, L., & Miniero, R. (2005). Serum ghrelin concentration and weight gain in healthy term infants in the first year of life. *Journal of Pediatric Gastroenterology and Nutrition*, *41*, 653–659.

Schachter, S. (1968). Obesity and eating – internal and external cues differentially affect eating behavior of obese and normal subjects. *Science*, *161*, 751–756.

Schachter, S. (1971). Some extraordinary facts about obese humans and rats. *American Psychologist*, *26*, 129–144.

Schachter, S., Goldman, R., & Gordon, A. (1968). Effects of fear, food deprivation, and obesity on eating. *Journal of Personality and Social Psychology*, *10*, 91–97.

Serlachius, A., Hamer, M., & Wardle, J. (2007). Stress and weight change in university students in the United Kingdom. *Physiology and Behavior*, *92*, 548–553.

Shunk, J.A., & Birch, L.L. (2004). Girls at risk for overweight at age 5 are at risk for dietary restraint, disinhibited overeating, weight concerns, and greater weight gain from 5 to 9 years. *Journal of the American Dietetic Association*, *104*, 1120–1126.

Silverman, B.L., Rizzo, T.A., Cho, N.H., & Metzger, B.E. (1998). Long-term effects of the intrauterine environment. The Northwestern University Diabetes in Pregnancy Center. *Diabetes Care*, *21*, 142–149.

Sleddens, E.F., Kremers, S.P., & Thijs, C. (2008). The Children's Eating Behaviour Questionnaire: factorial validity and association with Body Mass Index in Dutch children aged 6-7. *International Journal of Behavioral Nutrition and Physical Activity*, *5*, 49.

Snoek, H.M., van Strien, T., Janssens, J., & Engels, R. (2007). Emotional, external, restrained eating, and overweight in Dutch adolescents. *Scandinavian Journal of Psychology*, *48*, 23–32.

Speakman, J.R., Rance, K.A., & Johnstone, A.M. (2008). Polymorphisms of the FTO gene are associated with variation in energy intake, but not energy expenditure. *Obesity*, *16*, 1961–1965.

Spiegel, T.A. (2000). Rate of intake, bites, and chews – the interpretation of lean-obese differences. *Neuroscience and Biobehavioral Reviews*, *24*, 229–237.

Steinle, N.I., Hsueh, W.C., Snitker, S., Pollin, T.I., Sakul, H., St Jean, P.L., Bell, C.J., Mitchell, B.D., & Shuldiner, A.R. (2002). Eating behavior in the Old Order Amish: heritability analysis and a genome-wide linkage analysis. *American Journal of Clinical Nutrition*, *75*, 1098–1106.

Stratigopoulos, G., Padilla, S.L., Leduc, C.A., Watson, E., Hattersley, A.T., McCarthy, M.I., Zeltser, L.M., Chung, W.K., & Leibel, R.L. (2008). Regulation of Fto/Ftm gene expression in mice and humans. *American Journal of Physiology-Regulatory Integrative and Comparative Physiology*, *294*, 1185–1196.

Striegel-Moore, R.H., Morrison, J.A., Schreiber, G., Schumann, B.C., Crawford, P.B., & Obarzanek, E. (1999). Emotion-induced eating and sucrose intake in children: the NHLBI Growth and Health Study. *International Journal of Eating Disorders*, *25*, 389–398.

Stunkard, A.J., & Messick, S. (1985). The three-factor eating questionnaire to measure dietary restraint, disinhibition and hunger. *Journal of Psychosomatic Research*, *29*, 71–83.

Stunkard, A.J., Harris, J.R., Pedersen, N.L., & McClearn, G.E. (1990). The body-mass index of twins who have been reared apart. *New England Journal of Medicine*, *322*, 1483–1487.

Stunkard, A.J., Berkowitz, R.I., Schoeller, D., Maislin, G., & Stallings, V.A. (2004). Predictors of body size in the first 2y of life: a high-risk study of human obesity. *International Journal of Obesity*, *28*, 503–513.

Sullivan, S.A., & Birch, L.L. (1990). Pass the sugar, pass the salt – experience dictates preference. *Developmental Psychology*, *26*, 546–551.

Sullivan, S.A., & Birch, L.L. (1994). Infant dietary experience and acceptance of solid foods. *Pediatrics*, *93*, 271–277.

Taylor, P.D., & Poston, L. (2007). Developmental programming of obesity in mammals. *Experimental Physiology*, *92*, 287–298.

Temple, J.L., Giacomelli, A.M., Roemmich, J.N., & Epstein, L.H. (2007). Overweight children habituate slower than non-overweight children to food. *Physiology and Behavior*, *91*, 250–254.

Temple, J.L., Legierski, C.M., Giacomelli, A.M., Salvy, S.J., & Epstein, L.H. (2008). Overweight children find food more reinforcing and consume more energy than do non overweight children. *American Journal of Clinical Nutrition*, *87*, 1121–1127.

Tholin, S., Rasmussen, F., Tynelius, P., & Karlsson, J. (2005). Genetic and environmental influences on eating behavior: the Swedish young male twins study. *American Journal of Clinical Nutrition*, *81*, 564–569.

Timpson, N.J., Emmett, P.M., Frayling, T.M., Rogers, I., Hattersley, A.T., McCarthy, M.I., & Davey Smith, G. (2008). The fat mass- and obesity-associated locus and dietary intake in children. *American Journal of Clinical Nutrition*, *88*, 971–978.

van den Bree, M.B., Eaves, L.J., & Dwyer, J.T. (1999). Genetic and environmental influences on eating patterns of twins aged ≥ 50 y. *American Journal of Clinical Nutrition, 70*, 456–465.

van Strien, T., & Oosterveld, P. (2008). The childrens DEBQ for assessment of restrained, emotional, and external eating in 7- to 12-year-old children. *International Journal of Eating Disorders, 41*, 72–81.

van Strien, T., Frijters, J., Bergers, G., & Defares, P.B. (1986). The Dutch Eating Behavior Questionnaire (DEBQ) for assessment of restrained, emotional, and external eating behavior. *International Journal of Eating Disorders, 5*, 295–315.

Vauthier, J.M., Lluch, A., Lecomte, E., Artur, Y., & Herbeth, B. (1996). Family resemblance in energy and macronutrient intakes: the Stanislas Family Study. *International Journal of Epidemiology, 25*, 1030–1037.

Vereecken, C.A., Keukelier, E., & Maes, L. (2004). Influence of mother's educational level on food parenting practices and food habits of young children. *Appetite, 43*, 93–103.

Viana, V., Sinde, S., & Saxton, J.C. (2008). Children's Eating Behaviour Questionnaire: associations with BMI in Portuguese children. *British Journal of Nutrition, 100*, 445–450.

Vickers, M.H., Breier, B.H., Cutfield, W.S., Hofman, P.L., & Gluckman, P.D. (2000). Fetal origins of hyperphagia, obesity, and hypertension and postnatal amplification by hypercaloric nutrition. *American Journal of Physiology – Endocrinology and Metabolism, 279*, 83–87.

Wade, J., Milner, J., & Krondl, M. (1981). Evidence for a physiological regulation of food selection and nutrient intake in twins. *American Journal of Clinical Nutrition, 34*, 143–147.

Wardle, J., & Gibson, E.L. (2001). Impact of stress on diet: process and implications. In S. Stansfield & M.G. Marmot (Eds.), *Stress and heart disease* (pp. 35–40). London: British Medical Journal Books.

Wardle, J., Marsland, L., Sheikh, Y., Quinn, M., Fedoroff, I., & Ogden, J. (1992). Eating style and eating behaviour in adolescents. *Appetite, 18*, 167–183.

Wardle, J., Guthrie, C.A., Sanderson, S., & Rapoport, L. (2001a). Development of the children's eating behaviour questionnaire. *Journal of Child Psychology and Psychiatry and Allied Disciplines, 42*, 963–970.

Wardle, J., Guthrie, C., Sanderson, S., Birch, L., & Plomin, R. (2001b). Food and activity preferences in children of lean and obese parents. *International Journal of Obesity, 25*, 971–977.

Wardle, J., Cooke, L.J., Gibson, E.L., Sapochnik, M., Sheiham, A., & Lawson, M. (2003a). Increasing children's acceptance of vegetables; a randomized trial of parent-led exposure. *Appetite, 40*, 155–162.

Wardle, J., Herrera, M.L., Cooke, L., & Gibson, E.L. (2003b). Modifying children's food preferences: the effects of exposure and reward on acceptance of an unfamiliar vegetable. *European Journal of Clinical Nutrition, 57*, 341–348.

Wardle, J., Carnell, S., Haworth, C.M., & Plomin, R. (2008a). Evidence for a strong genetic influence on childhood adiposity despite the force of the obesogenic environment. *American Journal of Clinical Nutrition, 87*, 398–404.

Wardle, J., Carnell, S., Haworth, C., Farooqi, I.S., O'Rahilly, S., & Plomin, R. (2008b). Obesity associated genetic variation in *FTO* is associated with diminished satiety. *Journal of Clinical Endocrinology & Metabolism, 93*, 3640–3643.

Wardle, J., Llewellyn, C., Sanderson, S., & Plomin, R. (2009). The *FTO* gene and measured food intake in children. *International Journal of Obesity, 33*, 42–45.

Waxman, M., & Stunkard, A.J. (1980). Caloric-intake and expenditure of obese boys. *Journal of Pediatrics, 96*, 187–193.

Webber, L., Hill, C., Saxton, J., Van Jaarsveld, C.H., & Wardle, J. (2009). Eating behaviour and weight in children. *International Journal of Obesity, 33*, 21–28.

Whitaker, R.C., Wright, J.A., Pepe, M.S., Seidel, K.D., & Dietz, W.H. (1997). Predicting obesity in young adulthood from childhood and parental obesity. *New England Journal of Medicine, 337*, 869–873.

Willer, C.J., Speliotes, E.K., Loos, R.J., Li, S., Lindgren, C.M., Heid, I.M., Berndt, S.I., Elliott, A.L., Jackson, A.U., & Lamina, C. (2009). Six new loci associated with body mass index highlight a neuronal influence on body weight regulation. *Nature Genetics, 41*, 25–34.

Wright, C., & Birks, E. (2000). Risk factors for failure to thrive: a population-based survey. *Child Care, Health and Development, 26*, 5–16.

Yang, W., Kelly, T., & He, J. (2007). Genetic epidemiology of obesity. *Epidemiologic Reviews, 29*, 49–61.

Chapter 26
Childhood Obesity: Etiology - Synthesis Part II

Luis A. Moreno, Iris Pigeot, and Wolfgang Ahrens

Introduction

The rapid increase in the prevalence of obesity in children and adolescents raises concerns about the main determinants of this phenomenon. From a life course perspective, determinants of obesity development appear early in life (Fig. 26.1). Depending on the timing and the complex interplay of multiple exposures, the excess of body fat and obesity related complications, mainly the metabolic ones, will develop. Obesity and its related complications are responsible for, in the short and long term, chronic morbidity, including cardiovascular diseases, type 2 diabetes and cancer, amongst others, and result in excess mortality later in life (Fig. 26.1). For these reasons, primary prevention of obesity beginning in childhood or even earlier during pregnancy should be a public health priority.

At the individual level, genetic susceptibility strongly determines the ability to develop obesity. At the population level, non-genetic factors are the main drivers of obesity development. These factors are very different in nature: epigenetics, early nutrition, food patterns and eating behavior, physical (in-)activity, psychological, social, and environmental factors. The increased availability of palatable, energy dense foods and the reduced requirement for physical exertion during working and domestic life as well as during leisure time contribute to a sustained state of positive energy balance and are critical factors underlying the obesity pandemic. The relative impact of the obesity risk factors and their interactions are still not fully understood.

This chapter highlights the current knowledge on the most important factors, their interplay and their impact on the development of obesity with assessment of their evidence. It will give an integrative assessment of the key factors contributing to the obesity epidemic and by this it will summarize the state-of-the art presented in the chapters of Part II of this book.

L.A. Moreno (✉)
GENUD (Growth, Exercise, Nutrition and Developement) Research Group,
E.U. Ciencias de la Salud, Universidad de Zaragoza, Zaragoza, Spain
e-mail: lmoreno@unizar.es

I. Pigeot and W. Ahrens
Bremen Institute for Prevention Research and Social Medicine (BIPS), University Bremen,
Achterstrasse 30, 28359, Bremen, Germany

L.A. Moreno et al. (eds.), *Epidemiology of Obesity in Children and Adolescents*,
Springer Series on Epidemiology and Public Health 2, DOI 10.1007/978-1-4419-6039-9_26,
© Springer Science+Business Media, LLC 2011

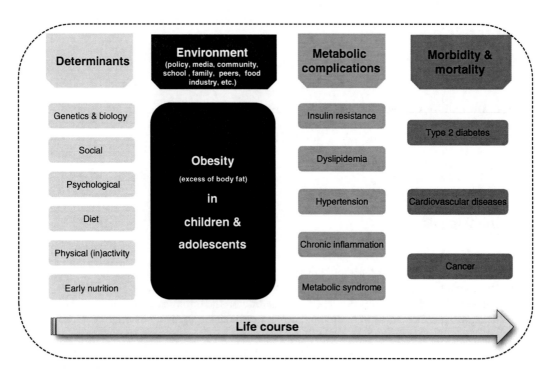

Fig. 26.1 Factors influencing the risk of obesity and related metabolic consequences and health outcomes in a life course perspective

Genetics, Epigenetics and Nutrigenomics

The most widely accepted theories attribute the current worldwide increase of obesity, both in adults and in children, to the interaction between a genetic predisposition favoring efficient energy storage, and an obesogenic environment (Chapter 14 by Russo et al.). Our understanding of the complex interaction between genetic determinants and environmental factors in the rapid global increase of obesity has been challenged by the need to integrate the role of epigenetic adaptation (Stoger 2008). Epigenetic effects are frequently invoked as potentially important mechanisms for associations of prenatal risk factors with a range of later life outcomes. However, as yet there is insufficient research in humans to draw definite conclusions about the nature and importance of these effects (Chapter 17 by Lawlor et al.).

The study of the genetic basis of polygenic obesity is basically the same in the different stages of life, including childhood and adolescence. Nowadays, information has been accumulated regarding the molecular constituents of physiological pathways controlling energy balance and body fat content. Analysis of these pathways has identified possible candidate genes whose variation – in terms of DNA sequence and/or epigenetic markers – might underlie the genetic basis of variation in body fat mass and distribution. DNA sequence variants may influence an individual's susceptibility to obesity and related syndromes.

Palou et al. (Chapter 15) present an overview of main genes whose variations have been related to monogenic and complex forms of obesity in humans. They present obesity-related genes, in connection with the biochemical process in which their encoded protein products are likely to be involved. However, lack of replication of findings is more the rule than the exception in genetic association studies regarding the etiology of human obesity. Lack of replication can be due to poor study design, differences in the demographic or behavioral characteristics of the studied populations, and differences in the phenotype studied.

In recent years, the advent of the genome wide association studies has changed the perspective of gene discoveries in the field of complex diseases. The integration of different "omics" disciplines (transcriptomics, proteomics, metabolomics and nutrigenomics) will help to elucidate the molecular basis of obesity.

There is a complex and dynamic interaction between nutrition and the human genome. This interaction determines gene expression and the metabolic response, which ultimately affects an individual's health status and/or predisposition to disease (Chapter 15). The gene-environment interaction may be defined as the conditional effect of environmental exposures acting through the individual genotype on the phenotype. For example, apolipoprotein A5 gene variation can modulate the effects of dietary fat intake on BMI and obesity risk (Corella et al. 2007).

Dietary compounds may act as regulators of gene expression at multiple levels, involving nutrigenomic effects, nutrigenetic interactions and modulation of intracellular signaling pathways (Chapter 15). Cells have several sensory systems that detect energy and metabolic status and adjust flux through metabolic pathways accordingly. Nutrients play a key role as signaling molecules and regulators of intermediary metabolism adjusting in an integrated manner nutrient availability and energy status at both the cellular and whole-body levels and then to regulate whole-body energy homeostasis.

Early Nutrition Programming

Childhood and adult obesity are considered to be programmed by early life nutrition. Several mechanisms have been proposed that may account for programming of adiposity, including disruptions in pancreatic structures and function, leading to alterations in insulin secretion and sensitivity, increases in the number and/or size of fat cells or alterations in adipose tissue function, and alterations in the development of the central nervous system, leading to an impairment in the feeding control (Martorell et al. 2001).

The association between maternal obesity with or without gestational diabetes and body composition of the developing child through adulthood requires further studies. Maternal diabetes during pregnancy is associated with higher birth weight and greater fetal adiposity (Catalano et al. 2003). In addition, there is increasing evidence that the offspring of women with gestational diabetes is at increased risk of obesity (Dabelea 2007). Several mechanisms may explain this, including genetic predisposition, shared familial socio-economic and lifestyle factors, as well as specific intrauterine effects. The developmental over nutrition hypothesis (also known as fetal teratogenesis) suggests a possible intrauterine mechanism for the association of maternal pregnancy diabetes with offspring adiposity (Dabelea 2007).

Several studies have shown an association of maternal obesity with excessive fetal growth and adiposity independent of gestational diabetes (Baeten et al. 2001). Others have also found a positive association between maternal pre-pregnancy or early pregnancy BMI and offspring BMI or obesity in later life (Laitinen et al. 2001). A number of studies have also examined the association between maternal weight gain during pregnancy and later BMI or obesity in offspring, finding an association between greater weight gain during pregnancy and greater mean BMI or increased risk of obesity in offspring (Mamun et al. 2009).

Evidence to date suggests that birth weight is positively associated with BMI and total fat and lean mass, but whether there is an inverse association with central adiposity remains unclear (Labayen et al. 2006). Rapid weight gain in the first few months of life has been inconsistently related to obesity in later life. The impact of rate of weight gain in early infancy on later risk of adiposity may vary depending upon the underlying nutritional status of the infants being studied (Chapter 17). This issue requires further investigation.

There is increasing epidemiological evidence suggesting that breastfeeding compared to infant formula confers protection against obesity later in life. Existing studies on duration of breastfeeding strongly support a dose-dependent association between a longer duration of breastfeeding and a decrease in the risk of becoming overweight (Harder et al. 2005). Breastfeeding is known to be associated with multiple social, behavioral and biological exposures that are themselves correlated with obesity. The evidence for long-term protective effects of breastfeeding on obesity is largely observational and not experimental. In addition to the differences in the caloric content and macronutrients (mainly proteins) between breast milk and infant formula, it is possible that the protective effect of breast milk against the development of obesity in later life could be due to a particular component of the milk. For instance, leptin is naturally present in breast milk but is not present in infant formula (Palou et al. 2008).

Neuroendocrine Regulation

Despite the almost daily variation in food intake and energy expenditure, body weight remains relatively constant. Only when small differences in energy expenditure/intake are integrated over long periods of time, an increase in adiposity is produced. A complex network of hormones, neuropeptides and metabolites involved in the regulation of appetite and metabolism has been identified (Chapter 16 by Barrios et al.). Current evidence suggests that the primary cause of peripheral fat accumulation could involve modifications at the level of the central nervous system (Schwartz et al. 2000). The hypothalamus regulates energy homeostasis by integrating numerous input signals. Thus, obesity may result in changes at the hypothalamic level or the disturbance of homeostatic processes at this level may result in obesity.

Neuropeptide Y (NPY)/agouti-related protein (AgRP) and proopiomelanocortin (POMC)/cocaine- and amphetamine-regulated transcript (CART) are two neuronal populations involved in metabolic control of appetite and metabolism. In the hypothalamus, NPY/AgRP neurons integrate multiple signals to then send out signals to increase food intake and decrease metabolism. In contrast, POMC/CART neurons within the hypothalamic arcuate nucleus have the opposite function, decreasing appetite and increasing metabolic turnover. Many circulating hormones reach these neuronal populations, either by active or passive transport into the brain, to modulate their output signals and control eating behavior and metabolic rate.

Exogenous obesity is normally associated with a decrease in the sensitivity to leptin and insulin signaling (Chapter 16). Leptin and insulin have overlapping effects in the arcuate nucleus, with defects in their signaling resulting in disordered energy homeostasis (Niswender and Schwartz 2003). Hypothalamic alterations in leptin and/or insulin signaling cause increased body weight (Pelleymounter et al. 1995).

The gastrointestinal (GI) tract and the pancreas also produce several peptides related to satiation (the feeling of fullness which terminates eating) and satiety (the prolongation of the interval between meals), with the exception of gastric derived ghrelin, which is known to be a powerful orexigenic signal (Woods and D'Alessio 2008).

Food Patterns and Eating Behavior

Among all risk factors that are known to modulate obesity development and its persistence into adulthood, diet composition and food patterns are among the main environmental determinants of energy balance through different periods of life (Chapter 18 by Rodríguez et al.). Accurate assessment of dietary intake in children is of major concern in population-based nutrition research. Little is known on how to obtain accurate measures of dietary intake in obese and normal weight children. While a general underreporting bias exists in free-living subjects describing their diets, regardless of weight status, all evidence points to this problem being magnified in the obese, including children and adolescents.

Multifactorial obesity develops when energy intake exceeds energy expenditure during long periods of time, leading to slow accumulation of body fat. Even a minor positive daily energy imbalance maintained over longer periods will result in significant weight gain. Excessive global energy intake due to easy and continuous food accessibility, consumption of energy-dense foods, excessive percentage of energy intake from fats or proteins, contemporary eating patterns (elevated consumption of bakery foods, sweetened beverages, sweets or low-quality foods, the low consumption of fruit and vegetables, big portion sizes, daily meal patterns and daily energy intake distribution) are all considered potential contributors to the obesity epidemic (Chapter 18). Scientific evidence is increasing about some dietary factors associated with obesity, specifically a low meal frequency, skipping breakfast and a high consumption of sugar sweetened beverages (Moreno et al. 2010).

Nowadays, dietary intake is strongly influenced by multiple factors like environmental, sociocultural and economic ones. People eat frequently away from home, there are time limitations with respect to eating and meal preparation, children eat alone without family supervision (sometimes watching television) and children with both parents at work eat in school canteens.

In modern environments where highly palatable food is abundant and cheap, high external responsiveness could lead to over-eating and weight gain, especially if it is not buffered by strong satiety sensitivity (Chapter 25 by Llewellyn et al.). Certain eating behaviors which can be seen early in childhood are associated with adiposity, including lower sensitivity to satiety, food-cue responsiveness, a higher "reinforcing" value of food, and preferences for energy-dense foods. There is reasonable evidence for the broad spectrum heritability for several eating behaviors in adults, but less research has been carried out with children. Heritability estimates are known to change over the lifespan; therefore, it is important to understand the relative influences of genes and shared and non-shared environments. Family environmental influences have been shown to also play a role, some of which are modifiable, including early over- or under-nutrition, parental feeding style, and parental behaviors, all of which may modify the expression of genetically determined behavioral tendencies.

Research into taste preferences has indicated the importance of early exposure to many different kinds of foods for taste preferences later on. These findings suggest it may be helpful to limit foods high in sugar and fat during the early years, and to offer fruits and vegetables as early as possible (Chapter 25). It may also be possible to influence early preferences for fruit and vegetables through modeling by parents and older siblings.

Consumer Behavior

A multilevel approach can distinguish four different dimensions of factors influencing health behavior among children: intrapersonal, interpersonal, community, and societal level (Chapter 24 by Reisch et al.). The intrapersonal level represents individual factors, incorporating psychological factors and lifestyle aspects such as meal and activity patterns. Concerning the interpersonal level, social learning theory assumes that young children learn mainly by imitating dietary habits, food preferences, eating habits, and physical activities from their immediate environment. At the community level, the emphasis is on the availability and accessibility of healthy food and opportunities for physical activity; the community level comprises the immediate pre-school/school environment as well as restaurants, supermarkets, and playgrounds. Information on children's buying power and "pester power" as well as on media exposure and media literacy enters the model on the societal level. Pester power describes the influence children have on their parents' buying behavior, while buying power is the money that is directly available for children.

Children as consumers represent three markets in one: the classical children's market where they spend their own money; the second market where children influence the purchases of their parents; and the third market, the future market where children become potential adult customers. There are four main socialization agents: parents, caretakers, peers, and media. Parents are the key agents in children's early food socialization by forming their nutritional habits and preferences. Parents exert a powerful influence on their children via role modeling, communication models, and parenting styles; however, the socialization process is not the same in all families. On entering pre-school and school, caretakers and teachers as individuals and as representatives of their institutions (and hence following the institutions' rules) influence children's dietary behavior and physical activity.

Children spend a good deal of their day within the childcare/school system and, at least in British and Scandinavian settings eat, on average, at least one meal and one snack per day (Edmunds et al. 2001). In childcare settings, meals play an important role by structuring the day, offering breaks, forming eating habits, experimenting with new tastes, likes and dislikes, and offering the possibility of spending time together outside the play or class room.

Media's influential potential as well as children's buying power make children a very appealing target for marketers who use all kinds of media channels to transmit their messages. The media are quite influential in forming children's food habits. Food and drink advertisements are heavily focused on less healthy product choices: Most television spots promote sweet, fatty, or salty snacks or drinks. Besides the classical tool of television advertising, companies use more subtle forms of advertising such as product placement in TV programs, internet websites, games, and communities, toys or games created in partnerships with food companies, in-school marketing activities such as vending machines, sponsoring, or supply of educational material (Story and French 2004). Despite the spread of the internet and other types of media, television remains the major promotional channel for food producers, retailers, and restaurants to advertise their products to children. However, the studies available on the relationship between advertisements and childhood obesity are controversial.

Children often take an interest in food shopping and want to participate in the decision processes. It was observed that conflict potential is fairly high in supermarket shopping environments (Nicholls and Cullen 2004). While nutritional considerations are the most important determinant of the parental decision of what food to buy, preferences of their children are the second determinant of parental food choice (Spungin 2004). There is an increased supply of processed food and ready-made meals which contain more energy per food or drink unit and an increasing marketing of larger package sizes over the last 2–3 decades (Young and Nestle 2003). Hence, food industry is accused of facilitating obesogenic dietary behavior in order to realize higher profits (Procter 2007).

Physical (In-)Activity and Physical Fitness

The current literature agrees that association between physical activity and obesity is stronger for vigorous physical activity than for moderate physical activity (Chapter 19 by Jiménez-Pavón et al.). When the children are exercising at a higher intensity, the total energy expenditure associated with that activity is higher than for a similar time effort at moderate intensity. The question whether is it really the intensity what matters or whether it is the total amount of energy expenditure remains to be answered. For example, whether 30 min of moderate-intensity physical activity and 10 min of vigorous-intensity physical activity (assuming that both would have the same energy cost) have different effects on body composition indexes remains to be elucidated. Evidence from intervention studies supports that physical activity in children and adolescents reduces central body fat (Chapter 19).

Longitudinal data have shown a significant relationship between children's cardio-respiratory fitness and later body fatness, where higher cardio-respiratory fitness levels are associated with lower body fat levels (Ara et al. 2006). Several studies corroborated that cardio-respiratory fitness in childhood and adolescence is a predictor of excess of overall and central body fat later in life (Chapter 19).

Concerning sedentary behaviors, most of the studies on the one hand report a positive association between television viewing and adiposity, mainly in children younger than ten at baseline, suggesting that TV viewing is a risk factor for the development of overweight/obesity in children (Chapter 20 by Rey-López et al. 2008). In addition, duration of television viewing is often associated with a higher intake of sweetened drinks and high energy-dense food (Vereecken et al. 2006). On the other hand, the use of video games (video games console) and the use of computers (playing computer games, browsing the internet, etc.) seem not to be associated with obesity risk.

Environmental Factors

The current environment is characterized by a situation in which minimal physical activity is required for daily life and food is inexpensive, high in energy density and widely available (Chapter 22 by Huybrechts et al.). In our modern environment, people who are not devoting substantial conscious efforts to manage their body weight are likely to gain weight. The globally rising obesity prevalence suggests that the environment has changed in such a way that fewer and fewer people manage to maintain a healthy body weight by relying on their own biology and "instinctive" mechanisms to protect themselves (Peters et al. 2002).

Important environmental changes that contribute to the obesity epidemic are for instance an ever-increasing number of energy-dense foods, packaged in large portions, conveniently available at low cost (Berg et al. 2009). Furthermore, modern technologies allow people to be less active in their daily labor. All modern conveniences have eliminated the need for individuals to perform much of the physical activity that was once required for daily tasks at work and at home. In addition, also safety issues in the environment might stimulate those unhealthy lifestyle habits and decisions. For example, a person may not only choose not to walk to the store or to work because of laziness or convenience, but just because of a lack of alternatives and for safety reasons.

The most important factors concerning environmental barriers for energy expenditure are new technological developments, reduction of physical education classes at school, increase of sedentary pastimes, lack of safety, and reduction of walkability of neighborhoods, and reduced access to physical activity facilities (Chapter 22). Many environmental factors have been suggested to affect total energy intake: fast food restaurants, increased portion sizes, unhealthy school environments, unhealthy foods and drinks advertised via the media, availability and access to healthy foods, food availability 24 h a day, and good taste and palatability of the food products (Chapter 22).

Direct measurement through environmental audits has only been used in a few studies with obesity as the primary outcome (Giles-Corti and Donovan 2003). Measurements included the type of street and the presence of sidewalks. These measures were not sophisticated enough to capture relevant characteristics of the built environment to adequately account for all environmental factors that may influence obesity, such as street connectivity, safety and density of daily life facilities like shops, attractive playgrounds, physicians and spaces stimulating physical activity available in the living environment.

It is important to note that the relatively weak evidence found thus far for the association between environmental factors and obesity may not be interpreted as absence of a relationship between "the environment" and obesity-related behaviors. There is still a lack of high-quality studies and of study replications. Most of the available research was focused on only a part of the environment, especially micro-level factors in the socio-cultural and physical environment. Studies on macro-sized environmental factors are largely lacking. Furthermore, many potentially relevant environmental factors have not been studied at all (Brug et al. 2006).

Social and Psychological Factors

A large number of studies examined the cross-sectional association between socio-economic status (SES) and risk of childhood adiposity or obesity in different populations (Chapter 21 by Johnson et al.). In developing countries, a fairly consistent association was seen, with greater adiposity in children from higher SES backgrounds. However, recent data indicate that this is changing, particularly in urban areas. In many developing countries urban dwellers are further removed from the traditional lifestyle of their rural compatriots, and the inhabitants of cities often adopt more westernized diets and sedentary occupations.

In developed countries, the pattern is reverse. Of a total of 45 studies, 19 (42%) found an inverse association, linking low SES with greater adiposity, while 12 (27%) found no association (Shrewsbury and Wardle 2008). The magnitude of the association was assessed in 24 studies which revealed a summary odds of obesity in the lowest SES group around twice as compared to the highest SES group. Studies analyzed provided little evidence that sex is a strong moderator of the link between adiposity and SES in school-aged children (Shrewsbury and Wardle 2008). Socio-economic factors are associated with body weight from birth onwards, although the association between SES and weight in very young children is not straightforward. An inverse association between SES and obesity was found more frequently in children (10 of 18 studies) than in adolescents. Recent results show that while the overall increase of the prevalence of obesity in children appears to level off, this is not true for children from the lowest SES families (Lioret et al. 2009).

Several mechanisms explaining the association between SES and obesity in children have been suggested. In developing countries, the direct association between SES and adiposity is likely to be due to food shortages, but also due to the perception of overweight as a sign of wealth and healthiness. The prevailing picture is that as countries move away from food shortages, obesity starts to become more prevalent overall and the traditional association between higher SES and obesity begins to disappear and ultimately reverses as obesity rates rise faster in lower SES groups.

There is evidence to support an association between depression during childhood/adolescence and excess weight gain or the onset of obesity. This association may be mediated by a number of behavioral factors that are being investigated. Research also suggests an association between childhood adverse events and excess weight gain or the development of obesity (Chapter 23 by Sgrenci and Faith).

Childhood behavioral problems have also been found to be associated with the development of obesity in childhood and adulthood. It seems as if obesity develops more often in young adulthood for those with behavioral problems. However, the link between concurrent obesity and behavioral problems question which factor precedes the other, since it is possible that excess weight may precede behavioral problems as well.

Childhood obesity may lead to the following outcomes: body dissatisfaction, low self-esteem, poorer peer relationships, poor quality of life, stigmatization, and suicidal behaviors and thoughts. There is increasing evidence indicating that obese children and adolescents are significantly affected by stigmatization, as they are judged by others to be "unattractive, ugly, lazy, and dumb" (Allon 1981). These attitudes have not changed over the past several decades. Weight stigma and teasing are also associated with disordered eating patterns, drug use, and alcohol use. One of the most disconcerting consequences of childhood obesity is an increased risk of suicidal behaviors. Obese adolescents are more likely to endorse suicidal thoughts and to attempt suicide than normal weight peers (Ackard et al. 2003). Obesity impacts detrimentally on children's health related quality of life (Kolotkin et al. 2006). Strauss and Pollack (2003) also found that overweight adolescents were more likely to be socially isolated compared to normal weight adolescents.

Conclusions

The different etiologic factors considered in the second part of this book all affect the development of obesity in children. Interactions between them have been observed and should be clarified in the future to better quantify the relative contribution of each of the various risk factors. Complementary research approaches, integrating different scientific disciplines, are needed to identify the critical windows in childhood growth and development when the different factors could influence obesity incidence. The new research should identify the main drivers of obesity development in children and adolescents in order to propose new effective prevention and treatment strategies.

References

Ackard, D.M., Neumark-Sztainer, D., Story, M., & Perry, C. (2003). Overeating among adolescents: prevalence and associations with weight-related characteristics and psychological health. *Pediatrics, 111(1)*, 67–74.

Allon, N. (1981). The stigma of overweight in everyday life. In B.J. Wolman (Ed.), *Psychological Aspects of Obesity: A Handbook.* New York: Van Nostrand.

Ara, I., Vicente-Rodriguez, G., Perez-Gomez, J., Jimenez-Ramirez, J., Serrano-Sanchez, J.A., Dorado, C., & Calbet, J.A. (2006). Influence of extracurricular sport activities on body composition and physical fitness in boys: a 3-year longitudinal study. *International Journal of Obesity, 30*, 1062–1071.

Baeten, J.M., Bukusi, E.A., & Lambe, M. (2001). Pregnancy complications and outcomes among overweight and obese nulliparous women. *American Journal of Public Health, 91*, 436–440.

Berg, C., Lappas, G., Wolk, A., Strandhagen, E., Toren, K., Rosengren, A., Thelle, D., & Lissner, L. (2009). Eating patterns and portion size associated with obesity in a Swedish population. *Appetite, 52*, 21–26.

Brug, J., van Lenthe, F.J., & Kremers, S.P. (2006). Revisiting Kurt Lewin: how to gain insight into environmental correlates of obesogenic behaviors. *American Journal of Preventive Medicine, 31*, 525–529.

Catalano, P.M., Thomas, A., Huston-Presley, L., & Amini, S.B. (2003). Increased fetal adiposity: a very sensitive marker of abnormal in utero development. *American Journal of Obstetrics and Gynecology, 189*, 1698–1704.

Corella, D., Lai, C.Q., Demissie, S., Cupples, L.A., Manning, A.K., Tucker, K.L., & Ordovas, J.M. (2007). APOA5 gene variation modulates the effects of dietary fat intake on body mass index and obesity risk in the Framingham Heart Study. *Journal of Molecular Medicine, 85*, 119–128.

Dabelea, D. (2007). The predisposition to obesity and diabetes in offspring of diabetic mothers. *Diabetes Care, 30*, 169–174.

Edmunds, L, Waters, E., & Elliot, E.J. (2001). Evidence based management of childhood obesity. *British Medical Journal, 323(7318)*, 916–619.

Giles-Corti, B., & Donovan, R.J. (2003). Relative influences of individual, social environmental, and physical environmental correlates of walking. *American Journal of Public Health, 93*, 1583–1589.

Harder, T., Bergmann, R., Kallischnigg, G., & Plagemann, A. (2005). Duration of breastfeeding and risk of overweight: a meta-analysis. *American Journal of Epidemiology, 162*, 397–403.

Kolotkin, R.L., Zeller, M., Modi, A.C., Samsa, G.P., Quinlan, N.P., Yanovski, J.A., Bell, S.K., Maahs, D.M., de Serna, D.G., & Roehrig, H.R. (2006). Assessing weight related quality of life in adolescents. *Obesity, 14(3)*, 448–457.

Labayen, I., Moreno, L.A., Blay, M.G., Blay, V.A., Mesana, M.I., Gonzalez-Gross, M., Bueno, G., Sarria, A., & Bueno, M. (2006). Early programming of body composition and fat distribution in adolescents. *Journal of Nutrition, 136*, 147–152.

Laitinen, J., Power, C., & Jarvelin, M.R. (2001). Family social class, maternal body mass index, childhood body mass index, and age at menarche as predictors of adult obesity. *American Journal of Clinical Nutrition, 74*, 287–294.

Lioret, S., Touvier, M., Dubuisson, C., Dufour, A., Calamassi-Tran, G., Lafay, L., Volatier, J.L., & Marie, B. (2009). Trends in child overweight rates and energy intake in France from 1999 to 2007: relationships with socioeconomic status. *Obesity (Silver Spring), 17*, 1092–1100.

Mamun, A.A., O'Callaghan, M., Callaway, L., Williams, G., Najman, J., & Lawlor, D.A. (2009). Associations of gestational weight gains with offspring body mass index and blood pressure at 21 years: evidence from a birth cohort study. *Circulation, 119*, 1720–1727.

Martorell, R., Stein, A.D., & Schroeder, D.G. (2001). Early nutrition and later adiposity. *The Journal of Nutrition, 131*, 874S–880S.

Moreno, L.A., Rodriguez, G., Fleta, J., Bueno-Lozano, M., Lazaro, A., & Bueno, G. (2010). Trends of dietary habits in adolescents. *Crit Rev Food Sci Nutr, 50*, 106–112.

Nicholls, A.J., & Cullen, P. (2004). The child-parent purchase relationship: 'pester power', human rights and retail ethics. *Journal of Retailing and Consumer Services, 11(2)*, 75–86.

Niswender, K.D., & Schwartz, M.W. (2003). Insulin and leptin revisited: adiposity signals with overlapping physiological and intracellular signaling capabilities. *Frontiers in Neuroendocrinology, 24*, 1–10.

Palou, A., Oliver, P., Sanchez, J., Priego, T., & Pico, C. (2008). The role of breast milk leptin in the prevention of obesity and related medical complications in later life. In M. Cerf (Ed.), *Developmental Programming of Diabetes and Metabolic Syndrome* (pp. 39–49). India: Kerala.

Pelleymounter, M.A., Cullen, M.J., Baker, M.B., Hecht, R., Winters, D., Boone, T., & Collins, F. (1995). Effects of the obese gene product on body weight regulation in ob/ob mice. *Science, 269*, 540–543.

Peters, J.C., Wyatt, H.R., Donahoo, W.T., & Hill, J.O. (2002). From instinct to intellect: the challenge of maintaining healthy weight in the modern world. *Obesity Reviews, 3*, 69–74.

Procter, K.L. (2007). The aetiology of childhood obesity: a review. *Nutrition Research Reviews, 20(1)*, 29–45.

Rey-López, J.P., Vicente-Rodríguez, G., Biosca, M., & Moreno, L.A. (2008). Sedentary behaviour and obesity development in children and adolescents. *Nutrition, Metabolism and Cardiovascular Diseases, 18*, 242–251.

Schwartz, M.W., Woods, S.C., Porte, D. Jr., Seeley, R.J., & Baskin, D.G. (2000). Central nervous system control of food intake. *Nature, 404*, 661–671.

Shrewsbury, V., & Wardle, J. (2008). Socioeconomic status and adiposity in childhood: a systematic review of cross-sectional studies 1990-2005. *Obesity (Silver.Spring), 16*, 275–284.

Spungin, P. (2004). Parent power, not pester power. *Young Consumers, 5(3)*, 37–40.

Stoger, R. (2008). Epigenetics and obesity. *Pharmacogenomics, 9*, 1851–1860.

Story, M., & French, S. (2004). Food advertising and marketing directed at children and adolescents in the US. *International Journal of Behavioral Nutrition and Physical Activity, 1(1)*, 3.

Strauss, R.S., & Pollack, H.A. (2003). Social marginalization of overweight children. *Archives of Pediatric & Adolescent Medicine, 157*, 746–752.

Vereecken, C.A., Todd, J., Roberts, C., Mulvihill, C., & Maes, L. (2006). Television viewing behaviour and associations with food habits in different countries. *Public Health Nutrition, 9*, 244–250.

Woods, S.C., & D'Alessio, D.A. (2008). Central control of body weight and appetite. *The Journal of Clinical Endocrinology and Metabolism, 93*, S37–S50.

Young, L.R., & Nestle, M.S. (2003). Expanding portion sizes in the US marketplace: implications for nutrition counselling. *Journal of the American Dietetic Association, 103(2)*, 231–234.

Index